Lippincott's Illustrated Q&A Review of

Pharmacology

Stanley Zaslau, MD
Professor and Chief, Division of Urology
Urology Residency Program Director
Course Director, Urology Rotation
West Virginia University
Morgantown, West Virginia

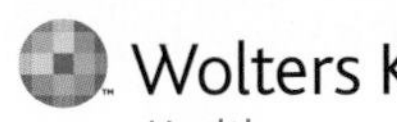

Wolters Kluwer Health | Lippincott Williams & Wilkins
Philadelphia • Baltimore • New York • London
Buenos Aires • Hong Kong • Sydney • Tokyo

Acquisitions Editor: Susan Rhyner
Product Manager: Catherine Noonan
Marketing Manager: Joy Fisher-Williams
Designer: Doug Smock
Compositor: Absolute Service, Inc.

First Edition

351 West Camden Street
Baltimore, MD 21201

Two Commerce Square
2001 Market Street
Philadelphia, PA 19103

Printed in China

9 8 7 6 5 4 3 2 1

Library of Congress Cataloging-in-Publication Data

Zaslau, Stanley.
Lippincottt's illustrated Q&A review of pharmacology / Stanley Zaslau.—1st ed.
p. ; cm.
Illustrated Q&A review of pharmacology
Includes index.
ISBN 978-1-4511-8286-6
I. Title. II. Title: Illustrated Q&A review of pharmacology.
[DNLM: 1. Pharmacology—Examination Questions. 2. Pharmaceutical Preparations—Examination Questions. QV 18.2]

615.1076—dc23

2012046819

DISCLAIMER

Care has been taken to confirm the accuracy of the information present and to describe generally accepted practices. However, the authors, editors, and publisher are not responsible for errors or omissions or for any consequences from application of the information in this book and make no warranty, expressed or implied, with respect to the currency, completeness, or accuracy of the contents of the publication. Application of this information in a particular situation remains the professional responsibility of the practitioner; the clinical treatments described and recommended may not be considered absolute and universal recommendations.

The authors, editors, and publisher have exerted every effort to ensure that drug selection and dosage set forth in this text are in accordance with the current recommendations and practice at the time of publication. However, in view of ongoing research, changes in government regulations, and the constant flow of information relating to drug therapy and drug reactions, the reader is urged to check the package insert for each drug for any change in indications and dosage and for added warnings and precautions. This is particularly important when the recommended agent is a new or infrequently employed drug.

Some drugs and medical devices presented in this publication have Food and Drug Administration (FDA) clearance for limited use in restricted research settings. It is the responsibility of the health care provider to ascertain the FDA status of each drug or device planned for use in their clinical practice.

To purchase additional copies of this book, call our customer service department at (800) 638-3030 or fax orders to (301) 223-2320. International customers should call (301) 223-2300.

Visit Lippincott Williams & Wilkins on the Internet: http://www.lww.com. Lippincott Williams & Wilkins customer service representatives are available from 8:30 am to 6:00 pm, EST.

RRS1212

Preface

This compendium of pharmacology questions was created for the medical students to be able to test their knowledge of the subject. Questions are clinically based and divided by body system. Explanations are provided for correct and incorrect answers. This will allow the students to use the question guide to prepare for medical school course examinations as well as more comprehensive end-year exams and for licensure examinations. Furthermore, students will find the clinical nature of the questions useful for review in their third- and fourth-year rotations as well. Significant contributions to this text were made by medical students who are very familiar with the important concepts in pharmacology that are necessary to master for success on examinations. I am grateful for their contributions to this book.

Acknowledgments

The author would like to acknowledge the outstanding efforts of the following contributing authors: Chad Morley, MD and Jared Manwaring, BA. Dr. Morley completed his medical education at West Virginia University and is currently enrolled in the Urology Residency at West Virginia University Hospitals. He has contributed a significant number of questions for this publication. Jared Manwaring, BA, is a fourth-year medical student at West Virginia University. He, with his tireless work ethic, also contributed a significant number of questions for this publication.

Medical students make great teachers. The efforts of the aforementioned students during their medical education have taught their teacher, me, a great deal about how students think and process when faced with examination questions. The product of our efforts is reflected in this publication, which we sincerely hope is beneficial to the study of pharmacology.

Contents

Chapter 1

Principles of Pharmacology

QUESTIONS

Select the single best answer.

1 A 79-year-old man with end-stage Alzheimer's disease and dysphagia is taking multiple medications. Physical examination reveals xerostomia and a limited gag reflex. Which of the following routes of medication administration would provide the lowest serum drug concentration?

(A) Enteral
(B) Intramuscular
(C) Intrathecal
(D) Intravenous
(E) Transdermal

2 A 28-year-old man with seborrheic dermatitis is prescribed a topical corticosteroid crème by his dermatologist in hopes of alleviating the chronic rash and erythema on the cheeks. Which of the following steps is most critical to achieve a therapeutic drug concentration in plasma?

(A) Absorption
(B) Distribution
(C) Elimination
(D) Glycosylation
(E) Metabolism

3 A 31-year-old man is brought to the emergency department complaining of dyspnea. He has a history of asthma and has had multiple asthma attacks requiring intubation for airway maintenance. He is noncompliant with his medications prescribed for this condition. Physical examination reveals a young man in acute distress. His room air oxygen saturation is 87%. In addition to administration of oxygen, immediate drug administration of albuterol should be administered by which of the following routes?

(A) Inhalation
(B) Intranasal puff metered dose
(C) Subcutaneous
(D) Sublingual
(E) Topical

4 A 27-year-old female with vulvovaginal candidiasis is given a one-time 100 mg dose of oral fluconazole. She has no other pertinent medical problems and takes no prescription medications. Administration of the medication results in a peak plasma concentration of 20 μg/mL. What is the apparent volume of drug distribution?

(A) 0.5 L
(B) 1 L
(C) 3 L
(D) 5 L
(E) 50 L

5 A 48-year-old-man with end-stage liver disease is hospitalized on the intensive care unit. Review of his blood work reveals elevated liver function tests to five times the normal rate. The patient is receiving multiple intravenous medications. Which of the following medications is likely to be therapeutic for this patient?

(A) Epinephrine
(B) Erythromycin
(C) Nifedipine
(D) Rifampin
(E) Verapamil

6 A 29-year-old man presents to his primary care physician complaining of dysuria, urgency, and painful ejaculation. The patient has a past medical history of allergic rhinitis. Physical examination reveals a tender prostate. The patient is given a prescription of sulfamethoxazole to be taken daily (q 12 h) for 30 days. The half-life is 12 h. How long will it take for the medication to reach 90% of its final steady state level?

(A) 10 h
(B) 20 h
(C) 30 h
(D) 40 h
(E) 50 h

7 A hospitalized patient with systemic candidiasis is receiving intravenous antifungal medications. He also has hepatic and renal insufficiency. Which of the following drug administration schemes would allow for the most steady state amount of drug in the body over a 2-week hospitalization period where medication administration will be necessary?

(A) Continuous IV infusion
(B) Once weekly IV injection
(C) Single daily IV injection
(D) Twice daily IV injection
(E) Twice weekly IV injection

8 A 27-year-old man with HIV disease and hepatic insufficiency presents to his primary care physician complaining of rectal pain and bleeding with bowel movements. Physical examination reveals several internal and external hemorrhoids. The patient would like to avoid surgical therapy for this condition. Which of the following routes of drug administration would be preferred in this patient?

(A) Enteral
(B) Intramuscular
(C) Intravenous
(D) Rectal
(E) Transdermal

9 A hospitalized patient with systemic infection is receiving intravenous antibiotics. He also has hepatic and renal insufficiency. After receiving medications for 5 days, he is found by nursing staff to be jaundiced. Drug toxicology profile is obtained and indicated drug levels of 10 times the acceptable value. Which of the following drug administration schemes is most likely to explain this situation?

(A) Continuous IV infusion
(B) Once weekly IV injection
(C) Single daily IV injection
(D) Twice daily IV injection
(E) Twice weekly IV injection

10 A patient receives a single dose of antibiotics following a prostate needle biopsy. He takes 500 mg of ciprofloxacin immediately after completion of the procedure. The half-life of the medication is 8 h. At approximately how many half-lives will it take for 90% of the drug to be excreted from the body?

(A) 1.0
(B) 2.0
(C) 3.0
(D) 3.3
(E) 5.0

11 The P-glycoprotein is a multidrug transmembrane transporter protein that transports medications across cell membranes. Functions of this protein include

(A) Pumping drugs into the urine for excretion
(B) Transport of drugs into liver hepatocytes
(C) Transport of drugs into fetal circulation for fetal treatment
(D) Transport of drugs from the intestinal lumen to the circulation
(E) Transport of drugs from the bloodstream into brain cells

12 A researcher is studying the bioavailability of commonly used antimuscarinics to treat irritable bowel syndrome. Medication A is administered in a 100 mg daily dose orally and 60 mg of the drug is absorbed from the gastrointestinal tract unchanged. Thus, the bioavailability of Medication A is

(A) 50%
(B) 60%
(C) 70%
(D) 80%
(E) 90%

13 A 40-year-old man is brought to the emergency department after suffering a cardiac arrest while in a shopping mall. His blood pressure is 70/40 mm Hg and his pulse is 40 beats/minute. He is given a dose of intravenous epinephrine. Which of the following reactions is necessary to induce a biologic response of increased heart rate?

(A) Detrusor contraction
(B) Drug-receptor complex formation
(C) Hepatic oxidation reaction
(D) Renal arteriolar contraction
(E) Splanchnic nerve stimulation

14 A 59-year-old female with diabetes presents to her primary care physician for routine follow-up. Her current medications include insulin. Her fasting blood sugars are in the range of 80 to 120 mg/dL. The intracellular effects of this medication are likely caused by which of the following mechanisms of action?

(A) Changes in ionic concentration within the cell
(B) Changes in membrane potential
(C) Protein phosphorylation
(D) Protein and receptor phosphorylation
(E) Receptor destruction

15 The therapeutic index of a drug is the ratio of the dose that produces toxicity to the dose that produces an efficacious response. By this definition, which of the following medications has the largest therapeutic index?

(A) Diazepam
(B) Digoxin
(C) Gentamicin
(D) Lithium
(E) Theophylline

16 A medical student is doing a summer research project studying five antibiotics to determine potency using the EC50. Antibiotics are placed in plated culture wells with 100,000 CFU of *Escherichia coli*. The EC50 results for the five antibiotics are shown in the following choices. Based on the results, the most potent antibiotic is

(A) Antibiotic A EC50 = 100
(B) Antibiotic B EC50 = 2
(C) Antibiotic C EC50 = 80
(D) Antibiotic D EC50 = 20
(E) Antibiotic E EC50 = 50

17 A drug that binds to a receptor and produces a biological response that mimics the response to the endogenous ligand is known as

(A) Agonist
(B) Antagonist
(C) Functional antagonist
(D) Partial agonist
(E) Partial antagonist

18 A 47-year-old HIV positive male with hepatic insufficiency and renal insufficiency presents to his primary care physician complaining of dysuria. Urine culture reveals greater than 100,000 CFU/mL of *Escherichia coli* pan-sensitive to all antibiotics. Which of the following would be the most appropriate treatment for this patient?

(A) Chloramphenicol
(B) Erythromycin
(C) Gentamicin
(D) Penicillin
(E) Rifampin

19 A researcher for a pharmaceutical company is studying a new medication to treat parkinsonism. The medication is dosed at 10 mg and causes improvement in bradykinesia and cogwheel rigidity in 99% of patients. However, 100 mg of this medication causes toxicity manifested as seizures in 1% of the population treated with this medication. What is the standard margin of safety of this medication?

(A) 100
(B) 300
(C) 500
(D) 700
(E) 900

20 A 67-year-old hospitalized patient with a deep venous thrombosis of the left calf and pulmonary embolism is currently on intravenous heparin on an hourly drip. Unfortunately, because of a calculation error, the heparin drip is running at 100 times the rate it should be running at. Protamine sulfate is immediately given intravenously. This agent works by which of the following mechanisms of action?

(A) Agonist
(B) Chemical antagonist
(C) Functional agonist
(D) Partial agonist
(E) Partial antagonist

21 A 61-year-old man is taking over-the-counter pseudoephedrine for cold and flulike symptoms. Over the course of the next few days, he experiences improvement in his rhinitis but should be concerned about the possibility of which of the following problems?

(A) Contraction of the iris causing visual changes
(B) Constriction of the bronchioles causing increased pulmonary secretions
(C) Erectile function improvement
(D) Thinning of his salivary glandular secretions
(E) Urinary retention

22 A 22-year-old woman who is afraid of running into her former boyfriend actually meets him unexpectedly in a shopping mall. Her fears are because their former relationship was marked by physical and mental abuse. Memories of him are met with increased anxiety and fear. Which of the following physiologic responses would this woman be expected to exhibit at this time of seeing this man?

(A) Bradycardia
(B) Diarrhea
(C) Hypertension
(D) Sweating
(E) Tracheal deviation

23 A 15-year-old boy who has diabetes and is insulin dependent is brought to the emergency department after collapsing at a baseball game. His blood sugar is 463 mg/dL by finger stick. Which of the following routes of administration would be most efficacious for medications to bring the blood sugar down?

(A) Intramuscular
(B) Intravenous
(C) Oral
(D) Subcutaneous
(E) Sublingual

24 A 16-year-old male high school football player takes 800 mg of ibuprofen after morning practice for a sore knee. Ibuprofen has a half-life of about 2 h. What percentage of the original plasma load of ibuprofen will remain in his blood when afternoon practice starts in 4 h?
(A) 0%
(B) 12.5%
(C) 25%
(D) 50%
(E) 75%

25 A 27-year-old woman takes phenytoin to control focal seizures. Most of the phenytoin in her blood is plasma-protein bound, and only the free fraction is pharmacologically active. The free fraction must diffuse through many barriers to reach its site of action. Many characteristics influence a drug's ability to diffuse across biologic membranes. Which of the following possible drug characteristics would aid such diffusion?
(A) Hydrophilicity
(B) Large molecular size
(C) Weak acid with a pKa of 7
(D) Weak base with a pKa of 7

26 You receive a call from a frantic mother whose 3-year-old son ate a handful of her amitriptyline (a weak acid). You instruct the mother to take her son to the emergency department where he is given bicarbonate (in addition to other measures). What is the most likely explanation for bicarbonate administration in this case?
(A) Bicarbonate should not have been given; a weak acid such as ammonium chloride should have been given instead
(B) Bicarbonate traps amitriptyline in the blood to keep it from reaching its active site
(C) Ion trapping the amitriptyline in the urine to hasten elimination is accomplished by giving bicarbonate
(D) Weak acids such as amitriptyline are chemically inactivated by bicarbonate

27 An 80-year-old male nursing home resident is hospitalized on a morphine drip to control pain for his terminal metastatic pancreatic cancer. Morphine undergoes phase I and phase II metabolism in the liver as well as being metabolized by other enzymes. Some of these metabolic reactions decrease with age. Which of the following metabolic reactions is likely still intact in this patient?
(A) Glucuronidation
(B) Hydrolysis
(C) Oxidation
(D) Reduction
(E) Unmasking of a functional group

28 A 34-year-old female insists on drinking a cup of grapefruit juice every morning for "body cleansing." Grapefruit juice is known to interfere with the cytochrome P450 system, disrupting levels of certain drugs. The cytochrome P450 system includes dozens of enzymes. Which is the most abundant CYP enzyme in human livers?
(A) CYP1A2
(B) CYP2A6
(C) CYP2D6
(D) CYP2E1
(E) CYP3A4

29 Researchers interested in studying a certain cytochrome P450 enzyme wish to isolate the enzyme of interest from the many other proteins in the cells. One of their initial steps is to lyse the cells and isolate the organelle which carries the enzyme they want to study. Which organelle will they isolate to find CYP enzymes?
(A) Golgi apparatus
(B) Lysosomes
(C) Mitochondria
(D) Peroxisomes
(E) Smooth endoplasmic reticulum

30 A 19-year-old female has a history of absence seizures. She currently takes ethosuximide to control her symptoms. The process of eliminating this drug involves multiple steps of metabolism followed by excretion. Many organs take part in both metabolism as well as excretion of drugs. Which of the following describes a step of metabolism?
(A) Acetaminophen glucuronidation by enterocytes
(B) Digoxin actively transported from hepatocytes into bile
(C) Ethanol passing from the blood into the alveoli
(D) Pancuronium being filtered in the kidney

31 An 18-year-old man is scheduled to have four wisdom teeth removed. The procedure is done under general anesthetic and there are no postoperative complications. He is discharged home with a prescription for codeine for pain control. Three days later, he contacts his physician and complains of difficulty moving his bowels. This type of adverse drug reaction is most similar to which of the following?
(A) A desquamating rash in a 36-year-old male receiving trimethoprim–sulfamethoxazole
(B) Aplastic anemia in a 12-year-old girl taking chloramphenicol
(C) Dizziness in a 65-year-old man after taking nitroglycerin
(D) Rhabdomyolysis in a 43-year-old male taking lovastatin
(E) Urticaria develops in a 7-year-old female after receiving a dose of penicillin

32 A 17-year-old pregnant female asks her doctor what she can do about her acne. The doctor prescribes a topical benzoyl peroxide preparation, but the patient is unsatisfied with the results. She has a close friend taking a vitamin A–based acne control product, and her friend often tells her how well it works. She begins taking her friend's pills and is pleased with the reduction in her acne. During which prenatal period is her unborn child at greatest risk for developing a birth defect?

(A) Before conception, because the drug described is known to cause mutations in the maternal germ cell line
(B) Days 1 to 17 after conception
(C) Days 18 to 55 after conception
(D) Days 56 to birth
(E) Vitamin A is a natural substance and therefore poses no risk of ill effects

33 A 24-year-old primigravid female's water breaks at 39 weeks gestation. Twenty-four hours later, she is having regular contractions 3 min apart. Her labor lasts 8 h. At the hospital, she gives birth to a baby boy, who initially appeared healthy. Within the next 12 h, the baby boy begins to have temperature fluctuations, difficulty breathing, and reduced movements. You suspect neonatal sepsis, so IV gentamicin plus ampicillin is started. Gentamicin and ampicillin are commonly used together because the combined effect is greater than the additive effects of both alone. This increased effectiveness is an example of what principle?

(A) Agonism
(B) Anergy
(C) Symbiosis
(D) Synergy

34 A 44-year-old black male is brought to the emergency department with 6 h of worsening lethargy and confusion. Past medical history is significant for easy bruising, 3 months of bone pain, and frequent pneumococcal infections. Labs were ordered, revealing serum calcium of 17 mg/dL (normal: 9.0 to 10.5 mg/dL). To rapidly lower his serum calcium, you administer calcitonin. However, calcitonin alone is insufficient because it is known to rapidly and suddenly lose its effectiveness within 2 to 3 days of repeated dosing. For this reason, a bisphosphonate, which take 2 to 3 days to become effective, is added simultaneously. What is the term for the rapid decrease in response to calcitonin?

(A) Anaphylaxis
(B) Prophylaxis
(C) Tachyphylaxis
(D) Tolerance

35 An 18-year-old college student is hanging shelves in his dorm room. He accidently hits his thumb with the hammer, which subsequently becomes swollen and red. He takes some acetaminophen for the pain. Many proteins are activated in response to injury leading to inflammation. Which of the following proteins is a transcription factor?

(A) COX-2
(B) HAT
(C) IκB
(D) iNOS
(E) NF-κB

36 A 24-year-old woman presents to her primary care physician complaining of feeling sleepy all the time. She has a history of hay fever since the age of 9 years. She is currently taking an antihistamine but cannot remember the name. She says it controls her hay fever symptoms well. You suspect that her medication is causing her to feel sleepy. First generation antihistamines can cause drowsiness because they cross the blood–brain barrier and act on which receptor?

(A) H_1
(B) H_2
(C) H_3
(D) H_4

37 A 21-year-old man presents to his primary care physician complaining of a single, painless ulcer on his penis, which he first noticed a few days ago. He admits to multiple sexual partners. You want to treat him for syphilis with penicillin G, but his history includes an itchy rash following amoxicillin treatment as a child. What must first occur in the body for a penicillin to become allergenic?

(A) First-pass metabolism in the liver creates a toxic metabolite
(B) It must bind to a larger molecule, resulting in a complex that the body sees as a foreign antigen
(C) Nothing additional needs to happen—simple exposure to penicillin can cause sensitization, which leads to a hypersensitivity reaction in subsequent exposures
(D) Penicillin is not allergenic—injection of penicillin simply causes histamine release by a mechanism not involving IgE or other immunoglobulin

38 A 66-year-old woman with chronic bronchitis who has smoked two packs of cigarettes per day for 50 years would like to quit. She has tried to quit five times in the past but felt she could not go long without a cigarette. The nicotine in her cigarettes stimulates many cells in her body by binding certain receptors. Which describes the response when nicotine binds its target receptor?

(A) A channel opens and negative ions flow into the cell
(B) A channel opens and positive ions flow into the cell
(C) Adenylyl cyclase is activated to increase intracellular cAMP
(D) Adenylyl cyclase is inhibited leading to decreased intracellular cAMP
(E) Phospholipase C is activated to increase intracellular IP_3 and DAG

39 A medical student is evaluating the effects of two α_1-adrenergic agonist in a rat-based model. Agent A is a short-acting agent with a half-life of 4 h. Agent B is a long-acting agent with a half-life of 12 h. Which of the following effects would be most likely to be observed at 2 h after administration of both agents?
(A) Decreased peripheral resistance
(B) Hypotension
(C) Miosis
(D) Urethral sphincter closure
(E) Vasodilation

40 A 54-year-old man hurt his lower back while lifting his garage door a month ago. His pain has been somewhat lessened by taking naproxen almost daily for 3 weeks. He began to have epigastric pain with meals 3 days ago. Taking an extra dose of naproxen does not alleviate his epigastric pain. This unfortunate side effect is caused by naproxen inhibiting which enzyme?
(A) COX-1
(B) COX-2
(C) Lipoxygenase
(D) Phospholipase A_2
(E) Thromboxane synthase

41 A 52-year-old woman with multiple endocrine neoplasia syndromes has a large pancreatic tumor and bilateral adrenal tumors. She is hospitalized on the medicine service. The tumor is considered inoperable. Her blood pressure is 180/100 mm Hg. In addition to intravenous fluids, this patient may benefit from which of the following interventions?
(A) Analgesics, oral route
(B) Analgesics, transdermal route
(C) Phenoxybenzamine, intravenous route
(D) Phentolamine, intravenous route
(E) Tolterodine, oral route

42 A 59-year-old man with decreased urinary stream and hypertension is prescribed doxazosin in hopes that both problems will be treated. He begins dose escalation with 1 mg given for one week, 2 mg given for 2 weeks, and 4 mg given for maintenance. He returns to his primary care physician saying that this medication is not helping. To determine whether or not the patient is taking the medication, it would be useful to look at the excreted concentration of medication in which of the following areas?
(A) Blood
(B) Feces
(C) Liver hepatocyte extract
(D) Skin
(E) Urine

43 A medical student is involved in a summer research project evaluating the excitatory and inhibitory effects of five neurotransmitters. Following as choices are the five neurotransmitters and their excitatory and inhibitory status. Which of the following neurotransmitters is likely to be serotonin?
(A) Neurotransmitter A; excitatory
(B) Neurotransmitter B; excitatory
(C) Neurotransmitter C; excitatory and inhibitory
(D) Neurotransmitter D; inhibitory
(E) Neurotransmitter E; generally inhibitory

44 A 19-year-old G1P0 woman lost her eyeglasses for a day. Constant squinting causes her to develop a headache, for which she takes ibuprofen. Which of the following poses the greatest risk to her fetus?
(A) Acute tubular necrosis
(B) Decreased pulmonary surfactant at birth
(C) Loss of physiologic heart shunt
(D) Low birth weight
(E) No risk—ibuprofen is a safe drug for pregnancy

45 A 63-year-old man with debilitating Parkinson's disease is currently taking levodopa. His primary care physician adds carbidopa to his treatment regimen. One week later, the patient presents to the emergency department complaining of anorexia, nausea, and vomiting. What is the most likely explanation for these findings?
(A) Drug toxicity
(B) Idiosyncratic drug reaction
(C) Stimulation of the chemoreceptor trigger zone
(D) Underlying infection
(E) Undiagnosed malignancy

46 When treating patients with Parkinson's disease, there are three dopamine agonists: pramipexole, ropinirole, and rotigotine. Regarding the pharmacokinetics of these agents, which of the parameters might suggest favorable clinical efficacy for pramipexole?

(A) Bioavailability
(B) Half-life
(C) Hepatic excretion capability
(D) Volume of distribution

47 A 33-year-old pregnant woman begins taking a new drug, Drug X, for morning sickness. Drug X has not been found to have adverse maternal or fetal effects in animal models, but no human studies have been done. Under which FDA Pregnancy Category would Drug X fall?
(A) A
(B) B
(C) C
(D) D
(E) X

48 A 56-year-old alcoholic male consumes a six-pack of beer before going to bed. After being absorbed from his gut, blood carries the alcohol through the portal vein into the liver where it can be metabolized. Phase I metabolism of ethanol is carried out by cytochrome P450 2E1. Which of the following is true of phase I metabolism?
(A) Always precedes phase II metabolism
(B) Are carried out largely in the plasma
(C) Examples are oxidation and reduction reactions
(D) Includes such reactions as glucuronidation and sulfation
(E) Produces very polar metabolites

49 A 74-year-old man with moderate stage Alzheimer's disease is seeing his primary care physician. He takes various medications and all are prescription items. He has just begun on memantine 6 months ago and his family notes no difference in his symptoms. What is the most likely explanation for these findings?
(A) Drug toxicity
(B) Expected side effect profile
(C) Interaction with antacids
(D) Interaction with vitamins
(E) Underlying tinnitus

50 A potential beneficial effect of a long-acting benzodiazepine, flurazepam, may have a cost-effective property beneficial to the development of a generic form. This could be related to which of the following areas?
(A) Adverse effects
(B) Efficacy
(C) Timing of administration
(D) Tonicity
(E) Toxicity

51 A 72-year-old man is going to undergo a left hemicolectomy. The anesthesiologist is preparing to anesthetize him and plans to use inhalational anesthetic agents. Which of the following factors will make the patient require more anesthetic agent to achieve the desired response?
(A) Chronic alcohol abuse
(B) Diet
(C) Immunodeficiency state
(D) Hypothermia
(E) Weight

52 A medical student is involved in a supper research project involving a mouse endothelial surface to determine which mediators are involved in platelet aggregation. The results of such studies will indicate an important role for which of the following substances?
(A) Cyclic AMP
(B) Cyclic ATP
(C) Cyclic GMP
(D) Cyclic GTP
(E) Progesterone

53 A 54-year-old man with insulin-dependent diabetes mellitus is treated with daily glargine. His blood sugars are typically in the range of 100 to 180 mg/dL. The rationale behind the use of this agent and its success as demonstrated in this patient involve which of the following?
(A) Degradation by gastric juice
(B) Low isoelectric point
(C) Hepatic metabolism
(D) Oral administration
(E) Renal excretion

54 A 78-year-old woman with vaginal vault stenosis and urinary burning is prescribed topical estrogen, which is applied to the anterior vaginal wall every other day. Physical examination reveals a mild cystocele. Which of the following statements is correct about this agent?
(A) Hydroxylated in the kidney
(B) Metabolized by sulfation
(C) Metabolites excreted in the urine
(D) Reabsorption occurs in the lungs
(E) Toxicities are greater than that for oral preparations

55 A 22-year-old woman presents to the student health clinic inquiring about a progesterone-only birth control pill. She is concerned that taking an estrogen preparation will cause her to have bloating and swelling. The rationale against the use of progesterone by itself as a birth control agent is because of

(A) Bad taste in the mouth
(B) Cost
(C) Dosing biweekly
(D) Low bioavailability
(E) Slow metabolism

56 A 58-year-old man is recovering in the hospital following a heart attack. He is started on clopidogrel. The initial dose, also known as the loading dose, is higher than his normal daily dose, also known as the maintenance dose. Which of the following represents the calculation for a maintenance dose?
(A) $= 0.7 \times Vd/t_{1/2}$
(B) = amount of drug in body/drug plasma concentration
(C) $= Cp \times CL/F$
(D) $= Cp \times Vd/F$
(E) $= U \times V/P$

57 A 24-year-old woman complains of irritability, restlessness, and trouble sleeping. She says that she worries about everything. The physician prescribes diazepam to help calm her anxiety. Diazepam must cross the blood–brain barrier to be effective. Which of the following characteristics would help a drug molecule cross this barrier?
(A) Hydrophilicity
(B) Large size
(C) Lipid solubility
(D) Weak acid with pKa of 4
(E) Weak base with pKa of 9

58 A 47-year-old man with AIDS is hospitalized for a fever of unknown origin. He is placed in a combination of antibiotics including a β-lactam and an aminoglycoside. The rationale behind the use of multiple antibiotics includes which of the following?
(A) Hepatotoxicity
(B) Nephrotoxicity
(C) Synergism
(D) Toxicity

59 A 12-year-old male with Type-1 diabetes mellitus takes an insulin preparation before his meals to avoid hyperglycemia. Once glucose molecules enter his cells, they are phosphorylated. Phosphorylated glucose is unable to leave the cell. Two enzymes that can phosphorylate glucose are glucokinase and hexokinase. Glucokinase is found primarily in the liver and has a lower affinity for glucose but a greater capacity to phosphorylate glucose than hexokinase, which is found in other body tissues. Compared to glucokinase, which of the following differences in enzyme kinetics will hexokinase display?
(A) Higher Km and higher V_{max}
(B) Higher Km and lower V_{max}
(C) Lower Km and higher V_{max}
(D) Lower Km and lower V_{max}
(E) There will be no difference in the enzyme kinetics hexokinase compared to glucokinase

60 A 47-year-old woman who has been diagnosed with bipolar disorder needs a refill on her lithium prescription. She also has hypertension that is well controlled with an ACE inhibitor. Lithium has a narrow therapeutic index. Which of the following describes a narrow therapeutic index?
(A) The chance of toxicity is remote at the therapeutic dose
(B) The ratio of TD50 to ED50 equals 1
(C) The ratio of TD50 to ED50 is less than 1
(D) The therapeutic dose approaches the toxic dose
(E) The therapeutic dose is much greater than the toxic dose

61 A 23-year-old woman with a history of bacterial vaginosis is prescribed oral metronidazole. On the third day of treatment, she calls her physician complaining of a metallic taste in her mouth. What is the most appropriate course of action for her physician to take?
(A) Administer Benadryl, oral
(B) Administer Benadryl, topical
(C) Discontinue medication
(D) Prednisone
(E) Watchful waiting

62 A 46-year-old woman with infiltrating ductal carcinoma of the breast undergoes radical mastectomy and axillary node dissection. Pathology reveals that the cancer has spread to the regional lymph nodes. Systemic chemotherapy is considered for this patient. Which of the following statements about this therapy is true?
(A) Cells in the G0 phase are susceptible to chemotherapeutic agents
(B) Rapidly dividing cells are sensitive to the cytotoxic effects
(C) Slowly dividing cells are susceptible to chemotherapeutic agents
(D) Unimodal therapy is most often advocated for treatment of breast cancer
(E) Watchful waiting is the best course of action for this patient

63 A 13-year-old girl with abnormal menses presents to her primary care physician for treatment. She has a history of inguinal hernia repairs in the past. Her physician begins therapy with oral micronized estradiol in order to regulate menses. Which of the following is true regarding this therapy?

(A) Limited bioavailability
(B) Limited first-pass metabolism
(C) Minimally available
(D) Nephrotoxicity at low doses
(E) Neuromuscular blockade likely

64 A 59-year-old man is going to undergo a prostate needle biopsy by his urologist. As a preparation for the procedure, he is required to take a fleet enema per rectum and a one time dose of ciprofloxacin 500 mg prior to the procedure. He has a prior medical history of diabetes mellitus, which is controlled with diet. Administration of the medication results in a peak plasma concentration of 20 μg/mL. What is the apparent volume of drug distribution?

(A) 0.5 L
(B) 1 L
(C) 5 L
(D) 15 L
(E) 25 L

65 A 17-year-old woman who is a college freshman presents to the student health clinic complaining of a creamy discharge from her vagina. She is not sexually active. Physical examination reveals an intact hymenal ring with no evidence of pelvic prolapse. The patient is given a prescription of fluconazole to be taken daily (q 12 h) for 3 days. The half-life is 12 h. How long will it take for the medication to reach 90% of its final steady state level?

(A) 10 h
(B) 20 h
(C) 30 h
(D) 40 h
(E) 50 h

66 A 49-year-old man receives a single dose of antibiotics following a colonoscopy with biopsy of several polypoid lesions. The patient has a family history of colorectal polyps. He has a past medical history of hypertension. He takes 500 mg of levofloxacin immediately after completion of the procedure. The half-life of the medication is 20 h. At approximately how many half-lives will it take for 90% of the drug to be excreted from the body?

(A) 1.5
(B) 2.5
(C) 3.0
(D) 3.3
(E) 5.5

67 A researcher is attempting to develop a cholinomimetic agent to use in patients with colonic motility syndrome. This agent will serve as a procolonic agent by increasing muscular contractions in the sigmoid colon and rectum. The medication is known as Agent X112A. The medication is administered in a 100 mg daily dose orally and 50 mg of the drug is absorbed from the gastrointestinal tract unchanged. Thus, the bioavailability of this drug is

(A) 50%
(B) 70%
(C) 80%
(D) 85%
(E) 95%

68 A 22-year-old man presents with a painless penile ulcer. His social history is significant for multiple sexual contacts. The physician prescribes benzathine penicillin G, which is renally excreted. Which of the following relationships describes clearance?

(A) $= 0.7 \times Vd/t_{1/2}$
(B) = Amount of drug in the body/plasma drug concentration
(C) $= Cp \times Cl/F$
(D) $= Cp \times Vd/F$
(E) $= pKa + \log([A^-]/[HA])$

69 A 39-year-old man takes a 100 mg dose of medication X. This drug is taken orally and becomes biotransformed by metabolism in the liver and secondary metabolism in the kidneys. This defines which of the following processes?

(A) Absorption
(B) Catabolism
(C) Distribution
(D) Elimination
(E) Metabolism

70 A 49-year-old man with a history of chronic headaches takes over-the-counter aspirin. He complains of mid-epigastric pain. His primary care physician switches him to enteric coated aspirin. His epigastric pain resolves. Which of the following is the most likely explanation for this finding?

(A) The enteric component is basic and stable
(B) The enteric component protects the drug from jejunal acid
(C) The enteric component dissolves in the small intestine
(D) The enteric component is fluid sensitive

71 A 49-year-old man with diabetes mellitus takes subcutaneous insulin for his insulin-dependent diabetes mellitus. He takes 4 U of regular insulin every 12 h to maintain his blood sugar in the range of 80 to 140 mg/dL. This route of administration allows for absorption of insulin by which of the following processes?

(A) Active transport
(B) Facilitated transport
(C) Osmosis
(D) Passive transport
(E) Simple diffusion

72 A 6-month-old male infant is hospitalized for nausea, vomiting, fevers, and failure to tolerate oral medications. He is placed on Phenergan per rectum once daily to treat the nausea and vomiting. Which of the following statements is true about this route of administration?

(A) Allows destruction of the medication by gastric enzymes
(B) Maximal biotransformation of the drug by the liver
(C) Rectal administration of medications is well accepted
(D) Rectal irritation following administration is uncommon
(E) Useful if patient is unconscious or vomiting

73 Medication AB has efficacy in animal studies to improve the symptoms of systemic diseases. Its function is mediated by the P-glycoprotein system. Which of the following functions would likely be unaffected by this system?

(A) Limitation of drug access to the brain
(B) Reduction of absorption of drugs in the spleen
(C) Transport of drugs into bile for elimination
(D) Transport of drugs into the intestinal lumen
(E) Transport of drugs from fetal to maternal systems

74 A patient takes an oral sympathomimetic agent for regulation of heart rate. This agent is taken orally. Which of the following systemic effects is likely a result of this medication?

(A) Bronchoconstriction
(B) Hypotension
(C) Pupillary constriction
(D) Tachycardia
(E) Urinary frequency

75 A 17-year-old pregnant woman asks her doctor what she can do about her acne. The doctor prescribes a topical benzoyl peroxide preparation, but the patient is unsatisfied with the results. She has a close friend taking isotretinoin for acne control, and her friend often tells her how well it works. She begins taking her friend's pills and is pleased with the reduction in her acne. In which FDA Pregnancy Category does this drug belong?

(A) Category A
(B) Category B
(C) Category C
(D) Category D
(E) Category X

76 A 57-year-old man with a history of knee trauma undergoes a total knee replacement. Postoperatively, he is given warfarin for deep vein thrombosis prophylaxis. Warfarin helps by preventing the γ-carboxylation of certain clotting factors, which renders them ineffective. Warfarin prevents the γ-carboxylation of which of the following clotting factors?

(A) Factor I
(B) Factor V
(C) Factor VIII
(D) Factor IX
(E) Factor XII

77 Compound XY is a novel agent that will improve bladder contractility through its ability to bind to receptors on the bladder wall. Which of the following drug bonds is most important in drug–receptor associations for this compound to be effective?

(A) Covalent interactions
(B) Hydrogen bonds
(C) Ionic bonds
(D) Van der Waals interactions

78 Compound AQ1 is a novel agent that will mimic the function of endogenous thyroid hormone and be useful in the treatment of hypothyroidism. The compound will bind to its receptor at target sites. The molecular structure in this compound will dictate its physical properties. Which of the following properties is unlikely to influence its ability to function effectively?

(A) Chemical name
(B) Conformation
(C) Hydrophobicity
(D) Ionization state
(E) Stereochemistry

79 Drug XA12 is a novel antibiotic agent that is renally excreted. The drug enters the kidney through the renal arteries and ultimately into Bowman's space. Which of the following indicators will have the smallest effect on elimination of this drug from the body?

(A) Glomerular filtration rate of 60 mL/min
(B) Glomerular filtration rate of 100 mL/min
(C) Lipid solubility
(D) Plasma binding of drug reduced by 50%
(E) Renal plasma flow of 200 mL/min

80 A 28-year-old man is hospitalized after a fall from a cliff. His current medical problems include cardiogenic shock, heart failure, renal disease, and cirrhosis from chronic alcoholism. Because of weight loss, he is felt to be somewhat hypermetabolic. Which of the following factors will have the most significant effect to decrease drug half-life of medications administered to him?

(A) Cardiogenic shock
(B) Cirrhosis
(C) Heart failure
(D) Hypermetabolic state
(E) Renal disease

81 A 55-year-old man with chronic cardiac failure currently takes multiple medications, including digoxin. He is brought to the emergency department because of slurred speech and inappropriate behavior. It turns out that he has not taken his digoxin for the last 2 weeks. The physician gives 125 μg as standard dose. Twenty-four hours later, his serum levels were reported to be 2 ng/mL (2 μg/L). The target therapeutic level is 0.8 ng/mL. What dose of digoxin should he receive?

(A) 25 μg
(B) 50 μg
(C) 75 μg
(D) 100 μg
(E) 125 μg

82 A 44-year-old man with a sacral spinal cord injury has atonia of the sigmoid colon and rectum. Despite sacral nerve root stimulation, no normal colorectal function is able to be achieved. Which of the following is true concerning the postganglionic receptors at the distal colon and rectum?

(A) Exogenous ligand formation is taking place
(B) The active and inactive receptor states are in irreversible equilibrium
(C) The receptors are likely in a transient state
(D) The drugs occupying the receptor are producing conformational change in the receptor

83 Ligand-gated ion channels allow for fast flow of ions across cell membranes via binding of the ligand to the channel. Based on this information, the most likely location of these channels in a 35-year-old man with no pertinent medical or surgical history is in which of the following areas?

(A) Cardiac muscle
(B) Cerebellum
(C) Pancreas
(D) Spleen
(E) Thyroid gland

84 A 39-year-old man with chronic abdominal pain takes prescription narcotic medication (hydrocodone) for pain control. He currently takes eight pills per day but still complains of pain. Previously, the same dose would relieve his pain but now there appears to be a diminished effect. What is the most likely explanation for this finding?

(A) Receptor denervation
(B) Receptor depolarization
(C) Receptor desensitization
(D) Receptor hypersensitivity
(E) Receptor telescopic transformation

85 A novel cholinomimetic agent is being designed to improve salivary glandular secretions in patients with xerostomia. This agent will increase the uptake of choline into cells. This will combine with acetyl coenzyme A which is found in which of the following locations?

(A) Cytosol
(B) Golgi apparatus
(C) Mitochondria
(D) Rough endoplasmic reticulum
(E) Smooth endoplasmic reticulum

86 Regarding the use of a daily baby aspirin, oral fiber supplements, and a daily "water" pill in an 89-year-old man with hypertension and coronary artery disease, which of the following statements is true regarding pharmacology in the elderly patient?

(A) Coexisting disease states are unlikely to produce additive impairment
(B) Elderly patients are less sensitive to drug effects
(C) Elderly patients are less sensitive to drug side effects
(D) Elimination of drugs becomes impaired with age
(E) Responses to compensate for drug accumulation are satisfactory

87 A medical student is doing a summer research project evaluating the percentage of drug absorbed orally in a mouse model. Several characteristics of the agents are evaluated such as acid/base status, solubility, and size of side chains. Characteristics of the studied agent that would be best absorbed following oral administration in the tested mice would most likely include
(A) Bulky charged side chains
(B) Lipid solubility
(C) Strong acid
(D) Strong base
(E) Water solubility

88 A 37-year-old man is in the intensive care unit with sepsis. He is receiving intravenous (IV) vasopressors to maintain his blood pressure. During morning rounds, you notice his IV has extravasated and the skin around the IV site is cool and pale. What should be done?
(A) Atropine should be injected
(B) Dopamine should be injected
(C) Nothing
(D) Phentolamine should be injected
(E) Topical prednisone should be given

89 A 29-year-old woman cuts her arm when her steak knife slips while cutting a steak at a barbeque dinner. She sustains a 4-cm laceration of the lateral aspect of her left arm that will require sutures. A 2% lidocaine is infiltrated prior to suture placement. Which of the following will have an effect on the onset and duration of action of this medication?
(A) Blood pH
(B) Lidocaine pH
(C) Lipid solubility of the tissue
(D) Nerve diameter
(E) pKa of the drug

90 When comparing the administration of local anesthesia in a 4-year-old healthy boy to an 80-year-old man with a history of hypertension, cirrhosis, and diabetes, which of the following statements is likely to be true?
(A) Liver failure is less likely a problem in the older patient
(B) Maximal dose of anesthetic must be calculated
(C) Older patients require higher doses of anesthetic
(D) Older patients will have a better response to anesthetic
(E) Younger patients will have a better response to anesthetic

91 A 28-year-old man is an unrestrained driver in a motor vehicle accident. He suffers a compound fracture of the right femur and is currently undergoing fixation in the operating room. The surgery is not completed and anesthesia is not being administered at this time. Recovery from IV induction agents is caused by
(A) Ionization
(B) Liver metabolism
(C) Plasma clearance
(D) Protein binding
(E) Redistribution from sites in the CNS

92 Drug A and Drug B are of equal magnitude. If Drug A and Drug B are combined together, this would be an example of which of the following?
(A) Additive effects
(B) Neutralization
(C) Potentiation
(D) Synergism

93 A 77-year-old woman with metastatic breast cancer suffers from chronic pain. She is on end-of-life care with home hospice. She is given scheduled morphine injections to keep her comfortable. Which of the following statements regarding the mechanism of this agent is correct?
(A) Depolarization of nerve cells
(B) Inhibition of nerve firing
(C) Presynaptic stimulation of transmitter release
(D) Substance P abundant concentrations and release
(E) Stimulation of excitatory neurotransmitter release

94 Which of the following drug equations exemplifies the concepts of potentiation?
(A) Drug AB > Drug A + Drug B
(B) Drug AB = Drug A = Drug B
(C) Drug AB < Drug A < Drug B
(D) Drug AB = Drug B > Drug A

95 Regarding the prescription of controlled substances, drugs that have a low abuse potential, may or may not require a prescription, and are subject to state and local regulation describe which of the following classifications?
(A) CII
(B) CIII
(C) CIV
(D) CV

96 A new vasopressor in development, Drug X, is a partial agonist at α_1-adrenergic receptors. Epinephrine is a full agonist at these same receptors. What will be the level of α_1-receptor stimulation if both of these drugs (Drug X and epinephrine) are given simultaneously?

(A) It is impossible to tell from the information given
(B) They will be stimulated at a higher level than when epinephrine is given alone
(C) They will be stimulated but at a lower level than when epinephrine is given alone
(D) They will be stimulated at the same level as when epinephrine is given alone
(E) They will result in no net stimulation

97 A new vasopressor in development, Drug X, is a partial agonist at α_1-adrenergic receptors. Epinephrine is a full agonist at these same receptors. Which of the following statements is true regarding the potency of Drug X compared to epinephrine?

(A) Drug X and epinephrine are equally potent because they act on the same receptors
(B) Drug X is more potent because it is a partial agonist
(C) Epinephrine is more potent because it is a full agonist
(D) Epinephrine is more potent because it is an endogenous neurotransmitter
(E) Relative potency cannot be determined from the information given

98 Referring to the following figure regarding the pharmacokinetics of prototype Drug X-100A, a novel chemotherapeutic agent to treat breast cancer, which of the following letters represents the process of elimination?

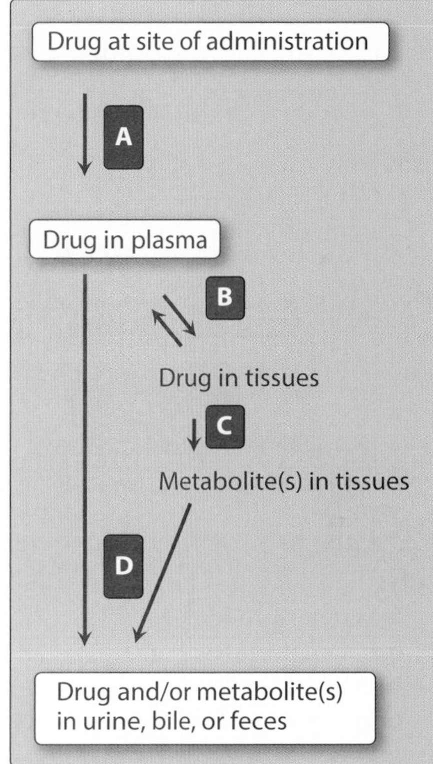

(A) Letter A
(B) Letter B
(C) Letter C
(D) Letter D

99 A 47-year-old man with schizophrenia is hospitalized for an exacerbation of baseline psychotic symptoms. He is found to be agitated and is disoriented. Haloperidol can be administered by Injection #1 or Injection #2 in the following figure. Furthermore, this injection should be given into which of the following skin layers?

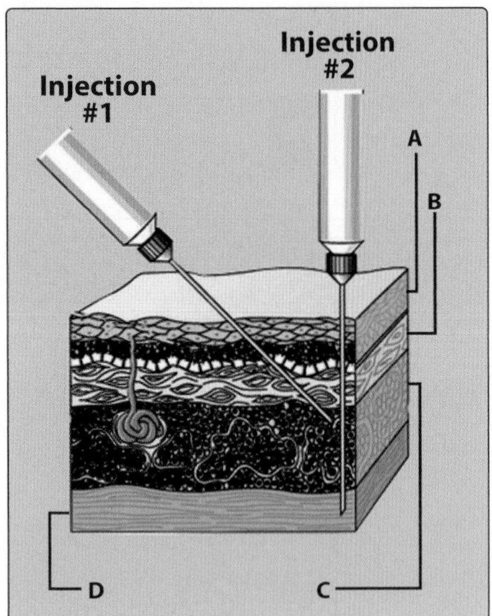

(A) Injection #1 to level A
(B) Injection #2 to level A
(C) Injection #2 to level B
(D) Injection #2 to level C
(E) Injection #2 to level D

100 A 55-year-old woman with overactive bladder complains of urinary frequency of approximately 15 times per day. She is seen by her primary care physician who prescribes a transdermal patch containing an anticholinergic agent. The following figure represents a picture of the patch formulation of this medication. The drug reservoir is contained in which of the following letters of the figure?

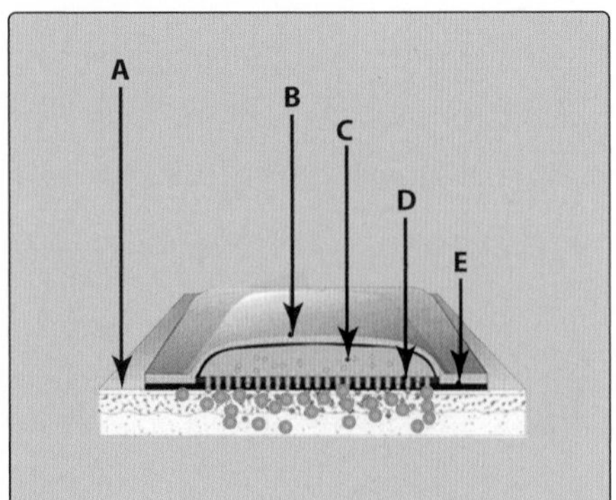

(A) Letter A
(B) Letter B
(C) Letter C
(D) Letter D
(E) Letter E

101 A novel medication designed to treat lymphoma can be administered via injection or orally. If the drug is given orally, an estimation of the area under the curve for this dose may be represented by which of the following letters in the following figure?

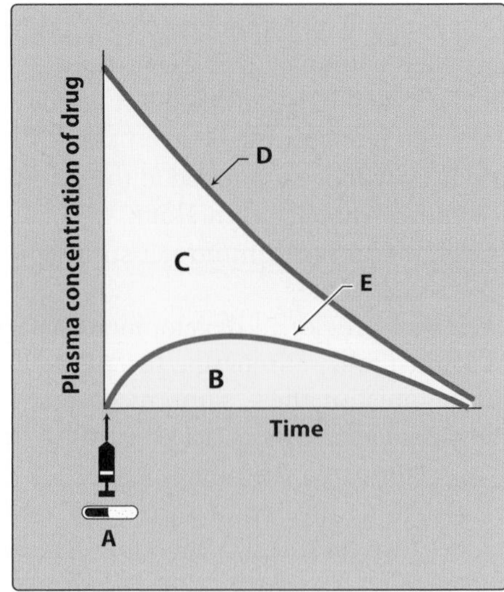

(A) Letter A
(B) Letter B
(C) Letter C
(D) Letter D
(E) Letter E

102 An orally administered medication is eliminated by the kidney. Passive reabsorption of the drug occurs because it is lipid soluble and un-ionized. At which of the following locations in the kidney will this reabsorption occur?

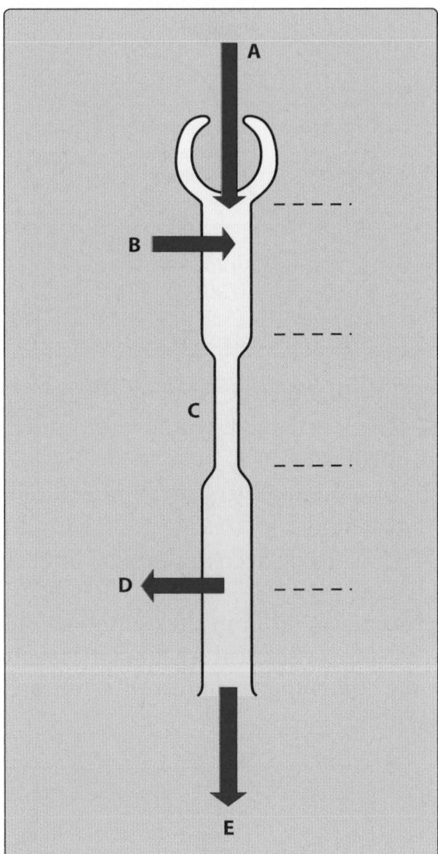

(A) Letter A
(B) Letter B
(C) Letter C
(D) Letter D
(E) Letter E

103 A 55-year-old man with a systemic infection is given an intravenous antibiotic at a high rate of infusion. A graph of plasma concentration of drug versus time is presented next. Which of the following letters represents the steady state region?

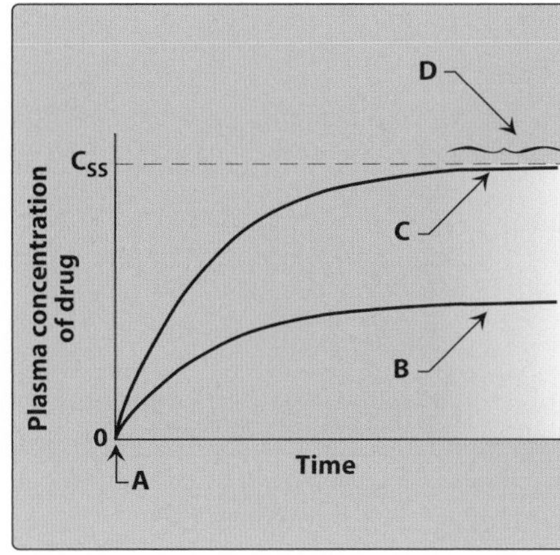

(A) Letter A
(B) Letter B
(C) Letter C
(D) Letter D

104 A 54-year-old man is hospitalized with an infection. He is being treated with an intravenous injection of antibiotics. The following figure represents different doses of drug administration based on various pharmacokinetics. Which of the following curves would produce the largest amount of drug available in the body?

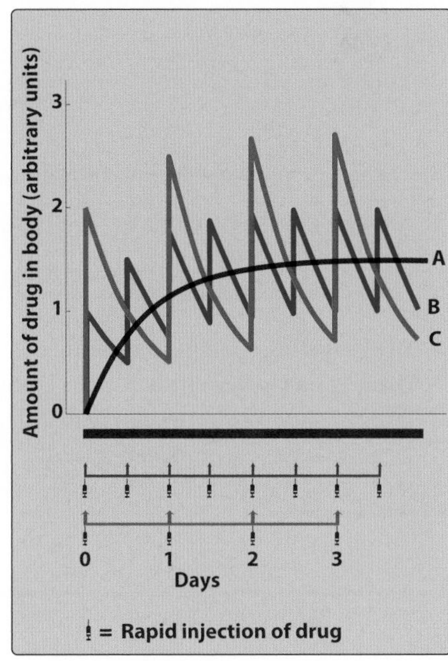

(A) Curve A
(B) Curve B
(C) Curve C
(D) Cannot be determined

105 Two drugs are shown in the following figure. Both are antibiotics used to treat bacterial pneumonia. Which of the following statements is correct about the figure shown next?

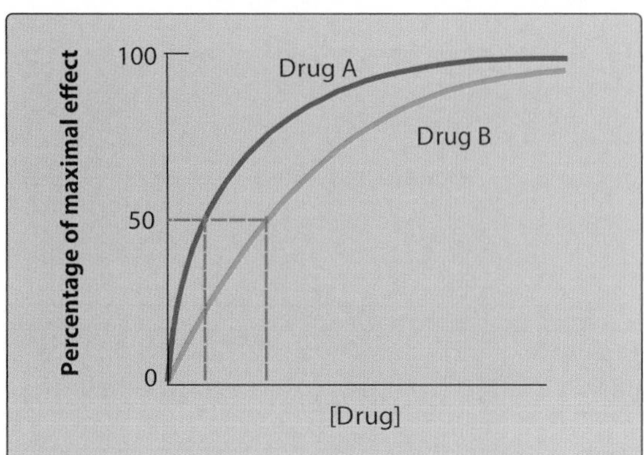

(A) Drug A has a lower EC50
(B) Drug B has a lower EC50
(C) Drug A is less potent than Drug B
(D) Drug B should be given intramuscularly
(E) Drug A should be given intravenously

106 Three novel drugs to treat Alzheimer's disease have undergone phase I trials. A graph of the biologic effect versus log drug concentration is plotted in the following graph. Which of the following statements is true?

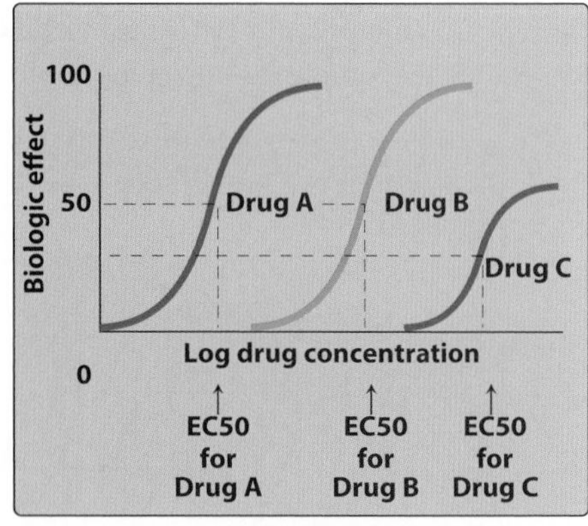

(A) Drug A is less potent than Drug B
(B) Drug A has lower efficacy than Drug B
(C) Drug C shows lower potency than Drugs A and B
(D) Drug C is best administered orally
(E) Drug C is most likely to be approved for use

107 A graph of the therapeutic index of warfarin is shown in the following figure. Which of the following statements is true?

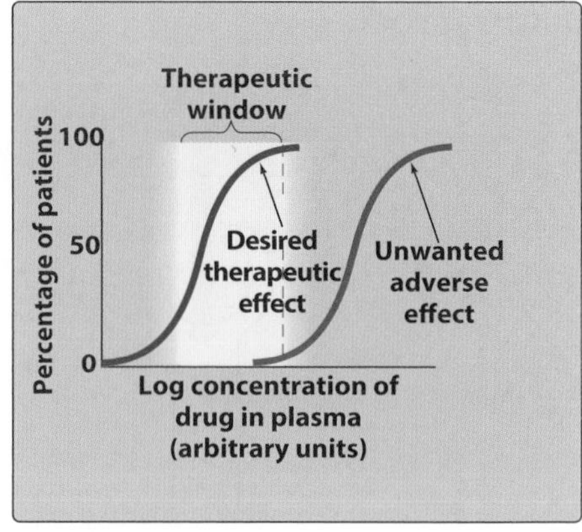

(A) The therapeutic window is large
(B) There is a small window of desired effect of this medication
(C) Unwanted adverse events are unlikely with this agent
(D) Unwanted adverse events are unlikely dose related

108 Neurotransmission in the autonomic nervous system is related to chemical signaling between cells. Which of the following examples illustrates direct contact signaling?

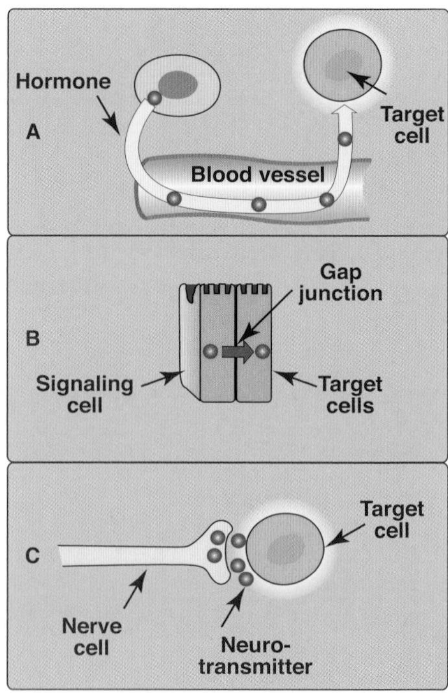

(A) Letter A
(B) Letter B
(C) Letter C
(D) Cannot be determined

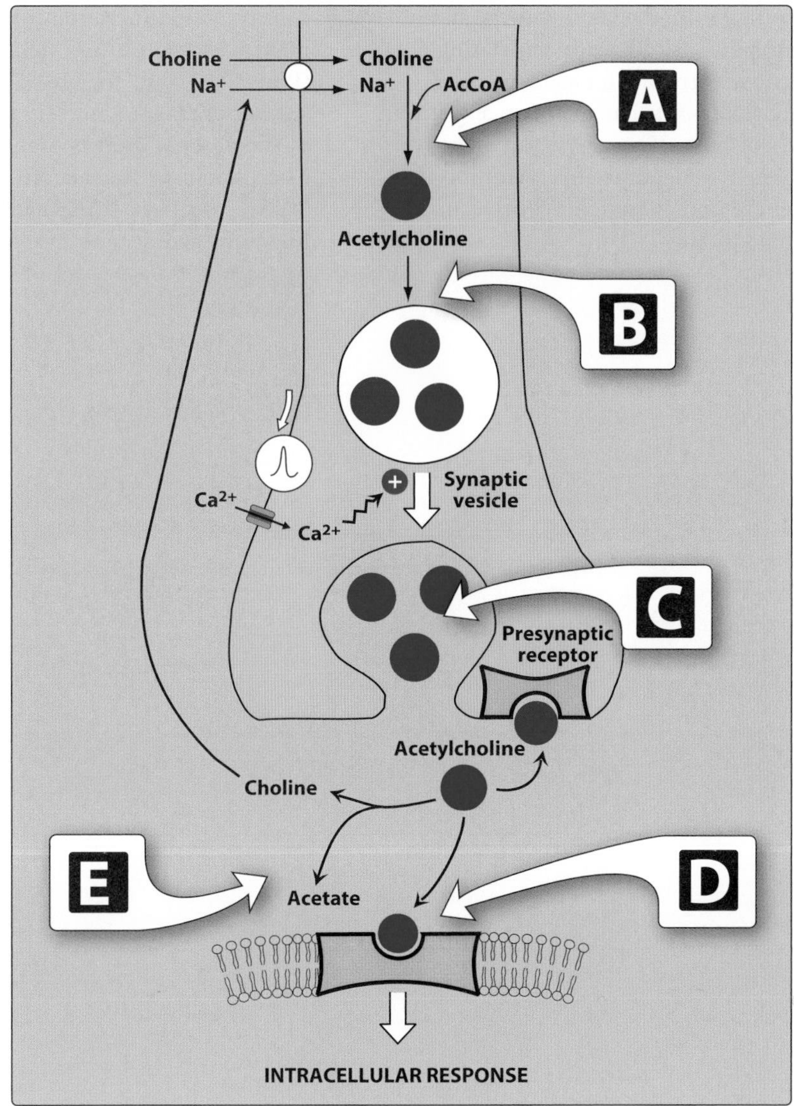

109 Alzheimer's disease is thought to result from an imbalance in the synthesis and release of acetylcholine from the cholinergic neuron. Above is a diagram of this process. In which of the following steps is acetylcholine taken up into storage vesicles?

(A) Letter A
(B) Letter B
(C) Letter C
(D) Letter D
(E) Letter E

110 A 78-year-old woman is hospitalized with a methicillin resistant bacterial infection with bacteremia. She has previously demonstrated resistance to multiple antibiotics and has not begun on a course of intravenous tigecycline. Despite therapy for 3 days, she continues to spike fevers daily. What is the most likely explanation for this finding?

(A) Antibiotic susceptibility pattern
(B) Drug–drug interaction
(C) Rapid distribution to body tissues
(D) Subtherapeutic dosing
(E) Supratherapeutic dosing

111 A 52-year-old female with diabetes presents to the ambulatory care clinic for follow-up. She has no complaints and is tolerating her metformin well. Her hemoglobin A_{1c} is 13.5. Her urine analysis shows microalbuminuria. She is started on captopril, which competitively inhibits angiotensin-converting enzyme. What effect does a competitive inhibitor have on enzyme kinetics?

(A) Decreases K_m
(B) Decreases V_{max}
(C) Increases K_m
(D) Increases V_{max}
(E) No effect on K_m or V_{max}

112 A 68-year-old man presents to the ambulatory care clinic with the complaint of difficulty urinating. He has difficulty starting his stream and feels his bladder is still full after he urinates. He has to get up about four times a night to urinate. The physician starts him on finasteride, which noncompetitively inhibits 5α-reductase. What effect does a noncompetitive inhibitor have on enzyme kinetics?

(A) Decreases K_m
(B) Decreases V_{max}
(C) Increases K_m
(D) Increases V_{max}
(E) No effect on K_m or V_{max}

113 A 33-year-old man presents to the emergency department with pain in his right buttock. The pain is constant, 8/10, and increases when he sits down. A CT scan confirms the presence of an abscess. Gram stain of the abscess fluid is gram-positive cocci in clusters. The patient is started on vancomycin for a possible MRSA infection. If the half-life of vancomycin is 5 h, how long will it take to reach clinical steady state?

(A) 10 h
(B) 12 h
(C) 15 h
(D) 18 h
(E) 23 h

ANSWERS

1 **The answer is A: Enteral.** This patient has dysphagia and Alzheimer's disease. These conditions would make drug administration by mouth difficult and limit direct absorption via the stomach. This route of drug administration would give the lowest serum drug concentrations for the reasons described previously. (B) Intramuscular administration, although painful for the patient, would give acceptable serum drug concentrations. (C) Intrathecal administration would give acceptable therapeutic drug concentrations but would be limited to CNS disease states. (D) Intravenous administration would provide medications via vein and therapeutic drug concentrations. It could be used for various medications. (E) Transdermal administration applies medications to the skin and could achieve therapeutic drug concentrations.

2 **The answer is A: Absorption.** Drug absorption from the site of administration, in this case via the topical route, allows the medication to enter into the skin and then into the plasma. Following this step, the medication can distribute into tissues and also be metabolized in tissues. (B) Distribution occurs following absorption of the drug from the site of administration. (C) Elimination involves removal of the drug from the body via urine, bile, or feces. (D) Glycosylation is not a step in the process of drug pharmacokinetics. (E) Metabolism of drugs occurs in the kidneys or liver after the drug has achieved adequate levels in tissues.

3 **The answer is A: Inhalation.** Inhalation provides rapid delivery of a drug across a large surface area of the respiratory tract and is the route of administration of choice in a patient with an airway disease such as asthma. Inhaled albuterol is commonly administered in this manner. (B) Intranasal puff metered dose would only deliver a small amount of drug to the patient and would not be recommended in this acutely ill patient. (C) Subcutaneous administration is a slow route of administration and is not preferred in this acutely ill patient. (D) Sublingual, although allowing the medication to enter the circulation would be less preferred than the inhalation route in this acutely ill patient. (E) Topical administration would only achieve a local effect of the drug and is contraindicated in this acutely ill patient.

4 **The answer is D: 5 L.** The volume of distribution is calculated by dividing the total amount of drug in the body by the plasma concentration of the drug. In this case, Vd = 100 mg fluconazole/20 μg/mL which is the peak plasma concentration. Thus, the volume of distribution of fluconazole is 5 L.

5 **The answer is A: Epinephrine.** This patient has end-stage liver disease. This ability to metabolize medications through the cytochrome system of the liver is impaired. Drugs that are metabolized in this fashion will not be properly broken down and will accumulate to toxic levels. Epinephrine is not metabolized by the cytochrome system and can be used with caution in this patient. (B) Erythromycin is an antibiotic metabolized by the hepatic cytochrome system. (C) Nifedipine is an antihypertensive metabolized by the hepatic cytochrome system. (D) Rifampin is used in the treatment of tuberculosis and is also metabolized by the hepatic cytochrome system. (E) Verapamil is a calcium channel blocker and is also metabolized by the hepatic cytochrome system.

6 **The answer is D: 40 h.** To figure out how long it will take a medication to reach 90% of its final steady state, use the formula: $(3.3) \times (t_{1/2})$. In this case, the half-life is 12 h. Thus, $(3.3) \times (12)$ is approximately 40 h. Of note, because of poor penetration into prostate tissues, despite achieving 90% steady state levels in 40 h, patients with this condition often need to take antibiotics for approximately 3 to 4 weeks for cure.

7 **The answer is A: Continuous IV infusion.** Continuous IV infusion results in a less rapid influx of drug into the body initially. However, within a short time, a steady state of drug level in the body will be achieved. Although the drug level will achieve steady state, injection of drugs several times daily will result in higher drug amounts initially after dosing but will decrease according to half-life. (B) Once weekly IV injection will result in a peak and trough level of the drug with initially high concentrations and will decrease to almost no drug in the system. (C) Single daily IV injections result in lower amounts of drug in the body with peaks and troughs. (D) Twice daily IV injections will result in the highest amounts of drug in the body but will also have peaks and troughs. (E) Twice weekly IV injections will result in higher amounts of drug in the body as compared with once weekly IV injections.

8 **The answer is D: Rectal.** This patient has hemorrhoids, and a topical route of administration of medication is preferred. This route avoids the hepatic first pass effect so the patient's liver insufficiency would not likely be problematic with this route of administration. (A) Enteral route administration will be unlikely to achieve an adequate therapeutic response in a patient with hemorrhoids. (B) Intramuscular route administration is an ineffective therapy for rectal diseases. (C) Intravenous administration is an ineffective therapy for rectal diseases such as hemorrhoids. (E) Transdermal administration achieves systemic effects through systemic absorption of medication. It is not effective for internal hemorrhoids.

9 **The answer is D: Twice daily IV injection.** Twice daily drug administrations cause the highest amounts of drug available in the body. In a patient with hepatic and renal insufficiency, drug metabolism is compromised; and within a few doses using this administration scheme, high levels of drug in the body will be noted. (A) Continuous IV infusion results in steady state drug levels on the body. (B) Once weekly IV injections result in lower amounts of drug in the body with peaks and troughs. (C) Single daily IV injections result in lower amounts of drug in the body but will also have peaks and troughs. (E) Twice weekly IV injections will result in higher amounts of drug in the body as compared with twice daily IV injections.

10 **The answer is D: 3.3.** At the first half-life, 50% of the drug will be eliminated from the body. At the second half-life, 75% of the drug will be eliminated from the body. At the third half-life, 87.5% of the drug will be eliminated from the body. Finally, at 3.3 half-lives, 90% of the drug will be eliminated from the body.

11 **The answer is A: Pumping drugs into the urine for excretion.** The P-glycoprotein is a multidrug transmembrane transport protein that transports medication across cell membranes. In the kidney, responsibilities include pumping drugs into the urine for excretion. (B) This protein excretes drugs into bile for excretion in feces. (C) This protein transports drugs out of fetal circulation via the placenta into the maternal circulation. (D) This protein transports drugs from the circulation into the intestinal lumen. (E) This protein transports blood out of the brain cells to protect them from drug toxicities.

12 **The answer is B: 60%.** Medication A has a bioavailability of 60%. Bioavailability is the fraction of administered drug that reaches the systemic circulation. In this example, if 100 mg of Medication A is administered orally, and 60 mg of this drug is absorbed unchanged, the bioavailability is 0.6, or 60%. Determining bioavailability is important for calculating drug dosages for various routes of administration other than the intravenous route.

13 **The answer is B: Drug-receptor complex formation.** The epinephrine must be recognized by a receptor to induce a biologic response. The drug will bind to the receptor. In this case, these are β-adrenergic receptors. A drug-receptor complex is formed. A biologic response is achieved. In this case, the biologic response is increased heart rate and blood pressure. (A) Epinephrine does not cause detrusor muscle contraction. (C) Epinephrine is not metabolized by hepatic oxidation reactions. (D) While renal arteriolar contraction occurs with epinephrine, this is not the basis of its cardiac effects. (E) Splanchnic nerve stimulation is not the basis of tachycardia induced by epinephrine.

14 **The answer is D: Protein and receptor phosphorylation.** This patient has diabetes and takes insulin. This medication (hormone) functions via insulin receptors. The transmembrane signaling mechanism for insulin involves protein and receptor phosphorylation. (A) Cholinergic nicotinic receptors signal via changes in ionic concentration within the cell. (B) Cholinergic nicotinic receptors signal via changes in membrane potential. (C) α-Adrenergic receptors signal via protein phosphorylation. (E) Receptor destruction is not a mechanism of transmembrane signaling.

15 **The answer is A: Diazepam.** Diazepam has a large therapeutic index. A large number of patients achieve therapeutic effects that are desired and a much smaller percentage of patients have adverse effects. (B) Digoxin has a narrow therapeutic index and requires frequent drug level monitoring to limit adverse effects associated with use. (C) Gentamicin has a narrow therapeutic index. Frequent peak and trough levels are drawn during therapy to minimize potential toxicities. (D) Lithium has a narrow therapeutic index and requires close monitoring of levels to limit toxicities. (E) Theophylline has a narrow therapeutic index and requires frequent monitoring of levels to limit adverse events.

16 **The answer is B: Antibiotic B EC50=2.** The EC50 is the drug dose that shows a 50% maximal response. When several drugs are studied, this would allow the investigator to determine the relative potencies. The lower the EC50, the more potent the drug is. Thus, Antibiotic B is the most potent of the choices given because its EC50 is 2. (A) Antibiotic A has the highest EC50 and is the least potent of the antibiotics presented in this question. (C) Antibiotic C has the second highest EC50 and is the second least potent of the antibiotics presented in this question. (D) Antibiotic D has the second lowest EC50 and would be considered the second most potent of the antibiotics presented in this question. (E) Antibiotic E has an EC50 of 50, which places it in the middle of the relative potencies of the five antibiotics presented in this question.

17 **The answer is A: Agonist.** The definition of an agonist is the biologic response produced by a drug binding to its receptor. For example, the α-adrenergic agonist phenylephrine when it binds to its receptor produces responses similar to the endogenous ligand. (B) Antagonists are drugs that decrease the actions of another drug or the endogenous ligand. (C) Functional antagonists may act at a separate receptor and oppose those effects of the agonist. (D) Partial agonists have activities somewhere between the full agonist and no agonistic activity. (E) Partial antagonists have activities somewhere between the full antagonist and no antagonistic activity.

18 The answer is D: Penicillin. Penicillin is the best choice antibiotic in this patient because of its large therapeutic index. It is safe and common to give large doses greater than the minimal required doses even in patients with hepatic and renal insufficiency. (A) Chloramphenicol would have a narrow therapeutic index in patients with hepatic insufficiency. (B) Erythromycin would induce the cytochrome system in a patient with hepatic insufficiency and induce toxicity. (C) Gentamicin is a nephrotoxic antibiotic and should be avoided in a patient with renal insufficiency. (E) Rifampin is metabolized by the cytochrome system and should be avoided in patients with hepatic insufficiency.

19 The answer is E: 900. The standard margin of safety is a ratio of the LD1 (lethal dose to 1% of the population) divided by the ED99 (the dose effective in 99% of the population) minus 1 × 100. In this case, the LD1 is 100 and the ED99 is 10. Thus, (100/10) − 1 × 100 = 900. Thus, the dose that is effective in 99% must be increased to 900% to be toxic to 1% of the population.

20 The answer is B: Chemical antagonist. A chemical antagonist prevents the actions of an agonist by modifying or sequestering the agonist so that it is incapable of binding to and activating its receptor. Protamine sulfate is a chemical antagonist for heparin. (A) Agonist is the biologic response produced by a drug binding to its receptor. (C) Functional antagonists can act at separate receptors than traditional antagonists. (D) Partial agonists have activities somewhere between the full agonist and no agonistic activity. (E) Partial antagonists have activities somewhere between the full antagonist and no antagonistic activity.

21 The answer is E: Urinary retention. Pseudoephedrine is a sympathomimetic agent that can cause relaxation of the detrusor and contraction of the external urethral sphincter. This can result in urinary retention, an important concern to warn older men about who take this over-the-counter agent. (A) α-Agonists will cause dilation of the pupils. (B) α-Agonists cause bronchodilation. (C) α-Agonists stimulate ejaculation. (D) α-Agonists cause thickening of the salivary gland secretions.

22 The answer is C: Hypertension. This patient is exhibiting features of the "fight-or-flight" response, which is triggered by sympathetic activation. The cardiac effects include increased heart rate, contractility, and blood pressure. Skeletal muscle blood vessels dilate while skin blood vessels vasoconstrict. (A) This patient will exhibit tachycardia. (B) This patient will exhibit increased gastrointestinal sphincter tone. (D) This patient will have vasoconstriction of the skin and mucous membranes. (E) Tracheal dilation, not deviation occurs in the "fight-or-flight" response.

23 The answer is B: Intravenous. Insulin (as most drugs) needs to enter the bloodstream for maximal effect; IV infusion will result in the fastest and highest peak blood insulin concentration. There are many formulations of insulin for intramuscular or subcutaneous injection, but even the fastest have no effect until the insulin reaches the systemic blood circulation. There is no way to make insulin absorption into the blood from intramuscular or subcutaneous injection faster than injecting directly into the blood. The same can be said for inhaled and sublingual insulin preparations. (A) Intramuscular insulin can be given in rapidly acting formulations, but even this is not as fast as IV insulin. (C) Insulin given orally would be broken down and rendered ineffective by peptidases in the gut. (D) Subcutaneous insulin can be given in rapidly acting formulations, but even this is not as fast as IV insulin. (E) Insulin is not normally given sublingually, and sublingual absorption is slower than IV infusion.

24 The answer is C: 25%. Half-life refers to the time it takes for half of the drug to be eliminated from the body. Half-life is a term used for drugs that follow first-order elimination. This means that the rate of elimination of drug is proportional to the concentration of drug (as opposed to zero-order elimination—as in phenytoin, ethanol, and aspirin—in which the rate of elimination is constant regardless of the drug concentration). If a drug follows first-order elimination, half of the amount present in the body will be eliminated after each half-life. For example, the concentration of a drug with a half-life of 2 h will drop to 50% after 2 h, 25% after 4 h, 12.5% after 6 h, and 6.25% after 8 h. (A) Even after 8 h, 6.25% of the original dose of ibuprofen will still be in his blood. (B) After 6 h, the plasma concentration will be 12.5%. (D) After 2 h (1 half-life) the plasma concentration will be 50%. (E) The plasma concentration would never be higher than 50% of the original after at least one half-life has past.

25 The answer is D: Weak base with a pKa of 7. Characteristics that aid diffusion across biologic membranes include hydrophobicity (uncharged, nonpolar) and small size. A weak base with a pKa of 7 at a pH of 7 would exist as half RNH2 and half RNH3$^+$. Increasing the pH to 7.4 means decreasing the [H$^+$], so the equilibrium for the reaction RNH3$^+$ → RNH2 + H$^+$ would be shifted to the right. A base with a pKa of 7 then would be mostly in the RNH2 state (not ionized RNH3$^+$ state) at physiologic pH. This uncharged state (RNH2) is conducive to diffusion across biologic membranes. (A) Hydrophobicity aids diffusion across membranes, not hydrophilicity. (B) Small molecular size, not large, aids diffusion across membranes. (C) A weak acid with a pKa of 7 would exist as half ionized RCOO$^-$ and half un-ionized RCOOH. As pH increases, more RCOOH will give up their H^+ to become $RCOO^-$. At physiologic pH, 7.4, more of this compound would be in the ionized $RCOO^-$ state than in the uncharged RCOOH. Charges and polarity hinder a molecule's ability to diffuse across biologic membranes.

26 **The answer is C: Ion trapping the amitriptyline in the urine to hasten elimination is accomplished by giving bicarbonate.** Excess bicarbonate is rapidly excreted in the urine, raising the urine pH. Any weak acid, such as amitriptyline, that enters this basic urine will become ionized. Once ionized, it is not reabsorbed and so is effectively trapped for excretion in the urine. The reaction is RCOOH (in blood) → $RCOO^- + H^+$ (in the urine). (A) A weak acid lead to acidic urine. Acidic urine would cause amitriptyline to be less ionized and therefore more effectively reabsorbed. (B) Bicarbonate is rapidly excreted in the urine to maintain physiologic pH in the blood. It is not therapeutically reasonable to manipulate the blood pH for the purpose of ion trapping. (D) Weakly acidic medications are not generally inactivated by bases.

27 **The answer is A: Glucuronidation.** Morphine is metabolized by P-glycoprotein on enterocytes, by cytochrome P450 3A4 enzymes (phase I), and by glucuronidation (phase II). Phase I metabolism usually involves oxidation, but may involve reduction or hydrolysis, and results in the unmasking or addition of functional groups such as -OH, −COOH, −SH, −NH2. The goal of phase I metabolism is to render the molecule more water soluble. If after phase I the drug is sufficiently water soluble, it is excreted. If not, it may additionally pass through phase II, which involves conjugation with a highly polar moiety. In some cases, a phase I reaction may follow a phase II reaction; but often, the phase I reaction provides the functional group needed for conjugation (phase II). Phase I metabolism is generally decreased in the elderly, whereas phase II remains intact. Of the options listed, only glucuronidation is a phase II reaction. We would expect the other reactions to be decreased in this patient. (B) Hydrolysis is a phase I reaction, which would likely be decreased. (C) Oxidation is a phase I reaction, which would likely be decreased. (D) Reduction is a phase I reaction, which would likely be decreased. (E) Unmasking a functional group is the result of phase I metabolism, which would likely be decreased.

28 **The answer is E: CYP3A4.** Cytochrome P450 3A4 (CYP3A4) accounts for roughly 30% of human liver CYP enzymes. CYP1A2 makes up about 15%, CYP2A6 about 4%, CYP2D6 about 5%, and CYP2E1 about 10%. Many drugs are metabolized by this enzyme, including cyclosporine, protease inhibitors, and benzodiazepines. CYP3A4 activity is also modulated by many substances that it does not metabolize, including grapefruit juice (inhibition) and St. John's wort (induction). (A) CYP1A2 makes up about 15% of human liver CYP enzymes. (B) CYP2A6 makes up about 4% of human liver CYP enzymes. (C) CYP2D6 makes up about 5% of human liver CYP enzymes. (D) CYP2E1 makes up about 10% of human liver CYP enzymes.

29 **The answer is E: Smooth endoplasmic reticulum.** The cytochrome enzymes are involved in oxidation and reduction reactions and contain heme groups. All cytochrome P450 enzymes are found in the smooth endoplasmic reticulum (SER). Functions of the SER include lipid and steroid synthesis, drug metabolism, and regulation of intracellular calcium concentration. The Golgi apparatus, lysosomes, and peroxisomes contain no cytochrome enzymes. Mitochondria contain cytochrome C but no cytochrome P450. (A) The Golgi apparatus is involved in protein trafficking and glycosylation. It has no cytochrome enzymes. (B) Lysosomes contain hydrolytic enzymes, which work at a low pH. The inside of a lysosome is acidified to activate these enzymes. Lysosomes contain no cytochrome enzymes. (C) Mitochondria do have cytochrome C (involved in the electron transport chain of oxidative phosphorylation) but do not contain cytochrome P450 enzymes. (D) Peroxisomes are involved in the metabolism of very long chain fatty acids (>22 carbons) and have no cytochrome enzymes.

30 **The answer is A: Acetaminophen glucuronidation by enterocytes.** Many steps are involved in the elimination of most drugs from the body. Ethosuximide, for example, undergoes phase I metabolism (hydroxylation) followed by phase II metabolism (glucuronidation) in the liver. The metabolites are then excreted in the urine. Steps in metabolism involve chemical changes to a molecule's structure, whereas excretion is simply moving a drug molecule from inside the body to outside the body (no change in chemical structure is made). Of the options listed, only glucuronidation is a type of metabolism. The other responses are all methods of excretion. (B) The passage of digoxin from hepatocytes into bile involves no chemical change to digoxin. This is an example of excretion. (C) Ethanol diffusing from the blood into the alveoli involves no chemical change to the ethanol. This is an example of excretion. (D) Pancuronium filtration in the kidney involves no chemical change to pancuronium. This is an example of excretion.

31 **The answer is C: Dizziness in a 65-year-old man after taking nitroglycerin.** Adverse drug reactions (ADRs) are broadly categorized into two types: A and B. Type A describes reactions that are either an exaggeration of the drug's primary effect (such as headache following nitroglycerin because of its vasodilatation effect) or because of another pharmacological effect of the drug (such as opioids causing constipation as well as pain relief). Type B describes reactions that are unusual or unexpected, including allergic reactions. Type A reactions are often foreseeable and correlate well with drug dose. Type B is usually much more rare and unforeseeable. (A) A desquamating rash in a patient receiving a sulfa drug may be Stevens–Johnson syndrome, a rare but serious side effect. This is not caused by the expected effects of trimethoprim–sulfamethoxazole, so it is a type B reaction. (B) Aplastic anemia is a rare but serious side effect of chloramphenicol administration. This is not caused by the expected effects of chloramphenicol, so it is a type B reaction. (D) Rhabdomyolysis is a rare side effect of all statins. It is not caused by the expected effects of statins, so it is a type B reaction. (E) Urticaria in a patient following administration of penicillin is likely caused by an allergic reaction to penicillin. This is not caused by the expected effects of penicillin, so it is a type B reaction.

32 **The answer is C: Days 18 to 55 after conception.** Development can be divided into three periods based on reaction to teratogens. The first period, which includes implantation, starts at fertilization (day 1) and goes to about day 17. Insults during this period have an "all-or-nothing" effect. This is because at this stage, cells are still totipotent, so either so many cells are lost that a spontaneous abortion results or enough cells are spared that can replace destroyed cells completely so no defect is seen in the newborn. The next stage is the embryonic period, days 18 to 55. Organogenesis takes place during this stage, so any insults to the rapidly dividing, differentiated cells during this period easily lead to malformations. This is the period of development in which an unborn child is at greatest risk for a birth defect. Days 56 to parturition comprise the fetal period. Insults during this period generally cause only a reduction in cell number in the growing organs (not structural defects to the organs themselves). (A) Vitamin A is not known to cause mutations in the maternal germ cell line leading to birth defects. (B) Insults during days 1 to 17 after conception usually have either no lasting effect or lead all the way to a spontaneous abortion. (D) Insults during days 56 to birth can cause growth retardation (particularly in the CNS), but the embryo is much more susceptible to teratogens during days 18 to 55. (E) Vitamin A at the high levels present in acne medication is known to be teratogenic. Whether a substance is natural or synthetic has no bearing on its teratogenicity.

33 **The answer is D: Synergy.** Synergy is a term used to describe a situation when the combined effect of two or more drugs simultaneously is greater than can be explained by arithmetically adding the individual effects. A fine example is the synergistic effect when penicillin such as ampicillin is combined with an aminoglycoside such as gentamicin. (A) An agonist is a molecule that elicits a response from a receptor by binding to it. The term can refer to endogenous or exogenous compounds. (B) Anergy refers to a lack of the body's immune system to mount a normal response to an antigen. It does not describe cooperation between drugs. (C) Symbiosis refers to a mutually beneficial relationship between organisms. It is not used to describe interactions between medications.

34 **The answer is C: Tachyphylaxis.** Tachyphylaxis describes a scenario in which the response to a drug rapidly decreases. Tachyphylaxis resembles tolerance in that the response to the drug cannot be restored by increasing the dose. There are some important differences between tolerance and tachyphylaxis, however. Tolerance is a slow decrease in response to a drug, whereas tachyphylaxis is rapid. Tolerance comes from the target cells or tissue modifying its physiology to compensate for the effect of a drug. Tachyphylaxis occurs when something disrupts the drug itself from functioning, such as internalization of receptors or uncoupling of signal transduction. (A) Anaphylaxis is a manifestation of a type I hypersensitivity reaction mediated by mast cells and preformed antibody. It does not lead to a decreased response in a drug's action. (B) Prophylaxis refers to measures taken to prevent disease rather than treat disease once it occurs. It does not describe changes in response to a drug. (D) Tolerance and tachyphylaxis both refer to a decreased response to a drug, but tolerance has a slower onset and relates to changes in physiology to compensate for the drug's effect.

35 **The answer is E: NF-κB.** Inflammation is a cellular response with many triggers. Some examples are infection, chemical stress, and (as in this case) physical stress. The first step is phosphorylation of IκB, an inhibitory protein whose role is to bind NF-κB and keep it inactive in the cytoplasm. Phosphorylation of IκB causes dissociation from NF-κB. NF-κB then enters the nucleus where it activates histone acetyltransferase (HAT) and acts as a transcription factor for COX-2 and iNOS. COX-2 and iNOS are enzymes that produce mediators that lead to the signs and symptoms of inflammation. (A) COX-2 is an enzyme induced by NF-κB and is responsible for the sustained production of inflammatory prostaglandins following injury. (B) HAT can be activated by NF-κB. By acetylating histones, it promotes a more open configuration of DNA thereby facilitating transcription of genes. (C) When IκB is bound to NF-κB, IκB hides the nuclear localization signal domain on NF-κB to keep it inactive in the cytoplasm. (D) iNOS is another enzyme inducible by NF-κB. iNOS produces nitric oxide (NO), which is a potent vasodilator.

36 **The answer is A: H_1.** Blockade of H_1 receptors in the CNS are thought to be the reason for drowsiness caused by first generation antihistamines. H_1 receptors are found in many cell types, including sensory neurons, CNS neurons, and endothelial cells. Histamine acting on these cells cause itching, wakefulness, and vasodilatation, respectively. First-generation antihistamines cross the blood–brain barrier more readily than second-generation antihistamines. Once in the CNS, first-generation antihistamines block H_1 receptors to decrease wakefulness. (B) H_2 receptors are known for their location on gastric parietal cells. H_2 antagonists can be used to treat GERD by decreasing acid secretion. Blocking H_2 receptors does not ameliorate symptoms of hay fever or cause changes in wakefulness. (C) H_3 receptors are located presynaptically in the CNS and work as auto receptors via negative feedback to decrease histamine release. Stimulation would cause increased histamine release, resulting in increased wakefulness. (D) H_4 receptors are found on such cells as eosinophils and neutrophils and mediate chemotaxis. They are not known to influence wakefulness.

37 **The answer is B: It must bind to a larger molecule, resulting in a complex that the body sees as a foreign antigen.** Although many patients inaccurately report an allergy to penicillin, a patient who developed urticaria following exposure to penicillin likely does have an allergy and should not be exposed again without being tested first. The penicillin molecule by itself is too small to be allergenic. According to the hapten hypothesis, such drugs likely bind to proteins or other macromolecules that the body then recognizes as foreign. (A) The liver plays only a minor role in the elimination of penicillin. Most is excreted unchanged in the urine. The metabolites that are formed are not known to be particularly toxic. (C) This is not correct because penicillin itself does not cause an immune reaction. Only after binding to a macromolecule does penicillin become allergenic. (D) Morphine is an example of a drug that causes histamine release not involving immunoglobulin. This has not been demonstrated with penicillin.

38 **The answer is B: A channel opens and positive ions flow into the cell.** Nicotinic cholinergic receptors are ligand-gated positive ion channels. They are so named because they are the receptors that the drug nicotine binds. They are found on muscles at the neuromuscular junction (NM type) and in postganglionic neurons in the autonomic ganglia (NN type). When acetylcholine or nicotine binds the receptor, the channel pore opens and positive ions flow through it. Although some K^+ ions leave the cell, far more Na^+ ions enter the cell and the net effect is depolarization. (A) This answer describes GABA channels in the brain, which open to allow Cl^- to enter the neuron causing hyperpolarization. (C) This answer describes β-adrenergic receptors. (D) This answer describes α_2-adrenergic receptors. (E) This answer describes α_1-adrenergic and cholinergic muscarinic receptors.

39 **The answer is D: Urethral sphincter closure.** α_1-Adrenergic agonists have the following effects: closure of the urethral sphincter and increasing peripheral resistance. This will lead to an increase in blood pressure (hypertension). The ophthalmic effects of this agent include mydriasis. (A) Peripheral resistance will increase with α_1-adrenergic agonist. (B) Hypertension occurs because of increase in peripheral vascular resistance. (C) Mydriasis, not miosis, occurs with an α_1-adrenergic agonist. (E) Vasoconstriction, not vasodilation, will result from α_1-adrenergic agonist.

40 **The answer is A: COX-1.** Gastric mucosa is protected in part by the actions of prostaglandins produced from arachidonic acid in part by COX-1. COX-1 is constitutively active (not activated by inflammation). Both COX-1 and COX-2 make prostaglandin H_2, the direct precursor for other prostaglandins as well as thromboxane. Prostaglandins act on gastric mucosa to decrease acid secretion and increase mucus production. COX-2 is responsible for prostaglandin production during inflammation and is the intended target of NSAIDs, but most NSAIDs (including naproxen) inhibit both COX-1 and COX-2. (B) COX-2 is inhibited by naproxen, but this enzyme is the primary target. Inhibiting COX-2 does not constitute a side effect in this case. (C) Lipoxygenase uses arachidonic acid to make leukotrienes. This enzyme is not inhibited by NSAIDs. (D) Phospholipase A_2 cleaves membrane phospholipids to provide arachidonic acid for the COX, lipoxygenase, and thromboxane synthase enzymatic reactions. It is inhibited by glucocorticoids. (E) Thromboxane synthase is found in platelets. This enzyme itself is not inhibited by NSAIDs, but NSAIDs do block production of thromboxane synthase's substrate, prostaglandin H_2, by inhibiting COX enzymes.

41 **The answer is C: Phenoxybenzamine, intravenous route.** Phenoxybenzamine is used in the treatment of pheochromocytoma, a catecholamine-secreting tumor of cells derived from the adrenal medulla. Prior to surgical removal of the tumor, patients are treated with phenoxybenzamine to preclude the hypertensive crisis that can result from manipulation of the tissue. This drug is also useful in the chronic management of these tumors, particularly when the catecholamine-secreting cells are diffuse and, therefore, inoperable. This medication should be given intravenously. (A) This patient should have immediate treatment of her hypertension. (B) Transdermal administration is not the preferred method of administration in this patient. (D) Phentolamine is the preferred agent for short-term treatment of pheochromocytoma. (E) Tolterodine is indicated in men with benign prostate hyperplasia.

42 **The answer is B: Feces.** Metabolism leads to inactive products that are excreted in urine except for those of doxazosin, which appear in feces. Doxazosin is the longest acting of these drugs used to treat benign prostate hyperplasia. Doxazosin has added benefit in that it can also treat mild hypertension. (A) Doxazosin is not excreted into the blood. (C) Doxazosin is not measured through liver hepatocyte extract. (D) Doxazosin is not excreted through the skin. (E) Alfuzosin and tamsulosin are excreted into the urine.

43 **The answer is C: Neurotransmitter C; excitatory and inhibitory.** Serotonin is a biogenic amine, which has postsynaptic effects that are both excitatory and inhibitory. This neurotransmitter has effects on feeding, body temperature control, regulation of mood and emotions, and sleepiness/wakefulness. (A) Neurotransmitter A could be acetylcholine. (B) Neurotransmitter B could be acetylcholine or norepinephrine. (D) Neurotransmitter D could be GABA or glycine. (E) Neurotransmitter E is likely to be met-enkephalin.

44 **The answer is C: Loss of physiologic heart shunt.** Ibuprofen is a nonsteroidal anti-inflammatory drug (NSAID), which inhibit cyclooxygenase enzymes to block prostaglandin synthesis. This is useful for mild pain management because prostaglandins are pain sensitizers and cause inflammation. But prostaglandins serve other functions as well, one of which is to maintain a patent ductus arteriosus in the fetus. NSAIDs are contraindicated in pregnancy because they will inhibit production of fetal PGE_2, allowing this physiologic shunt to close prematurely. (A) Ibuprofen can cause acute tubular necrosis because of inhibition of vasodilatory prostaglandins, but this is more a concern for patients with underlying renal disease. (B) NSAIDs are not known to have a negative impact on pulmonary surfactant production. (D) NSAIDs are not known to lead to low birth weights. (E) Ibuprofen is contraindicated in pregnancy because of the risk of premature ductus arteriosus closure.

45 **The answer is C: Stimulation of the chemoreceptor trigger zone.** One of the adverse effects of carbidopa is nausea and vomiting. This can occur because of stimulation of the chemoreceptor trigger zone of the medulla. This is not a drug toxicity nor is it an unexpected idiosyncratic drug reaction. (A) There is no evidence to suggest drug toxicity in this case. (B) This is not an unexpected reaction. It is an important side effect of carbidopa to realize. (D) There is no evidence in the history of this patient to suggest infection. (E) There is no evidence in the history of this patient to suggest underlying malignancy.

46 **The answer is A: Bioavailability.** Pharmacokinetic properties of dopamine agonists of pramipexole, ropinirole, and rotigotine are evaluated in this question. Pramipexole has the highest percentage of bioavailability of the three agents at >90%. (B) The half-lives are similar for all three agents at approximately 6 to 8 h. (C) All three agents are excreted via the kidney. (D) Rotigotine has the largest volume in distribution but the lowest bioavailability (45%).

47 **The answer is B: B.** Pregnancy Category A contains drugs that have shown no risk to the fetus in the first trimester of pregnancy in well-controlled human studies. Category B is for drugs that have either had no well-controlled human studies but show no risk in animal studies, or drugs that show risk in animal studies but not in well-controlled human studies. Category C is for drugs that show risk in animal models and have had no well-controlled human studies. Category D is for drugs that are known to pose a risk to the fetus but the benefits may outweigh the risks. Category X is for drugs absolutely contraindicated in pregnancy. Category X drugs pose such a great risk to the fetus that no benefit is seen to outweigh the risk. (A) Category A drugs have undergone well-controlled human studies and are shown to be safe in pregnancy. (C) Category C drugs have shown risk to fetus in animal models. (D) Category D is known to pose a risk to the human fetus. (E) Category X is known to pose a risk to the human fetus.

48 **The answer is C: Examples are oxidation and reduction reactions.** Drug metabolism is grouped into two categories: phase I and phase II. Phase I metabolism is carried out by cytochrome P450 enzymes in the liver and includes oxidation, reduction, and hydrolysis reactions. Phase II metabolism conjugates the metabolite with a highly polar moiety to facilitate their excretion in the urine. Phase I is not a chronologic term; often, phase II metabolism precedes phase I. (A) Phase II metabolism can precede phase I metabolism. (B) Most phase I reactions are carried out in the liver by the cytochrome P450 enzymes found in hepatocytes. (D) Glucuronidation and sulfation are examples of conjugation with polar moieties, which describe phase II metabolism. (E) Phase I metabolites are generally somewhat more polar than the starting compound, but not as highly polar as phase II metabolites.

49 **The answer is B: Expected side effect profile.** Memantine is well tolerated, with few dose-dependent adverse events. Expected side effects, such as confusion, agitation, and restlessness, are indistinguishable from the symptoms of Alzheimer's disease. Given its different mechanism of action and possible neuroprotective effects, memantine is often given in combination with an AChE inhibitor. (A) There is no evidence in this question that there is a toxic effect from the drug. (C) This patient is not taking antacids. (D) This patient is not taking vitamins. (E) This patient has no otologic symptoms.

50 **The answer is B: Efficacy.** This long-acting benzodiazepine significantly reduces both sleep-induction time and the number of awakenings, and it increases the duration of sleep. Flurazepam has a long-acting effect and causes little rebound insomnia. With continued use, the drug has been shown to maintain its effectiveness for up to 4 weeks. Flurazepam and its active metabolites have a half-life of approximately 85 h, which may result in daytime sedation and accumulation of the drug. (A) This agent does have some significant adverse effects and this does not help its ability to have a generic form. (C) Timing of administration is not standard for this medication. (D) Tonicity is unrelated to this medication becoming a generic form. (E) This agent does have some significant toxic effects because of accumulation of the drug.

51 **The answer is A: Chronic alcohol abuse.** The more lipid soluble an anesthetic, the lower the concentration of anesthetic needed to produce anesthesia and thus the higher the potency of the anesthetic. Factors that can increase minimum alveolar concentration (MAC) (and make the patient less sensitive) include hyperthermia (greater than 42°C), drugs that increase CNS catecholamines, and chronic ethanol abuse. (B) Diet will not affect MAC. (C) Immunodeficiency state will not affect MAC. (D) Hyperthermia will increase MAC. (E) Weight will not affect MAC.

52 **The answer is A: Cyclic AMP.** Chemical mediators, such as prostacyclin and nitric oxide, are synthesized by intact endothelial cells and act as inhibitors of platelet aggregation. Prostacyclin (prostaglandin I_2) acts by binding to platelet membrane receptors that are coupled to the synthesis of cyclic adenosine monophosphate (cAMP), an intracellular messenger. (B) Cyclic AMP is an intracellular messenger. (C) Cyclic AMP is an intracellular messenger. (D) Cyclic AMP is an intracellular messenger. (E) Prostacyclin binds to the platelet membrane with cyclic AMP as the messenger.

53 **The answer is B: Low isoelectric point.** The isoelectric point of insulin glargine is lower than that of human insulin, leading to precipitation at the injection site and extending its action. It is slower in onset than NPH insulin and has a flat, prolonged hypoglycemic effect with no peak. Like other insulin, it must be given subcutaneously. (A) Degradation by gastric juice would prolong the hyperglycemic state and not treat this patient effectively. (C) Hepatic metabolism occurs with this agent, but this has nothing to do with its blood glucose–lowering properties. (D) This agent is administered subcutaneously. (E) This agent is metabolized in the liver.

54 **The answer is B: Metabolized by sulfation.** The estrogen preparations may be administered via the transdermal route (patch, topical gel, topical emulsion, or spray), intravaginally (tablet, cream, or ring), or by injection. They are hydroxylated in the liver to derivatives that are subsequently glucuronidated or sulfated. The parent drugs and their metabolites undergo excretion into bile and are then reabsorbed through the enterohepatic circulation. Inactive products are excreted in urine. (A) This agent is hydroxylated in the liver. (C) The metabolites of estrogen are broken down in the liver and inactive products are excreted in the urine. (D) Reabsorption occurs in the liver. (E) Toxicities are less than that for oral preparations.

55 **The answer is D: Low bioavailability.** Progesterone by itself is not used widely as a contraceptive therapy because of its rapid metabolism, resulting in low bioavailability. Synthetic progestogens (i.e., progestins) used in contraception are more stable to first-pass metabolism, allowing lower doses when administered orally. (A) This pill is swallowed whole but can have a bad taste if bitten. (B) Cost is not the reason why this agent is an ineffective birth control method. (C) The dosing for this agent would be daily. (E) Metabolism of progesterone is rapid, which results to low bioavailability.

56 **The answer is C: = Cp × CL/F.** The maintenance dose is the amount of drug that must be given to maintain that drug's plasma concentration at a predetermined target level. The equation that describes this relationship is maintenance dose = Cp × CL/F. Cp means the desired plasma concentration of the drug, CL stands for clearance of the drug, and F stands for bioavailability, or how much of a given dose will reach the plasma. Bioavailability depends more on the route of administration than on the specific drug. For example, a drug given by IV has a bioavailability of 1. Given orally, the same drug would have a bioavailability <1. (A) This is an equation describing the clearance of a substance, or how rapidly it is removed from the plasma. Vd is the volume of distribution and $t_{1/2}$ is the half-life. (B) This relationship describes the Vd of a drug. A low Vd corresponds to a drug that stays mostly in the blood. A high Vd corresponds to a drug that distributes widely in other body tissues. (D) This equation describes the loading dose. Cp is the desired plasma

concentration, Vd is the volume of distribution, and F is the bioavailability. It closely resembles the calculation for maintenance dose except that it depends on volume of distribution rather than clearance. (E) This equation describes a specific pathway of clearance—namely, renal clearance. U stands for the concentration of the substance in the urine, P stands for the concentration of the substance in the plasma, and V refers to the urine flow rate.

57 **The answer is C: Lipid solubility.** The blood–brain barrier is made up of many layers of cell membrane from multiple cell types. The common physical characteristic of these many membranes is their high lipid content. This means that small size and lipophilicity are drug characteristics favorable for diffusion across the barrier. Hydrophilicity, large size, and positive and negative charges all decrease the ability of a molecule to cross the blood–brain barrier. (A) Hydrophilicity impedes a molecule's diffusion across the blood–brain barrier. (B) Large size can also impede a molecule's diffusion across the blood–brain barrier. (D) Most of a weak acid with a pKa of 4 would have lost its proton at physiologic pH (~7.4) and would be found in the ionized form. Ionized molecules have greater difficulty crossing the blood–brain barrier than nonionized molecules. (E) Most of a weak base with a pKa of 9 would have gained a proton at physiologic pH (~7.4) and would be found in the ionized form. Ionized molecules have greater difficulty crossing the blood–brain barrier than nonionized molecules.

58 **The answer is C: Synergism.** Certain combinations of antibiotics, such as β-lactams and aminoglycosides, show synergism; that is, the combination is more effective than either of the drugs used separately. Because such synergism among antimicrobial agents is rare, multiple drugs used in combination are only indicated in special situations—for example, when an infection is of unknown origin. (A) Hepatotoxicity can occur with combination therapy and this is not a beneficial rationale for such use. (B) Nephrotoxicity can certainly occur with combination therapy and this must be monitored by the treating physician. (D) Increased toxicity can occur with combination therapy with antibiotics.

59 **The answer is D: Lower Km and lower V_{max}.** Hexokinase has a lower Km and lower V_{max} than glucokinase. Km refers to the concentration of substrate (glucose, in this case) needed for the reaction rate to reach 1/2 V_{max}. Glucokinase and hexokinase both carry out the same reaction on glucose; but because hexokinase has a higher affinity, a lower concentration of glucose is needed for it to reach 1/2 V_{max}. However, glucokinase has a higher capacity. At high concentrations of glucose, glucokinase actually works faster than hexokinase so glucokinase has a higher V_{max}. (A) Hexokinase has a lower Km and a lower V_{max} than glucokinase. (B) Hexokinase has a lower Km and a lower V_{max} than glucokinase. (C) Hexokinase has a lower Km and a lower V_{max} than glucokinase. (E) Hexokinase has a lower Km and a lower V_{max} than glucokinase.

60 **The answer is D: The therapeutic dose approaches the toxic dose.** The therapeutic index refers to the relationship between the dosage of a drug that is toxic to 50% of the population (TD50) and the dose that is effective in 50% of the population (ED50). A narrow therapeutic index means that the TD50 is not much greater than the ED50. When the TD50 and ED50 approach each other in this way, toxicity is more likely because it takes only a relatively small increase in drug concentration. (A) This response describes a wide therapeutic index. A drug with a wide therapeutic index has a low chance of causing toxicity at the therapeutic dose. (B) This scenario describes a drug in which the effective dose in 50% of the population equals the toxic dose in 50% of the population. This drug would not be useful therapeutically. (C) This response describes a scenario in which the effective dose in 50% of the population is greater than the toxic dose in 50% of the population. This drug would not be useful therapeutically. (E) In this scenario, toxicity precedes the clinical effect and this drug would not be useful clinically.

61 **The answer is E: Watchful waiting.** The most common adverse effects of metronidazole are those associated with the gastrointestinal tract, including nausea, vomiting, epigastric distress, and abdominal cramps. An unpleasant, metallic taste is commonly experienced. Other effects include oral moniliasis (yeast infection of the mouth) and, rarely, neurotoxicologic problems, such as dizziness, vertigo, and numbness or paresthesias in the peripheral nervous system. (A) This is not a true allergic reaction and thus, Benadryl is not likely to be of benefit. (B) Topical Benadryl is unlikely to be of benefit because this reaction is not a true allergy. (C) This medication can be continued in this patient. (D) Corticosteroids are unlikely to be of benefit to this patient.

62 **The answer is B: Rapidly dividing cells are sensitive to the cytotoxic effects.** The fraction of tumor cells that are in the replicative cycle ("growth fraction") influences their susceptibility to most cancer chemotherapeutic agents. Rapidly dividing cells are generally more sensitive to anticancer drugs, whereas slowly proliferating cells are less sensitive to chemotherapy. In general, nonproliferating cells (those in the G0 phase) usually

survive the toxic effects of many of these agents. (A) Cells in the G0 phase are resistant to chemotherapeutic agents. (C) Slowly dividing cells are resistant to chemotherapeutic agents. (D) Multimodal therapy is more effective than unimodal therapy. (E) Watchful waiting is ill advised for patients with metastatic breast cancer.

63 **The answer is B: Limited first-pass metabolism.** These agents and their esterified or conjugated derivatives are readily absorbed through the gastrointestinal tract, skin, and mucous membranes. Taken orally, estradiol is rapidly metabolized (and partially inactivated) by the microsomal enzymes of the liver. Micronized estradiol is available and has better bioavailability. Although there is some first-pass metabolism, it is not sufficient to lessen the effectiveness when taken orally. (A) Micronized estradiol has better bioavailability. (C) These agents are maximally available. (D) Nephrotoxicity occurs at high doses. (E) Neuromuscular blockade is highly unlikely.

64 **The answer is E: 25 L.** The volume of distribution is calculated by dividing the total amount of drug in the body by the plasma concentration of the drug. In this case, Vd = 500 mg ciprofloxacin/20 μg/mL, which is the peak plasma concentration. Thus, the volume of distribution of ciprofloxacin is 25 L.

65 **The answer is D: 40 h.** To figure out how long it will take a medication to reach 90% of its final steady state, use the formula: $(3.3) \times (t_{1/2})$. In this case, the half-life is 12 h. Thus, $(3.3) \times (12)$ is approximately 40 h. Of note, because of poor penetration into tissues, despite achieving 90% steady state levels in 40 h, patients with this condition often need to take antibiotics for approximately 3 to 4 weeks for cure.

66 **The answer is D: 3.3.** At the first half-life, 50% of the drug will be eliminated from the body. At the second half-life, 75% of the drug will be eliminated from the body. At the third half-life, 87.5% of the drug will be eliminated from the body. Finally, at 3.3 half-lives, 90% of the drug will be eliminated from the body.

67 **The answer is A: 50%.** Agent X112A has a bioavailability of 50%. Bioavailability is the fraction of administered drug that reaches the systemic circulation. In this example, if 100 mg of Agent X112A is administered orally, and 50 mg of this drug is absorbed unchanged, the bioavailability is 0.5, or 50%. Determining bioavailability is important for calculating drug dosages for various routes of administration other than the intravenous route.

68 **The answer is A: $= 0.7 \times Vd / t_{1/2}$.** Clearance refers to the rate at which a drug is excreted, or cleared, from the body in relation to the drug's plasma concentration. Mathematically, clearance equals the rate of elimination divided by the plasma concentration. Another equation relates clearance to the half-life—clearance also equals the volume of distribution divided by the half-life multiplied by the constant 0.7. (B) This equation describes the volume of distribution, Vd. The Vd is small for drugs that remain confined to the plasma and large for drugs that distribute widely in the body's tissues. (C) This equation is used to calculate the maintenance dose of a drug. Cp is the target drug concentration, Cl is the drug's clearance, and F refers to the bioavailability of the drug. (D) This equation is used to calculate the loading dose of a drug. Cp is the target drug concentration, Vd is the drug's volume of distribution, and F refers to the bioavailability of the drug. (E) This relationship comes from the Henderson-Hasselbalch equation and is used to calculate the pH of an acid in solution when the concentrations of the acid and its conjugate base as well as the acid's pKa are known.

69 **The answer is E: Metabolism.** This is the definition of metabolism. Metabolism is the third step in the process of drug delivery and utilization. The drug may be biotransformed by metabolism by the liver or other tissues. (A) Absorption: First, drug absorption from the site of administration permits entry of the therapeutic agent (either directly or indirectly) into plasma. (B) Catabolism involves breakdown of substances by the body. (C) Distribution: Second, the drug may then reversibly leave the bloodstream and distribute into the interstitial and intracellular fluids. (D) Elimination: Finally, the drug and its metabolites are eliminated from the body in urine, bile, or feces.

70 **The answer is C: The enteric component dissolves in the small intestine.** An enteric coating is a chemical envelope that resists the action of the fluids and enzymes in the stomach but dissolves readily in the upper intestine. Such coating is useful for certain groups of drugs (e.g., omeprazole) that are acid unstable. Enteric coatings protect the drug from stomach acid, delivering them instead to the less acidic intestine, where the coating dissolves and allows the drug to be released. Similarly, drugs that have an irritant effect on the stomach, such as aspirin, can be coated with a substance that will dissolve only in the small intestine, thereby protecting the stomach. (A) The enteric component is acid unstable. (B) The enteric component protects the drug from gastric acid. (D) The enteric component is resistant to fluid and enzymes.

71 **The answer is E: Simple diffusion.** The subcutaneous (SC) route of administration, like IM injection, requires absorption via simple diffusion and is somewhat slower than the IV route. SC injection minimizes the risks of hemolysis or thrombosis associated with IV injection and may provide constant, slow, and sustained effects. This route should not be used with drugs that cause tissue irritation because severe pain and necrosis may occur. (A) Active transport requires enzymes and energy to complete this process. (B) Facilitated transport does not require energy to complete this process. (C) Osmosis is the diffusion of water through a membrane and does not require energy to complete the process. (D) Passive transport does not require energy to complete this process.

72 **The answer is E: Useful if patient is unconscious or vomiting.** Because 50% of the drainage of the rectal region bypasses the portal circulation, the biotransformation of drugs by the liver is minimized with rectal administration. Like the sublingual route of administration, the rectal route has the additional advantage of preventing the destruction of the drug by intestinal enzymes or by low pH in the stomach. The rectal route is also useful if the drug induces vomiting when given orally, if the patient is already vomiting, or if the patient is unconscious. A side effect of rectal administration of medication is rectal irritation. Rectal administration of medications is not a well-accepted route. (A) The oral route of administration allows destruction of the medication by gastric enzymes. (B) Biotransformation of drugs by the liver is minimized with rectal administration. (C) Rectal administration of medications is not well accepted. (D) Rectal irritation following administration is common.

73 **The answer is B: Reduction of absorption of drugs in the spleen.** P-glycoprotein is a multidrug transmembrane transporter protein responsible for transporting various molecules, including drugs, across cell membranes. It is expressed throughout the body, and its functions include the following: In the liver: transporting drugs into bile for elimination. In kidneys: pumping drugs into urine for excretion. In the placenta: transporting drugs back into maternal blood, thereby reducing fetal exposure to drugs. In the intestines: transporting drugs into the intestinal lumen and reducing drug absorption into the blood. In the brain capillaries: pumping drugs back into blood, limiting drug access to the brain. (A) The P-glycoprotein system will limit drug access to the brain. (C) The P-glycoprotein system will allow transport of drugs into bile for elimination. (D) The P-glycoprotein system will allow transport of drugs into the intestinal lumen. (E) The P-glycoprotein system will allow for exchange of blood between the fetal and maternal systems.

74 **The answer is D: Tachycardia.** The effect of sympathetic output is to increase heart rate (tachycardia) and blood pressure, to mobilize energy stores of the body, and to increase blood flow to skeletal muscles and the heart while diverting flow from the skin and internal organs. Sympathetic stimulation results in dilation of the pupils and the bronchioles. It also affects GI motility and the function of the bladder and sexual organs. (A) Bronchodilation will result from sympathetic stimulation. (B) Hypertension and tachycardia result from sympathetic stimulation. (C) Pupillary dilation will result from sympathetic stimulation. (E) Urinary retention can result from sympathetic stimulation.

75 **The answer is E: Category X.** Pregnancy Category A contains drugs that have shown no risk to the fetus in the first trimester of pregnancy in well-controlled human studies. Category B is for drugs that either have had no well-controlled human studies but show no risk in animal studies, or drugs that show risk in animal studies but not in well-controlled human studies. Category C is for drugs that show risk in animal models and have had no well-controlled human studies. Category D is for drugs that are known to pose a risk to the fetus but the benefits may outweigh the risks. Category X is for drugs absolutely contraindicated in pregnancy. Category X drugs pose such a great risk to the fetus that no benefit is seen to outweigh the risk. Isotretinoin is a Category X drug. (A) Category A drugs have undergone well-controlled human studies and are shown to be safe in pregnancy. Prenatal vitamins are an example. (B) Category B is for drugs that either have had no well-controlled human studies but show no risk in animal studies or drugs that show risk in animal studies but not in well-controlled human studies. Penicillins and cephalosporins are an example. (C) Category C drugs have shown risk to fetus in animal models. Rifampin is an example. (D) Category D drugs are known to pose a risk to the human fetus, but their benefits to the mother (and therefore to the pregnancy) may outweigh the risks to the pregnancy. Tetracycline and phenytoin are examples.

76 **The answer is D: Factor IX.** γ-Carboxylation of factors of factors II, VII, IX, and X (as well as proteins C and S) allows their calcium-mediated adhesion to platelet cell membranes. Vitamin K is a cofactor in the γ-carboxylation reaction and is usually recycled by the enzyme vitamin K epoxide reductase. Warfarin is a vitamin K analog and inhibits epoxide reductase so vitamin K cannot be recycled and the γ-carboxylation reaction of factors II, VII, IX, and X does not occur. (A) Factor I is more commonly referred to by its name, fibrinogen. It does not require γ-carboxylation and so is not influenced by warfarin. (B) Factor V is a cofactor with factor X to increase X's ability to convert prothrombin into thrombin. It does not require γ-carboxylation and so is not influenced by warfarin. (C) Factor VIII is a cofactor with factor IX to activate factor X. It does not require γ-carboxylation and so is not influenced by warfarin. (E) Factor XII activates factor XI, which in turn activates factor IX. Factor XII does not require γ-carboxylation and so is not influenced by warfarin.

77 **The answer is B: Hydrogen bonds.** Hydrogen bonds have substantial strength and are important in drug–receptor interactions. This involves interaction between positively and negatively charged atoms. On a molecular level, nitrogen and oxygen are most likely involved. (A) Covalent bonds result from sharing a pair of electrons between two atoms. (C) Ionic bonds are strong bonds that result from interactions between positively and negatively charged atoms. (D) Van der Waals forces are weak interactions between drugs and their receptors caused by electron density shifts.

78 **The answer is A: Chemical name.** The chemical name of this compound does not affect its ability to bind to its target receptor. The drug's conformation, hydrophobicity, ionization state, and stereochemistry will effect its ability to bind to target receptors. Receptor binding pockets for drugs are specific, and small changes in these properties can have large effects on drug efficacy. Chemical name has no effect on these properties. (B) Conformation will have an effect on drug–receptor binding. (C) Hydrophobicity will have an effect on drug–receptor binding. (D) Ionization state will have an effect on drug–receptor binding. (E) Stereochemistry will have an effect on drug–receptor binding.

79 **The answer is C: Lipid solubility.** Drugs enter the kidney through renal arteries, which divide to form a glomerular capillary plexus. Free drug (not bound to albumin) flows through the capillary slits into Bowman's space as part of the glomerular filtrate. The glomerular filtration rate (125 mL/min) is normally about 20% of the renal plasma flow (600 mL/min). Lipid solubility and pH do not influence the passage of drugs into the glomerular filtrate. However, varying the glomerular filtration rate and plasma binding of the drugs may affect this process. (A) Glomerular filtration rate will affect drug elimination. (B) Decreasing the glomerular filtration rate will have a significant effect on drug elimination. (D) Alteration of plasma binding of drug will affect renal elimination of this medication. (E) Normal renal plasma flow should be 200 mL/min. Changes to renal plasma flow will change drug elimination.

80 **The answer is D: Hypermetabolic state.** It is important to be able to predict in which patients a drug is likely to have a change in half-life. The half-life of a drug is increased by (1) diminished renal plasma flow or hepatic blood flow, for example, in cardiogenic shock, heart failure, or hemorrhage; (2) decreased ability to extract drug from plasma, for example, as seen in renal disease; and (3) decreased metabolism, for example, when another drug inhibits its biotransformation or in hepatic insufficiency, as with cirrhosis. Increased metabolism will decrease the half-life of a drug. (A) Cardiogenic shock will increase drug half-life. (B) Cirrhosis will increase drug half-life. (C) Heart failure will decrease renal plasma flow to increase drug half-life. (E) Renal disease decreases the kidney's ability to extract drug from plasma, which will increase drug half-life.

81 **The answer is B: 50 μg.** Vd = dose/C = 125 μg/2 μg/L = 62.5 L. Vd (C2 − C1) = dose to be received = 62.5 (0.8 μg/L − 2 μg/L) = −75 μg. Subtract this dose from standard dose. New dose to be administered = 125 μg − 75 μg = 50 μg.

82 **The answer is D: The drugs occupying the receptor are producing conformational change in the receptor.** More recent information suggests that receptors exist in at least two states: inactive (R) and active (R*) states that are in reversible equilibrium with one another. In the absence of an agonist, R* typically represents a small fraction of the total receptor population (i.e., the equilibrium favors the inactive state). Drugs occupying the receptor can stabilize the receptor in a given conformational state. (A) Some drugs may cause similar shifts in equilibrium between R and R* as an endogenous ligand. (B) The active and inactive receptor states are in reversible equilibrium. (C) Equilibrium of the receptors favors an inactive state, not a transient state.

83 **The answer is A: Cardiac muscle.** Ligand-gated ion channels are responsible for regulation of the flow of ions across cell membranes. The activity of these channels is regulated by the binding of a ligand to the channel. Response to these receptors is very rapid, enduring for only a few milliseconds. These receptors mediate diverse functions, including neurotransmission, cardiac conduction, and muscle contraction. (B) Ligand-gated ion channels are found in tissues that can complete a rapid response to stimulation. (C) The pancreas is both an exocrine and endocrine gland that responds slower than nerve and muscle tissue. (D) The spleen is not capable of rapid receptor responses. (E) Thyroid tissue responds slower than muscle and heart tissue to cellular conduction.

84 **The answer is C: Receptor desensitization.** Several mechanisms have evolved to protect a cell from excessive stimulation. When repeated administration of a drug results in a diminished effect, the phenomenon is called tachyphylaxis. The receptor becomes desensitized to the action of the drug. In this phenomenon, the receptors are still present on the cell surface but are unresponsive to the ligand. (A) The receptor is likely still functional and active but does not respond to stimulation by the ligand. (B) The receptor is still capable of normal neural function but may require a different ligand. (D) Receptor hypersensitivity can occur in cases of neural injury such as spinal cord injury. (E) This does not represent an example of receptor telescopic transformation.

85 **The answer is A: Cytosol.** The uptake of choline is the rate-limiting step in ACh synthesis. Choline acetyltransferase catalyzes the reaction of choline with acetyl coenzyme A (CoA) to form ACh (an ester) in the cytosol. Acetyl CoA is derived from the mitochondria and is produced by the pyruvate oxidation and fatty acid oxidation. (B) The Golgi apparatus does not produce acetylcholine. (C) The mitochondria produce acetyl CoA. (D) The rough endoplasmic reticulum does not produce acetyl CoA. (E) The smooth endoplasmic reticulum produces steroids and participates in detoxification reactions.

86 **The answer is D: Elimination of drugs becomes impaired with age.** Patients of advanced age consume most of the drugs that are prescribed. Although no drugs are specifically contraindicated in the elderly, exercise particular caution when prescribing drugs to this group. In particular, be aware that the elderly are often more sensitive to both the effects and adverse effects of a drug. There are many reasons for this. Drug elimination becomes progressively impaired with age, causing drug accumulation. In addition, the adverse effects of many drugs are blunted by physiological compensatory responses. These compensatory responses are less efficient in the elderly. Elderly patients are more likely to have coexisting disease that may alter their response to drugs. (A) Coexisting diseases produce additive impairment of organ function in the elderly patient. (B) Elderly patients are more sensitive to drug effects. (C) Elderly patients are more sensitive to drug side effects. (E) Responses to compensate for drug accumulation become impaired with age.

87 **The answer is B: Lipid solubility.** Although oral administration of a pharmacologic agent is convenient and economical, the drug must possess several characteristics for maximal absorption. In the stomach, drugs that are lipid soluble and that are weak acids can be readily absorbed. In the small intestine, drugs that are either weak acids or weak bases are able to be absorbed. (A) Medications with bulky side chains are not well absorbed following oral administration. (C) Strong acids are not well absorbed following oral administration. (D) Strong bases are not well absorbed following oral administration. (E) Water solubility can affect absorption rates of orally administered medications.

88 **The answer is D: Phentolamine should be injected.** Extravasation of α-adrenergic agonists into surrounding tissue is a serious problem. The paleness and coolness of the skin around his IV site is caused by constriction of the vasculature in his skin. The vasoconstriction caused by vasopressors can lead to tissue necrosis. An α-antagonist should be injected into the affected tissue as soon as possible to counteract the vasopressor that has extravasated. Phentolamine can be used to restore blood flow to the affected area. (A) Atropine is a muscarinic cholinergic antagonist. The receptors being stimulated in this patient's case are α_1-adreneric receptors. Atropine would not reverse the vasopressor effect. (B) Dopamine itself is an α_1-agonist and is used as a vasopressor. Injection of dopamine would worsen the situation. (C) Doing nothing will likely result in irreversible tissue necrosis. Phentolamine should be injected to counteract the vasopressor. (E) Prednisone is a glucocorticoid, which has little effect on vasculature except to indirectly inhibit vasodilation during inflammation. Phentolamine should be injected to counteract the vasopressor.

89 **The answer is E: pKa of the drug.** Onset and duration of action of local anesthetics are influenced by several factors. These include tissue pH, pKa of the drug, nerve morphology, concentration, and lipid solubility of the drug. Of these, the most important are pH of the tissue and pKa of the drug. At physiologic pH, these compounds are charged. The ionized form interacts with the protein receptor of the sodium channel to inhibit its function and, thereby, achieve local anesthesia. The pH may drop in sites of infection, which causes onset to be delayed or even prevented. (A) Tissue pH is more significant than blood pH. (B) pKa of the drug is a significant factor. (C) Lipid solubility of the drug is a significant factor. (D) Nerve morphology is a significant factor.

90 **The answer is B: Maximal dose of anesthetic must be calculated.** Before administering local anesthetic to a child, the maximum dose based on the child's weight should be calculated to help prevent inadvertent overdose. There are no significant differences in the response to local anesthetics between younger and older adults, and the doses required for each block are the same regardless of patient age. However, it is prudent to stay well below the maximum recommended doses

in elderly patients who often have some compromise in liver function. (A) Liver failure will be a problem in the older patient because he has a history of cirrhosis. (C) Older patients require the same doses for block regardless of age. (D) Older patients and younger patients have the same response to anesthetic. (E) Older patients and younger patients have the same response to anesthetic.

91 **The answer is E: Redistribution from sites in the CNS.** Following initial flooding of the CNS with nonionized molecules, the drug diffuses into other tissues. With secondary tissue uptake, plasma concentration falls, allowing the drug to diffuse out of the CNS. This initial redistribution of drug into other tissues leads to the rapid recovery seen after a single dose of an IV induction drug. (A) Ionization affects rate of transfer. (B) Liver metabolism affects rate of transfer. (C) Plasma clearance affects rate of transfer. (D) Protein binding affects rate of transfer.

92 **The answer is A: Additive effects.** The additive effects of drugs occur when two drugs with the same effect are added together and produce an effect that is equal in magnitude to the sum of the effects when the two drugs are given individually. (B) Neutralization occurs when two drugs combine with another to form an inactive compound. (C) Potentiation occurs if a drug lacking an effect of its own increases the effect of a second active drug. (D) Synergism occurs if two drugs with the same effect, when given together, produce an effect that is in greater magnitude than the sum of the effects when the drugs are given individually.

93 **The answer is B: Inhibition of nerve firing.** The mechanism of action of opioids is complex. Opioids exert their major effects by interacting with opioid receptors in the CNS and in other anatomic structures, such as the GI tract and the urinary bladder. Opioids cause hyperpolarization of nerve cells, inhibition of nerve firing, and presynaptic inhibition of transmitter release. Morphine acts at κ receptors in laminae I and II of the dorsal horn of the spinal cord and it decreases the release of substance P, which modulates pain perception in the spinal cord. Morphine also appears to inhibit the release of many excitatory transmitters from nerve terminals carrying nociceptive (painful) stimuli. (A) Morphine causes hyperpolarization of nerve cells. (C) Morphine causes presynaptic inhibition of transmitter release. (D) Decrease of release of substance P is caused by morphine. (E) Excitatory neurotransmitter release is inhibited.

94 **The answer is A: Drug AB > Drug A + Drug B.** Potentiation occurs if a drug lacking an effect of its own increases the effect of a second active drug. As shown next: Drug AB > Drug A + Drug B. (B) This is an example of equal drug efficacy. (C) This is an example of Drug B showing stronger potency. (D) This is an example of Drug AB and B being more potent than drug A.

95 **The answer is D: CV.** Class CV medications have a low abuse potential, may or may not require a prescription, and are subject to state and local regulation. (A) CII medications have a high potential for abuse and can lead to psychological and physical dependence. (B) CIII medications may lead to moderate or low physical dependence or high psychological dependence. (C) CIV medications have low abuse potential and use may lead to limited physical or psychological dependence.

96 **The answer is C: They will be stimulated but at a lower level than when epinephrine is given alone.** Stimulation of α_1-receptors by epinephrine occurs when epinephrine molecules bind at a specific site on the receptor's surface. Drug X and epinephrine both bind to the same receptor but elicit responses—Drug X does not elicit as great a maximum response as epinephrine so it results in less stimulation than epinephrine when used alone. Because they both bind to the same place on the same receptor, Drug X and epinephrine would compete for available receptors when administered together. This would result in an overall level of stimulation less than when epinephrine is given alone. (A) A partial α_1-adrenergic agonist such as Drug X would compete with epinephrine for binding sites. Some sites would be occupied by Drug X and others by epinephrine, so the result would be a level of stimulation less than that when epinephrine is given alone. (B) A partial α_1-adrenergic agonist such as Drug X would compete with epinephrine for binding sites. Some sites would be occupied by Drug X and others by epinephrine, so the result would be a level of stimulation less than that when epinephrine is given alone. (D) A partial α_1-adrenergic agonist such as Drug X would compete with epinephrine for binding sites. Some sites would be occupied by Drug X and others by epinephrine, so the result would be a level of stimulation less than that when epinephrine is given alone. (E) Of course there would be some amount of α_1-adrenergic stimulation because both drugs stimulate the receptors to some degree. When given together, some sites would be occupied by Drug X and others by epinephrine, so the result would be a level of stimulation less than that when epinephrine is given alone.

97 **The answer is E: Relative potency cannot be determined from the information given.** Potency is the measure of a substance's ability to evoke a response in relation to the substance's concentration. A compound with a low potency will only evoke a response in high

concentrations. In contrast, a compound with a high potency can evoke a response at a low concentration. The property of potency is largely independent of the compound's efficacy, which is a measure of the maximum response that a substance can elicit. We know Drug X has a lower maximum efficacy because it is classified as a partial agonist. However, we cannot tell whether Drug X has higher, lower, or equal potency as compared to epinephrine. (A) Acting on the same receptors is no guarantee of equal potency. Drug X may have higher, lower, or equal potency compared to epinephrine, but this property cannot be deduced from the information given. (B) A substance's potency is not directly related to its efficacy. Drug X may have higher, lower, or equal potency compared to epinephrine, but this property cannot be deduced from the information given. (C) A substance's potency is not directly related to its efficacy. Drug X may have higher, lower, or equal potency compared to epinephrine, but this property cannot be deduced from the information given. (D) Whether a substance is endogenous or synthetic has no bearing on its potency. Drug X may have higher, lower, or equal potency compared to epinephrine, but this property cannot be deduced from the information given.

98 **The answer is D: Letter D.** Elimination is represented by letter D. The drug and its metabolites are eliminated from the body in urine, bile, or feces. (A) Letter A represents the process of drug absorption from the site of administration. (B) Letter B represents the process of drug distribution ultimately into the interstitial and intracellular fluids. (C) Letter C represents the metabolism of the drug in the liver or other tissues.

99 **The answer is E: Injection #2 to level D.** This figure shows two different types of injection. Injection #1 is subcutaneous, whereas injection #2 is intramuscular. Haloperidol is typically given intramuscularly into the muscle layer, which is represented by level D in the figure. (A) Injection #1 is a subcutaneous injection that goes to level C, the subcutaneous tissue. (B) Injection #2 is an intramuscular injection and should be injected into level D. (C) Injection #2 is the correct injection to be given to this patient; but in this choice, the injection is going into the dermis. (D) Injection #2 is the correct injection to be given to this patient; but in this choice, the injection is going into the subcutaneous tissue.

100 **The answer is C: Letter C.** The transdermal route of administration allows achievement of therapeutic effects through the use of a patch. Several components of the patch are critical for drug delivery and should be understood by clinicians. The drug reservoir is illustrated by letter C in the diagram. (A) The skin is represented by letter A. (B) The clear backing of the patch is represented by letter B. (D) The drug-release membrane of the patch is represented by letter D. (E) The contact adhesive of the patch is represented by letter E.

101 **The answer is B: Letter B.** Letter B represents the area under the curve (AUC) for oral administration of this agent. Letter C represents the AUC for injection of this agent. The ratio of Letter B to Letter C is the bioavailability of this agent. (A) Letter A is the drug administered. (C) Letter C is the area under the curve for injection of this agent. (D) Letter D is the drug injected degradation curve plotted against time. (E) Letter E is the drug given orally degradation curve plotted against time.

102 **The answer is D: Letter D.** Passive reabsorption occurs at level D, which is the distal tubule/collecting duct. Here, passive reabsorption of lipid-soluble, unionized drug can undergo reabsorption. (A) Letter A represents free drug entering the glomerular filtrate. (B) Letter B represents active secretion into the proximal tubule. (C) Letter C represents the loop of Henle. (E) Letter E represents the ionized lipid-insoluble drug in the urine.

103 **The answer is D: Letter D.** The graph shows the effect of infusion rate on the steady state concentration of drug in plasma. Letter D represents the steady state region which is reached only when the drug is given at a high rate of infusion. (A) Letter A represents the start of the infusion. (B) Letter B represents the drug when given at a low rate of infusion. (C) Letter C represents the drug when given at a high rate of infusion.

104 **The answer is C: Curve C.** Curve C represents injection of 2U of the medication once per day. This results in the highest peak concentration of drug in the body. (B) Curve B represents injection of 1U of drug twice per day. This curve is similar to the drug concentration that would be observed if continuous infusion of 2U of drug per day were infused. (C) Curve C represents continuous infusion of 2U of drug per day. (D) Curve C represents the highest peak concentration of drug in the body.

105 **The answer is A: Drug A has a lower EC50.** The figure shows that drug A has a lower EC50. The EC50 is the concentration of drug that produces a response equal to 50% of the maximal response. (B) Drug A has a lower EC50. (C) Drug A is likely to be more potent than Drug B. (D) One cannot determine the best dosing method from the information given in this question. (E) One cannot determine the best dosing method from the information given in this question.

106 The answer is C: Drug C shows lower potency than Drugs A and B. Drug C shows lower potency than Drugs A and B. This information is easily discerned from the figure earlier. (A) Drug A is more potent than Drug B, but both show the same efficacy. (B) Drug A and B have the same efficacy. (D) One cannot determine how this drug should be administered from the information provided. (E) One cannot determine potential for approval for clinical trials based on the information provided.

107 The answer is B: There is a small window of desired effect of this medication. The figure shows the therapeutic index for warfarin. There is a narrow window of desired therapeutic effect. Thus, at higher drug concentrations, there is a higher likelihood of unwanted adverse effects. (A) The therapeutic window is small. (C) Unwanted adverse effects are likely with this agent. (D) Unwanted adverse events are likely to be dose related with this agent.

108 The answer is B: Letter B. Direct contact involves gap junctions between cells. There is a signaling cell and a target cell in this scenario. (A) Letter A illustrates endocrine signaling with hormone acting on a target cell. (C) Letter C illustrates synaptic signaling between a nerve cell, a neurotransmitter that is released, and a target cell which will elicit a response.

109 The answer is B: Letter B. Letter B represents the update into storage vesicles. Acetylcholine is protected from degradation in the vesicle. (A) Letter A represents the synthesis of acetylcholine. (C) Letter C represents release of the neurotransmitter. (D) Letter D represents binding to the receptor. (E) Letter E represents degradation of acetylcholine by acetylcholinesterase in the synaptic cleft.

110 The answer is C: Rapid distribution to body tissues. Following a 30- to 60-min intravenous infusion every 12 h, tigecycline rapidly distributes into the body tissues and thus should never be used to treat bacteremia. It does not undergo significant liver metabolism, but it is primarily eliminated via biliary/fecal excretion. No dose adjustment is necessary for patients with renal impairment. However, dose adjustment is needed in severe hepatic dysfunction. (A) This antibiotic is rather broad in its spectrum. (B) This is a drug distribution effect, not a drug–drug interaction. (D) The dosing strategy for this patient is correct. (E) The dosing strategy for this patient is correct.

111 The answer is C: Increases K_m. A competitive inhibitor increases the K_m. This means the affinity of the substrate for the enzyme decreases. A competitive inhibitor binds to the enzyme at the active site. (A) Competitive inhibitors increase K_m, not decrease it. (B) Competitive inhibitors have no effect on V_{max}. (D) Competitive inhibitors have no effect on V_{max}. (E) Competitive inhibitors have no effect on V_{max}, but they do increase K_m.

112 The answer is B: Decreases V_{max}. Noncompetitive inhibits decrease the V_{max}. Noncompetitive inhibitors block enzyme activity with or without substrates bound, therefore the affinity is unaffected. The V_{max} decreases because when the inhibitor is bound, it decreases the amount of active sites available for the substrate. (A) Noncompetitive inhibitors have no effect on K_m. (C) Noncompetitive inhibitors have no effect on K_m. (D) Noncompetitive inhibitors decrease, not increase V_{max}. (E) Noncompetitive inhibitors have no effect on K_m, but they do decrease V_{max}.

113 The answer is E: 23 h. It takes four to five half-lives to reach clinical steady state, and therefore, 23 h in this case. Clinical steady state is reached when the concentration is more than 94%. At four half-lives, the concentration is 93.75%. (A) The concentration is 75% after two half-lives. (B) The concentration at 12 h would be about 80%. (C) The concentration is 87.5% after three half-lives. (D) The concentration at 18 h would be about 90%.

Chapter 2

Principles of Neuropharmacology

QUESTIONS

Select the single best answer.

1 Commonalities of the sympathetic, parasympathetic, and somatic nervous systems involve which of the following neuroeffector transmitters?
(A) Acetylcholine
(B) Dopamine
(C) Epinephrine
(D) Norepinephrine
(E) Serotonin

2 There are major differences in the anatomical arrangement of neurons, which lead to variations of the functions in each division of the nervous system. Which of the following features describes the parasympathetic nervous system?
(A) Diffuse response
(B) Extensive preganglionic fiber branching
(C) Ganglia close to the spinal cord
(D) Short postganglionic fibers
(E) Wide distribution

3 A 47-year-old woman presents to the emergency department complaining of blurry vision, vomiting, and excessive sweating after splashing herself with carbamate insecticide while gardening. Her condition improves after administration of atropine. Which of the following is true of competitive antagonists?
(A) Decrease efficacy of proteins they bind to
(B) Decrease potency of proteins they bind to
(C) For enzymes, K_m is unchanged
(D) Cannot be overcomed by high concentrations of the protein's native ligand or substrate
(E) Usually bind somewhere other than the protein's native ligand or substrate binding site

4 A 47-year-old man is given atropine to decrease dental secretions during a root canal procedure. This agent is most likely to have an effect on which of the following target organs/glands?
(A) Adrenal medulla
(B) Kidney
(C) Pilomotor muscles
(D) Salivary glands
(E) Sweat glands

5 A 42-year-old woman is sunbathing on a very warm day. She falls asleep on the beach and then awakens with chills and sweats. She has no pertinent past medical or surgical history. Paramedics on the scene record a blood pressure of 80/40 mm Hg. Reflex responses of the autonomic nervous system would include which of the following?
(A) Decreased blood pressure
(B) Decreased cardiac output
(C) Decreased cardiac contractility
(D) Increased peripheral resistance
(E) Stimulation of the parasympathetic nervous system

6 A researcher who is interested in creating an anticholinergic agent that would be useful in patients with irritative bladder symptoms would be interested in targeting which of the following receptors?
(A) M_1
(B) M_2
(C) M_3
(D) M_4
(E) M_5

7 A 38-year-old woman presents to the ophthalmologist for a routine eye examination. She is given intraocular pilocarpine. She was supposed to be administered two drops in each to dilate the eyes for the examination. Unfortunately, the eyedrops were administered by a new technician who inadvertently administered 10 drops of pilocarpine in each eye. Which of the following agents should be immediately given to the patient?
(A) Atropine
(B) Carbachol
(C) Donepezil
(D) Galantamine
(E) Rivastigmine

8 A 58-year-old woman with a history of myasthenia gravis presents to the emergency department complaining of generalized abdominal pain. Her current medications include nifedipine and neostigmine. Her caretaker reports that her bottle of neostigmine is empty but was full earlier in the day. Which of the following findings is likely in this patient?

(A) Bronchodilation
(B) Constipation
(C) Dizziness
(D) Hypotension
(E) Xerostomia

9 A 79-year-old man with Alzheimer's disease is found to have significant elevation of liver function tests on routine follow-up examination. Which of the following medications should be maintained at current doses in this patient?

(A) Donepezil
(B) Galantamine
(C) Rivastigmine
(D) Tacrine
(E) Tacrolimus

10 A 52-year-old woman with end-stage multiple sclerosis who is currently taking several medications including prednisone and neostigmine is seen by a new physician. After examination, the patient has begun on dalfampridine. What is the most likely mechanism of action for this medication?

(A) Calcium channel blocker
(B) Cholinesterase inhibitor
(C) Permeability enhancer
(D) Potassium channel blocker
(E) Sodium channel blocker

11 A 71-year-old man will undergo a prostate needle biopsy under anesthesia because of his low pain tolerance and high level of anxiety. The procedure is estimated to take approximately 10 min to complete. Which of the following is the most appropriate anesthetic agent for the patient to receive?

(A) Doxacurium
(B) Mivacurium
(C) Pancuronium
(D) Rocuronium
(E) Tubocurarine

12 A medical student is performing a summer research project evaluating the pharmacologic effects of atropine at varying doses. Doses are extrapolated from normal human doses of this agent. Slow infusion of this agent to a steady state dose of 0.5 mg would be expected to produce which of the following effects?

(A) Bradykinesia
(B) Coma
(C) Dilation of the pupils
(D) Dry mouth
(E) Tachycardia

13 A 61-year-old woman is going on a cruise and is afraid that she will develop motion sickness during the trip. She is given a prescription for scopolamine patch. She has no other medical problems and has never had surgery. On the first day of the trip, the boat is rocking heavily, and the patient is nauseous and she applies the patch. Instead of being sedated, she actually became very excited and agitated. What is the most likely explanation for these findings?

(A) Patient also drank four beers in addition to using the scopolamine patch
(B) Patient did not follow proper medication directions
(C) Underlying hepatic insufficiency
(D) Underlying renal insufficiency
(E) Underlying urinary tract abnormality

14 A 43-year-old man is stabbed in the chest and is brought to the emergency department for evaluation. Because of hemodynamic instability, he is brought to the operating room for thoracotomy. An adequate anesthesia history could not be obtained from the patient. No family member was present at the time of surgery. Upon induction of anesthesia with succinylcholine, the patient's heart rate increased to 150 beats/minute and experienced muscular rigidity. What is the most appropriate treatment for this patient?

(A) Dantrolene
(B) Rapid warming with blanket
(C) Sodium bicarbonate administered intravenously
(D) Succinylcholine intravenous drip at steady state
(E) Tubocurarine intravenous bolus

15 A 79-year-old man undergoes a hip replacement procedure under general anesthesia and is unable to be weaned from the ventilator postoperatively. Review of the anesthesia records indicated that he received the following agents: succinylcholine, diazepam, rocuronium, and fentanyl. He spends the next 5 days on a ventilator in the intensive care unit. Which of the following is the most likely explanation for this situation?

(A) Diaphragm paralysis
(B) Hypokalemia
(C) Hyponatremia
(D) Hypocalcemia
(E) Underlying digitalis toxicity

16 An 8-month-old girl is brought to the emergency department by her parents because she has been "acting funny." They say she has been weaker than normal. She is afebrile but appears lethargic. While talking with the parents, you discover that they sometimes give her honey to calm her down and gave her a spoonful yesterday. What is the mechanism of the toxin likely causing her symptoms?

(A) Preventing acetylcholine release
(B) Preventing acetylcholine synthesis
(C) Preventing glycine release
(D) Preventing norepinephrine release
(E) Preventing norepinephrine synthesis

17 A medical student is involved in a summer research project evaluating the potencies of the α-adrenergic agonists at different receptor sites. Which of the following α-adrenergic agonists would be expected to have the strongest potency at the α-receptor?

(A) Acetylcholine
(B) Epinephrine
(C) Isoproterenol
(D) Metanephrine
(E) Norepinephrine

18 A 73-year-old man presents to his primary care physician complaining of a weak stream and nocturia four times at night. He is very sensitive to the medication side effects and is reluctant to take medications for this reason. Physical examination reveals a mildly enlarged prostate. Treatment of this condition may involve the use of which of the following agents to minimize side effects?

(A) Alfuzosin
(B) Doxazosin
(C) Prazosin
(D) Tamsulosin
(E) Terazosin

19 A group of teenage boys comes to the emergency department after ingesting a plant they heard would make them high. One member of the group still had some plant parts in his pocket, which you use to identify deadly nightshade that contains compounds metabolized to atropine. Which of the following is an effect of atropine?

(A) Bronchospasm
(B) Lacrimation
(C) Mydriasis
(D) Salivation
(E) Urination

20 A 62-year-old retired small business owner has had slowly increasing intraocular pressure bilaterally. You start him on drug used to treat his open-angle glaucoma, which also happens to cross the blood–brain barrier better than other drugs in its class. Which of the following drugs is this?

(A) Echothiophate
(B) Edrophonium
(C) Neostigmine
(D) Physostigmine
(E) Pyridostigmine

21 A 28-year-old man is hospitalized on the trauma service with multiple organ system failure after sustaining multiple fractures and internal injuries. His most recent CT scan of the abdomen does not reveal any visceral organ injury. He is currently on an intravenous epinephrine drip to maintain his blood pressure and heart rate. His most recent laboratory studies reveal a blood glucose level of 425 mg/dL. What is the most likely explanation of this finding?

(A) Hepatic glycogenolysis
(B) Hepatic gluconeogenesis
(C) Pancreatic failure
(D) Pancreatic infarct from trauma
(E) Splenic rupture

22 A 37-year-old woman with a history of asthma is brought to the emergency department suffering from an attack. She takes no medications other than her inhaler for asthma. Her room air pulse oximetry is 86% and her lips are blue. Intravenous epinephrine and intranasal albuterol are given immediately. She becomes unresponsive a few minutes later then becomes pulseless and apneic. She expires despite resuscitative efforts. What is the most likely explanation for her demise?

(A) Cardiac arrest
(B) Cardiac arrhythmia
(C) Cerebral hemorrhage
(D) Pulmonary embolism
(E) Tension headache

23 A 37-year-old woman with hyperthyroidism and asthma has frequent asthma attacks, requiring inhalational albuterol and epinephrine. Her attacks are occurring several times per week. Her most recent blood tests reveal elevated T_3 and T_4 levels twice the normal values. These levels significantly increased from her last laboratory studies 6 months ago. What is the most likely explanation for these findings?

(A) Hypersensitivity vasculature response
(B) Goiter formation
(C) Neoplastic transformation
(D) Thyroid gland infarct
(E) Supratherapeutic levels of exogenous thyroid hormone

24 A 68-year-old man presents to the emergency department with worsening chest pain. He has a history of congestive heart failure and currently takes digoxin. Physical examination reveals an acutely ill man who is tachypneic. His room air pulse oximetry is 90%. Pulmonary auscultation reveals bilateral wheezing. Neck examination reveals jugular venous distension. Which one of the following is the most appropriate treatment for this patient?
(A) Albuterol via nebulizer
(B) Dobutamine
(C) Epinephrine via nebulizer
(D) Norepinephrine
(E) Phenylephrine

25 A 32-year-old man presents to his primary care physician because of a 2-week history of nasal stuffiness, cough, and sinus pain. He is prescribed with phenylephrine. He must be aware of which of the following potential adverse effects?
(A) Constipation
(B) Diarrhea
(C) Epistaxis
(D) Hypertension
(E) Tinnitus

26 A 49-year-old man who smokes three packs of cigarettes per day for the last 20 years (60 pack years) is currently taking an oral nicotine agent to stop smoking as well as clonidine. Approximately 3 days ago, he stopped taking his clonidine and now complains of a pounding headache. What is the most likely explanation for this finding?
(A) Development of portal hypotension
(B) Development of subclinical diabetes
(C) Development of rebound hypertension
(D) Receptor hypersensitivity

27 A 70-year-old man with hypertension and decreased urinary flow presents to his primary care physician for treatment of his urinary symptoms. His current medications include a calcium channel blocker. Physical examination reveals a 20-g prostate without nodules. Which of the following is the most efficacious treatment for this patient with minimal potential for adverse events?
(A) Alfuzosin
(B) Doxazosin
(C) Phenoxybenzamine
(D) Phentolamine
(E) Tamsulosin

28 A 58-year-old man with cardiac dysfunction is placed on propranolol. Over the ensuing days, he develops worsening pedal edema, and review of his serum electrolyte reveals a serum sodium of 151 mEq/L. What is the most appropriate treatment for this patient?
(A) Furosemide
(B) Potassium chloride intravenous fluid bolus
(C) Sodium chloride intravenous fluid bolus
(D) Triamterene
(E) Watchful waiting

29 In patients with Parkinson's disease, histologic studies suggest an imbalance in brain neurotransmitters. In contrast to normal individuals, the patients with Parkinson's disease have an abundance of which of the following neurons and associated neurotransmitters?
(A) Acetylcholine
(B) Dopamine
(C) Epinephrine
(D) Norepinephrine
(E) Serotonin

30 A 59-year-old man with Parkinson's disease begins a course of bromocriptine in hopes of improving his significant symptoms of cogwheel rigidity and bradykinesia. After being on the medication for 6 months, a renal ultrasound is obtained that reveals bilateral hydronephrosis and elevation of his serum creatinine to 2.5 mg/dL. What is the most likely explanation for these findings?
(A) Drug toxicity
(B) Renal artery stenosis
(C) Renal artery thrombosis
(D) Renal vein thrombosis
(E) Retroperitoneal fibrosis

31 A 72-year-old woman with Parkinson's disease is taking a medication that increases release of dopamine, blockade of cholinergic receptors, and inhibiting the *N*-methyl-D-aspartate receptor. This describes which of the following agents?
(A) Amantadine
(B) Bromocriptine
(C) Pramipexole
(D) Rotigotine
(E) Tolcapone

32 A 67-year-old man with early onset of Alzheimer's disease is being seen by his primary care physician. Consideration is being made to begin preemptive therapy with an anticholinesterase inhibitor. The patient and family are made aware of such side effects as nausea, vomiting, diarrhea, and muscle cramps. The mechanism of action of these effects likely involves which of the following?

(A) Adrenergic transmission
(B) Cholinergic transmission
(C) Purine metabolism impairment
(D) Transaminase enzyme elevation
(E) Uremia

33 A 24-year-old male comes to the clinic complaining of vague abdominal pain, headaches, sweating, and unintentional weight loss. Urinalysis reveals elevated levels of catecholamine metabolites. Which of the following is a metabolite specific to the breakdown of epinephrine?
(A) Dihydroxyphenylalanine
(B) Dihydroxymandelic acid
(C) Homovanillic acid
(D) Metanephrine
(E) Vanillylmandelic acid

34 A 60-year-old man presents to his primary care physician. During his interview, it is discovered that he is taking several outdated drugs for his medical condition. One of his medical conditions is hypertension, for which he takes a drug that prevents neurotransmitter uptake into vesicles. This prevents neurons from being able to concentrate and store certain neurotransmitters such as norepinephrine. Which of the following drugs is this?
(A) Clonidine
(B) Methyldopa
(C) Reserpine
(D) Scopolamine
(E) Tyramine

35 A 58-year-old woman with multiple sclerosis presents to her primary care physician for follow-up. She ambulates well and has few issues with her disease. Which of the following agents may be beneficial in slowing the progression of this disease?
(A) Dalfampridine
(B) Fingolimod
(C) Mitoxantrone
(D) Vitamin A
(E) Vitamin E

36 A 62-year-old woman with mild MS has some mild difficulty with walking. She is interested in becoming more active with walking and is considering walking a 3.1-mile event with her daughter. Which of the following agents may be beneficial in assisting her with improved ambulation?
(A) Dalfampridine
(B) Fingolimod
(C) Mitoxantrone
(D) Prednisone
(E) Prednisolone

37 A 42-year-old man with ALS presents to his primary care physician for follow-up. He has not had any issues in the last few years and does not need supplemental oxygen. Which of the following agents may be beneficial to delay the need for ventilator support in this patient?
(A) Memantine
(B) Metronidazole
(C) Prednisone
(D) Prednisolone
(E) Riluzole

38 Five patients present to their primary care physician with various complaints and problems. Which of the following patients would have the most limited response to their symptoms if given a prescription for diazepam?
(A) A 24-year-old woman with chronic pelvic pain
(B) A 36-year-old man with chronic anxiety
(C) A 42-year-old man with seizure disorder
(D) A 45-year-old woman with seizure disorder
(E) A 52-year-old man with spinal cord pain from an accident

39 A 40-year-old man with chronic anxiety and alcohol abuse has difficulty getting to sleep. He has no other medical problems. Physical examination of the heart, lungs, and abdomen are within normal limits. Which of the following is the best agent to help this patient get to sleep?
(A) Clonazepam
(B) Diazepam
(C) Flurazepam
(D) Temazepam
(E) Triazolam

40 An 83-year-old woman with Parkinson's disease is currently being treated with carbidopa/levodopa, but her Parkinson's symptoms are worsening. She has normal liver function and no history of liver disease. The physician adds tolcapone to her regimen on tolcapone. How does tolcapone help in Parkinson's disease?
(A) Increased norepinephrine synthesis
(B) Inhibition of COMT
(C) Inhibition of MAO
(D) Stimulation of acetylcholine release
(E) Stimulation of norepinephrine release

41 A 7-year-old boy is brought to the emergency department by his parents after being stung by a bee. The parents say that he is allergic to bee stings, and the patient is having great difficulty breathing. Epinephrine is administered immediately. His symptoms improve as molecules of epinephrine bind to β_2-receptors in bronchial smooth muscle. Which of the following describes a feature of β_2-receptors?

(A) Contains a domain that passes through the cell membrane seven times
(B) Forms a dimer and autophosphorylates intracytoplasmic residues
(C) Ligand-gated chloride channel
(D) Physically attached to smooth endoplasmic reticulum, causing release of intracellular calcium stores
(E) Reside in the cytoplasm, not the cell surface

42 In review of the benzodiazepine class, which of the following agents has the longest duration of action and may be useful in the treatment of a 39-year-old patient with spinal cord injury and with skeletal muscle spasticity?

(A) Diazepam
(B) Lorazepam
(C) Oxazepam
(D) Temazepam
(E) Triazolam

43 A 38-year-old man with chronic anxiety and agitation is currently being treated with a long-acting benzodiazepine. He is having challenges with sleep and is referred to a sleep center for a 24-h sleep study to further ascertain his difficulties. Which of the following is the most likely abnormality to be noted on this study?

(A) Calming effect during sleep induction
(B) Hourly awakening from sleep
(C) Hypnotic effect with dreams
(D) Improved slow-wave sleep
(E) Shortened stage 2 non-REM sleep

44 Five patients are seen by their primary care physician because of chronic anxiety. Benzodiazepines are being considered for each of the patients. Which of the following patients would be best suited for this medication?

(A) A 31-year-old woman who is 16 weeks pregnant
(B) A 32-year-old woman with alcoholic liver disease and HIV disease
(C) A 36-year-old man with gastroesophageal reflux disorder
(D) A 39-year-old man with alcoholic liver disease
(E) A 62-year-old man with narrow-angle glaucoma

45 A 28-year-old woman complains of fatigue that increases throughout the day. At the end of her workday, she says her eyes feel "heavy" and "droopy," although she does not feel particularly tired. Pyridostigmine is prescribed to treat her myasthenia gravis. Which of the following is a potential side effect of this therapy?

(A) Constipation
(B) Diaphoresis
(C) Mydriasis
(D) Tachycardia
(E) Urinary retention

46 A 78-year-old man with generalized anxiety disorder and mild dementia is being seen by his primary care physician. Physical examination of the heart, lungs, and abdomen are within normal limits. Which of the following would be the best treatment option for his generalized anxiety disorder?

(A) Alprazolam
(B) Buspirone
(C) Flumazenil
(D) Temazepam
(E) Triazolam

47 A 47-year-old man with a history of intermittent panic disorders presents to his primary care physician desiring therapy. He has no other pertinent past medical or surgical history. Physical examination of the heart, lungs, and abdomen are within normal limits. What is the most appropriate treatment for this patient?

(A) Alprazolam
(B) Lorazepam
(C) Temazepam
(D) Triazolam
(E) Zolpidem

48 A 35-year-old man who serves as a chief operating officer of a local bank consumes 14 cups of coffee per day as a means of dealing with his stressful job. He presents to his primary care physician as a checkup to be established as a patient. Which of the following signs might the physician observe in this patient?

(A) Anxiety
(B) Depression
(C) Fatigue
(D) Memory loss
(E) Tinnitus

49 A 52-year-old man who depends upon his three cups of coffee per day, which he purchases at his place of work, suddenly finds that the coffee stand has closed. He now is unable to drink his three cups of coffee per day. Which of the following effects might he exhibit at work?

(A) Enhanced penmanship
(B) Facile ability with calling clients
(C) Facile ability with writing letters
(D) Tiredness toward midmorning

50 A 19-year-old college student has come to the conclusion that smoking one cigarette per day may help him excel in his classes. Note: This behavior is not endorsed by the American Medical Association. The student's belief in having one cigarette per day may actually improve which of the following performance areas?
(A) Attention
(B) Differentiation of colors
(C) Skill in essay writing
(D) Tactile sensation
(E) Word finding

51 A 38-year-old man who is an inpatient in prison is serving a life sentence because of murder in the first degree. He is interested in suicide, but his only means is to overdose on coffee, which he has free access. The lethal dose of caffeine in grams and the estimated number of cups of coffee to achieve this is which of the following?
(A) 2 g, 20 cups
(B) 4 g, 40 cups
(C) 8 g, 80 cups
(D) 10 g, 100 cups
(E) 20 g, 200 cups

52 A 34-year-old woman with chronic irritable bowel syndrome with predominance of diarrhea and left lower quadrant pain begins smoking in response to the numerous stresses in her personal and professional life. She smokes one pack per day. She presents to her primary care physician for treatment of her irritable bowel syndrome. The physician expects a change in which of the following symptoms of her irritable bowel syndrome?
(A) Diarrhea
(B) Muscle aches
(C) Right lower quadrant pain
(D) Right upper quadrant pain
(E) Temporomandibular joint dysfunction

53 A 45-year-old man with attention-deficit/hyperactivity disorder presents to his primary care physician for evaluation and treatment. Physical examination of the heart, lungs, and abdomen are within normal limits. The patient has begun on atomoxetine. Which of the following underlying disorders must the treating physician be aware of?
(A) Anxiety
(B) Bipolar disease
(C) Bleeding disorders
(D) Chronic diarrhea
(E) Glaucoma

54 A 21-year-old college student is brought to the emergency department by his roommate after getting high on LSD after receiving a poor grade on a final examination. Physical examination by the triage nurse is performed. Which of the following findings would be expected in this patient?
(A) Constricted pupils
(B) Hypotension
(C) Hypothermia
(D) Piloerection
(E) Sinus drainage

55 A 48-year-old man with schizophrenia on thioridazine for 20 years develops bilateral facial and jaw movements and rhythmic motions of his tongue. Physical examination of the heart, lungs, and abdomen are unremarkable. What is the most likely aberration on a neurotransmitter level?
(A) Acetylcholine
(B) Dopamine
(C) Epinephrine
(D) Norepinephrine
(E) Serotonin

56 A 27-year-old hospital worker has access to the pharmacy when no other workers are around. He is able to find morphine and inject himself with supratherapeutic dose of morphine. He then collapses and is found dead by coworkers 24 h later. What is the most likely explanation for his death?
(A) Cardiac arrest
(B) Cardiac ischemia
(C) Cardiomyopathy
(D) Respiratory depression and arrest
(E) Transient cerebral ischemic attack and subsequent stroke

57 A 39-year-old man with recurrent epileptic seizures presents to his primary care physician for follow-up. He has no pertinent past medical, surgical, or family history in relation to his seizures. CT scan of the head reveals normal cerebral and cerebellar structures. There is no evidence of hydrocephalus. What is the most likely explanation of this patient's seizures?
(A) Alcohol induced
(B) Iatrogenic
(C) Idiopathic
(D) Neoplastic
(E) Traumatic

58 A 34-year-old man suffers a seizure while in a shopping mall. Witnesses tell the paramedics that the individual lost consciousness and then had rapid contraction and relaxation of his extremities. He then awoke and was confused. What is the most likely diagnosis?

(A) Absence seizures
(B) Febrile seizures
(C) Myoclonic seizures
(D) Status epilepticus
(E) Tonic-clonic seizures

59 A 42-year-old woman presents to her primary care physician in follow-up from a visit to the emergency department for a treatment of a seizure. The patient has had seizures approximately every other month for the last 6 months. Consideration is now being given to beginning an antiseizure medication. Which of the following indications will play the lowest role in the physician's mind as to which antiseizure agent to start in this patient?
(A) Comorbid conditions
(B) Cost of the medication
(C) Lifestyle of the patient
(D) Personal preference
(E) Race of the patient

60 A 53-year-old woman with seizure disorder, bipolar disorder, and trigeminal neuralgia presents to her primary care physician for follow-up and treatment. She has no new complaints. Which of the following medications may serve to treat all of her earlier mentioned problems?
(A) Carbamazepine
(B) Ethosuximide
(C) Felbamate
(D) Gabapentin
(E) Lacosamide

61 A mother brings her unconscious 14-year-old son to the emergency department. He was found unresponsive in his bedroom. His respirations are 10 breaths per minute. The mother suspects that her son has been abusing her prescription diazepam, showing her empty pill bottle. What should be given to him to counteract the diazepam?
(A) Amphetamine
(B) Epinephrine
(C) Flumazenil
(D) Phenobarbital
(E) Theophylline

62 A 55-year-old woman with schizophrenia has been taking fluphenazine for 10 years to control her symptoms. At her regular 6-month checkup today, she complains of uncontrollable lip puckering movements. What is the next step the physician should take?
(A) Add another neuroleptic that will help fluphenazine control the twitches
(B) Ask about illicit drug use
(C) Consider discontinuing her medication
(D) Increase the dose of fluphenazine
(E) No change is necessary

63 A 57-year-old man with a seizure disorder takes antiepileptic medications. His physician would like to use a medicine that is metabolized only by the CYP1A2 receptor. Which of the following agents would be preferred?
(A) Carbamazepine
(B) Divalproex
(C) Felbamate
(D) Phenobarbital
(E) Phenytoin

64 A 47-year-old man with seizure disorder presents to his primary care physician for follow-up. Because of a recent exacerbation in his seizures, he is prescribed with lacosamide. Which of the following is the most likely mechanism of action of this medication?
(A) Binds to collapsing response mediator protein-2
(B) Binds to GABA receptors
(C) Blockade of calcium channels
(D) Blockade of sodium channels
(E) Blockade of both sodium and calcium channels

65 A 19-year-old man with a significant seizure history has various seizures including partial onset seizures, myoclonic seizures, and, occasionally, primary generalized tonic-clonic seizures. His physician prescribed levetiracetam. This agent likely works on which of the following structures?
(A) Calcium channel modulation
(B) Collapsing response mediator protein-2
(C) GABA receptors
(D) Sodium channels
(E) Synaptic vesicle protein

66 A 78-year-old man with a long history of seizure disorder controlled with phenytoin presents to his dentist for routine follow-up. Which of the following findings must the dentist be concerned about and evaluate for?
(A) Dental caries
(B) Exposed nerve roots
(C) Jaw bone exposure
(D) Gingival overgrowth
(E) Teeth erosion

67 A 54-year-old man with seizure disorder and chronic neuropathic pain presents to his primary care physician for follow-up. Review of his laboratory studies indicates elevated liver function tests to four times the normal levels. Which of the following agents would be preferred to manage this patient?

(A) Carbamazepine
(B) Phenobarbital
(C) Phenytoin
(D) Pregabalin

68 A 16-year-old boy is brought to the urgent care clinic after suffering an episode of lip smacking followed by stiffness and convulsions. His mother explains that this is the third such attack in the past 2 years and that each attack has lasted about a minute. The pediatrician prescribes carbamazepine to control his seizures. What is the mechanism of action of this agent?

(A) Inhibition of calcium channels
(B) Inhibition of potassium channels
(C) Inhibition of sodium channels
(D) Potentiation of GABA receptors
(E) Stimulation of chloride channels

69 A 72-year-old man is brought to his physician by his son. The son complains that this patient has been becoming forgetful, confused, moody, and aggressive over the past few months. Which of the following neurotransmitter changes is characteristic of Alzheimer's disease?

(A) Decreased acetylcholine
(B) Decreased dopamine
(C) Decreased norepinephrine
(D) Increased acetylcholine
(E) Increased dopamine

70 A 62-year-old man presents with cogwheel rigidity, resting tremor, and bradykinesia. He is diagnosed with Parkinson's disease. His medications include a monoamine oxidase (MAO) inhibitor and a catechol-*O*-methyltransferase (COMT) inhibitor. The intent of inhibiting these enzymes is to increase synaptic dopamine, although many amine neurotransmitters are substrates for both of these enzymes. Which of the following is a substrate for MAO only?

(A) Acetylcholine
(B) Epinephrine
(C) γ-Aminobutyric acid
(D) Norepinephrine
(E) Serotonin

71 A 59-year-old man presents to his primary care physician with an extremely sore shoulder following an accident at work. He is not found to have any fractures or tears and is treated with an injection of prednisolone for bursitis. He smokes and is currently taking levothyroxine because of a thyroidectomy, a β-blocker for mild heart failure, and prazosin for benign prostatic hyperplasia. His medications and the nicotine in his cigarettes each act on a different receptor. Activation of which of the following receptors produces the fastest cellular response?

(A) α_1-Adrenergic receptor
(B) β_1-Adrenergic receptor
(C) Glucocorticoid hormone receptor
(D) Nicotinic cholinergic receptor
(E) Thyroid hormone receptor

72 A 3-year-old boy who is suffering from convulsions is brought to the emergency department by his parents. They report finding him eating a rodenticide, which they brought with them for identification. The active ingredient in this brand of poison is strychnine. How does strychnine work?

(A) Agonist of α_1-adrenergic receptors
(B) Agonist of GABA receptors
(C) Agonist of nicotinic cholinergic receptors
(D) Antagonist of glutamate receptors
(E) Antagonist of glycine receptors

73 A 31-year-old female is brought to the emergency department by friends who said she has been "taking drugs." They did not know specifically what she had taken. She presents with respiratory depression and dysphoria. Stimulation of which receptor is likely causing her dysphoria?

(A) Cannabinoid receptor
(B) GABA receptor
(C) κ-Opioid receptor
(D) μ-Opioid receptor
(E) Serotonin receptor

74 A 21-year-old man complains of depressed mood, lack of pleasure in activities he previously enjoyed, and lack of energy. This has been going on for 2.5 years now. His physician prescribes fluoxetine. Which of the following side effects is most likely to occur in this patient?

(A) Abdominal pain
(B) Peptic ulcers
(C) Impotence
(D) Loss of taste
(E) Pancreatitis

75 A 35-year-old man who is employed as a salesman complains of fatigue. He also mentions that he no longer likes to fly his model airplanes, which has been a hobby of his since childhood and was a major occupier of his free time. The physician prescribes the antidepressant bupropion. What else is bupropion commonly used for?
(A) Alcoholism
(B) Anxiety
(C) Delirium tremens
(D) Opioid overdose
(E) Smoking cessation

76 A 22-year-old man presents to his primary care physician with progressively worsening hallucinations and delusions. His friends describe him as less interested in certain activities and less talkative than he used to be. The physician prescribes clozapine for schizophrenia. Which of the following symptoms will be helped most by clozapine?
(A) Attention deficit
(B) Delusions
(C) Flat affect
(D) Lack of motivation
(E) Poverty of speech

77 A 53-year-old woman with schizophrenia managed for years with chlorpromazine complains of a dry mouth, constipation, blurred vision, and feeling tired. Low-potency typical antipsychotics such as chlorpromazine are known to interfere with many neurotransmitter receptors aside from their target. Which of the following type of receptors is spared from antagonism by chlorpromazine?
(A) α-Adrenergic receptors
(B) β-Adrenergic receptors
(C) Dopamine receptors
(D) Histamine receptors
(E) Muscarinic cholinergic receptors

78 A 44-year-old man with schizophrenia is being treated with a low-potency typical antipsychotic. He complains that his medication's side effects are more than he can handle and wants to try another medication. If he was to switch from a low-potency to a high-potency antipsychotic drug, which of the following side effects would likely diminish?
(A) Anticholinergic effects
(B) Parkinsonism
(C) Perioral tremor
(D) Tardive dyskinesia
(E) Torticollis

79 A 35-year-old man who is an immigrant has been taking prazepam for anxiety for 10 years. This drug is not available in the United States, so he goes to see a physician about a drug that would be a good replacement. What might happen to this patient if he was unable to replace his prazepam and abruptly quit taking it?
(A) Adrenal insufficiency
(B) Convulsions and hallucinations
(C) Fever and muscle rigidity
(D) Myocardial infarction
(E) Respiratory depression

80 A 26-year-old man complains of tremors, tachycardia, and diaphoresis when speaking in public. He has started a new job that requires him to give frequent presentations to large audiences and is worried he would not be able to work effectively. His physician prescribes propranolol. How will propranolol help with this patient's anxiety?
(A) CNS sedation
(B) CNS stimulation
(C) Patients with anxiety usually have comorbid heart disease
(D) Propranolol is not used to treat anxiety
(E) Symptomatic relief

81 A 47-year-old woman is recovering from a hysterectomy. Her physician prescribes an opioid analgesic as needed for postoperative pain. Opioids can cause many effects in addition to analgesia including constipation, respiratory depression, euphoria, miosis, and drowsiness. With prolonged use, tolerance develops to most of these effects. Which of the following effects persists in spite of tolerance leading to a decrease in the other effects?
(A) Analgesia
(B) Constipation
(C) Drowsiness
(D) Euphoria
(E) Nausea and vomiting

82 A 21-year-old male college student complains of difficulty falling asleep at night. He asks if there is anything "mild" he can take to help him get to sleep. Which of the following hypnotics mimics an endogenous hormone?
(A) Diazepam
(B) Lorazepam
(C) Phenobarbital
(D) Ramelteon
(E) Zolpidem

83 A 29-year-old woman who has been diagnosed with multiple sclerosis presents to her primary care physician with muscle rigidity and spasms. She also complains of difficulty sleeping, heartburn, and muscle pain. One of the drugs her physician prescribes is baclofen. Which of the following will baclofen do for this patient?

(A) Anti-inflammatory to decrease muscle pain
(B) Decrease heartburn
(C) Relieve muscle spasms
(D) Reverse the progression of MS
(E) Sleep aid

84 A 34-year-old woman with multiple sclerosis presents with uncontrollable muscle spasms. The physician prescribes tizanidine to help control the spasms. Tizanidine's mechanism of action is most similar to which of the following drugs?

(A) Amlodipine
(B) Clonidine
(C) Dantrolene
(D) Lorazepam
(E) Phenobarbital

85 A 54-year-old man is elected to undergo a total knee replacement following a knee arthroscopy. He arrives the day of the surgery in good health. The anesthesiologist induces sedation using phenobarbital. Which of the following parameter changes may be evident in this patient because of the phenobarbital?

(A) Decreased AST/ALT
(B) Decreased serum bilirubin
(C) Increased serum amylase
(D) Increased serum bilirubin
(E) Increased serum CK

86 An 83-year-old man is brought to the clinic by his family with complaints stating he can no longer perform his daily activities or be trusted to live on his own. During his neurological exam, he presents with moderate memory loss, apraxia, and anomia. Also, he displays aggressive behaviors throughout the physical exam. He was diagnosed to be in an early stage of Alzheimer's disease. What class of drugs would be most helpful in treating the patient?

(A) Cholinesterase stimulants
(B) Cholinesterase inhibitors
(C) Dopamine agonists
(D) Muscarinic receptor inhibitors
(E) NMDA glutamate receptor agonists

87 A 56-year-old man came to the clinic with complaints of tremor, bradykinesia, and "a feeling of persistent restlessness" after beginning a new antipsychotic regimen 2 months ago. The patient has a history of schizophrenia and depression. He is afraid he may have Parkinson's syndrome. The doctor recommended cessation of the new regimen and assures the patient the symptoms will clear after a few weeks or months after withdrawal. What antipsychotic was the most likely to have caused the patient's symptoms?

(A) Aripiprazole
(B) Clozapine
(C) Haloperidol
(D) Olanzapine
(E) Ziprasidone

88 Researchers are studying the intracellular effects of certain hormones and neurotransmitters on their respective receptors. After exposing a culture of cells to a catecholamine solution, they saw an increase in the intracellular calcium concentration. Stimulation of which of the following receptors would cause this?

(A) α_1-Adrenergic
(B) α_2-Adrenergic
(C) β_1-Adrenergic
(D) β_2-Adrenergic
(E) Dopaminergic-1 (D_1)

89 A 53-year-old woman is on a cruise to the Caribbean. The waters are somewhat choppy, and she fears that she will have motion sickness. She presents to the ship physician who gives her scopolamine to take to prevent motion sickness. This agent works in which of the following pathways?

(A) Blockade of β_1-receptors
(B) Blockade of β_2-receptors
(C) Blockade of H_2 receptors
(D) Blockade of M receptors
(E) Stimulation of the CTZ receptors

90 A 72-year-old man is brought to his physician by his son. The son complains that this patient has been becoming forgetful, confused, moody, and aggressive over the past few months. One drug that may be used to treat this patient's symptoms is donepezil. Which of the following describes an effect of donepezil?

(A) Decreases synaptic acetylcholine
(B) Decreases synaptic dopamine
(C) Decreases synaptic norepinephrine
(D) Increases synaptic acetylcholine
(E) Increases synaptic dopamine

91 A 64-year-old man presents with a shuffling gait, cogwheel rigidity, and a resting tremor. His physician prescribes levodopa and his symptoms greatly improve, supporting a diagnosis of Parkinson's disease. How does levodopa help this patient's symptoms?
(A) Increase dopamine production
(B) Inhibit acetylcholinesterase
(C) Stimulate acetylcholine receptors
(D) Stimulate dopamine receptors
(E) Stimulate release of preformed dopamine

92 Regarding differences between the sympathetic and parasympathetic nervous systems in a healthy 29-year-old graduate student athlete, which of the following is a feature of the sympathetic nervous system?
(A) Discrete response
(B) Ganglia located near target organs
(C) Limited distribution
(D) Short preganglionic fibers
(E) Thoracolumbar region of the spinal cord

93 A novel medication to treat gastric motility disorders will act at the terminal step in the synthesis/breakdown of acetylcholine. Which of the following is the terminal step in the synthesis and release of acetylcholine?
(A) Degradation
(B) Release of neurotransmitter
(C) Recycling of choline
(D) Synthesis
(E) Uptake into storage vesicles

94 Which of the following statements is correct about the normal functioning of the nicotinic receptors in a 19-year-old man college student athlete from the college baseball team?
(A) Nicotine at high doses stimulates the receptor
(B) Nicotinic receptors are located in the adrenal cortex
(C) Nicotinic receptors are located in the autonomic ganglia
(D) Nicotinic receptors located at the neuromuscular junction are known as NN receptors

95 A 29-year-old man with spinal cord injury and with chronic gastric immotility syndrome has failed therapy with numerous cholinomimetic agents. He has begun on therapy with physostigmine. Unfortunately, a supratherapeutic dose is administered to the patient. Which of the following effects must the treating physician be aware of?
(A) Convulsions
(B) Flaccid paralysis
(C) Pulmonary embolism
(D) Sinus tachycardia
(E) Tetralogy of Fallot

96 A 7-year-old boy is brought to the clinic by his mother for a well-child checkup. Physical exam is normal, and he is in no acute distress. A few months ago, he started taking atomoxetine for attention-deficit/hyperactivity disorder. His mother has been pleased with the results but has one complaint that the physician immediately recognizes as a common side effect of atomoxetine. Which of the following is most likely the mother's complaint?
(A) Appetite suppression
(B) Diarrhea
(C) Pruritic rash
(D) Urinary incontinence
(E) Weight gain

97 A 37-year-old man is preparing to undergo functional endoscopic sinus surgery. In the operating room, he is given intravenous succinylcholine. This agent will initially produce which of the following responses?
(A) Apnea
(B) Ganglionic blockade
(C) Muscle fasciculations
(D) Vascular smooth muscle relaxation
(E) Urinary bladder paralysis

98 A 15-year-old boy attempts suicide and is brought to the emergency department by the local rescue squad. He was found in the garage with an opened spray bottle of insecticide nearby. He has lost consciousness. His heart rate is 45 beats/minute, and his blood pressure is 80/40 mm Hg. He is sweating and salivating profusely. What is the most appropriate treatment for this patient?
(A) Atropine
(B) Edrophonium
(C) Norepinephrine
(D) Physostigmine
(E) Trimethaphan

99 An individual lacks the ability to synthesize dopamine in the axoplasm of the adrenergic neuron. Should the problem occur at the rate-limiting step of this conversion, which of the following substances will accumulate?
(A) Dopamine
(B) L-dopa
(C) Norepinephrine
(D) Testosterone
(E) Tyrosine

100 After norepinephrine is released, it binds to receptors on the target organs. Then, it must be removed from the synaptic space. Which of the following mechanisms describes correct removal of norepinephrine from the synaptic space?

(A) ATPase pump is stimulated by cocaine
(B) ATPase pump is stimulated by imipramine
(C) Diffusion from the general circulation back into the synaptic space
(D) Metabolism to O-methylated derivatives in the synaptic space
(E) Pump system pumps norepinephrine out of the neuron

101 A 21-year-old woman presents to her primary care physician complaining of "feeling sleepy all the time." Physical exam is normal, but she has a history of hay fever since she was 14 years old. You discover that she is currently taking medicine for her allergy but cannot remember the name. She says it controls her hay fever symptoms well. You suspect that her medication is causing her to feel sleepy. Which of the following would be most likely to cause drowsiness?
(A) Amantadine
(B) Cimetidine
(C) Doxylamine
(D) Famotidine
(E) Fexofenadine

102 A 67-year-old man with hypertension is treated with guanethidine. He has been taking this medication for years. His blood pressure is 130/86 mm Hg. Which of the following adverse effects must this patient be aware of?
(A) Erectile dysfunction
(B) Hepatitis
(C) Hypertension
(D) Pheochromocytoma
(E) Pulmonary infection

103 Which of the following changes occur at the neurotransmitter/synaptic space when an excitatory postsynaptic potential is generated?
(A) Increased stimulation of excitatory neurons promoting further neurotransmitter release
(B) Neurotransmitter release, alanine
(C) Neurotransmitter release, aspartic acid
(D) Repolarization
(E) Transient increase in potassium permeability

104 Stimulation of inhibitory neurons causes which of the following effects at the postsynaptic membrane?
(A) Binding of GABA at the postsynaptic membrane
(B) Depolarization
(C) Stimulation of epinephrine
(D) Transient decrease in permeability of chloride
(E) Transient decrease in permeability of potassium

105 A 56-year-old man who is hospitalized for viral encephalitis develops pill-rolling tremors of the hands and cogwheel rigidity. He is thought to have parkinsonian symptoms that developed because of an underlying secondary cause. Which of the following is the most likely etiology of this condition?
(A) Carotid arterial atherosclerosis
(B) Large brain aneurysm
(C) Viral encephalitis
(D) Use of cocaine
(E) Use of isoniazid

106 A 68-year-old man with a 6-month history of progressive pill-rolling tremors of the hands, urinary incontinence, and cogwheel rigidity presents to his primary care physician for evaluation. Physical examination confirms the earlier findings. Which of the following is a therapeutic goal for this condition?
(A) Antagonizing the excitatory effect of cholinergic neurons
(B) Dynamic physical and occupational therapy
(C) Lower concentrations of CNS dopamine
(D) Restore dopamine concentration in the cerebellum
(E) Restore epinephrine concentration in the cerebrum

107 A 65-year-old man develops new onset of symptoms of urinary incontinence and cogwheel muscle rigidity. Evaluation of bladder function reveals sphincter bradykinesia. He has begun on treatment with levodopa. Which of the following effects should the physician warn this patient of?
(A) Bradycardia
(B) Hypertension
(C) Increased appetite
(D) Miosis
(E) Salivary gland secretion discoloration

108 Favorable characteristics of pramipexole as a dopamine agonist for treatment of parkinsonism in a 72-year-old man would include which of the following?
(A) Extensive metabolism
(B) Favorable bioavailability
(C) Hepatic excretion
(D) Short half-life
(E) Transdermal administration

109 A 71-year-old man with gradual impairment in short-term memory and speech is thought to have Alzheimer's disease. His primary care physician begins him on rivastigmine. This agent will most likely cause which of the following effects?
(A) Improved long-term memory capability
(B) Improved speech and language function
(C) Reduced rate of loss of cognitive function
(D) Tremors similar to that seen with parkinsonism

110 A 73-year-old woman with Alzheimer's disease is in a long-term care facility. She also has a history of hypertension, diabetes mellitus, and mild anxiety. Modest improvement in the memory of patients with Alzheimer's disease may occur with drugs that increase transmission at which of the following receptors?

(A) Adrenergic
(B) Cholinergic
(C) Dopaminergic
(D) GABAergic
(E) Serotonergic

111 A 54-year-old man with multiple medical problems and anxiety is placed on diazepam. He has been taking the medication for 6 months. He is concerned that he is having changes in his memory as a result of being on this medication. Which of the following memory effects are likely?

(A) Anterograde amnesia
(B) Long-term memory loss
(C) Loss of ability to taste
(D) Loss of prior negative memories
(E) Short-term memory loss

112 A 28-year-old alcoholic man is brought to the emergency department after a binge drinking. The treating physician is concerned about the risk of alcohol withdrawal and associated risk of withdrawal seizures. Which of the following medications would be most helpful in this patient to decrease these risks?

(A) Alcohol
(B) Clonazepam
(C) Lorazepam
(D) Oxazepam
(E) Tramadol

113 A physician has a choice in benzodiazepines to prescribe for patients. A particular patient (a 53-year-old man with anxiety) has a difficult time with compliance to medications. The physician is concerned about the patient going into withdrawal because of abrupt discontinuation of the antianxiety medication. Which of the following medications would have the least severe withdrawal reaction?

(A) Diazepam
(B) Flurazepam
(C) Temazepam
(D) Triazolam

114 A 66-year-old woman who has smoked two packs of cigarettes per day for 50 years has chronic bronchitis. She has tried to quit five times in the past but felt she could not go long without a cigarette. The nicotine in her cigarettes stimulates many cells in her body by binding certain receptors. Which of the following drugs blocks nicotinic receptors?

(A) Atropine
(B) Bethanechol
(C) Hexamethonium
(D) Metoprolol
(E) Phentolamine

115 A 19-year-old man is brought to the emergency department after being found by his roommate to have snorted cocaine several times in the past few days, the last time being 10 h previously. He was given a drug that sedated him, and he fell asleep. The drug that was used to counter this patient's apparent cocaine withdrawal was very likely which of the following?

(A) Cocaine
(B) Fluoxetine
(C) Hydroxyzine
(D) Lorazepam
(E) Phenobarbital

116 An 8-year-old boy presents to the emergency department after seizure-like activity. During class, the teacher noted that the boy stare off for about 45 s. He has done this three times in the past. He would not respond to her during the episode and was confused for about 1 min following it. What is the most appropriate first-line therapy for this child?

(A) Carbamazepine
(B) Ethosuximide
(C) Lamotrigine
(D) Phenytoin
(E) Valproic acid

117 A 15-year-old boy presents to clinic for follow-up for his tonic-clonic seizures. He reports that he has not had a seizure in the past 6 months. However, he has been more tired recently and is unsure why. A complete blood count is performed and shows megaloblastic anemia. The physician told the patient that this was most likely a side effect of his antiseizure medication. What is the most likely medication he was taking?

(A) Carbamazepine
(B) Ethosuximide
(C) Phenobarbital
(D) Phenytoin
(E) Valproic acid

118 A 60-year-old man presents to his primary care physician for a new patient appointment. He is taking several drugs for his medical conditions. One of his medical conditions is hypertension, for which he takes a drug that acts on α_2-receptors to lower blood pressure. Which of the following drugs is this?
(A) Clonidine
(B) Metoprolol
(C) Reserpine
(D) Scopolamine
(E) Tyramine

119 An 83-year-old woman with Parkinson's disease is currently being treated with carbidopa/levodopa, but her Parkinson's symptoms are worsening. She has normal liver function and no history of liver disease. Selegiline is added to her regimen. How does selegiline help in Parkinson's disease?
(A) Increased norepinephrine synthesis
(B) Inhibition of COMT
(C) Inhibition of MAO
(D) Stimulation of acetylcholine release
(E) Stimulation of norepinephrine release

120 A physician is preparing to suture a wound in a 19-year-old man who sustains a laceration of his left leg while playing in a baseball game. The physician is injecting 1% lidocaine to anesthetize the wound. He aspirates back prior to injection. If he did not do this and the lidocaine got into the systemic circulation, which of the following effects would be possible?
(A) CNS depression
(B) Muscle spasticity
(C) Muscle tetany
(D) Peripheral neurapraxia
(E) Swallowing disorder

121 A 68-year-old woman with a long history of sadness, gloom, and weight loss presents to her primary care physician for treatment. She is treated with a selective serotonin reuptake inhibitor. Which of the following statements is true?
(A) Maximum benefit may require 1 year
(B) Most patients require three antidepressants
(C) Twenty percent of patients with adequate doses for 8 weeks respond to therapy
(D) Two weeks of therapy are required for mood improvement

122 A 62-year-old woman with a history of mental decline, impaired physical activity, and significant mood impairment is seen by her primary care physician. Treatment with a tricyclic antidepressant has begun. Which of the following statements regarding this therapeutic option is true?
(A) Mental alertness is unlikely to change
(B) Mood elevation is likely
(C) Morbid preoccupation will unlikely change
(D) Physical dependence will occur
(E) Psychological dependence will occur

123 A 58-year-old man with Parkinson's disease presents to the clinic for follow-up. Recently, he has experienced an increase in his resting tremor and rigidity. He was wondering if there is a medication that could help these symptoms. What anticholinergic is the most appropriate treatment?
(A) Benztropine
(B) Bromocriptine
(C) Ipratropium
(D) Scopolamine
(E) Tropicamide

124 A 33-year-old woman who takes diazepam for anxiety disorder is currently enrolled in an online master's degree program in accounting. She states that she has attended all classes and studied for a final examination. She has never had this type of problem before. However, when she took the examination, she remembered nothing that she studied. What is the most likely explanation for this finding?
(A) Depression
(B) Pharmacologic effect
(C) Underlying learning disorder
(D) Underlying psychiatric disorder
(E) Uremia caused by supratherapeutic doses

125 A 43-year-old woman with a history of fibromyalgia and depression presents to her primary care physician for treatment. She complains of feeling sad and worthless in addition to multiple somatic complaints. Which of the following treatments would be best for this patient?
(A) Duloxetine
(B) Fluoxetine
(C) Mirtazapine
(D) Sertraline
(E) Watchful waiting

126 A 62-year-old woman with symptoms of feeling blue, sad, and without feelings presents to her primary care physician for treatment. She has a prior medical history of narrow-angle glaucoma. Which of the following treatments should be avoided in this patient?
(A) Amitriptyline
(B) Bupropion
(C) Fluvoxamine
(D) Mirtazapine
(E) Sertraline

127 A 42-year-old woman with feelings of sadness, despair, and tearfulness presents to her primary care physician for management. She has no prior medical or surgical history. Therapy with bupropion has begun. The treating physician must be aware of which of the following contraindications?

(A) Anorexia
(B) Depression
(C) Seasonal affective disorder
(D) Seasonal affective disorder with mania
(E) Transient ischemic attacks

128 An 18-year-old woman presents to clinic because of difficulty with school. She recently started college and is living on her own for the first time. She is constantly preoccupied with wondering if the door is locked. She checks the lock at least 20 times before she is able to leave her apartment. This often makes her late for class. She had been on selective serotonin reuptake inhibitors in the past, but they are ineffective. What is the most appropriate treatment for this patient?

(A) Amitriptyline
(B) Clomipramine
(C) Lithium
(D) Quetiapine
(E) Venlafaxine

129 A 28-year-old woman secretary complains of fatigue that increases throughout the day. At the end of her workday, she says her eyes feel "heavy" and "droopy," although she does not feel particularly tired. Pyridostigmine is prescribed to treat her myasthenia gravis. How does pyridostigmine work?

(A) Blocks acetylcholine degradation
(B) Blocks dopamine degradation
(C) Stimulates acetylcholine release
(D) Stimulates muscarinic cholinergic receptors
(E) Stimulates nicotinic cholinergic receptors

130 A 53-year-old man comes to clinic for depression. He has had decreased interest and a depressed mood for the past 6 months. He also smokes half a pack of cigarettes a day and thinks that if he could quit, that would help his mood as well. What is the most appropriate treatment for his depression and cessation of smoking?

(A) Bupropion
(B) Clomipramine
(C) Imipramine
(D) Mirtazapine
(E) Sertraline

131 A 63-year-old man with a history of Parkinson's disease and generalized anxiety is placed on a first-generation antipsychotic medication. Characteristics of this class of medications include which of the following?

(A) Competitive agonists
(B) Considered atypical antipsychotic agents
(C) Dopamine D_2-receptor blockers
(D) Highly considered for patients with dementia

132 A 49-year-old man with long-standing schizophrenia is hospitalized for a symptom exacerbation. His primary care physician places him on a second-generation antipsychotic agent. Characteristics of this agent include which of the following?

(A) Considered to be typical antipsychotic agents
(B) Have fewer extrapyramidal symptoms than first-generation agents
(C) Low risk of development of diabetes mellitus
(D) Low risk of development of hypercholesterolemia
(E) Low risk of development of weight gain

133 A 53-year-old man with long-standing schizophrenia has failed therapy with both first- and second-generation antipsychotic agents. He still has significant problems with mood, delusions, and hallucinations. He is placed on clozapine. Which of the following effects must the treating physician be aware of?

(A) Agranulocytosis
(B) Cholelithiasis
(C) Pancreatitis
(D) Pituitary adenoma
(E) Polycythemia

134 A 53-year-old man with schizophrenia presents to his primary care physician for follow-up. He has been treated with multiple different antipsychotic agents during his lifetime. Which of the following antipsychotic agents has the highest affinity for the D_2 receptors?

(A) Clozapine
(B) Olanzapine
(C) Quetiapine
(D) Risperidone
(E) Tramadol

135 A 21-year-old male has recently begun pimozide therapy for Tourette's disorder. His parents bring him to the emergency department. They describe that he has been having "different appearing tics" than before, such as prolonged contraction of the facial muscles. While being examined, he experiences opisthotonus (type of extrapyramidal spasm of the body in which the head and heels are bent backward and the body is bowed forward). Which of the following drugs would be beneficial in reducing these symptoms?

(A) Benztropine
(B) Bromocriptine
(C) Lithium
(D) Prochlorperazine
(E) Risperidone

136 A 43-year-old man who is a heroin addict is placed on methadone therapy to wean him off of heroin. Which of the following statements is true regarding the pharmacology of this agent?
(A) Best absorbed following intravenous administration
(B) Biotransformed in the liver and excreted in urine
(C) Lipophilic causing accumulation in tissues
(D) Metabolism dependent in single cytochromes in the liver
(E) Short half-life

137 Four patients with chronic low back pain are being considered for treatment with a centrally acting analgesic. Tapentadol is the agent being considered for use. Which of the following challenging patients would best benefit from this agent?
(A) A 21-year-old man with AIDS and end-stage liver disease
(B) A 30-year-old woman with multiple sclerosis and hepatitis
(C) A 34-year-old man with renal insufficiency and moderate back pain
(D) A 45-year-old man with metastatic liver cancer to lungs, brain, and bone

138 A 9-year-old boy is sent for neurologic evaluation because of episodes of apparent confusion. Over the past year, the child has experienced episodes during which he develops a blank look on his face and fails to respond to questions. Moreover, it appears to take several minutes before the boy recovers from the episodes. Which one of the following best describes this patient's seizures?
(A) Absence
(B) Complex partial
(C) Myoclonic
(D) Simple partial
(E) Tonic-clonic

139 A 48-year-old woman with refractory seizure disorder has failed every antiseizure medication on her local pharmacy formulary. She is considered to be truly refractory to medical therapy and undergoes vagal nerve stimulation. The most plausible mechanism of action of this therapy is which of the following?
(A) Blockade of potassium channels
(B) Blockade of sodium channels
(C) Depolarization of neuronal circuits
(D) Stimulation of seizure foci
(E) Unknown

140 A 27-year-old man is prescribed with an antidepressant for seasonal affective disorder. This particular antidepressant may also help him quit smoking. Which of the following antidepressants is he likely taking?
(A) Bupropion
(B) Duloxetine
(C) Imipramine
(D) Sertraline
(E) Trazodone

141 A 45-year-old woman with chronic anxiety presents to her primary care physician for follow-up. She currently takes Librium 10 mg three times per day. Important warning considerations for use of this medication include which of the following?
(A) Anxiety
(B) Grand mal seizures
(C) Manic depression
(D) Suicidal tendencies
(E) Tinnitus

142 A 44-year-old woman with social anxiety disorder is found to have an ovarian mass lesion. She is scheduled for exploratory laparoscopy. Her current medications include paroxetine. Important considerations for the treating anesthesiologist include screening for which of the following conditions?
(A) Dizziness
(B) Insomnia
(C) Neuroleptic malignant syndrome
(D) Nervousness
(E) Slowing of the heart rate

143 A 49-year-old man with manic depression has been maintained on lithium for long-term therapy. However, because of worsening of symptoms, he is placed on ziprasidone. The patient must be warned about which of the following adverse effects?
(A) Asthenia
(B) Erectile dysfunction
(C) Hypertension
(D) Slowing of heart rate
(E) Visual changes (improved color vision)

144 A medical student is involved in a summer research project involving an animal model of heart failure. Digitalis is administered intrathecally to the animal. Which of the following parameters will change as a result of this medication?
(A) Decrease in end-diastolic volume
(B) Decrease in myocardial contraction
(C) Decrease in myocardial circulation
(D) Decrease in vagal tone
(E) Increase in sympathetic activity

145 A 16-year-old boy is brought to the pediatrician after suffering an episode of lip smacking followed by stiffness and convulsions. His mother explains that this is the third such attack in the past 2 years and that each attack has lasted about a minute. The pediatrician prescribes diazepam to control his seizures. Which of the following describes diazepam's mechanism of action?

(A) Inhibition of calcium channels
(B) Inhibition of potassium channels
(C) Inhibition of sodium channels
(D) Potentiation of GABA receptors
(E) Potentiation of glutamate receptors

146 A 3-year-old girl was found by her mother chewing on some weeds in their flower garden. The mother rushed her to the hospital along with a portion of the weed. The emergency department physician identifies the weed as deadly nightshade, which contains atropine. Which of the following drugs might a physician give as an antidote to atropine?

(A) Dopamine
(B) Epinephrine
(C) Physostigmine
(D) Pralidoxime
(E) Scopolamine

147 A 31-year-old man who is a construction worker presents to the emergency department after cutting his hand with a utility knife. The 4-cm laceration is about a centimeter deep but did not cut any tendons. He has no numbness or tingling in his fingers and has full range of motion. He is given lidocaine for local anesthesia while suturing occurs. Which of the following nerve fibers is blocked first by lidocaine?

(A) Large diameter myelinated
(B) Large diameter unmyelinated
(C) Medium diameter myelinated
(D) Small diameter myelinated
(E) Small diameter unmyelinated

148 A 25-year-old woman with a history of drug abuse presents to the ambulatory care clinic for follow-up of her anxiety. She has not been doing well and states she is anxious most of the time. Her nerves are not allowing her to concentrate, and she has been told she may lose her job soon if she does not stop making mistakes. She is very worried and looks disheveled. She has been using buspirone, and now the physician would like to switch her to a benzodiazepine. However, the physician wants to avoid anything with strong addictive potential. What is the most appropriate medication for this patient?

(A) Clonazepam
(B) Alprazolam
(C) Lorazepam
(D) Oxazepam
(E) Triazolam

149 A 78-year-old woman with Alzheimer's disease presents to her primary care physician for a routine visit. She is brought in by her daughter, who reports her mother has become more forgetful. The patient is alert to person and place but is unsure of the year. The physician would like to add memantine to her regimen of donepezil and vitamin E. What is the mechanism of action of memantine?

(A) Acetylcholine receptor inhibitor
(B) Acetylcholinesterase inhibitor
(C) Increase dopamine release
(D) NMDA receptor agonist
(E) NMDA receptor antagonist

150 A 63-year-old man with Parkinson's disease presents to his primary care physician for follow-up. Over the past 6 months, his tremor has worsened and his gait has become more unstable. He noticed his symptoms have been progressively worsening, and he wants a medication that could make them better. He already takes levodopa. The physician adds a MAO_B inhibitor. What is the most likely medication added to his regimen?

(A) Amantadine
(B) Benztropine
(C) Carbidopa
(D) Selegiline
(E) Tolcapone

151 A 19-year-old woman with anorexia presents to her primary care physician for follow-up. She weighs 82 lb with a BMI of 16.2. She says she tries to eat but is just not happy enough to eat. She has been feeling depressed for quite a while. The physician decides to start her on medication that will increase her weight and improve her mood. What is the most appropriate treatment for this patient?

(A) Bupropion
(B) Maprotiline
(C) Mirtazapine
(D) Trazodone
(E) Venlafaxine

152 A 67-year-old woman complains of "wetting herself" occasionally. With further questioning, the physician learns that she feels sudden urges to urinate and can rarely make it to a restroom in time. She does not complain of urinating with coughing or sneezing. The physician prescribes darifenacin to help with her symptoms. Which of the following is a property of darifenacin?

(A) Blocks muscarinic cholinergic receptors
(B) Blocks nicotinic cholinergic receptors
(C) Increases sphincter tone
(D) Inhibits α-adrenergic receptors
(E) Inhibits β-adrenergic receptors

153 A 34-year-old woman with depression presents to the ambulatory care clinic with altered mental status. She is confused and unsure where she is. Her blood pressure is 240/152 mm Hg. Her Cr is 2.93 mg/dL, which is above her baseline of 0.90 mg/dL. Her husband says she never had a problem with high blood pressure before. Everything was normal 3 h ago prior to her having three glasses of wine and cheese at a party. She recently started a new medication for her depression. What is the most likely medication she started?

(A) Amitriptyline
(B) Duloxetine
(C) Fluoxetine
(D) Phenelzine
(E) Trazodone

154 A 32-year-old woman with change in vision presents to the ambulatory care clinic complaining of dry eye and visual field changes. She is seen by the on-call ophthalmologist who wants to evaluate the eye with a funduscopic examination. The following figure shows two medications that could be given to facilitate the examination. Which of the following statements is true?

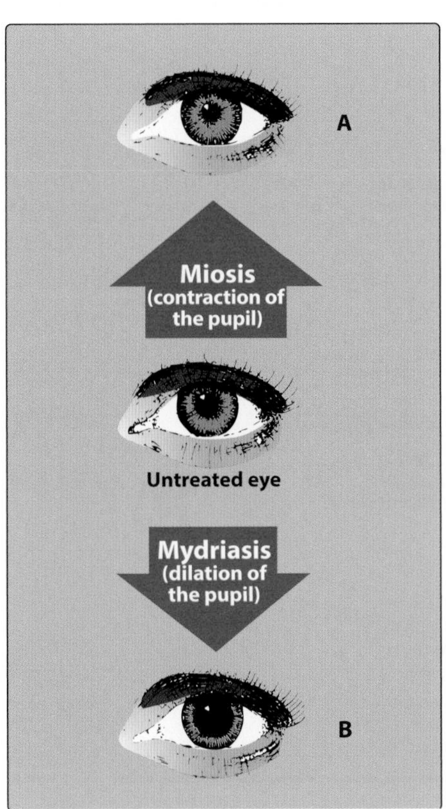

(A) Atropine is represented by letter B
(B) Carbachol is represented by letter A
(C) Mydriasis would challenge visualization during the examination
(D) The untreated eye is appropriate for examination

155 The following figure represents the dose-dependent effects of atropine. This medication is given intravenously into an animal model. If a dose of >10 mg is given, which of the following effects will occur?

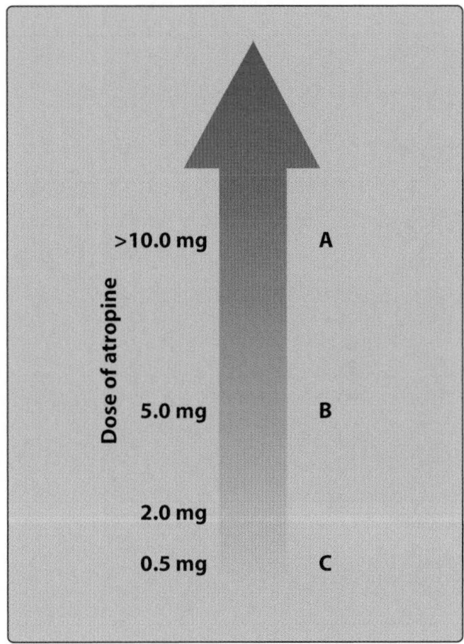

(A) Coma
(B) Dilation of pupil
(C) Near vision changes
(D) Sweating becomes difficult

156 Pheochromocytoma is thought to result from an imbalance in the synthesis and release of norepinephrine from the adrenergic neuron. The following is a diagram of this process. In which of the following steps is norepinephrine binding to receptors?

(A) Letter A
(B) Letter B
(C) Letter C
(D) Letter D
(E) Letter E

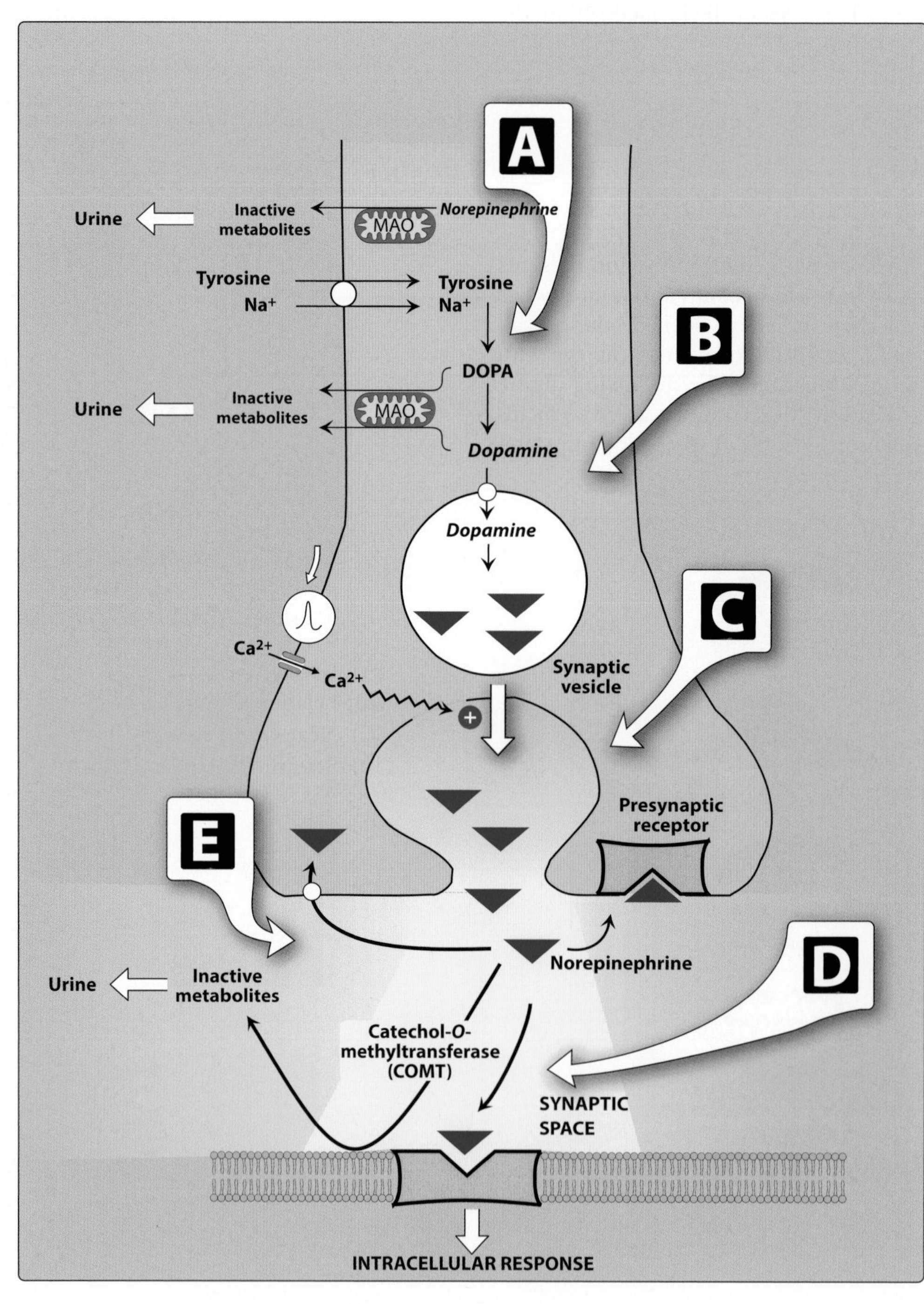

157 A 58-year-old man with long-standing depression presents to his primary care physician for follow-up. He has begun on therapy with duloxetine. This agent works at which of the following points in the succeeding diagram?

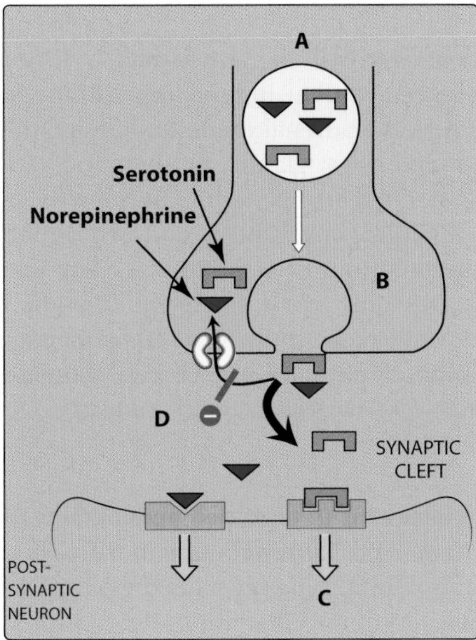

(A) Letter A
(B) Letter B
(C) Letter C
(D) Letter D

158 A 58-year-old man with long-standing schizophrenia presents to his primary care physician for follow-up. He has begun on therapy with a dopamine receptor blocker. This agent works at which of the following points in the succeeding diagram?

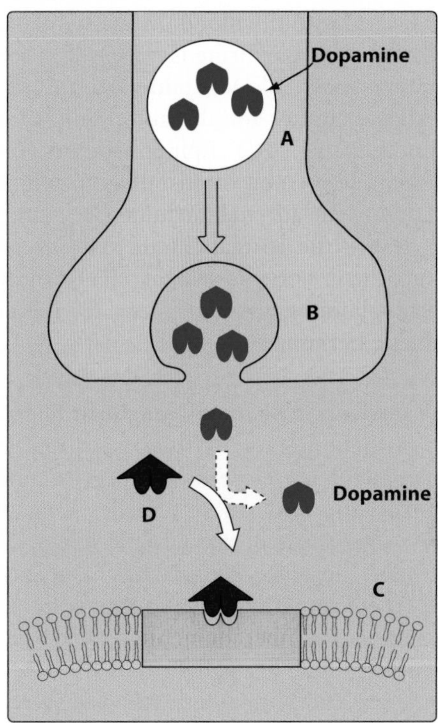

(A) Letter A
(B) Letter B
(C) Letter C
(D) Letter D

159 A 25-year-old woman has been taking an antiepileptic drug for a seizure disorder for 1 year. She now complains of episodes of blurred vision and diplopia. Which of the following antiepileptic drugs has she most likely been taking?

(A) Carbamazepine
(B) Ethosuximide
(C) Lorazepam
(D) Phenobarbital
(E) Valproic acid

ANSWERS

1 **The answer is A: Acetylcholine.** In the somatic and autonomic nervous system, the common neuroeffector transmitter is acetylcholine. However, in sympathetic stimulation of the adrenal medulla, epinephrine is released into the blood. In the sympathetic nervous system, norepinephrine is released by the postganglionic neurons. (B) Dopamine is a not a preganglionic neurotransmitter for the autonomic or somatic nervous systems. (C) Epinephrine is released as a postganglionic neurotransmitter in sympathetic stimulation of the adrenal medulla. (D) Norepinephrine is released as the postganglionic neurotransmitter of the sympathetic nervous system. (E) Serotonin is a not a preganglionic neurotransmitter for the autonomic or somatic nervous systems.

2 **The answer is D: Short postganglionic fibers.** The parasympathetic nervous system has a discrete response. The ganglia are close to the target organs. The parasympathetic nervous system has long preganglionic fibers and short postganglionic fibers. (A) The sympathetic nervous system has a diffuse response. (B) The sympathetic nervous system has extensive preganglionic fiber branching. (C) The sympathetic nervous system has ganglia that are close to the spinal cord. (E) The sympathetic nervous system has a wide distribution.

3 **The answer is B: Decrease potency of proteins they bind to.** Potency is defined as the amount of drug it takes to have a certain effect. Efficacy is defined as the greatest effect a drug can possibly have. Imagine two drugs, A and B. We will say Drug A has a maximal effect at a concentration of 1 mg/mL. Giving more Drug A past this level produces no increase in response. Now, let us say Drug B produces the same maximal effect but at a concentration of 0.01 mg/mL. Giving more Drug B past this level will have no increase in response. Although both drugs have the same maximal effect, Drug B exerts that effect at a much lower concentration than Drug A. We can say then that Drug A and Drug B have the same efficacy, but Drug B is more potent than Drug A. In the presence of competitive inhibition, more native ligand or substrate is needed to achieve any given effect. Therefore, potency is decreased with competitive inhibition. (A) Efficacy is defined as the greatest effect a drug can have (at its highest concentration). Under competitive inhibition, more native ligand or substrate is needed to overcome the competition. But once overcome, the maximal effect is the same as without inhibition so efficacy is not decreased. (C) In enzyme kinetics, the K_m is the substrate concentration needed to achieve 1/2 V_{max}. Under competitive inhibition, more native substrate is needed to achieve 1/2 V_{max} so K_m is increased. (D) Competitive inhibitors are overcomed by high concentrations of native ligand or substrate. (E) Competitive inhibitors usually bind a protein at the same site as the native ligand or substrate. Noncompetitive inhibitors usually bind elsewhere and exert their influence allosterically.

4 **The answer is D: Salivary glands.** Although most tissues receive dual innervation, some effector organs, such as the adrenal medulla, kidney, pilomotor muscles, and sweat glands, receive innervation only from the sympathetic system. The salivary glands receive cholinergic innervation and would be affected by administration of atropine. (A) The adrenal medulla receives only sympathetic innervation. (B) The kidney only receives sympathetic innervation. (C) The pilomotor muscles only receive sympathetic innervation. (E) The sweat glands only receive sympathetic innervation.

5 **The answer is D: Increased peripheral resistance.** This patient is probably dehydrated from staying out in the sun too long. This caused a drop in blood pressure as sensed by reduced stretch in the baroreceptors in the aortic arch. Efferent reflex impulses to this situation include increase in blood pressure, cardiac output, and cardiac contractility. Peripheral resistance will also increase. (A) Blood pressure will increase. (B) Cardiac output will increase. (C) Cardiac contractility will increase. (E) The sympathetic nervous system will be stimulated.

6 **The answer is C: M_3.** The M_3 receptor is felt to be bladder specific. However, this receptor is also found on exocrine glands such as salivary glands and smooth muscle. Specifically, although all five subtypes have been found on neurons, M_1 receptors are also found on gastric parietal cells and M_2 receptors on cardiac cells and smooth muscle. (A) M_1 receptors are found on gastric parietal cells. (B) M_2 receptors are found on cardiac cells and smooth muscle. (D) M_4 receptors are found on neurons. (E) M_5 receptors are found on neurons.

7 **The answer is A: Atropine.** Pilocarpine is applied topically to the eyes and produces rapid miosis and contraction of the ciliary muscle. This patient received too much medication. Atropine, an ocular muscarinic blocker, should be administered immediately. (B) Carbachol is an anticholinergic agent that works on the cardiovascular and gastrointestinal systems. (C) Donepezil is an anticholinergic agent that may have promise in the treatment of Alzheimer's disease. (D) Galantamine is an anticholinergic agent being studied for the treatment of Alzheimer's disease. (E) Rivastigmine is an anticholinergic agent that has been shown to delay progression of Alzheimer's disease.

8 **The answer is D: Hypotension.** This patient is currently taking neostigmine for treatment of myasthenia gravis. She has apparently overdosed on this medication. Adverse effects can include salivation, flushing, hypotension, nausea, abdominal pain, diarrhea, and bronchospasm. (A) Bronchospasm would be expected in this patient. (B) Diarrhea would be expected in this patient. (C) CNS effects are not expected with neostigmine. (E) Salivation would be expected in this patient.

9 **The answer is C: Rivastigmine.** Rivastigmine is hydrolyzed by AChE to a carbamylate metabolite and has no interactions with drugs that alter the activity of cytochrome P450–dependent enzymes. Thus, it can be maintained at routine doses in patients with elevated liver function tests. (A) Donepezil should be dose adjusted in this patient with hepatic insufficiency. (B) Galantamine is a substrate for cytochrome P450 and needs to be dose adjusted in this patient. (D) Tacrine has been replaced by other anticholinesterases because of its significant hepatotoxicity. (E) Tacrolimus is used in the renal transplant patient.

10 **The answer is D: Potassium channel blocker.** Dalfampridine, a potassium channel blocker administered orally, improves walking speeds versus placebo. It is the first drug approved for this use. Currently approved MS drugs are indicated to decrease relapse rates or, in some cases, to prevent accumulation of disability. (A) Nifedipine is an example of a calcium channel blocker. (B) Pyridostigmine is an example of a cholinesterase inhibitor. (C) Anticholinergic agents do not work through enhancement of permeability. (E) Anticholinergic agents do not work through blockade of sodium channels.

11 **The answer is B: Mivacurium.** Mivacurium has a rapid onset of action of about 2 min and requires a maximum of 16 min for patients to recover. Thus, this is a very good agent to use for a short surgical procedure such as prostate needle biopsy, which takes about 10 min to perform. (A) Doxacurium has a slow onset of action (6 min) and requires nearly 90 min for patients to recover. (C) Pancuronium has a rapid onset of action (3 min) and requires nearly 90 min for patients to recover. (D) Rocuronium has a very rapid onset of action (1 min) and requires 45 min for patients to recover. (E) Tubocurarine has a rapid onset of action (2 min) and requires approximately 40 min for patients to recover.

12 **The answer is D: Dry mouth.** Low doses of atropine will produce dry mouth and inhibition of sweating. Higher doses such as those greater than 1 mg will produce cardiac effects. Higher doses can produce tachycardia, delirium, hallucinations, and coma. (A) Bradycardia can result when atropine is given at low doses. (B) Coma can occur when doses of atropine >10 mg are given. (C) Dilation of the pupils occurs when doses of atropine >5 mg are given. (E) Tachycardia can occur when doses of atropine >5 mg are given.

13 **The answer is B: Patient did not follow proper medication directions.** In contrast to atropine, scopolamine produces sedation, but at higher doses, it can produce excitement instead. Scopolamine may produce euphoria and is susceptible to abuse. It turns out that this patient actually inadvertently applied two patches instead of one because of her fear of motion sickness. Furthermore, this agent does not treat motion sickness but prevents it. (A) Alcohol would likely produce sedative effects in this patient. (C) This patient has no evidence of hepatic insufficiency given that she is otherwise healthy. (D) This patient has no evidence of renal insufficiency given that she is otherwise healthy. (E) There is no reason to suspect an underlying urinary tract abnormality in this patient.

14 **The answer is A: Dantrolene.** When halothane is used as an anesthetic, administration of succinylcholine has occasionally caused malignant hyperthermia (with muscular rigidity, metabolic acidosis, tachycardia, and hyperpyrexia) in genetically susceptible people. This is treated by rapidly cooling the patient and by administration of dantrolene, which blocks release of Ca^{2+} from the sarcoplasmic reticulum of muscle cells, thereby reducing heat production and relaxing muscle tone. (B) This patient is hyperthermic and needs rapid cooling. (C) This patient needs to have the succinylcholine infusion stopped immediately. (D) This patient has a genetic condition of malignant hyperthermia from succinylcholine administration, which must be stopped immediately. (E) Although tubocurarine could be given to this patient, he needs immediate treatment with dantrolene to stop the malignant hyperthermic process.

15 **The answer is A: Diaphragm paralysis.** Administration of succinylcholine to a patient who is genetically deficient in plasma cholinesterase or who has an atypical form of the enzyme can lead to prolonged apnea caused by paralysis of the diaphragm. The rapid release of potassium may also contribute to prolonging apnea in patients with electrolyte imbalances who receive this drug. (B) Hyperkalemia is possible in patients who receive succinylcholine. (C) This patient is likely to have normal serum sodium levels. (D) This patient may have hypercalcemia, not hypocalcemia. (E) There is no evidence to suggest digitalis toxicity in this patient.

16 **The answer is A: Preventing acetylcholine release.** Lower motor neurons activate skeletal muscle by releasing acetylcholine stored in synaptic vesicles onto nicotinic cholinergic receptors on muscle cells. Honey may contain *Clostridium botulinum* spores, which can germinate in the GI tract of infants younger than 12 months old. The bacteria produce a toxin that enters synaptic knobs of lower motor neurons and cleaves a protein necessary for vesicle fusion, preventing acetylcholine release. (B) Botulinum toxin does not prevent the synthesis of acetylcholine. (C) Glycine is an inhibitory neurotransmitter in the spinal cord. Tetanus toxin blocks glycine release in the same manner that botulinum toxin blocks acetylcholine release—by cleaving proteins necessary for vesicle fusion. (D) Botulinum toxin does not affect norepinephrine synthesis or release. (E) Botulinum toxin does not affect norepinephrine synthesis or release.

17 **The answer is B: Epinephrine.** The α-adrenoceptors show a weak response to the synthetic agonist isoproterenol, but they are responsive to the naturally occurring catecholamines: epinephrine and norepinephrine. For receptors, the rank order of potency is epinephrine < norepinephrine < isoproterenol. (A) Acetylcholine is a cholinomimetic agent. (C) Isoproterenol is the least potent receptor agonist. (D) Metanephrine is a breakdown product of catecholamines. (E) Norepinephrine has intermediate potency at the α-receptor sites.

18 **The answer is D: Tamsulosin.** Tamsulosin is a selective α_1-antagonist that is used to treat benign prostate hyperplasia. The drug is clinically useful because it targets α_1-receptors found primarily in the urinary tract and prostate gland. (A) Alfuzosin is a nonselective α-blocker, which has increased side effects compared with selective α-blockers. (B) Doxazosin is a nonselective α-blocker that has to be dose titrated for efficacy and thus has a significant side-effect profile. (C) Prazosin is not used in the treatment of benign prostate hyperplasia. (E) Terazosin is a nonselective α-blocker, which has to be dose titrated for efficacy and also has a significant side-effect profile at higher doses.

19 **The answer is C: Mydriasis.** The sympathetic and parasympathetic nervous systems often work simultaneously on the same organ. The net effect on an organ is determined by which branch of the autonomic nervous system is most active at any given time. The sympathetic nervous system's effector neurotransmitter is generally norepinephrine, whereas the parasympathetic nervous system's is acetylcholine. Atropine is a cholinergic antagonist. Exposure to atropine would result in a clinical picture in which the parasympathetic nervous system (PNS) appeared to be missing, leaving control to the sympathetic nervous system (SNS). The PNS would normally push equilibrium toward bronchospasm, lacrimation, meiosis, salivation, and urination. Leaving the SNS in control then would lead to bronchodilation; mydriasis; and decreased lacrimation, salivation, and urination. (A) Bronchospasm is induced by the parasympathetic nervous system. (B) Lacrimation is inhibited by atropine. (D) Salivation is induced by the parasympathetic nervous system. (E) Urination (bladder contraction) is controlled by the parasympathetic nervous system.

20 **The answer is D: Physostigmine.** All of the drugs listed inhibit acetylcholinesterase, but physostigmine best crosses the blood–brain barrier. These drugs increase the effects of endogenous acetylcholine by inhibiting acetylcholinesterase, which increase the half-life of acetylcholine in the synaptic cleft. Physostigmine decreases intraocular pressure by stimulating contraction of the ciliary muscle, which opens the trabecular meshwork, increasing outflow of the aqueous humor. (A) Echothiophate is an acetylcholinesterase inhibitor that can also be used for glaucoma but does not cross the blood–brain barrier. (B) Edrophonium was historically used to diagnose myasthenia gravis. It is very short acting and is not used for glaucoma nor does it cross the blood–brain barrier. (C) Neostigmine is often used after surgeries to hasten recovery from anesthesia. It does not cross the blood–brain barrier. (E) Pyridostigmine is used to treat myasthenia gravis. It does not cross the blood–brain barrier.

21 **The answer is A: Hepatic glycogenolysis.** Epinephrine has a significant hyperglycemic effect because of increased glycogenolysis in the liver, increased release of glucagon, and a decreased release of insulin. These effects are mediated via the cAMP mechanism. (B) This patient will produce very little glucose from gluconeogenesis. (C) Pancreatic failure in this patient is unlikely. Cardiac failure is more likely because of blood loss. (D) There is no reason to suggest pancreatic infarct in this patient. (E) There is no reason to suggest splenic infarct in this patient.

22 **The answer is C: Cerebral hemorrhage.** This patient received epinephrine intravenously, which has some significant adverse effects. Epinephrine can produce adverse CNS effects that include anxiety, fear, tension, headache, and tremor. The drug may induce cerebral hemorrhage as a result of a marked elevation of blood pressure. Epinephrine can trigger cardiac arrhythmias, particularly if the patient is receiving digoxin. Pulmonary edema: Epinephrine can induce pulmonary edema. (A) Epinephrine should stimulate heart rate and blood pressure increase in this patient. (B) Cardiac arrhythmia is likely in patients taking digoxin. This patient is only taking an inhaler for asthma. (D) Pulmonary edema, not pulmonary embolism is likely in this patient. (E) This drug can induce anxiety, fear, tension, headache, and tremor.

23 **The answer is A: Hypersensitivity vasculature response.** Epinephrine may have enhanced cardiovascular actions in patients with hyperthyroidism. If epinephrine is required in such an individual, the dose must be reduced. The mechanism appears to involve increased production of adrenergic receptors on the vasculature of the individual with hyperthyroidism, leading to a hypersensitive response. (B) Goiter formation is uncommon given this presentation. (C) Neoplastic transformation is unlikely to develop because epinephrine is not carcinogenic. (D) Thyroid gland infarct would not be expected given this presentation. (E) There is no indication that this patient is taking excessive amounts of her thyroid medications.

24 **The answer is B: Dobutamine.** Dobutamine increases cardiac output without significantly increasing heart rate, a complicating condition in heart failure. Because epinephrine can significantly increase heart rate, it is not typically used for acute heart failure. Both norepinephrine and phenylephrine have significant one-receptor–stimulating properties. The subsequent increase in blood pressure would worsen the heart. (A) This patient needs intravenous medications, not intranasal medications. (C) This patient needs intravenous medications, not intranasal medications, and this agent would worsen cardiac failure. (D) Norepinephrine would worsen cardiac failure in this patient. (E) Phenylephrine would not serve as an inotropic agent, which is most needed in this patient.

25 **The answer is D: Hypertension.** Phenylephrine is a vasoconstrictor that raises both systolic and diastolic blood pressures. It has no effect on the heart itself but rather induces reflex bradycardia when given parenterally. It is often used topically on the nasal mucous membranes and in ophthalmic solutions for mydriasis. Phenylephrine acts as a nasal decongestant (applied every 4 h) and produces vasoconstriction. The drug is used to raise blood pressure and to terminate episodes of supraventricular tachycardia (rapid heart action arising both from the AV junction and from atria). Large doses can cause hypertensive headache and cardiac irregularities. (A) This agent does not cause constipation. (B) This agent does not cause diarrhea. (C) Epistaxis is unlikely following administration of phenylephrine. (E) Tinnitus is unlikely following administration of phenylephrine.

26 **The answer is C: Development of rebound hypertension.** Clonidine acts centrally to produce inhibition of sympathetic vasomotor centers, decreasing sympathetic outflow to the periphery. The most common side effects of clonidine are lethargy, sedation, constipation, and xerostomia. These effects generally decrease with therapy progression or dose reduction. Abrupt discontinuance must be avoided to prevent rebound hypertension. (A) Portal hypertension can develop as a result of abrupt withdrawal of clonidine. (B) Subclinical diabetes should not develop in this patient. (D) Rebound hypertension, not receptor hypersensitivity, will develop following abrupt withdrawal of clonidine in this patient.

27 **The answer is E: Tamsulosin.** All of these agents decrease peripheral vascular resistance and lower arterial blood pressure by causing the relaxation of both arterial and venous smooth muscle. Tamsulosin has the least effect on blood pressure. These drugs, unlike phenoxybenzamine and phentolamine, cause minimal changes in cardiac output, renal blood flow, and the glomerular filtration rate. (A) Alfuzosin can have an effect in blood pressure in this patient. (B) Doxazosin can have an effect on blood pressure in this patient. (C) Phenoxybenzamine is not a recommended treatment for benign prostatic hyperplasia. (D) Phentolamine is not a recommended treatment for benign prostatic hyperplasia.

28 **The answer is A: Furosemide.** Reduced blood pressure causes a decrease in renal perfusion, resulting in an increase in Na^+ retention and plasma volume. In some cases, this compensatory response tends to elevate the blood pressure. For these patients, blockers are often combined with a diuretic to prevent Na^+ retention. In this case, administration of furosemide is the most appropriate treatment. (B) Intravenous fluid bolus will worsen this patient's peripheral edema. (C) Intravenous fluid bolus will worsen this patient's peripheral edema. (D) Triamterene would worsen the electrolyte abnormalities in this patient. (E) Watchful waiting will worsen the electrolyte abnormalities in this patient.

29 **The answer is A: Acetylcholine.** In addition to an abundance of inhibitory dopaminergic neurons, the neostriatum is also rich in excitatory cholinergic neurons that oppose the action of dopamine. Many of the symptoms of parkinsonism reflect an imbalance between the excitatory cholinergic neurons and the greatly diminished number of inhibitory dopaminergic neurons. (B) Dopaminergic neurons are decreased in patients with Parkinson's disease. (C) Epinephrine neurons are unchanged in patients with Parkinson's disease. (D) Norepinephrine neurons are unchanged in patients with Parkinson's disease. (E) Serotonergic neurons are unchanged in patients with Parkinson's disease.

30 **The answer is E: Retroperitoneal fibrosis.** Serious cardiac problems may develop, particularly in patients with a history of myocardial infarction. In patients with peripheral vascular disease, a worsening of the vasospasm occurs; and in patients with peptic ulcer, there is a worsening of the ulcer. Because bromocriptine

is an ergot derivative, it has the potential to cause pulmonary and retroperitoneal fibrosis. In this patient, the findings of hydronephrosis and renal insufficiency suggest this diagnosis. (A) There is no reason to suggest drug toxicity in this patient. (B) The ultrasound does not suggest renal artery stenosis and it would be uncommon in this patient presentation. (C) Renal artery thrombosis is unlikely given this patient presentation. (D) Renal vein thrombosis is unlikely given this patient presentation.

31 **The answer is A: Amantadine.** Amantadine has several effects on several neurotransmitters implicated in causing parkinsonism, including increasing the release of dopamine, blockading cholinergic receptors, and inhibiting the *N*-methyl-D-aspartate (NMDA) type of glutamate receptors. Current evidence supports an action at NMDA receptors as the primary action at therapeutic concentrations. (B) Bromocriptine is a dopamine receptor agonist used in advanced Parkinson's disease. (C) Pramipexole is a dopamine receptor agonist used in advanced Parkinson's disease. (D) Rotigotine is a dopamine receptor agonist used in the treatment of early Parkinson's disease. (E) Tolcapone is a nitrocatechol derivative that selectively and reversibly inhibit COMT.

32 **The answer is B: Cholinergic transmission.** Common adverse effects of anticholinesterase inhibitors to treat Alzheimer's disease include nausea, diarrhea, vomiting, anorexia, tremors, bradycardia, and muscle cramps, all of which are predicted by the actions of the drugs to enhance cholinergic neurotransmission. (A) Anticholinesterase inhibitors do not affect adrenergic transmission. (C) Purine metabolism is not impaired by anticholinesterase inhibitors. (D) Transaminase enzyme elevation is unlikely in patients taking anticholinesterase inhibitors. (E) There is no evidence to suggest uremia in this case.

33 **The answer is D: Metanephrine.** Three important catecholamines in the body are dopamine, epinephrine, and norepinephrine. Catecholamine synthesis starts with the amino acid tyrosine. Tyrosine is converted to dihydroxyphenylalanine, or L-dopa, by tyrosine hydroxylase. L-dopa is then converted to dopamine by dopa decarboxylase. Dopamine can be metabolized to homovanillic acid by a two-step process involving monoamine oxidase (MAO) and catechol-*O*-methyltransferase (COMT). Dopamine can also be converted to norepinephrine by dopamine β-hydroxylase. Epinephrine is made from norepinephrine by phenylethanolamine N-methyltransferase (PNMT). Both epinephrine and norepinephrine can be converted to dihydroxymandelic acid by MAO, which is then metabolized to vanillylmandelic acid by COMT. Alternatively, COMT can first convert epinephrine to metanephrine and norepinephrine to normetanephrine. Metanephrine and normetanephrine are then converted to vanillylmandelic acid by MAO. (A) Dihydroxyphenylalanine, or L-dopa, is a precursor to, not metabolite of, epinephrine. (B) Dihydroxymandelic acid is a metabolite of both epinephrine and norepinephrine. (C) Homovanillic acid is a metabolite of dopamine, not epinephrine. (E) Vanillylmandelic acid is a metabolite of both epinephrine and norepinephrine.

34 **The answer is C: Reserpine.** Neurotransmitters are synthesized and stored in vesicles at the presynaptic terminal, so they can be quickly released in large amounts when an action potential arrives. After being synthesized in the cytoplasm, norepinephrine, dopamine, and serotonin are transported into storage vesicles by the vesicular monoamine transporter (VMAT). Reserpine inhibits VMAT, impairing the neurons' ability to concentrate and store these neurotransmitters. These monoamine neurotransmitters are degraded by monoamine oxidase (MAO) and catechol-*O*-methyltransferase (COMT) when left in the cytoplasm. (A) Clonidine acts on α_2-adrenergic receptors in the central nervous system. These receptors normally provide negative feedbacks that allow norepinephrine to inhibit further norepinephrine release. (B) Methyldopa is converted into methylnorepinephrine in neurons, which binds preferentially to α_2-receptors. It does not inhibit VMAT. (D) Scopolamine is an anticholinergic, antimuscarinic drug. It does not block VMAT. (E) Tyramine is normally rapidly metabolized by MAO, but in the presence of MAO inhibitors, it can cause excess norepinephrine release. It does not inhibit VMAT.

35 **The answer is B: Fingolimod.** Fingolimod is the first oral drug that can slow the progression of disability and reduce the frequency and severity of symptoms in MS, offering patients an alternative to the currently available injectable therapies. Fingolimod alters lymphocyte migration, resulting in sequestration of lymphocytes in lymph nodes. (A) Dalfampridine, a potassium channel blocker administered orally, improves walking speeds versus placebo. (C) Mitoxantrone is a cytotoxic anthracycline analog, which can kill T cells. (D) Vitamin A therapy has not been shown to slow progression of MS. (E) Vitamin E therapy has not been shown to slow progression of MS.

36 **The answer is A: Dalfampridine.** Dalfampridine, a potassium channel blocker administered orally, improves walking speeds versus placebo. It is the first drug approved for this use. Currently approved MS drugs are indicated to decrease relapse rates or, in some cases, to prevent accumulation of disability. (B) Fingolimod can slow the progression of disability and reduce the frequency and severity of

symptoms in MS. (C) Mitoxantrone is a cytotoxic anthracycline analog, which can kill T cells. (D) Prednisone should be avoided in this patient because of toxicities. (E) Prednisolone should be avoided in this patient and is not a preferred treatment in this clinical scenario.

37 **The answer is E: Riluzole.** Riluzole blocks glutamate, sodium channels, and calcium channels. It may improve the survival time and delay the need for ventilator support in patients suffering from ALS. (A) Memantine is used in the treatment of Alzheimer's disease. (B) Metronidazole is an antibiotic used in the treatment of female pelvic infections. (C) Prednisone will not delay need for ventilator support in this patient. (D) Prednisolone will not delay need for ventilator support in this patient.

38 **The answer is A: A 24-year-old woman with chronic pelvic pain.** Diazepam is a benzodiazepine that works well in patients with chronic anxiety and seizure disorders. It will also work in a patient with spinal cord–related pain caused by an accident. These agents are less effective in patients with chronic pelvic pain, and in such a patient, her pain may not improve with this therapy. (B) This patient is likely to be helped with diazepam for his chronic anxiety. (C) This patient is likely to be helped with diazepam for his seizure disorder. (D) Diazepam is not contraindicated in men or women with seizure disorder and is equally effective. (E) Diazepam will be helpful in a patient with spinal cord–related pain.

39 **The answer is E: Triazolam.** Triazolam is a benzodiazepine that has a relatively short duration of action and, therefore, is used to induce sleep in patients with recurring insomnia. Whereas temazepam is useful for insomnia caused by the inability to stay asleep, triazolam is effective in treating individuals who have difficulty in going to sleep. (A) Clonazepam is useful in treatment of seizures. (B) Diazepam is not recommended in this patient because of its longer duration of action. (C) Flurazepam is a long-acting benzodiazepine and would cause sleep difficulties. (D) Temazepam is useful for insomnia caused by the inability to stay asleep.

40 **The answer is B: Inhibition of COMT.** The symptoms of Parkinson's disease appear to result primarily from insufficient dopamine release from the substantia nigra. Many drugs used to treat Parkinson's disease address this insufficiency. Tolcapone is a catechol-*O*-methyltransferase (COMT) inhibitor. Dopamine is normally metabolized by COMT and monoamine oxidase (MAO). Inhibition of these enzymes potentiates the effects of what little dopamine is released from the substantia nigra. (A) Tolcapone does not increase norepinephrine synthesis. (C) Tolcapone is not a MAO inhibitor. (D) Tolcapone does not stimulate acetylcholine release. (E) Tolcapone does not stimulate norepinephrine release.

41 **The answer is A: Contains a domain that passes through the cell membrane seven times.** The α- and β-adrenergic receptors are members of the G protein–coupled receptor (GPCR) class. These receptors are embedded in the cell membrane by a seven-pass transmembrane domain. They also have an extracellular ligand-binding domain and an intracellular domain that exchanges a GTP for a GDP in the associated G protein, activating the G protein to exert its downstream effects. (B) This describes a receptor tyrosine kinase. Insulin binds to this type of receptor. (C) This describes a GABA receptor. GABA binds allowing influx of chloride and hyperpolarization of the cell. (D) This describes the ryanodine receptor in skeletal muscle. (E) This describes glucocorticoid receptors.

42 **The answer is A: Diazepam.** Diazepam is a long-acting benzodiazepine. Diazepam is useful in the treatment of skeletal muscle spasms, such as muscle strain, and in treating spasticity from degenerative disorders, such as multiple sclerosis and cerebral palsy. Its duration of action can be 1 to 3 days. (B) Lorazepam is an intermediate-acting benzodiazepine. Its duration of action is approximately 10 to 20 h. (C) Oxazepam is a short-acting benzodiazepine. Its duration of action is approximately 3 to 8 h. (D) Temazepam is an intermediate-acting benzodiazepine. Its duration of action is approximately 10 to 20 h. (E) Triazolam is a short-acting benzodiazepine. Its duration of action is approximately 3 to 8 h.

43 **The answer is A: Calming effect during sleep induction.** This patient is likely to experience a calming effect during sleep induction. Not all benzodiazepines are useful as hypnotic agents, although all have sedative or calming effects. They tend to decrease the latency to sleep onset and increase stage 2 of nonrapid eye movement (non-REM) sleep. Both REM sleep and slow-wave sleep are decreased. In the treatment of insomnia, it is important to balance the sedative effect needed at bedtime with the residual sedation ("hangover") upon awakening. (B) This patient is unlikely to experience hourly awakening from sleep. (C) This patient is unlikely to experience a hypnotic effect with dreams. (D) This patient will experience a decrease in slow-wave sleep. (E) This patient will experience an increased stage 2 non-REM sleep.

44 **The answer is C: A 36-year-old man with gastroesophageal reflux disorder.** Benzodiazepines should be used cautiously in treating patients with liver disease. These drugs should be avoided in patients with acute

narrow-angle glaucoma. Alcohol and other CNS depressants enhance the sedative-hypnotic effects of the benzodiazepines. Benzodiazepines are, however, considerably less dangerous than the older anxiolytic and hypnotic drugs. As a result, a drug overdose is seldom lethal unless other central depressants, such as alcohol, are taken concurrently. (A) Benzodiazepines should be avoided in pregnancy. (B) Benzodiazepines should be avoided in patients with alcoholic liver disease and HIV. (D) Benzodiazepines should be avoided in patients with alcoholic liver disease. (E) Benzodiazepines should be avoided in patients with narrow-angle glaucoma.

45 **The answer is B: Diaphoresis.** Myasthenia gravis is characterized by muscle weakness caused by autoantibodies blocking nicotinic acetylcholine receptors on skeletal muscle. Pyridostigmine is an acetylcholinesterase inhibitor, potentiating the effects of acetylcholine released into the neuromuscular junction. This excess acetylcholine can overcome the effects of antibodies blocking some of the receptors. Pyridostigmine will block acetylcholinesterase throughout the body, however, not only at the neuromuscular junction. This can lead to cholinergic symptoms such as diaphoresis, miosis, diarrhea, bradycardia, and urination. (A) Constipation is a common side effect of opioids, but increasing acetylcholine with pyridostigmine use would cause increased GI motility leading to diarrhea. (C) This is an adrenergic side effect. (D) This is an adrenergic side effect. (E) This is an adrenergic side effect.

46 **The answer is B: Buspirone.** Buspirone is the best agent for this patient. The frequency of adverse effects is low, with the most common effects being headaches, dizziness, nervousness, and light-headedness. Sedation and psychomotor and cognitive dysfunction are minimal, and dependence is unlikely. It does not potentiate the CNS depression of alcohol. (A) Alprazolam could have CNS effects and should be avoided in this elderly patient with dementia. (C) Flumazenil is a short-acting agent and is not recommended for use in this elderly patient with dementia. (D) Temazepam could also have CNS effects and is not recommended in this patient. (E) Triazolam is a benzodiazepine and could have CNS effects. It is not recommended in this elderly patient.

47 **The answer is A: Alprazolam.** Alprazolam is a benzodiazepine that is effective in the treatment of panic disorder. The agent is administered orally and has side effects that may involve drowsiness and confusion. (B) Lorazepam is a benzodiazepine that does not require phase I metabolism and has few drug–drug interactions. (C) Temazepam is a benzodiazepine that does not require phase I metabolism and has few drug–drug interactions. (D) Triazolam is a benzodiazepine that causes rebound insomnia on withdrawal. (E) Zolpidem has no anticonvulsant or muscle-relaxing properties.

48 **The answer is A: Anxiety.** The caffeine contained in one to two cups of coffee (100 to 200 mg) causes a decrease in fatigue and increased mental alertness as a result of stimulating the cortex and other areas of the brain. Consumption of 1.5 g of caffeine (12 to 15 cups of coffee) produces anxiety and tremors. The spinal cord is stimulated only by very high doses (2 to 5 g) of caffeine. (B) This patient would experience anxiety and tremors. (C) This patient would not have fatigue but increased mental alertness. (D) This patient would not be expected to have memory loss. (E) This patient would not be expected to have tinnitus.

49 **The answer is D: Tiredness toward midmorning.** Tolerance can rapidly develop to the stimulating properties of caffeine, and withdrawal consists of feelings of fatigue and sedation. This patient has now exhibited signs and symptoms of caffeine withdrawal since his coffee stand has closed. (A) This patient may have poor penmanship because of fatigue. (B) This patient may have a less effective ability to work with and call clients. (C) This patient may have a less effective ability to write letters.

50 **The answer is A: Attention.** Cigarette smoking or administration of low doses of nicotine produces some degree of euphoria and arousal as well as relaxation. It improves attention, learning, problem solving, and reaction time. (B) Cigarette smoking will not improve differentiation of colors. (C) Cigarette smoking will not improve skill in essay writing. (D) Cigarette smoking will not improve tactile sensation. (E) Cigarette smoking will not improve word-finding skills.

51 **The answer is D: 10 g, 100 cups.** The lethal dose is 10 g of caffeine (about 100 cups of coffee), which induces cardiac arrhythmias. Death from caffeine is, therefore, highly unlikely. Lethargy, irritability, and headache occur in drinkers who routinely consumed more than 600 mg of caffeine per day (roughly six cups of coffee per day) and then suddenly stop.

52 **The answer is A: Diarrhea.** This patient would experience a worsening of diarrhea from smoking. Nicotine may also cause intestinal cramps, diarrhea, and increased heart rate and blood pressure. In addition, cigarette smoking increases the rate of metabolism for several drugs. (B) This patient has no evidence of muscle aches or pains. (C) This patient has left lower quadrant pain and this can worsen with smoking. (D) This patient has left lower quadrant pain and this can worsen with smoking. (E) This patient has no evidence of temporomandibular joint dysfunction.

53 **The answer is E: Glaucoma.** Atomoxetine is a nonstimulant drug approved for ADHD in children and adults. This drug should not be taken by individuals on MAO inhibitors and by patients with narrow-angle glaucoma. Unlike methylphenidate, which blocks dopamine reuptake, atomoxetine is a norepinephrine reuptake inhibitor. Therefore, it is not habit forming and is not a controlled substance. (A) Anxiety is not a contraindication to the use of atomoxetine. (B) Bipolar disease is not a contraindication to the use of atomoxetine as long as the patient is not taking an MAO inhibitor. (C) Bleeding disorders are not a contraindication to the use of atomoxetine. (D) Chronic diarrhea is not a contraindication to the use of atomoxetine.

54 **The answer is D: Piloerection.** Activation of the sympathetic nervous system occurs, which causes pupillary dilation, increased blood pressure, piloerection, and increased body temperature. Taken orally, low doses of LSD can induce hallucinations with brilliant colors. Mood alteration also occurs. Tolerance and physical dependence have occurred, but true dependence is rare. (A) Pupillary dilation occurs. (B) Hypertension would be expected in this patient. (C) Hyperthermia would be expected in this patient. (E) Sinus drainage would be unlikely in this patient.

55 **The answer is B: Dopamine.** Long-term treatment with antipsychotics can cause this motor disorder. Patients display involuntary movements, including bilateral and facial jaw movements and "fly-catching" motions of the tongue. A prolonged holiday from antipsychotics may cause the symptoms to diminish or disappear within a few months. However, in many individuals, tardive dyskinesia is irreversible and persists after discontinuation of therapy. Tardive dyskinesia is postulated to result from an increased number of dopamine receptors that are synthesized as a compensatory response to long-term dopamine receptor blockade. (A) Tardive dyskinesia is caused by overload of dopamine receptors. (C) Epinephrine receptors are not a component of the pathophysiology of tardive dyskinesia. (D) Norepinephrine receptors are not involved in tardive dyskinesia. (E) Serotonin receptors are uninvolved in this disease process.

56 **The answer is D: Respiratory depression and arrest.** Morphine causes respiratory depression by reduction of the sensitivity of respiratory center neurons to carbon dioxide. This can occur with ordinary doses of morphine in patients who are opioid-naïve and can be accentuated as the dose is increased until, ultimately, respiration eases. Respiratory depression is the most common cause of death in acute opioid overdoses. (A) Respiratory depression is the most likely cause of death in morphine overdose. (B) Cardiac ischemia is unlikely in a healthy 27-year-old man. (C) Cardiomyopathy is unlikely in a healthy 27-year-old man. (E) A 27-year-old man likely has intact cerebral circulation and would be at low risk for transient ischemic attacks.

57 **The answer is C: Idiopathic.** When no specific anatomic cause for the seizure, such as trauma or neoplasm, is evident, a patient may be diagnosed with idiopathic or cryptogenic (primary) epilepsy. These seizures may result from an inherited abnormality in the central nervous system (CNS). Patients are treated chronically with antiseizure drugs or vagal nerve stimulation. Most cases of epilepsy are idiopathic. (A) This patient has a negative social history suggesting that he does not smoke or drink alcohol. (B) This condition is not physician induced. (D) The CT scan of the head is normal, suggesting that there is no intracranial pathology. (E) This patient has no history of recent trauma.

58 **The answer is E: Tonic-clonic seizures.** Tonic-clonic seizures result in loss of consciousness, followed by tonic (continuous contraction) and clonic (rapid contraction and relaxation) phases. The seizure may be followed by a period of confusion and exhaustion caused by the depletion of glucose and energy stores. (A) Absence seizures involve a brief, abrupt, and self-limiting loss of consciousness. The onset generally occurs in patients at 3 to 5 years of age and lasts until puberty or beyond. (B) Febrile seizures: Young children may develop seizures with illness accompanied by high fever. This tendency may run in siblings. (C) Myoclonic seizures: These seizures consist of short episodes of muscle contractions that may recur for several minutes. They generally occur after wakening and exhibit as brief jerks of the limbs. (D) In status epilepticus, two or more seizures occur without recovery of full consciousness between them.

59 **The answer is E: Race of the patient.** Choice of drug treatment is based on the classification of the seizures, patient-specific variables (e.g., age, comorbid medical conditions, lifestyle, and personal preference), and characteristics of the drug (such as cost and interactions with other medications). Several of the antiseizure drugs may be equally effective. There is no racial predilection for medication selection in this class of medications. The toxicity of the agent and characteristics of the patient are major considerations in drug selection and treatment plan. In newly diagnosed patients, monotherapy is instituted with a single agent until seizures are controlled or toxicity. (A) Comorbid conditions will play a role in medication selection. (B) Medication cost as dictated by insurance coverage of the patient nearly always plays a role on medication selection. (C) Lifestyle of the patient will play a role in medication selection. (D) Personal preference of the patient and physician play a role in medication selection.

60 **The answer is A: Carbamazepine.** Carbamazepine is effective for treatment of partial seizures and, secondarily, generalized tonic-clonic seizures. It is also used to treat trigeminal neuralgia and bipolar disorder. Carbamazepine is absorbed slowly and erratically following oral administration and may vary from generic to generic, resulting in large variations in serum concentrations of the drug. (B) Ethosuximide reduces propagation of abnormal electrical activity in the brain, most likely by inhibiting T-type calcium channels. (C) Felbamate has a broad spectrum of anticonvulsant action. (D) Gabapentin is a GABA analog and can treat chronic neuropathic pain. (E) Lacosamide can treat chronic partial seizures.

61 **The answer is C: Flumazenil.** Diazepam belongs to the class of drugs called benzodiazepines. These drugs bind to GABA receptors in the brain. GABA receptors are ligand-gated ion channels. When GABA binds, chloride is allowed to enter the cell, resulting in hyperpolarization. Although benzodiazepines do not directly stimulate GABA receptors, they increase the frequency of the channel opening to potentiate the effect of endogenous GABA. Overactivation of these receptors leads to an overall depressed state in the brain. Flumazenil competes with benzodiazepines for the same binding site on GABA receptors, but flumazenil does not potentiate the effect of GABA. For this reason, flumazenil is used as an antidote for benzodiazepine overdose. (A) Amphetamine is a CNS stimulant but is not used in benzodiazepine toxicity. It can be prescribed for attention-deficit/hyperactivity disorder and narcolepsy. (B) Epinephrine is an adrenergic agonist. It stimulates the sympathetic nervous system and is used to treat anaphylactic shock. (D) Phenobarbital is a barbiturate. Barbiturates, like benzodiazepines, potentiate the effect of endogenous GABA. However, barbiturates work by increasing the duration of the chloride channel opening, not its frequency. (E) Theophylline is structurally similar to caffeine. It is used to treat and prevent bronchospasm.

62 **The answer is C: Consider discontinuing her medication.** This scenario is extremely worrisome for the possibility of the patient developing tardive dyskinesia as a result of her medication. Neuroleptics are known to potentially cause tardive dyskinesia, which is characterized by involuntary movements of the perioral, ocular, or extremity muscles. The proper treatment is to discontinue or at least decrease the medication. If not addressed, tardive dyskinesia will likely worsen and may become permanent. The risk of worsening her psychosis by decreasing or discontinuing her medication must be weighed against the risk of permanent dyskinesia. (A) Another neuroleptic may appear to help initially by decreasing symptoms but will likely exacerbate the underlying disorder caused by her medication. (B) Although she may be using illicit drugs, this patient's presentation is more worrisome and classic for tardive dyskinesia. (D) Increasing the dose of fluphenazine may appear to help initially by decreasing symptoms but will likely exacerbate the underlying disorder caused by her medication. (E) Unless the medication dose is discontinued or decreased, her tardive dyskinesia will likely worsen and may become permanent.

63 **The answer is A: Carbamazepine.** Carbamazepine is an antiseizure medication metabolized by the CYP1A2 and CYP2C8 receptors. This agent reduces the propagation of abnormal impulses in the brain by blocking sodium channels, thereby inhibiting the generation of repetitive action potentials in the epileptic focus and preventing their spread. (B) Divalproex is metabolized by the CYP2C9 receptor. (C) Felbamate is metabolized by the CYP2C19 receptor. (D) Phenobarbital is metabolized by the CYP2C19 receptor. (E) Phenytoin is metabolized by the CYP2C19 receptor.

64 **The answer is A: Binds to collapsing response mediator protein-2.** Lacosamide binds to collapsing response mediator protein-2 (CRMP-2), a phosphoprotein mainly expressed in the nervous system and involved in neuronal differentiation and control of axonal outgrowth. The role of CRMP-2 binding in seizure control is unknown. Lacosamide is approved for adjunctive treatment of partial seizures. In clinical trials, the drug caused euphoria similar to that produced by alprazolam. (B) Gabapentin is a GABA analog that acts at GABA receptors. (C) Lamotrigine blocks sodium channels and also calcium channels. (D) Lamotrigine blocks sodium channels and also calcium channels. (E) Lamotrigine blocks sodium channels and also calcium channels.

65 **The answer is E: Synaptic vesicle protein.** Levetiracetam is approved for adjunct therapy of partial onset seizures, myoclonic seizures, and primary generalized tonic-clonic seizures in adults and children. The exact mechanism of anticonvulsant action is unknown. It demonstrates high affinity for a synaptic vesicle protein (SV2A). In mice, this was associated with potent antiseizure action. (A) Lamotrigine modulates calcium channels. (B) Lacosamide acts at the collapsing response mediator protein-2. (C) Gabapentin is a GABA analog that acts at GABA receptors. (D) Oxcarbazepine acts at sodium channels.

66 **The answer is D: Gingival overgrowth.** Gingival hyperplasia (overgrowth) may cause the gums to grow over the teeth. Long-term use may lead to development of peripheral neuropathies and osteoporosis. Although phenytoin is the drug used most commonly worldwide for epilepsy because of its low cost per tablet, the cost of therapy may be much higher when the potential for

serious toxicity and adverse effects is weighed. (A) Phenytoin is not associated with an increased risk of dental caries. (B) Phenytoin is not associated with an increased risk of exposed nerve roots. (C) Phenytoin is not associated with jaw bone exposure. (E) Phenytoin is not associated with teeth erosion.

67 **The answer is D: Pregabalin.** Pregabalin is an antiseizure medication that works through voltage-gated calcium channels in the CNS, inhibiting excitatory neurotransmitter release. The exact role it plays in treatment is not known, but the drug has proven effects on partial onset seizures, neuropathic pain associated with diabetic peripheral neuropathy, postherpetic neuralgia, and fibromyalgia. More than 90% of pregabalin is eliminated renally, with no indication of CYP involvement. (A) Carbamazepine is eliminated by the liver and would accumulate in this patient. (B) Phenobarbital undergoes extensive hepatic metabolism and would not be the best choice in this patient with impaired liver function. (C) Phenytoin undergoes metabolism by the cytochrome system of the liver and is not a preferred choice for this patient with impaired liver function.

68 **The answer is C: Inhibition of sodium channels.** This patient presents with tonic-clonic seizures, which generally have an unknown cause. They are characterized by an overall hyperactive state in the brain in which the neurons rapidly depolarize and stimulate neighboring neurons to also depolarize resulting in an overabundance of excitatory action potentials. The depolarization occurs when sodium flows into the cell, raising its resting potential. Chloride channels (whose opening is mediated by GABA) allow chloride ions into the cell to lower its resting potential (hyperpolarization), making it less likely to fire. Similarly, potassium channels allow potassium to flow out of the cell leading to hyperpolarization. Carbamazepine inhibits sodium entry into cells, making them less likely to depolarize and thereby controlling the seizure. (A) Ethosuximide is a seizure medication that blocks calcium channels. It works in the thalamus and is used for absence seizures. (B) Blocking potassium channels would make the cell more likely to depolarize by inhibiting outward flow of positive ions. Potassium channel blockers would not help control a seizure. (D) GABA is the neurotransmitter that binds to chloride channels to hyperpolarize neurons. Benzodiazepines and barbiturates (and ethanol) work by potentiating the effects of GABA on chloride channels. (E) Carbamazepine is not known to affect chloride channels.

69 **The answer is A: Decreased acetylcholine.** Alzheimer's disease is associated with a degeneration of the basal nucleus of Meynert and a decrease in acetylcholine in the brain. The disease is characterized by amyloid plaques and neurofibrillary tangles, although the relationship between these lesions and the progression of the disease is unclear. Some drugs that increase acetylcholine in the brain include donepezil and rivastigmine, both acetylcholinesterase inhibitors. These drugs are used to treat symptoms of Alzheimer's disease but cannot reverse the disease's progression. (B) Decreased dopamine is associated with Parkinson's disease and depression. (C) Norepinephrine is decreased in depression. This is the rationale behind the use of SNRIs. SNRIs increase the amount of norepinephrine (and serotonin) in neural synapses. (D) Patients with Parkinson's disease also exhibit an increase in acetylcholine, prompting the use of benztropine (an acetylcholine antagonist) as one of the treatments of Parkinson's disease. (E) Dopamine is increased in schizophrenia. Antipsychotics such as haloperidol, clozapine, and olanzapine are potent antagonists of dopamine receptors. They work to counterbalance the increased dopamine levels.

70 **The answer is E: Serotonin.** MAO and COMT are both used in the metabolism of dopamine, epinephrine, and norepinephrine. Serotonin, also known as 5-hydroxytryptamine, is a monoamine but is not a catecholamine. It is, therefore, not a substrate for COMT. Oxidation by MAO is the first step in serotonin metabolism. The next step is carried out by aldehyde dehydrogenase and produces 5-hydroxyindoleacetic acid (5-HIAA), which is excreted by the kidneys. (A) Acetylcholine is a substrate for neither MAO nor COMT. It is broken down by acetylcholinesterase found in the synaptic cleft. (B) Epinephrine is a substrate of both MAO and COMT. Each neurotransmitter undergoes metabolism by each enzyme; whether first by MAO or first by COMT, it does not matter. (C) γ-Aminobutyric acid (GABA) is neither a substrate for MAO or COMT. GABA is broken down by GABA transaminase. This enzyme is the target of a medication called vigabatrin used to treat infantile spasms. (D) Norepinephrine is a substrate of both MAO and COMT. Each neurotransmitter undergoes metabolism by each enzyme; whether first by MAO or first by COMT, it does not matter.

71 **The answer is D: Nicotinic cholinergic receptor.** The actions of hormones and neurotransmitters depend on the downstream effects of the receptors they bind, not on the hormone or neurotransmitter itself. Receptors may open ion channels, increase or decrease second messengers such as cAMP, or act as transcription factors to regulate gene expression. The receptors that cause the most rapid cellular response are those that open ion channels. Nicotinic cholinergic receptors are an example of ligand-gated ion channels. (A) α_1-Adrenergic receptors are G_q G protein–coupled

receptors (GPCRs) that increase intracellular calcium and DAG as second messengers. They do not elicit as rapid a response as nicotinic cholinergic receptors. (B) β_1-Adrenergic receptors are G_s GPCRs that increase intracellular cAMP as a second messenger. They do not elicit as rapid a response as nicotinic cholinergic receptors. (C) Glucocorticoid hormone receptors act as transcription factors once their respective ligands bind. Their effects are evident only after RNA has been transcribed and translated and the resulting protein carries out its action. The effect of activating these receptors is much slower than the influx of ions following nicotinic cholinergic receptor activation. (E) Glucocorticoid hormone receptors act as transcription factors once their respective ligands bind.

72 **The answer is E: Antagonist of glycine receptors.** Strychnine works by blocking the glycine receptor in the spinal cord. Glycine is an inhibitory neurotransmitter, and the glycine receptor is a chloride channel. When glycine binds its receptor, chloride ions enter and hyperpolarize the cell. When strychnine blocks glycine receptors, stimulatory signals are unopposed. This leads to a spastic paralysis similar to tetanus (tetanus toxin blocks glycine release). (A) Agonist of α_1-adrenergic receptors would not lead to convulsions. These receptors are found on vascular smooth muscle cells, so an α_1-adrenergic agonist would cause hypertension. (B) Agonist of GABA receptors would have an overall inhibitory effect on the CNS. One of the treatments for strychnine poisoning involves a GABA agonist such as a barbiturate or benzodiazepine. (C) Succinylcholine is an agonist of nicotinic cholinergic receptors at the motor end plate. Although it initially causes fasciculations, succinylcholine's prolonged depolarization of skeletal muscle produces a flaccid paralysis because the muscle cells do not repolarize. (D) Glutamate is a stimulatory neurotransmitter of the CNS. Antagonist of glutamate receptors would have an overall inhibitory effect on the CNS and would not lead to convulsions. Strychnine is not an antagonist of glutamate receptors.

73 **The answer is C: κ-Opioid receptor.** Of the receptors listed, only stimulation of κ-opioid receptors leads to dysphoria. The endogenous opioid dynorphin normally binds κ-receptors. Stimulation of κ-receptors leads to analgesia, hypnosis, dysphoria, and respiratory depression, although κ-receptor stimulation causes less respiratory depression than μ-receptor stimulation. (A) Cannabinoid receptors are G protein–coupled receptors that are inhibitory in nature. Stimulation of cannabinoid receptors in the brain leads to euphoria, not dysphoria. (B) GABA receptors are chloride ion channels that cause hyperpolarization of neural cells. Stimulation of GABA receptors leads to CNS depression. Ethanol, barbiturates, and benzodiazepines stimulate GABA receptors. (D) μ-Opioid receptors share many effects with κ-opioid receptors except that μ-receptor stimulation leads to euphoria rather than dysphoria. Stimulation of either causes analgesia and respiratory depression. (E) Stimulation of serotonin receptors does not cause dysphoria. Many antidepressants rely on the production of excess serotonin stimulation, such as by inhibiting serotonin reuptake from the synapse (SSRIs and SNRIs).

74 **The answer is C: Impotence.** This patient's presentation suggests major depressive disorder. Fluoxetine can be used to treat depression. It is a selective serotonin reuptake inhibitor (SSRI) that improves mood by prolonging the actions of serotonin in the brain. It may take weeks of SSRI use before a patient notices improvements in symptoms, although side effects may appear more rapidly. SSRIs frequently cause sexual side effects, including impotence (erectile dysfunction), decreased libido, and ejaculatory dysfunction in males. (A) Abdominal pain may be caused by many drugs. Abdominal pain has even been reported with fluoxetine use, although this is very rare. Impotence is a more likely side effect. (B) Peptic ulcers may be caused by NSAIDs because these inhibit the formation of protective mucus by blocking prostaglandin synthesis. Peptic ulcers have been reported with fluoxetine use, although rarely. Impotence is a more likely side effect. (D) Loss of taste is an uncommon side effect of fluoxetine use. Sexual side effects such as impotence are more common. (E) Pancreatitis is rarely caused by fluoxetine. Many other drugs can cause pancreatitis, especially nucleotide reverse transcriptase inhibitors such as zalcitabine and zidovudine.

75 **The answer is E: Smoking cessation.** Bupropion is an antidepressant whose mechanism of action is not completely understood. It inhibits neuronal reuptake of dopamine; although at concentrations too low to interfere with dopamine reuptake, it still appears to have an antidepressant effect. Bupropion also inhibits norepinephrine reuptake but not as strongly as tricyclic antidepressants do. This is perhaps related to its ability to cause anxiety. Bupropion is also commonly used to help patients quit smoking. (A) Disulfiram is a drug used to combat alcoholism. Disulfiram inhibits aldehyde dehydrogenase, leading to a buildup of acetaldehyde that causes nausea and headaches if taken with alcohol. (B) Anxiety is a potential side effect of bupropion. Bupropion is not used to treat anxiety. (C) Delirium tremens occurs when a chronic alcoholic abruptly stops taking in alcohol. Inhibitory GABA receptors that were normally stimulated by alcohol experience a sudden drop in activity. This allows normal stimulatory signals to proceed unchecked,

leading to hallucinations and tremors. (D) Opioid overdose can be treated with naloxone or naltrexone. These drugs are similar, but only naltrexone is active orally. They are opioid receptor antagonists.

76 **The answer is B: Delusions.** Schizophrenia often manifests in late adolescence and early adulthood. Symptoms of schizophrenia are classified in two groups: positive and negative. Negative symptoms include a flat affect, lack of motivation, poverty of speech, and decreased attention; these refer to deficits in normal function that are seen in patients with schizophrenia. Positive symptoms include hallucinations and delusions; these are present in patients with schizophrenia but usually not experienced by people without schizophrenia. Antipsychotics such as clozapine have a greater effect on positive symptoms than negative. (A) Attention deficit is a negative symptom of schizophrenia. (C) Flat affect is a negative symptom of schizophrenia. (D) Lack of motivation is a negative symptom of schizophrenia. (E) Poverty of speech is a negative symptom of schizophrenia.

77 **The answer is B: β-Adrenergic receptors.** Chlorpromazine, like other antipsychotics, targets dopamine receptors in the brain. By antagonizing these receptors, chlorpromazine reduces many of the positive symptoms of schizophrenia. Chlorpromazine also antagonizes α-adrenergic receptors (causing sedation and orthostatic hypotension), histamine receptors (also causing sedation), and muscarinic cholinergic receptors (causing blurred vision, urine retention, constipation, dry mouth, and confusion). Of the receptors listed, only β-adrenergic receptors are spared from antagonism by chlorpromazine. (A) Although not chlorpromazine's target, these receptors are all antagonized to some degree by low-potency antipsychotics such as chlorpromazine. (C) Dopamine receptors (specifically D_2 receptors) are the target of antipsychotics such as chlorpromazine. The blockade of D_2 receptors decreases the positive symptoms of schizophrenia. (D) Although not chlorpromazine's target, these receptors are all antagonized to some degree by low-potency antipsychotics such as chlorpromazine. (E) Although not chlorpromazine's target, these receptors are all antagonized to some degree by low-potency antipsychotics such as chlorpromazine.

78 **The answer is A: Anticholinergic effects.** Low-potency antipsychotics cause more anticholinergic, antihistaminic, and antiadrenergic side effects than high-potency antipsychotics. However, high-potency antipsychotics cause more extrapyramidal side effects than low-potency antipsychotics. Extrapyramidal side effects include parkinsonism, perioral tremor, tardive dyskinesia, and torticollis (stiff neck from muscle spasms). If this patient switches to a high-potency antipsychotic, he would likely have less anticholinergic side effects but more extrapyramidal side effects. (B) Parkinsonism refers to symptoms that resemble Parkinson's disease such as akinesia, resting tremor, and rigidity. Parkinsonism can be a manifestation of extrapyramidal antipsychotic side effects, which are more likely with high-potency antipsychotics. (C) Perioral tremor can be a manifestation of extrapyramidal side effects. This effect would likely be worse with a high-potency antipsychotic. (D) Tardive dyskinesia is a late-onset extrapyramidal side effect. It may be irreversible. Tardive dyskinesia is more likely with high-potency antipsychotic therapy. (E) Torticollis is an extrapyramidal side effect. High-potency antipsychotics typically cause more extrapyramidal side effects than low-potency antipsychotics.

79 **The answer is B: Convulsions and hallucinations.** Prazepam is a benzodiazepine, which work by stimulating the inhibitory GABA receptors in the brain. Ethanol also stimulates these receptors. Abrupt discontinuation of a benzodiazepine can mimic delirium tremens following abrupt cessation of alcohol intake in a chronic alcoholic, possibly leading to convulsions and hallucinations. (A) Adrenal insufficiency may follow abrupt cessation of corticosteroid therapy. High levels of corticosteroids suppress ACTH secretion from the anterior pituitary leading to adrenal atrophy. If exogenous corticosteroids are suddenly halted, the adrenal glands are unable to respond with endogenous steroid production rapidly enough. (C) Fever and muscle rigidity occur in neuroleptic malignant syndrome. A similar syndrome may develop following abrupt cessation of levodopa therapy. (D) Myocardial infarction, arrhythmias, and hypertension may result from abrupt discontinuation of β-adrenergic antagonists such as atenolol. (E) Respiratory depression can follow opioid administration, especially in overdose. Abrupt cessation of prazepam would not cause respiratory depression.

80 **The answer is E: Symptomatic relief.** Systematic manifestations of performance anxiety include tremors, tachycardia, and diaphoresis. These end effects are mediated in part by the sympathetic nervous system. The sympathetic nervous system evokes a "fight-or-flight" response by the body. A β-adrenergic receptor blocker such as propranolol treats the symptoms of anxiety by blocking the ability of the sympathetic nervous system to cause the end effects. (A) Propranolol does cross the blood–brain barrier but does not treat anxiety by depressing the CNS. Barbiturates and benzodiazepines are used in this manner. (B) CNS stimulants are not used to treat anxiety. Most can cause anxiety as a side effect. Propranolol is not a CNS stimulant. (C) Comorbid heart disease is not the reason why propranolol is prescribed for anxiety.

Propranolol is used because it blocks the systemic end effects of a panic attack. (D) Propranolol is used to treat anxiety, although its possible side effects must be weighed against its benefits. It should be remembered that propranolol treats only the symptoms of anxiety.

81 **The answer is B: Constipation.** Tolerance means that a greater amount of drug than was previously effective is needed for the same effect. A major problem with opioids is that patients develop tolerance to their analgesic effects so the effective dose must be constantly increased. However, patients do not generally develop opioid tolerance to constipation. Constipation usually persists with a fixed dose even after the other effects have disappeared. (A) A major problem with opioids is the tolerance that develops to their analgesic effect. The same pain relief provided initially will wear off under a constant dose, and more opioid must be given to achieve the same effect. (C) Opioids may cause drowsiness, but this effect will generally wear off after several days. (D) Euphoria is the profound sense of well-being that can accompany opioid use. Tolerance will develop to the euphoria opioids produce. (E) Nausea and vomiting usually occur when an opioid is initially started or when switching to a new opioid. This effect often lasts only a few days before tolerance develops.

82 **The answer is D: Ramelteon.** A hypnotic is a drug that induces sleep. Many sedatives have a hypnotic effect. Their sedation is mediated by binding to GABA receptors. Ramelteon works instead by binding melatonin receptors, mimicking the effects of melatonin. Ramelteon does not appear to lead to dependence as do many GABA modulators. Rebound insomnia does not occur with ramelteon, and it is not a controlled substance. (A) Diazepam is a benzodiazepine. It mimics the neurotransmitter GABA but binds a different site on receptors than GABA. (B) Lorazepam is a benzodiazepine. It mimics the neurotransmitter GABA but binds a different site on receptors than GABA. (C) Phenobarbital is a barbiturate. It mimics the neurotransmitter GABA but binds a different site on receptors than GABA. (E) Zolpidem binds one of the three GABA subunits that benzodiazepines bind. Zolpidem causes a similar sedation to benzodiazepines but has less anxiolytic and muscle-relaxing effects, and it better preserves stages 3 and 4 sleep.

83 **The answer is C: Relieve muscle spasms.** Multiple sclerosis (MS) can manifest in various ways depending on which area of the brain is affected. One such presentation is muscle rigidity and spasms, as in this patient's case. Baclofen has been shown to reduce muscle spasticity in certain conditions, including that associated with MS. Baclofen's exact mechanism is unclear, but it does bind GABA receptors. (A) Baclofen is not anti-inflammatory in nature. Anti-inflammatory drugs include corticosteroids and nonsteroidal anti-inflammatory drugs (NSAIDs). Baclofen may help reduce this patient's muscle pain by inhibiting muscle spasticity, but it does not reduce inflammation. (B) Drugs that raise gastric pH are used to treat heartburn. Many drugs exist for this purpose; some impair block proacid signaling, some block acid production directly, and others are bases that chemically react with gastric acid to neutralize it. Baclofen has none of these properties. (D) Baclofen can be used to treat the muscle spasticity associated with MS, but this is only one possible symptom of the disease. Baclofen will not reverse or even halt the progression of MS. (E) Although it binds GABA receptors, baclofen does not produce sedation. Baclofen is not useful as a sleep aid.

84 **The answer is B: Clonidine.** Tizanidine is an α_2-adrenergic agonist. α_2-Adrenergic receptors are found on neurons. When stimulated, α_2-adrenergic receptors inhibit neurotransmitter release. Tizanidine causes a decreased release of excitatory neurotransmitters from interneurons. Although used for central hypertension rather than muscle spasms, clonidine also stimulates α_2-adrenergic receptors. (A) Amlodipine is a dihydropyridine calcium channel blocker. It impairs contraction of vascular smooth muscle and is used to treat hypertension. (C) Dantrolene blocks calcium release from the sarcoplasmic reticulum, preventing skeletal muscle contraction. It is used to treat malignant hyperthermia. (D) Lorazepam is a benzodiazepine. It causes sedation by stimulating inhibitory GABA receptors in the CNS. (E) Phenobarbital is a barbiturate. It also stimulates inhibitory GABA receptors in the CNS, leading to sedation.

85 **The answer is B: Decreased serum bilirubin.** Phenobarbital is a barbiturate commonly used for sedation induction. It can cause an increase in serum liver enzymes (AST and ALT) and also induces enzymes used in bilirubin conjugation. Phenobarbital can, therefore, cause a decrease in serum bilirubin. It can be used to decrease bilirubin concentrations in certain cases such as neonatal hyperbilirubinemia and chronic cholestasis, although these indications are not FDA-approved for phenobarbital. (A) Phenobarbital may cause an increase, not a decrease, in the liver enzymes AST and ALT. This is an uncommon side effect, especially with short-term doses. (C) Serum amylase will be increased in cases of pancreatitis. Phenobarbital is not known to cause pancreatitis. (D) Phenobarbital induces enzymes involved in bilirubin conjugation. This leads to a decrease, not an increase, in serum bilirubin. (E) Serum CK is elevated in cases of skeletal muscle injury. This may occur during therapy with an HMG-CoA reductase inhibitor

such as lovastatin, but phenobarbital is not known to cause skeletal muscle damage.

86 **The answer is B: Cholinesterase inhibitors.** Because of the evidence of loss of cholinergic neuron activity involved with Alzheimer's disease, cholinesterase inhibitors would allow the patient to have an increased level of acetylcholine and a longer duration of its action. (A) Cholinesterase stimulants would increase the breakdown of acetylcholine. This would result in further reduction the duration and level of the neurotransmitter. (C) Dopamine agonists are associated with the treatment of Parkinson's disease where there are reduced levels of dopamine. (D) Muscarinic receptor inhibitors or antimuscarinic drugs are usually used in the treatment of Parkinson's disease. Studies have shown that they may improve the tremor and rigidity. In a patient with Alzheimer's disease, this treatment would result in further reducing acetylcholine's function. (E) NMDA glutamate receptor agonists would enhance the development of the patient's disease because excitotoxic activation of NMDA glutamate receptors has been linked to the progression of Alzheimer's disease. NMDA glutamate receptor antagonists would be used, not agonists.

87 **The answer is C: Haloperidol.** Haloperidol belongs to the butyrophenone class of antipsychotics. Its mechanism of action is to block dopamine receptors. Under high dosages, the drugs can potentially produce a disorder similar to Parkinson's disease. In addition to haloperidol, reserpine, tetrabenazine, and the phenothiazines are all known to be associated with drug-induced parkinsonism. (A) Aripiprazole is a dihydrocarbostyril. It is a new drug whose toxicities are still unknown. However, it has the advantage of a lower weight gain and longer half-life than most antipsychotics. (B) Clozapine is a dibenzodiazepine. It is known to have little extrapyramidal toxicity, but it can be associated with agranulocytosis in up to 2% of patients and a dose-related lowering of seizure threshold. (D) Olanzapine is a thienobenzodiazepine. It is associated with little to no extrapyramidal system dysfunction; the drug can lead to weight gain and dose-related lowering of seizure threshold. (E) Ziprasidone is a dihydroindolone. It is shown to reduce weight gain but may cause a prolonged QTc.

88 **The answer is A: α_1-Adrenergic.** Catecholamines include epinephrine, norepinephrine, and dopamine. All of these receptors are G protein–coupled receptors (GPCRs), but only α_1-adrenergic receptors cause an increase in the intracellular calcium concentration. Stimulation of this receptor releases the G_q subunit, which in turn activates phospholipase C. Phospholipase C phosphatidylinositol 4,5-bisphosphate (PIP_2) into diacylglycerol (DAG) and inositol triphosphate (IP_3). One of the downstream effects of IP_3 is to bind calcium channels in the smooth endoplasmic reticulum to release stored calcium and raise the intracellular calcium concentration. (B) α_2-Adrenergic receptors involve the G_i subunit. Stimulation of this receptor causes a decrease in intracellular cAMP, not an increase in calcium. (C) β_1-Adrenergic receptors involve the G_s subunit. Stimulation of this receptor causes an increase in intracellular cAMP, not an increase in calcium. (D) β_2-Adrenergic receptors involve the G_s subunit. Stimulation of this receptor causes an increase in intracellular cAMP, not an increase in calcium. (E) D_1 receptors involve the G_s subunit. Stimulation of this receptor causes an increase in intracellular cAMP, not an increase in calcium.

89 **The answer is D: Blockade of M receptors.** Scopolamine is an effective agent for prevention of the symptoms of motion sickness. The antihistamines prevent or diminish vomiting and nausea mediated by both the chemoreceptor and vestibular pathways. The antiemetic action of these medications seems to be caused by their blockade of central H and muscarinic receptors. (A) Scopolamine blocks central H and muscarinic receptors. (B) Scopolamine is not a β_2-receptor blocker. (C) Scopolamine is not an H_2-receptor blocker. (E) Scopolamine inhibits the chemoreceptor and vestibular pathways.

90 **The answer is D: Increases synaptic acetylcholine.** Alzheimer's disease is associated with a degeneration of the basal nucleus of Meynert and a decrease in acetylcholine in the brain. The disease is characterized by amyloid plaques and neurofibrillary tangles, although the relationship between these lesions and the progression of the disease is unclear. Some drugs that increase acetylcholine in the synapses in the brain include donepezil and rivastigmine, both acetylcholinesterase inhibitors. These drugs are used to treat symptoms of Alzheimer's disease but cannot reverse the disease's progression. (A) Donepezil is an acetylcholinesterase inhibitor and so would increase synaptic acetylcholine. Acetylcholine depletion is one of the problems in patients with Alzheimer's disease; decreasing synaptic acetylcholine would make this patient's symptoms worse. (B) Decreased dopamine is associated with Parkinson's disease and depression. Donepezil does not decrease synaptic dopamine nor would this help the symptoms of Alzheimer's disease. (C) Norepinephrine is decreased in depression. This is the rationale behind the use of SNRIs, which increase the amount of norepinephrine (and serotonin) in neural synapses. Donepezil does not decrease synaptic norepinephrine. (E) Dopamine is decreased in Parkinson's disease. Drugs such as levodopa and tolcapone work to increase synaptic dopamine. Donepezil does not affect dopamine levels.

91 **The answer is A: Increase dopamine production.** The symptoms of Parkinson's disease are caused by depletion of dopamine from neurons in the substantia nigra. Many of the medications used to treat Parkinson's disease address this deficiency in various ways. Levodopa is the direct precursor to dopamine biosynthesis. Once in the bloodstream, it crosses the blood–brain barrier and leads to an increased production of dopamine. (B) Donepezil is an acetylcholinesterase inhibitor but is not used in the treatment of Parkinson's disease. Dopamine deficiency, not acetylcholine deficiency, is responsible for the symptoms of Parkinson's disease. (C) Levodopa is a precursor to dopamine synthesis, not an acetylcholine receptor agonist. Bethanechol is an example of an acetylcholine receptor agonist and is not used to treat Parkinson's disease. (D) Bromocriptine is a dopamine-receptor agonist. Levodopa is not a receptor agonist but a precursor to dopamine. (E) Levodopa does not stimulate the release of preformed dopamine. It serves as a precursor to dopamine to increase dopamine synthesis.

92 **The answer is E: Thoracolumbar region of the spinal cord.** The sympathetic nervous system originates from the thoracolumbar cord from T11 to L2. The parasympathetic nervous system originates from the brain and sacral spinal cord. Epinephrine and norepinephrine are typical neurotransmitters of the sympathetic nervous system. (A) Parasympathetic nervous system neurons have a discrete response. (B) Parasympathetic nervous system contains ganglia located near the target organs. (C) Parasympathetic nervous system neurons have a limited distribution. (D) Parasympathetic nervous system contains long preganglionic fibers and short postganglionic fibers.

93 **The answer is C: Recycling of choline.** Choline may be recaptured by a sodium-coupled, high-affinity uptake system that transports the molecule back into the neuron. There, it is acetylated into ACh that is stored until released by a subsequent action potential. (A) Degradation of acetylcholine: The signal at the postjunctional effector site is rapidly terminated because AChE cleaves ACh to choline and acetate in the synaptic cleft. (B) When an action potentially propagated by voltage-sensitive sodium channels arrives at a nerve ending, voltage-sensitive calcium channels on the presynaptic membrane open, causing an increase in the concentration of intracellular calcium. (D) Choline is transported from the extracellular fluid into the cytoplasm of the cholinergic neuron by an energy-dependent carrier system that cotransports sodium. (E) ACh is packaged and stored into presynaptic vesicles by an active transport process coupled to the efflux of protons.

94 **The answer is C: Nicotinic receptors are located in the autonomic ganglia.** Nicotine at low concentration stimulates the receptor and at high concentration blocks the receptor. Nicotinic receptors are located in the CNS, adrenal medulla, autonomic ganglia, and the neuromuscular junction (NMJ). Those at the NMJ are sometimes designated NM and the others, NN. The nicotinic receptors of autonomic ganglia differ from those of the NMJ. For example, ganglionic receptors are selectively blocked by hexamethonium, whereas NMJ receptors are specifically blocked by tubocurarine. (A) Nicotine at low doses stimulates the receptor and at high doses blocks the receptor. (B) Nicotinic receptors are located in the adrenal medulla. (D) Nicotinic receptors located at the neuromuscular junction are known as NM receptors.

95 **The answer is A: Convulsions.** The effects of physostigmine on the CNS may lead to convulsions when high doses are used. Bradycardia and a fall in cardiac output may also occur. Inhibition of AChE at the skeletal NMJ causes the accumulation of ACh and, ultimately, results in paralysis of skeletal muscle. However, these effects are rarely seen with therapeutic doses. (B) Skeletal muscle paralysis may occur as a toxic effect. (C) Thromboembolic disease is not a commonly observed effect of physostigmine toxicity. (D) Sinus bradycardia and a fall on cardiac output can result. (E) Tetralogy of Fallot is a congenital anomaly involving the heart.

96 **The answer is A: Appetite suppression.** Atomoxetine is a selective norepinephrine reuptake inhibitor. The exact mechanism by which inhibiting norepinephrine reuptake helps with the symptoms of ADHD is unclear. It appears to have no abuse potential and so is not a controlled substance, making it an attractive choice for the treatment of ADHD. It is not classified as stimulant but shares their side effect of suppressing the appetite. (B) Diarrhea is not a side effect of atomoxetine use. Atomoxetine is known to potentially cause constipation and xerostomia. (C) Hypersensitivity to atomoxetine could lead to a pruritic rash with use. This is not a common side effect, however. (D) Atomoxetine is not known to cause urinary incontinence. A possible side effect of atomoxetine is actually urinary retention or hesitancy. (E) Many antipsychotics can cause weight gain. Stimulants and atomoxetine, on the other hand, are known to cause appetite suppression and possibly weight loss.

97 **The answer is C: Muscle fasciculations.** Succinylcholine initially produces brief muscle fasciculations and a ganglionic block except at high doses, but it does have weak histamine-releasing action. Administering a small dose of nondepolarizing neuromuscular blocker prior to succinylcholine helps decrease or prevent

the fasciculations, which cause muscle soreness. Normally, the duration of action of succinylcholine is extremely short because this drug is rapidly broken down by plasma pseudocholinesterase. (A) Apnea is produced at higher doses with muscular blockade of the diaphragm. (B) Ganglionic blockade occurs at higher doses of succinylcholine. (D) Succinylcholine does not produce relaxation of vascular smooth muscle. (E) At higher doses of succinylcholine, urinary bladder relaxation will occur.

98 **The answer is A: Atropine.** The patient is exhibiting signs of cholinergic stimulation. Insecticide poisoning is a likely diagnosis. Thus, either intravenous or intramuscular doses of atropine are indicated to antagonize the muscarinic symptoms. (B) Edrophonium is a cholinesterase inhibitor and would exacerbate the problem. (C) Norepinephrine would not be effective in combating the cholinergic stimulation. (D) Physostigmine is a cholinesterase inhibitor and would exacerbate the problem. (E) Trimethaphan, being a ganglionic blocker, would also worsen the condition.

99 **The answer is E: Tyrosine.** Tyrosine will accumulate. Regarding the synthesis of norepinephrine, tyrosine is transported by a Na^+-linked carrier into the axoplasm of the adrenergic neuron, where it is hydroxylated to dihydroxyphenylalanine (dopa) by tyrosine hydroxylase. This is the rate-limiting step in the formation of norepinephrine. Dopa is then decarboxylated by the enzyme dopa decarboxylase (aromatic l-amino acid decarboxylase) to form dopamine in the cytoplasm of the presynaptic neuron. (A) Dopamine is an end product of this pathway and would be in low concentration. (B) L-dopa is a product of the rate-limiting step of this pathway and would be in low concentration. (C) Norepinephrine is an end product of this pathway and would also be in low concentration. (D) Testosterone is synthesized in the adrenal cortex and is not formed from precursor tyrosine.

100 **The answer is D: Metabolism to O-methylated derivatives in the synaptic space.** Removal of norepinephrine: Norepinephrine may (1) diffuse out of the synaptic space and enter the general circulation, (2) be metabolized to O-methylated derivatives by postsynaptic cell membrane–associated catechol-O-methyltransferase (COMT) in the synaptic space, or (3) be recaptured by an uptake system that pumps the norepinephrine back into the neuron. The uptake by the neuronal membrane involves a sodium- or potassium-activated ATPase that can be inhibited by tricyclic antidepressants, such as imipramine, or by cocaine. (A) The ATPase pump is inhibited by cocaine. (B) The ATPase pump is inhibited by imipramine and other tricyclic antidepressants. (C) Norepinephrine diffuses from the synaptic space back into the general circulation. (E) The pump system pumps norepinephrine back into the neuron.

101 **The answer is C: Doxylamine.** Blockade of H_1 receptors in the CNS are thought to be the reason for drowsiness caused by first-generation antihistamines. First-generation antihistamines cross the blood–brain barrier more readily than second-generation antihistamines. Of the options listed, only doxylamine is a first-generation H_1-receptor antagonist. H_1 receptors are found in many cell types, including sensory neurons, CNS neurons, and endothelial cells. Histamine acting on these cells cause itching, wakefulness, and vasodilation, respectively. (A) Amantadine is an old antiviral drug that is largely ineffective now because of resistance. Amantadine is not known for its ability to cause drowsiness. (B) Cimetidine blocks H_2 receptors found on gastric parietal cells. H_2 antagonists can be used to treat GERD by decreasing acid secretion. Blocking H_2 receptors does not ameliorate symptoms of hay fever or cause changes in wakefulness. (D) Famotidine blocks H_2 receptors found on gastric parietal cells. H_2 antagonists can be used to treat GERD by decreasing acid secretion. Blocking H_2 receptors does not ameliorate symptoms of hay fever or cause changes in wakefulness. (E) Fexofenadine is a second-generation H_1-receptor antagonist. It can be used to treat symptoms of hay fever but is not known to cause drowsiness.

102 **The answer is A: Erectile dysfunction.** Guanethidine blocks the release of stored norepinephrine as well as displaces norepinephrine from storage vesicles (thus producing a transient increase in blood pressure). This leads to gradual depletion of norepinephrine in nerve endings except for those in the CNS. Guanethidine commonly causes orthostatic hypotension and interferes with male sexual function. Supersensitivity to norepinephrine caused by depletion of the amine can result in hypertensive crisis in patients with pheochromocytoma. (B) Guanethidine does not cause hepatitis. (C) Guanethidine can cause orthostatic hypotension. (D) Guanethidine can cause hypertensive crisis in patients with pheochromocytoma. (E) Guanethidine is not associated with pulmonary infections.

103 **The answer is A: Increased stimulation of excitatory neurons promoting further neurotransmitter release.** These excitatory postsynaptic potentials (EPSPs) are generated by the following: (1) Stimulation of an excitatory neuron causes the release of neurotransmitter molecules, such as glutamate or acetylcholine, which bind to receptors on the postsynaptic cell membrane. This causes a transient increase in the permeability of sodium (Na^+) ions. (2) The influx of

Na^+ causes a weak depolarization, or EPSP, that moves the postsynaptic potential toward its firing threshold. (3) If the number of stimulated excitatory neurons increases, more excitatory neurotransmitter is released. (B) Stimulation of an excitatory neuron causes neurotransmitter molecule release such as glutamate. (C) Aspartic acid is not released as a consequence of excitatory neuron stimulation. (D) Excitatory postsynaptic potential causes depolarization. (E) Transient increase in sodium permeability will result.

104 **The answer is A: Binding of GABA at the postsynaptic membrane.** Stimulation of inhibitory neurons causes movement of ions that results in a hyperpolarization of the postsynaptic membrane. These inhibitory postsynaptic potentials (IPSP) are generated by the following: (1) Stimulation of inhibitory neurons releases neurotransmitter molecules, such as γ-aminobutyric acid (GABA) or glycine, which bind to receptors on the postsynaptic cell membrane. This causes a transient increase in the permeability of specific ions, such as potassium (K^+) and chloride (Cl^-) ions. (2) The influx of Cl^- and efflux of K^+ cause a weak hyperpolarization, or IPSP, that moves the postsynaptic potential away from its firing threshold. (B) Hyperpolarization results, which moves the postsynaptic potential away from its firing threshold. (C) Stimulation of inhibitory neurons causes release of GABA or glycine. (D) There is a transient increase in permeability of chloride. (E) There is a transient increase in permeability of potassium.

105 **The answer is C: Viral encephalitis.** Parkinsonian symptoms infrequently follow viral encephalitis or multiple small vascular lesions. Drugs such as the phenothiazines and haloperidol, whose major pharmacologic action is blockade of dopamine receptors in the brain, may also produce parkinsonian symptoms. These drugs should not be used in patients with Parkinson's disease. (A) Multiple small vascular lesions can cause secondary parkinsonism. (B) Small vessel cerebral disease can cause secondary parkinsonism. (D) Use of phenothiazines can block dopamine receptors of the brain and cause secondary parkinsonism. (E) Use of haloperidol can cause secondary parkinsonism.

106 **The answer is A: Antagonizing the excitatory effect of cholinergic neurons.** Many of the symptoms of parkinsonism reflect an imbalance between the excitatory cholinergic neurons and the greatly diminished number of inhibitory dopaminergic neurons. Therapy is aimed at restoring dopamine in the basal ganglia and antagonizing the excitatory effect of cholinergic neurons, thus reestablishing the correct dopamine/acetylcholine balance. Because long-term treatment with levodopa is limited by fluctuations in therapeutic responses, strategies to maintain CNS dopamine levels as constant as possible have been devised. (B) Although physical and occupational therapy are helpful in this patient, restoring the dopamine balance is foremost. (C) CNS dopamine concentrations must remain as constant as possible. (D) Dopamine must be restored in the basal ganglia. (E) Dopamine, not epinephrine, must be restored in the basal ganglia.

107 **The answer is E: Salivary gland secretion discoloration.** There are several side effects of levodopa to be concerned about. Peripheral effects: Anorexia, nausea, and vomiting occur because of stimulation of the chemoreceptor trigger zone of the medulla. Tachycardia and ventricular extrasystoles result from dopaminergic action on the heart. Hypotension may also develop. Adrenergic action on the iris causes mydriasis, and, in some individuals, blood dyscrasias and a positive reaction to the Coombs test are seen. Saliva and urine are a brownish color because of the melanin pigment produced from catecholamine oxidation. (A) Levodopa administration can cause tachycardia. (B) Tachycardia and hypotension can result. (C) Anorexia, nausea, and vomiting are possible side effects of levodopa. (D) Adrenergic action of levodopa causes mydriasis, not miosis.

108 **The answer is B: Favorable bioavailability.** Pramipexole has several favorable characteristics for use as a dopamine agonist. It is not extensively metabolized. It has favorable bioavailability. It is renally excreted. The half-life is 8 h. (A) Pramipexole does not undergo extensive metabolism. (C) Pramipexole is excreted by the kidneys. (D) Pramipexole has a half-life of 8 h. (E) Rotigotine is administered as a transdermal patch.

109 **The best answer is C: Reduced rate of loss of cognitive function.** At best, these compounds provide a modest reduction in the rate of loss of cognitive functioning in patients with Alzheimer's disease. Rivastigmine is hydrolyzed by AChE to a carbamylate metabolite and has no interactions with drugs that alter the activity of cytochrome P450–dependent enzymes. The other agents are substrates for cytochrome P450 and have a potential for such interactions. Common adverse effects include nausea, diarrhea, vomiting, anorexia, tremors, bradycardia, and muscle cramps, all of which are predicted by the actions of the drugs to enhance cholinergic neurotransmission. (A) Rivastigmine does not improve long-term memory capability. (B) Rivastigmine does not improve speech and language function. (D) Common adverse effects include nausea, diarrhea, vomiting, mild hand tremors, and bradycardia. Muscle cramps can also occur.

110 **The correct answer is B: Cholinergic.** Acetylcholinesterase inhibitors, such as rivastigmine, increase cholinergic transmission in the CNS and may cause a modest delay in the progression of Alzheimer's disease. (A) Adrenergic stimulation in the patient with Alzheimer's disease does not improve memory or prevent disease progression. (C) Dopaminergic stimulation will not benefit the patient with Alzheimer's disease. (D) GABAergic stimulation is not beneficial for Alzheimer's symptoms. (E) Serotonergic stimulation does not alter disease progression in the patient with Alzheimer's disease.

111 **The answer is A: Anterograde amnesia.** Anterograde amnesia can result from the use of benzodiazepines. The temporary impairment of memory with use of the benzodiazepines is also mediated by the α_1-GABAA receptors. This also impairs a person's ability to learn and form new memories. (B) Diazepam does not cause long-term memory loss. (C) Diazepam does not impair taste ability. (D) Diazepam does not cause loss of prior negative memories. (E) Diazepam does not cause short-term memory loss.

112 **The answer is D: Oxazepam.** Clonazepam is occasionally used in the treatment of certain types of epilepsy, whereas diazepam and lorazepam are the drugs of choice in terminating grand mal epileptic seizures and status epilepticus. Because of cross-tolerance, chlordiazepoxide, clorazepate, diazepam, and oxazepam are useful in the acute treatment of alcohol withdrawal and reducing the risk of withdrawal-related seizures. (A) Alcohol in this setting will not decrease risk of withdrawal and seizures. (B) Clonazepam is used to treat certain types of epilepsy. (C) Lorazepam is used in the treatment of grand mal seizures. (E) Tramadol is a pain reliever.

113 **The answer is B: Flurazepam.** Psychological and physical dependence on benzodiazepines can develop if high doses of the drugs are given over a prolonged period. Abrupt discontinuation of the benzodiazepines results in withdrawal symptoms, including confusion, anxiety, agitation, restlessness, insomnia, tension, and (rarely) seizures. Because of the long half-lives of some benzodiazepines, withdrawal symptoms may occur slowly and last several days after discontinuation of therapy. Benzodiazepines with a short elimination half-life, such as triazolam, induce more abrupt and severe withdrawal reactions than those seen with drugs that are slowly eliminated, such as flurazepam. (A) Diazepam has a relatively short elimination half-life. (C) Temazepam has a relatively short elimination half-life. (D) Triazolam has a relatively short elimination half-life.

114 **The answer is C: Hexamethonium.** Nicotinic cholinergic receptors are ligand-gated positive ion channels. They are so named because they are the receptors that the drug nicotine binds. They are found on muscles at the neuromuscular junction (NM type) and in postganglionic neurons in the autonomic ganglia (NN type). When acetylcholine or nicotine binds the receptor, the channel pore opens and positive sodium ions flow through it. Hexamethonium is an NN-type channel antagonist. (A) Atropine is a muscarinic cholinergic antagonist. It does not antagonize nicotinic cholinergic receptors. (B) Bethanechol is a muscarinic cholinergic agonist. It does not antagonize nicotinic cholinergic receptors. (D) Metoprolol is a β_1-adrenergic antagonist. It does not antagonize nicotinic cholinergic receptors. (E) Phentolamine is an α-adrenergic antagonist. It does not antagonize nicotinic cholinergic receptors.

115 **The correct answer is D: Lorazepam.** The anxiolytic properties of benzodiazepines, such as lorazepam, make them the drugs of choice in treating the anxiety and agitation of cocaine withdrawal. Lorazepam also has hypnotic properties. (A) Cocaine itself could counteract the agitation of withdrawal, but its use would not be proper therapy. (B) Fluoxetine is an antidepressant with no immediate effects on anxiety. (C) Hydroxyzine, an antihistamine, is effective as a hypnotic, and it is sometimes used to deal with anxiety, especially if emesis is a problem. (E) Phenobarbital has hypnotic properties, but its anxiolytic properties are inferior to those of the benzodiazepines.

116 **The answer is B: Ethosuximide.** The boy is having absence seizures. Ethosuximide is the first-line treatment of absence seizures. The mechanism of action of ethosuximide is blocking thalamic calcium channels. (A) Carbamazepine is a treatment option for tonic-clonic seizures. It is not used in the treatment of absence seizures. (C) Lamotrigine is a treatment of option for partial and tonic-clonic seizures. It is not used in the treatment of absence seizures. (D) Phenytoin is a treatment option for partial, tonic-clonic seizures, and status epilepticus. It is not used in the treatment of absence seizures. (E) Valproic acid is used in the treatment of absence seizures; however, it is not the first-line treatment.

117 **The answer is D: Phenytoin.** Phenytoin is used in the treatment of tonic-clonic seizures. Phenytoin has many side effects, like hirsutism, nystagmus, gingival hyperplasia, and megaloblastic anemia. (A) Common side effects of carbamazepine include ataxia and agranulocytosis, not megaloblastic anemia. (B) Common side effects of ethosuximide include GI distress and Stevens–Johnson's syndrome, not megaloblastic anemia. (C) Common side effects of phenobarbital include sedation and ataxia, not megaloblastic anemia. (E) Common side effects of valproic acid include GI distress and hepatotoxicity, not megaloblastic anemia.

118 **The answer is A: Clonidine.** Neurotransmitters are synthesized and stored in vesicles at the presynaptic terminal so they can be quickly released in large amounts when an action potential arrives. After being synthesized in the cytoplasm, norepinephrine is transported into storage vesicles by the vesicular monoamine transporter (VMAT). When released, norepinephrine binds to α_1-adrenergic receptors to stimulate the postsynaptic neuron as well as α_2-adrenergic receptors on the presynaptic neuron as a method of negative feedback to decrease the amount of norepinephrine released. Clonidine stimulates α_2-receptors in the CNS, lowering blood pressure by decreasing norepinephrine release. (B) Metoprolol is a β-adrenergic antagonist. It does not stimulate α_2-receptors. (C) Reserpine inhibits VMAT, preventing the accumulation of norepinephrine in synaptic vesicles. (D) Scopolamine is an anticholinergic, antimuscarinic drug. It does not stimulate α_2-receptors. (E) Tyramine is normally rapidly metabolized by MAO, but in the presence of MAO inhibitors, it can cause excess norepinephrine release. It does not stimulate α_2-receptors.

119 **The answer is C: Inhibition of MAO.** The symptoms of Parkinson's disease appear to result primarily from insufficient dopamine release from the substantia nigra. Many drugs used to treat Parkinson's disease address this insufficiency. Dopamine is normally metabolized by COMT and monoamine oxidase (MAO). Inhibition of these enzymes potentiates the effects of what little dopamine is released from the substantia nigra. Selegiline is a MAO inhibitor. (A) Selegiline does not increase norepinephrine synthesis. Selegiline works by inhibiting MAO to slow norepinephrine breakdown. (B) Selegiline is not a COMT inhibitor. Tolcapone, another drug used in Parkinson's disease, does inhibit COMT. (D) Selegiline does not stimulate acetylcholine release. Selegiline works by inhibiting MAO to slow norepinephrine breakdown. (E) Selegiline does not stimulate norepinephrine release. Selegiline works by inhibiting MAO to slow norepinephrine breakdown.

120 **The answer is A: CNS depression.** Toxic blood levels of the drug may be caused by repeated injections or could result from a single inadvertent IV injection. Aspiration before every injection is paramount to safety. The signs, symptoms, and timing of local anesthetic systemic toxicity are unpredictable. The most important step in treating local anesthetic toxicity is to consider the diagnosis in any patient with altered mental status or cardiovascular instability following injection of local anesthetic. CNS symptoms (either excitation or depression of the CNS) may be apparent but may also be subtle, nonspecific, or absent. (B) Muscle spasticity is less common than CNS or cardiovascular symptoms. (C) Muscle tetany is uncommon following lidocaine infiltration into a vessel. (D) Peripheral neurapraxia is an uncommon finding following lidocaine infiltration. (E) Swallowing disorder would not be expected in this patient.

121 **The answer is D: Two weeks of therapy are required for mood improvement.** Antidepressants, including SSRIs, typically take at least 2 weeks to produce significant improvement in mood, and maximum benefit may require up to 12 weeks or more. However, none of the antidepressants are uniformly effective. Approximately 40% of patients with depression treated with adequate doses for 4 to 8 weeks do not respond to the antidepressant agent. Patients who do not respond to one antidepressant may respond to another, and approximately 80% or more will respond to at least one antidepressant drug. (A) Maximum benefit may require up to 12 weeks or more. (B) Most patients respond to a single antidepressant drug. (C) Twenty percent of patients with depression treated with adequate doses for 4 to 8 weeks do not respond to the antidepressant agent.

122 **The answer is B: Mood elevation is likely.** The TCAs elevate mood, improve mental alertness, increase physical activity, and reduce morbid preoccupation in 50% to 70% of individuals with major depression. The onset of the mood elevation is slow, requiring 2 weeks or longer. These drugs do not commonly produce CNS stimulation or mood elevation in normal individuals. Physical and psychological dependence has been rarely reported; however, this necessitates slow withdrawal to minimize discontinuation syndromes and cholinergic rebound effects. These drugs, like all of the antidepressants, can be used for prolonged treatment of depression. (A) Mental alertness occurs with treatment of depression. (C) Morbid preoccupation will improve with treatment of depression. (D) Physical dependence is unlikely with tricyclic antidepressants. (E) Psychological dependence is unlikely with tricyclic antidepressants.

123 **The answer is A: Benztropine.** Benztropine is an anticholinergic that is used to treat the tremor and rigidity of Parkinson's disease by decreasing acetylcholine and decreasing the imbalance between acetylcholine and dopamine. Benztropine has no effect on the bradykinesia of Parkinson's disease. (B) Bromocriptine is a dopamine agonist used in the treatment of Parkinson's disease. It is not an anticholinergic. (C) Ipratropium is an anticholinergic that is used for asthma and COPD. It is not used for Parkinson's disease. (D) Scopolamine is an anticholinergic that is used for motion sickness, not for Parkinson's disease. (E) Tropicamide is an anticholinergic that is used to cause mydriasis. It is not used for Parkinson's disease.

124 The answer is B: Pharmacologic effect. Benzodiazepines can induce a temporary form of anterograde amnesia in which the patient retains memory of past events, but new information is not transferred into long-term memory. Therefore, important treatment information should be repeated to the patient after the effects of the drug have worn off. (A) There is no evidence to suggest that this patient has depression. (C) This patient by history has never has this problem before taking diazepam. (D) This patient has no evidence of a psychiatric disorder. (E) There is no evidence to suggest that this patient is taking a supratherapeutic dose of diazepam.

125 The answer is A: Duloxetine. Duloxetine is a serotonin/norepinephrine reuptake inhibitor that can be used for depression accompanied by neuropathic pain. Selective serotonin reuptake inhibitors (fluoxetine and sertraline), monoamine oxidase inhibitors (phenelzine), and atypical antidepressants (mirtazapine) have little activity against neuropathic pain. (B) Fluoxetine will treat depression but not neuropathic pain. (C) Mirtazapine will treat depression but not neuropathic pain. (D) Sertraline will only treat the depression in this patient. (E) This patient needs treatment so watchful waiting is not appropriate.

126 The answer is A: Amitriptyline. Because of its potent antimuscarinic activity, amitriptyline should not be given to patients with glaucoma because of the risk of acute increases in ocular pressure. (B) Bupropion is a good choice for this patient because it lacks significant anticholinergic activity. (C) Fluvoxamine is a realistic choice for this patient with glaucoma and depression. (D) Mirtazapine is a good choice for this patient with glaucoma and depression. (E) Sertraline is an SSRI that would be a good choice for this patient.

127 The answer is A: Anorexia. Bupropion is indicated in the treatment of depression and seasonal affective disorder. This agent is not recommended for patients younger than the age of 18 years. Contraindications include seizure disorders, anorexia, and bulimia. (B) Depression is an indication for bupropion. (C) Seasonal affective disorder is an indication for bupropion. (D) Seasonal affective disorder with mania may be improved with bupropion. (E) Transient ischemic attacks are not a contraindication for use of bupropion.

128 The answer is B: Clomipramine. This patient has obsessive-compulsive disorder. Clomipramine is a tricyclic antidepressant that is also used in the treatment of obsessive-compulsive disorder. It is used as a second-line treatment when selective serotonin reuptake inhibitors fail. (A) Amitriptyline is a tricyclic antidepressant that is used for major depression but not for obsessive-compulsive disorder. (C) Lithium is used for the treatment of bipolar disorder but not for obsessive-compulsive disorder. (D) Quetiapine is an atypical antipsychotic used for the treatment of schizophrenia but not for obsessive-compulsive disorder. (E) Venlafaxine is a serotonin and norepinephrine reuptake inhibitor used in the treatment of depression and generalized anxiety disorder but not for obsessive-compulsive disorder.

129 The answer is A: Blocks acetylcholine degradation. Myasthenia gravis is characterized by muscle weakness caused by autoantibodies blocking nicotinic acetylcholine receptors on skeletal muscle. Pyridostigmine is an acetylcholinesterase inhibitor, potentiating the effects of acetylcholine released into the neuromuscular junction. This excess acetylcholine can overcome the effects of antibodies blocking some of the receptors. (B) Selegiline and entacapone both block enzymes that break down dopamine and are useful in treating Parkinson's disease. Pyridostigmine does not inhibit dopamine breakdown and would not be useful to treat myasthenia gravis. (C) Stimulating acetylcholine release in theory may help treat the symptoms of myasthenia gravis, but this is not the mechanism of action of pyridostigmine. Pyridostigmine increases acetylcholine in the synapse by blocking its breakdown. (D) Bethanechol and pilocarpine are drugs that work by stimulating muscarinic receptors. Pyridostigmine does not directly stimulate muscarinic receptors. It inhibits acetylcholine breakdown. (E) Nicotine is a drug that stimulates the aptly named nicotinic receptors. Pyridostigmine does not directly stimulate cholinergic receptors, it prevents acetylcholine breakdown.

130 The answer is A: Bupropion. Bupropion is an antidepressant that is also used for smoking cessation. The mechanism of action is an increase in norepinephrine and dopamine. It is also used for those who do not want the sexual side effects of other antidepressants. (B) Clomipramine is a tricyclic antidepressant that can also be used for obsessive-compulsive disorder but not smoking cessation. (C) Imipramine is a tricyclic antidepressant that can also be used for bedwetting but not smoking cessation. (D) Mirtazapine is an atypical antidepressant. It could be used to treat his depression but does not aid in smoking cessation. (E) Sertraline is a selective serotonin reuptake inhibitor. It could be used to treat his depression but does not aid in smoking cessation.

131 The answer is C: Dopamine D_2-receptor blockers. The first-generation antipsychotic drugs (also called conventional, typical, or traditional antipsychotics) are competitive inhibitors at various receptors, but their antipsychotic effects reflect competitive blocking of D_2 receptors. First-generation antipsychotics are more likely to be associated with movement disorders, particularly for drugs that bind tightly to dopaminergic neuroreceptors, such as haloperidol, and less true of medications that bind weakly, such as chlorpromazine. No one drug is clinically more effective than another is. (A) First-generation antipsychotic agents are competitive inhibitors at various receptors. (B) These agents are called conventional, typical, or traditional antipsychotic agents. (D) These agents are highly appropriate for patients with movement disorders.

132 **The answer is B: Have fewer extrapyramidal symptoms than first-generation agents.** The second-generation antipsychotic drugs (also referred to as "atypical" antipsychotics) have fewer extrapyramidal symptoms (EPS) than the first-generation agents but are associated with a higher risk of metabolic side effects, such as diabetes, hypercholesterolemia, and weight gain. The second-generation drugs appear to owe their unique activity to blockade of both serotonin and dopamine (and, perhaps, other) receptors. (A) The second-generation antipsychotic agents are referred to as the atypical antipsychotic agents. (C) These agents have a high rate of development of diabetes mellitus. (D) These agents can cause hypercholesterolemia. (E) These agents can cause significant weight gain.

133 **The answer is A: Agranulocytosis.** Approximately 20% of patients with schizophrenia will have an insufficient response to all first- and second-generation antipsychotics. For these patients, clozapine has shown to be an effective antipsychotic with minimal risk of EPS. However, its clinical use is limited to refractory patients because of serious side effects. Clozapine can produce bone marrow suppression, seizures, and cardiovascular side effects. The risk of severe agranulocytosis necessitates frequent monitoring of white blood cell counts. (B) Clozapine is not associated with increased incidence of cholelithiasis. (C) Clozapine does not typically cause pancreatitis. (D) Clozapine is not associated with development of pituitary tumors. (E) Polycythemia is not a typical side effect of clozapine.

134 **The answer is C: Quetiapine.** Risperidone blocks 5-HT_{2A} receptors to a greater extent than it does D_2 receptors, as does olanzapine. The second-generation antipsychotic aripiprazole is a partial agonist at D_2 and 5-HT_{1A} receptors as well as a blocker of 5-HT_{2A} receptors. Quetiapine blocks D_2 receptors more potently than 5-HT_{2A} receptors but is relatively weak at blocking either receptor, and its low risk for EPS may also be related to the relatively short period of time it binds to the dopamine receptor. (A) Clozapine has high affinity for D_1, D_4, 5-HT_2, muscarinic, and adrenergic receptors, but it is also a weak dopamine D_2-receptor antagonist. (B) Olanzapine has high affinity for D_1, D_4, and serotonin receptors. (D) Risperidone blocks 5-HT_{2A} receptors to a greater extent than it does D_2 receptors. (E) Tramadol is an analgesic and does not work on D_2 receptors.

135 **The answer is A: Benztropine.** The patient is experiencing extrapyramidal symptoms because of pimozide, and a muscarinic antagonist such as benztropine would be effective in reducing the symptoms. The other drugs would have no effect or, in the case of prochlorperazine, might increase the symptoms. (B) Bromocriptine will not change symptoms. (C) Lithium will not change symptoms. (D) Prochlorperazine can increase these body spasms experienced by the patient. (E) Risperidone will not change symptoms.

136 **The answer is C: Lipophilic causing accumulation in tissues.** Methadone is readily absorbed following oral administration. The drug is biotransformed in the liver and is excreted almost exclusively in feces. It is important to understand the pharmacokinetics of methadone when using this medication because of multiple variables associated with it. Methadone is very lipophilic, leading to accumulation in the fat tissues. The slow release from these fat tissues causes the half-life to range from 12 to 40 h and has been reported to extend up to 150 h. The actual duration of analgesia ranges from 4 to 8 h. Upon repetitive dosing, methadone levels can accumulate caused by this long terminal half-life, thereby leading to toxicity. The metabolism is variable because it relies on multiple cytochrome P450 (CYP450) enzymes of equivalent doses of *heroin*, *buprenorphine*, and *methadone*. (A) This agent is best absorbed following oral administration. (B) Methadone is biotransformed in the liver and excreted in feces. (D) Methadone is metabolized by multiple cytochromes in the liver. (E) Methadone has a long half-life of up to 40 h.

137 **The answer is C: A 34-year-old man with renal insufficiency and moderate back pain.** Tapentadol is a centrally acting analgesic that binds the μ-opioid receptor and a norepinephrine reuptake inhibitor that is believed to create an additive effect to the opioid actions. It has been used to manage moderate to severe pain, both chronic and acute. Limited drug–drug interactions have been seen with tapentadol because of the pharmacokinetic profile. Tapentadol does not appear to inhibit or induce the CYP450 enzyme system because it is mainly metabolized by glucuronidation. Because tapentadol does not produce active metabolites, dosing adjustment is not necessary in mild to moderate renal impairment. (A) This patient has significant liver disease and would not be the best candidate for this treatment. (B) This patient has significant hepatitis and should not receive this medication. (D) This patient may experience only a limited therapeutic response to this medication.

138 **The answer is B: Complex partial.** The patient is experiencing episodes of complex partial seizures. Complex partial seizures impair consciousness and can occur in all age groups. Typically, staring is accompanied by impaired consciousness and recall. If you asked a question, the patient might respond with an inappropriate or unintelligible answer. Automatic movements are associated with most complex partial seizures and involve the mouth and face (lip smacking, chewing, tasting, and swallowing movements), upper extremities (fumbling, picking, tapping, or clasping movements), and vocal apparatus (grunts or repetition of words and phrases), as are complex acts (such as walking or mixing foods in a bowl). Subtle lateralizing signs (such as an asymmetric smile) may be present. (A) Absence seizures involve a brief, abrupt, and self-limiting loss of consciousness. (C) Myoclonic seizures consist of short episodes of muscle contractions that may recur for several minutes. (D) Simple partial seizures are caused by a group of hyperactive neurons exhibiting abnormal electrical activity, which are confined to a single locus in the brain. (E) Tonic-clonic seizures result in loss of consciousness, followed by tonic (continuous contraction) and clonic (rapid contraction and relaxation) phases.

139 **The answer is E: Unknown.** Vagal nerve stimulation (VNS) requires surgical implant of a small pulse generator with a battery and a lead wire for stimulus. The device is implanted and its lead wires wrapped around the patient's vagal nerve. This treatment was approved in 1997. The device is also approved for treatment of depression. The mechanism of action is unknown. Because it has diffuse involvement with neuronal circuits, there are various mechanisms by which it may exert its effect on seizure control. VNS has been effective in treatment of partial onset seizures and has enabled reduction of drug therapy in some cases. (A) Vagal nerve stimulation is a surgically implanted device with an unknown mechanism of action. (B) The mechanism of action of vagal nerve stimulation is unknown. (C) Vagal nerve stimulation does not involve depolarization of neuronal circuits. (D) Vagal nerve stimulation does not involve stimulation of seizure foci.

140 **The answer is A: Bupropion.** Bupropion is an antidepressant used to treat seasonal affective disorder (SAD) and used for smoking cessation. It is not chemically related to other known antidepressants. Although the mechanisms of action of bupropion for SAD and smoking cessation are not understood, it is known to inhibit dopamine reuptake. Interestingly, its antidepressant effect is seen even at doses too small to inhibit dopamine reuptake. (B) Duloxetine inhibits serotonin and norepinephrine reuptake. It is not indicated for SAD or for smoking cessation. (C) Imipramine is a tricyclic antidepressant. It can also be used in some cases of enuresis. It is not indicated for SAD or for smoking cessation. (D) Sertraline is a selective serotonin reuptake inhibitor. It is not indicated for SAD or for smoking cessation. (E) Although many antidepressants have been reported to cause priapism, trazodone is perhaps the antidepressant best known for it. It is not indicated for SAD or for smoking cessation.

141 **The answer is D: Suicidal tendencies.** Librium is a benzodiazepine antianxiety medication. There are several important warnings to be aware of. This agent can cause suicidal tendencies. Depression is possible as is psychosis and epilepsy. (A) Depression is more common than anxiety in patients taking Librium. (B) Grand mal seizures are unlikely to be seen in patients taking Librium. (C) Depression without mania can occur in patients taking Librium. (E) Tinnitus is unlikely in patients taking Librium.

142 **The answer is C: Neuroleptic malignant syndrome.** Paroxetine is useful in the treatment of panic disorder and social anxiety disorder. This medication has several important interactions. In this patient who is going to undergo surgery, the development of neuroleptic malignant syndrome is possible, and thus, this patient should discontinue this medication prior to surgery. (A) Dizziness is a possible adverse effect of paroxetine but should not change surgical considerations. (B) Insomnia is a common adverse event but will not change the surgical treatment plan for this patient. (D) Nervousness will not change the surgical treatment plan for this patient. (E) Tachycardia would be more likely to occur in this patient as compared to bradycardia.

143 **The answer is A: Asthenia.** Ziprasidone is a serotonin and dopamine antagonist used in the management of bipolar disorder. It can be used alone or in combination with lithium. Important side effects to be aware of include asthenia. (B) This agent can cause priapism in rare cases. (C) This agent can cause hypotension rather than hypertension. (D) Tachycardia is more likely to occur with ziprasidone than bradycardia. (E) This agent is associated with visual changes such as worsening of vision.

144 **The correct answer is A: Decrease in end-diastolic volume.** Administration of digitalis glycosides increases the force of cardiac contraction, causing the cardiac output to more closely resemble that of the normal heart. Increased myocardial contraction leads to a decrease in end-diastolic volume, thus increasing the efficiency of contraction (increased ejection fraction). The resulting improved circulation leads to reduced sympathetic activity, which then reduces peripheral resistance. Together, these effects cause a reduction in heart rate. Vagal tone is also enhanced, so the heart rate decreases and myocardial oxygen demand diminishes. (B) Myocardial contraction will increase in the presence of digitalis. (C) Myocardial circulation will increase in the presence of digitalis. (D) Vagal tone is enhanced. (E) Sympathetic activity is decreased, which reduced peripheral resistance.

145 **The answer is D: Potentiation of GABA receptors.** This patient presents with tonic-clonic seizures, which generally have an unknown cause. They are characterized by an overall hyperactive state in the brain in which the neurons rapidly depolarize and stimulate neighboring neurons to also depolarize resulting in an overabundance of excitatory action potentials. The depolarization occurs when sodium flows into the cell, raising its resting potential. Chloride channels (whose opening is mediated by GABA) allow chloride ions into the cell to lower its resting potential (hyperpolarization), making it less likely to fire. Similarly, potassium channels allow potassium to flow out of the cell leading to hyperpolarization. Benzodiazepines such as diazepam work by potentiating the effects of GABA on chloride channels leading to hyperpolarization and decreased rate of firing. (A) Ethosuximide is a seizure medication that blocks calcium channels. It works in the thalamus and is used for absence seizures. (B) Blocking potassium channels would make the cell more likely to depolarize by inhibiting outward flow of positive ions. Potassium channel blockers would not help control a seizure. (C) Carbamazepine is a drug that inhibits sodium entry into cells, making them less likely to depolarize and thereby controlling the seizure. Diazepam does not affect sodium channels. (E) Glutamate is an excitatory neurotransmitter. Potentiating the effects of glutamate would lead to hyperactivity, not seizure control.

146 **The answer is C: Physostigmine.** Atropine is an antimuscarinic, anticholinergic agent. Muscarinic receptors are found on the pupillary constrictor muscle, on gastrointestinal cells, on the sinoatrial (SA) node of the heart, and on many exocrine glands. The parasympathetic nervous system stimulates these receptors by releasing acetylcholine. Normally, acetylcholine release onto muscarinic receptors causes bradycardia, increased bronchial secretions, increased salivation, miosis, and increased gastric acid secretion. Atropine blocks these receptors leading to tachycardia, decreased bronchial secretions, decreased salivation, mydriasis, and decreased gastric acid secretion. Physostigmine inhibits acetylcholinesterase to increase acetylcholine in the synaptic cleft and could be used as an antidote for atropine poisoning. (A) Dopamine is often used for its vasopressive properties. It would not counteract the effects of atropine. (B) Epinephrine is a vasoconstrictor and bronchodilator. It would not counteract the effects of atropine. (D) Pralidoxime can be used in organophosphate poisoning to regenerate deactivated acetylcholinesterase. It would not counteract the effects of atropine. (E) Scopolamine is another antimuscarinic, anticholinergic drug. It would work with atropine and exacerbate this patient's symptoms.

147 **The answer is D: Small diameter myelinated.** The smaller the diameter of the nerve fiber, the faster it is affected by lidocaine. Myelinated nerves are blocked faster than unmyelinated. The diameter is the most important factor because small unmyelinated fibers will be affected before large myelinated fibers. (A) Small diameter nerve fibers are blocked before larger nerve fibers. (B) Small diameter nerve fibers are blocked before larger nerve fibers. (C) Small diameter nerve fibers are blocked before larger nerve fibers. (E) Myelinated nerve fibers are blocked before unmyelinated nerve fibers.

148 **The answer is A: Clonazepam.** Clonazepam is a long-acting benzodiazepine and therefore has the least addictive potential. It is commonly used to treat anxiety. In patients with a history of addiction, all short acting benzodiazepines should be avoided because of their higher addictive potential. (B) Alprazolam is short acting and therefore has higher addictive potential than clonazepam. (C) Lorazepam is intermediate acting and therefore would have a higher addictive potential than clonazepam. (D) Oxazepam is short acting and therefore has higher addictive potential than clonazepam. (E) Triazolam is short acting and therefore has higher addictive potential than clonazepam.

149 **The answer is E: NMDA receptor antagonist.** Memantine is an NMDA receptor antagonist used in the treatment of Alzheimer's disease. By antagonizing NMDA receptors, this inhibits the influx of calcium into neurons preventing the overexcitability thought to be found in neurons. (A) In Alzheimer's disease, acetylcholine levels are thought to be decreased, so inhibiting the acetylcholine receptor would not be appropriate treatment. (B) Donepezil is an acetylcholinesterase inhibitor used to treat Alzheimer's disease. (C) Amantadine increases the release of dopamine when used for the treatment of Parkinson's disease. (D) Memantine antagonizes the NMDA receptor, not agonize the receptor.

150 **The answer is D: Selegiline.** Selegiline is a selective inhibitor of MAO_B, which metabolizes dopamine. Dopamine is decreased in Parkinson's disease. Inhibiting MAO_B increases the amount of available dopamine. (A) Amantadine is an antiviral that is used in Parkinson's disease because it increases the release

of dopamine. (B) Benztropine is anticholinergic. In Parkinson's disease, cholinergic activity is increased. (C) Carbidopa is a dopa decarboxylase inhibitor that increases the amount of L-dopa. (E) Tolcapone is a COMT inhibitor that decreases the metabolism of L-dopa.

151 **The answer is C: Mirtazapine.** Mirtazapine is an atypical antidepressant that increases the release of norepinephrine and serotonin by α_2 antagonism. It is rarely used because of the side effects of increased appetite and weight gain. However, in the case of anorexia, this is beneficial for the patient. (A) Bupropion is an atypical antidepressant that is also used in smoking cessation. (B) Maprotiline is an atypical antidepressant used for depression, but it does not increase appetite and would not be beneficial in a patient with anorexia. (D) Trazodone is an atypical antidepressant that is also used for insomnia. (E) Venlafaxine is a serotonin and norepinephrine reuptake inhibitor that is used for anxiety, but it does not lead to increased appetite like mirtazapine.

152 **The answer is A: Blocks muscarinic cholinergic receptors.** This patient's presentation and history are consistent with overactive bladder (OAB). OAB is caused by detrusor hyperactivity and is often accompanied by urgency (a sudden onset feeling of the need to urinate) as in this patient's case. Urge incontinence (as in this case) is distinct from stress incontinence in which a decrease urethral tone allows sudden increases in intra-abdominal pressure (such as a cough, sneeze, or laugh) to force urine out of the bladder. Darifenacin can help in urge incontinence by blocking muscarinic cholinergic receptors on the bladder to decrease contraction signals from the autonomic nervous system. (B) Nicotinic cholinergic receptors are found on skeletal muscle cells and in autonomic ganglia but not on the bladder. Darifenacin blocks muscarinic, not nicotinic, receptors. (C) Some surgical procedures can artificially increase urethral tone, but darifenacin does not. It works by blocking muscarinic receptors on the bladder to decrease detrusor tone. (D) In males with BPH, an α-antagonist such as prazosin may help relax the prostatic smooth muscle and make voiding easier. This mechanism of action would not serve this patient nor does darifenacin work in this manner. (E) Inhibiting β-adrenergic receptors does not decrease bladder activity. Darifenacin blocks muscarinic cholinergic, not β-adrenergic receptors.

153 **The answer is D: Phenelzine.** Phenelzine is a monoamine oxidase inhibitor used in the treatment of depression. However, it is rarely used because of the risk of hypertensive crisis, which this patient has, after consuming tyramine-containing foods. Wine and aged cheeses are known for containing tyramine. (A) Amitriptyline is a tricyclic antidepressant that can cause anticholinergic side effects but not hypertensive crisis after consuming tyramine. (B) Duloxetine is a serotonin and norepinephrine reuptake inhibitor that can cause increased blood pressure, not hypertensive crisis, after consuming tyramine. (C) Fluoxetine is a selective serotonin reuptake inhibitor can cause serotonin syndrome when used with monoamine oxidase inhibitors but not hypertensive crisis after consuming tyramine. (E) Trazodone is an atypical antidepressant that can cause priapism, not hypertensive crisis, after consuming tyramine.

154 **The answer is A: Atropine is represented by letter B.** Atropine is a muscarinic blocker and will cause mydriasis. This dilation of the pupil facilitates ophthalmologic examination. (B) Pilocarpine is represented by letter A. This agent will cause contraction of the pupil. (C) Mydriasis would facilitate ophthalmologic examination. (D) The untreated eye has a narrow pupil which would not allow for complete examination of the fundus.

155 **The answer is A: Coma.** At a dose of atropine of >10 mg, hallucinations, delirium, and coma will result. This is represented by letter A in the diagram. (B) At an atropine dose of 5 mg, rapid heart rate, dry mouth, and pupil dilation will occur. This is represented by letter B in the diagram. (C) At an atropine dose of 0.5 mg, bradycardia and slight drying of the mouth occur. (D) Inhibition of sweating occurs at a dose of 0.5 mg of atropine. This is letter C of the diagram.

156 **The answer is D: Letter D.** Letter D represents the binding to the receptor. The postsynaptic receptor is activated by the binding of neurotransmitter. (A) Letter A represents the synthesis of norepinephrine. (B) Letter B represents the uptake of norepinephrine into storage vesicles. (C) Letter C represents the release of neurotransmitter via exocytosis. (E) Letter E represents the removal of norepinephrine through reuptake into the neuron.

157 **The answer is D: Letter D.** Duloxetine inhibits serotonin and norepinephrine reuptake at all doses. It is extensively metabolized in the liver to numerous metabolites. It acts at letter D in the diagram. (A) Letter A represents the presynaptic neuron. (B) Letter B represents the synaptic vesicle. (C) Letter C represents the postsynaptic area.

158 **The answer is D: Letter D.** Neuroleptics inhibit dopamine reuptake at all doses. It is extensively metabolized in the liver to numerous metabolites. It acts as letter D in the diagram. (A) Letter A represents the presynaptic neuron. (B) Letter B represents the synaptic vesicle. (C) Letter C represents the postsynaptic area.

159 **The answer is A: Carbamazepine.** There are many drugs used to control or limit seizure activity. Carbamazepine is a drug that may cause blurred vision and diplopia with use. Of the drugs listed, carbamazepine is the most likely culprit behind this patient's symptoms. Carbamazepine induces its own metabolism, so dosage adjustments early in therapy may be necessary. It is also used to treat trigeminal neuralgia. (B) Ethosuximide is one of the safer antiepileptic drugs. It is often used to treat absence seizures. It does not usually cause visual disturbances. (C) Lorazepam is a benzodiazepine that blocks seizure activity by lowering the seizure threshold. Its most common side effect is sedation and does not usually cause visual disturbances. (D) Phenobarbital is a barbiturate that blocks seizure activity by lowering the seizure threshold. Its most common side effect is sedation and does not usually cause visual disturbances. (E) Valproic acid blocks sodium channels to prevent the spread of seizure activity. Its most common side effect is gastrointestinal upset and does not usually cause visual disturbances.

Chapter 3

Cardiovascular Pharmacology

QUESTIONS

Select the single best answer.

1 A 61-year-old man with Parkinson's disease on bromocriptine dies suddenly of a cardiopulmonary arrest. Autopsy is performed at the request of the family. Sectioning of the lungs in this patient is most likely to reveal which of the following findings?

(A) Adenocarcinoma
(B) Pneumonia
(C) Pulmonary embolus
(D) Pulmonary fibrosis
(E) Squamous cell carcinoma

2 A medical student is doing a summer research project that involves administering β_2-receptor agonists to rats to determine the physiologic changes. Which of the following would be expected following steady state intravenous dosing of agent X, a β_2-receptor agonist?

(A) Bronchoconstriction
(B) Hyperglycemia
(C) Hypertension
(D) Uterine spasm
(E) Vasoconstriction

3 A 58-year-old woman who is obese presents to the emergency department with diaphoresis and crushing chest pain that radiates to her left arm. The physician orders an ECG and checks her cardiac enzymes to confirm his suspicion of myocardial infarction. Because of the quick response and intervention, she survives and is ultimately discharged with a prescription for low-dose daily aspirin to inhibit platelet aggregation. Two weeks after discharge, she takes ibuprofen for a tension headache. What is the effect of the ibuprofen on her anticoagulation regimen?

(A) Excessive antiplatelet activity because of a synergistic action between aspirin and ibuprofen on platelets
(B) Excessive antiplatelet activity because of ibuprofen's effects on endothelial cells combined with aspirin's effects on platelets
(C) Insufficient antiplatelet activity because ibuprofen induces liver cytochrome P450 metabolism of aspirin
(D) Insufficient antiplatelet activity because of inadequate platelet cyclooxygenase inhibition
(E) No change

4 The rationale behind the use of dopamine as a treatment of shock in a 38-year-old man who was a driver in a motor vehicle accident who was thrown from the vehicle is

(A) Impermeability to the blood–brain barrier
(B) Long duration of action
(C) Oral administration
(D) Potentiates hypotension
(E) Slow onset of action

5 A 28-year-old woman who is 24 weeks pregnant with her first child is admitted to the hospital for monitoring and intravenous fluid hydration. Which of the following agents prevents the development of preterm labor?

(A) Albuterol
(B) Isoproterenol
(C) Metaproterenol
(D) Metoprolol
(E) Terbutaline

6 Five patients with small pheochromocytomas are being prepared for surgical resection. All patients have tumors less than 3 cm in size and are confined to the adrenal gland. Phentolamine will be given to each patient. Which of the following patients would be most likely to suffer an adverse event related to this medication?

(A) A 33-year-old woman with hypertension
(B) A 41-year-old man with hypertension and kidney stones
(C) A 45-year-old man with hyperparathyroid adenoma and testicular cysts
(D) A 51-year-old man with angina who suffered a heart attack 2 years ago
(E) A 60-year-old woman with hypertension, kidney stones, and a left renal cyst

7 A 78-year-old man with Alzheimer's disease and hypertension is given oral propranolol to treat his hypertension because of a pharmacy clerical error. The patient has been taking the medication for 3 weeks and now presents to his primary care physician for follow-up. Which of the following effects would be most worrisome?
(A) Auditory hallucinations
(B) Excessive somnolence
(C) Muscular rigidity
(D) Short-term memory loss
(E) Urinary incontinence

8 A 63-year-old man with hypertension is currently taking carvedilol. He returns to his primary care physician for follow-up. His blood pressure is 130/70 mm Hg at this office visit. His cardiac, pulmonary, and abdominal examinations are within normal limits. Additional beneficial effects of this medication may be which of the following?
(A) Hypoglycemia
(B) Hyperglycemia
(C) Improved vascular wall thickening
(D) Increased lipid peroxidation
(E) Vasoconstriction

9 A 59-year-old black man with uncontrolled hypertension is brought to the urgent care center for evaluation. His blood pressure is 190/100 mm Hg. He currently takes no medications. Physical examination of the heart, lungs, and abdomen are noncontributory. Which of the following agents will have limited efficacy in the management of this patient?
(A) Labetalol
(B) Methyldopa
(C) Pindolol
(D) Triamterene
(E) Verapamil

10 A 47-year-old man with a 9-cm right adrenal tumor is going to undergo a laparoscopic surgical procedure to remove the tumor. It is anticipated that the procedure will take approximately 16 h. The patient has a history of hypertension controlled with a β-blocker. Which of the following agents, used intraoperatively, will provide efficacious blood pressure control for the duration of the procedure?
(A) Acebutolol
(B) Esmolol
(C) Metoprolol
(D) Nadolol
(E) Pindolol

11 A 78-year-old black male with hypertension is currently well controlled in terms of his blood pressure. He is presently taking an agent that blocks the Mg^{2+}/ATP-dependent transport of biogenic amines from the cytoplasm into storage vesicles in the adrenergic nerves. Which of the following medications is this patient most likely taking?
(A) Atenolol
(B) Esmolol
(C) Guanethidine
(D) Reserpine
(E) Timolol

12 A 43-year-old man with depression who has been in and out of the psychiatric unit because of noncompliance with medications decides to take intranasal cocaine on a regular basis. He notes that he feels better and thinks that this helps his depression. Through which of the following mediators does this effect likely occur?
(A) Dopamine
(B) Epinephrine
(C) Glutamine
(D) Norepinephrine

13 A 24-year-old man with myopia decides to undergo LASIK surgery to correct his vision. Prior to the procedure, the ophthalmologist dilates his pupils with phenylephrine, a sympathomimetic. Which of the following describes an effect of the sympathetic nervous system?
(A) Contraction of the detrusor muscle
(B) Decreasing heart rate
(C) Stimulating vascular smooth muscle in arterioles supplying the stomach
(D) Stimulating vascular smooth muscle in arterioles supplying the quadriceps femoris
(E) Stimulating bronchiolar smooth muscle

14 A 56-year-old man presents to his primary care physician complaining of difficulty urinating. Digital rectal exam reveals an enlarged prostate. The patient is started on a trial of terazosin, after which his symptoms improve dramatically. Which of the following describes terazosin's drug class?

(A) α_1-Adrenergic antagonist
(B) α_2-Adrenergic antagonist
(C) Anticholinergic
(D) β_2-Adrenergic agonist
(E) β_2-Adrenergic antagonist

15 A 64-year-old man is brought to the emergency department complaining of crushing chest pain radiating to his left arm. He is admitted, stabilized, and treated for an acute myocardial infarction. Later, he developed ventricular tachycardia and is treated with an antiarrhythmic. After a week of antiarrhythmic treatment, he began having difficulty breathing. A chest X-ray reveals pulmonary fibrosis. Which antiarrhythmic was he taking?

(A) Amiodarone
(B) Digoxin
(C) Lidocaine
(D) Procainamide
(E) Verapamil

16 A 58-year-old man undergoes open-heart surgery for a triple coronary artery bypass graft. His surgery goes smoothly, but the next day he develops chest palpitations. Metoprolol is started to keep his supraventricular tachycardia from interfering with ventricular rhythm. Under which Singh–Vaughan Williams class of antiarrhythmics does metoprolol fall?

(A) Class Ia
(B) Class Ib
(C) Class Ic
(D) Class II
(E) Class III
(F) Class IV

17 A 27-year-old woman presents to the emergency department complaining of right flank pain and hematuria. She has passed calcium oxalate stones in the past and likely has another stone. After treating her for the stone, which of the following diuretics could be started to prevent future calcium oxalate stones?

(A) Acetazolamide
(B) Furosemide
(C) Hydrochlorothiazide
(D) Mannitol
(E) Spironolactone

18 A 54-year-old man is mowing his lawn when his chest begins to hurt. The pain does not bother him too much, so he finishes his job and lies down to rest. The pain stops, so he disregards the episode entirely until the next day when he experiences a "funny feeling in his chest" and goes to the doctor at his wife's request. An ECG reveals atrial flutter, for which the doctor prescribes sotalol. The intended effect of sotalol involves modifying which phase of the cardiac myocyte action potential?

(A) Phase 0
(B) Phase 1
(C) Phase 2
(D) Phase 3
(E) Phase 4

19 A 35-year-old man presents to the emergency department complaining of a cough and runny nose of 1-week duration. While being evaluated, it is discovered that his blood pressure is 230/120 mm Hg. An antihypertensive is immediately administered. Later, he develops lactic acidosis, headache, vertigo, and confusion. Which antihypertensive was given to him?

(A) Enalapril
(B) Labetalol
(C) Losartan
(D) Nifedipine
(E) Nitroprusside

20 A 54-year-old woman with severe essential hypertension refractory to treatment switched to a new antihypertensive drug 1 month ago. Her blood pressure is currently well controlled. She now comes complaining of excessive hair growth. Which antihypertensive drug is she taking?

(A) Hydrochlorothiazide
(B) Isosorbide dinitrate
(C) Minoxidil
(D) Nifedipine
(E) Nitroglycerin

21 A 32-year-old woman experiences chest pain at rest. She reports having similar episodes in the past. It is determined that she is experiencing Prinzmetal angina or coronary artery vasospasm. She is given a prescription for nifedipine to relax her vascular smooth musculature. Which best describes a step on nifedipine's mechanism of action?

(A) Activation of adenylate cyclase
(B) Activation of guanylate cyclase
(C) Increasing NO
(D) Inhibition of cGMP phosphodiesterase
(E) Preventing calmodulin's activity

22 A 67-year-old man is hospitalized recovering from a left wall myocardial infarction. He begins to show signs of fluid retention. His doctors want to start a drug regimen for congestive heart failure, including either an ACE inhibitor or an angiotensin receptor blocker (ARB). ACE inhibitors and ARBs treat hypertension in a similar fashion and have similar side effects. Which of the following is a side effect of ACE inhibitors only?

(A) Dizziness
(B) Dry cough
(C) Erectile dysfunction
(D) Hypotension
(E) Tinnitus

23 A 42-year-old man is undergoing an office-based dental procedure using nitrous oxide as the anesthetic agent. His oxygen saturation is being monitored during the procedure by pulse oximetry. Which of the following physiologic effects of nitric oxide will be noted?

(A) Airway resistance increases apically
(B) Bronchodilation
(C) Hypotension
(D) Redirection of blood flow to the heart
(E) Spontaneous minute ventilation increases

24 Five trauma patients are undergoing surgery after being ejected from a bus that had rolled over off the side of the road. Each of the patients needs surgery for internal injuries. Which of the following patients will require the largest doses of inhalational anesthetic agents?

(A) Patient 1: blood pressure of 160/90 mm Hg, pulse = 120 beats/minute
(B) Patient 2: blood pressure of 150/80 mm Hg, pulse = 100 beats/minute
(C) Patient 3: blood pressure of 120/80 mm Hg, pulse = 120 beats/minute
(D) Patient 4: blood pressure of 100/60 mm Hg, pulse = 80 beats/minute
(E) Patient 5: blood pressure of 80/40 mm Hg, pulse = 60 beats/minute

25 A 45-year-old man with a family history of hyperlipidemia and heart disease presents to the emergency department diaphoretic with chest pain radiating to his left arm. An ECG shows ST segment elevation in leads II, III, and aVF. The doctor administers alteplase intravenously. Which of the following markers would you expect to be elevated in this patient's blood as a direct result of alteplase?

(A) AST
(B) CK-MB
(C) D-dimer
(D) Myoglobin
(E) Troponin I

26 A 62-year-old man has developed worsening hypertension despite therapy. His physician wants to prescribe an additional medication that will dilate his blood vessels to help lower his blood pressure. Which of the following is a calcium channel blocker that works primarily on vascular smooth muscle?

(A) Amlodipine
(B) Diltiazem
(C) Losartan
(D) Nitroprusside
(E) Verapamil

27 A 57-year-old man with hypertension presents to his primary care physician for a follow-up checkup. For the past two visits, his blood pressure has been 152/88 mm Hg and 150/86 mm Hg. Today, his blood pressure is 150/88 mm Hg. His past medical history is significant for a heart attack 2 years ago. His physician prescribes metoprolol. Which of the following parameters is most likely to change because of his metoprolol therapy?

(A) Blood calcium
(B) Blood potassium
(C) Blood lipids
(D) Creatinine clearance
(E) White blood cell count

28 A 60-year-old woman suffers an anterior wall myocardial infarction. She recovers well initially but soon develops left heart failure. Her physician prescribes multiple medications to treat different aspects of heart failure, including isosorbide dinitrate. What is the mechanism of action of this agent?

(A) Blocks the activity of angiotensin II at its receptor
(B) Causes excess fluid elimination
(C) Increases cardiac inotropy
(D) Inhibits production of angiotensin II
(E) Reduces preload

29 A 23-year-old baseball player has a normal heart rate and cardiac echocardiogram, suggesting normal cardiac contractility. This may be, in part, because of satisfactory intracellular concentrations of calcium within the heart. Which of the following sources of intracellular calcium plays the most minor role in cardiac contractility?

(A) Exchange with sodium
(B) Intracellular transport via voltage-sensitive channels
(C) Intracellular vacuolar release of calcium
(D) Mitochondria release of calcium
(E) Sarcoplasmic reticulum release of calcium

30 A 72-year-old man is having an electrocardiogram performed by his primary care physician to further evaluate intermittent chest pain. Regarding the phase 0 of the cardiac action potential, which of the following statements is true?
(A) Calcium channels open resulting in outward current
(B) Potassium channels rapidly open and close
(C) Sodium current can be blocked by quinidine in this phase
(D) Transient outward current develops
(E) This is called the rapid phase of repolarization

31 A 67-year-old chronic smoker with COPD and chronic heart failure presents to his primary care physician for follow-up. The patient takes multiple medications for these problems. Which of the following strategies may prove to have additional benefit in the treatment of this patient?
(A) Exercise program involving alternating running and walking on a daily basis
(B) Increase in dietary intake of sodium to 2,000 mg/d
(C) Stopping use of nonsteroidal anti-inflammatory agents
(D) Use of β-blockers at high doses
(E) Use of calcium channel blockers at high doses

32 A 67-year-old woman who is a chronic smoker with chronic congestive heart failure presents to her primary care physician for follow-up. She is currently taking captopril and hydrochlorothiazide. Which of the following changes would be expected as a result of this therapy?
(A) Increase in blood pressure
(B) Increase in exercise tolerance
(C) Increase in vascular resistance
(D) Increase in venous tone
(E) Increase in venous distension of the jugular vein

33 A 57-year-old man with congestive heart failure and hypertension presents to his primary care physician for follow-up. His current medications include digoxin and a calcium channel blocker. Serum electrolytes and a complete blood count are drawn. Which of the following blood indicators is most important to follow in this patient?
(A) Bicarbonate
(B) Chloride
(C) Glucose
(D) Potassium
(E) Sodium

34 A 62-year-old man with congestive heart failure and hypertension on digoxin takes an extra few pills because he is angry about his daughter being pregnant out of wedlock. He is found unconscious and brought to the emergency department for evaluation. If electrocardiogram is performed, which of the following would be most likely?
(A) Acute myocardial infarction
(B) Atrial conduction arrhythmia
(C) Pulmonary embolism
(D) Ventricular septal defect
(E) Ventricular tachycardia

35 A 67-year-old woman with a history of cardiac arrhythmias presents to her primary care physician for follow-up. Her current medications include amiodarone. She complains of a 4-week history of diarrhea, sweats, and muscle weakness. Her skin is normal. Which of the following is the most likely explanation for these findings?
(A) Hepatitis
(B) Hypertrophic cardiomyopathy
(C) Iatrogenic hyperthyroidism
(D) Iodine accumulation
(E) Systemic lupus-like syndrome

36 A 64-year-old man is discharged from the intensive care unit to home after suffering a myocardial infarction. He has a history of atrial arrhythmias. Which of the following agents would be best for this patient to prevent recurrence of arrhythmia and decrease his risk of mortality?
(A) Imipramine
(B) Mexiletine
(C) Procainamide
(D) Propafenone
(E) Sotalol

37 A 58-year-old male with diabetes comes to the clinic complaining of difficulty achieving an erection. He has a history of cardiovascular disease. The physician recommends sildenafil. What is the mechanism of action of this agent?
(A) Increasing intracellular cAMP
(B) Parasympathetic stimulation
(C) Sympathetic stimulation
(D) Vasodilation
(E) Vasoconstriction

38 A 67-year-old man is in the operating room undergoing a hip replacement. The procedure is going along uneventfully, and there is no indication of acute blood loss. Suddenly, the patient develops supraventricular tachycardia. Intravenous adenosine is administered and within 15 s, the electrocardiogram shows normal sinus rhythm. What is the most likely explanation for this normalization of the electrocardiogram?
(A) Development of hypotension
(B) Improved automaticity in the AV node
(C) Increase in conduction velocity
(D) Shortening of the refractory period
(E) The arrhythmia normalized spontaneously

39 A 74-year-old man presents to the emergency department complaining of chest pain that has increased in frequency, duration, and intensity. He also has shortness of breath. He is given nitroglycerin in the emergency department and still has chest pain. What is the most likely diagnosis?
(A) Classic angina
(B) Gastroesophageal reflux
(C) Prinzmetal angina
(D) Unstable angina

40 A 73-year-old woman with known angina has an attack of mild chest pressure and spasm while shopping at the mall. She takes a sublingual nitroglycerin tablet and within a few minutes has improvement in her symptoms. Which of the following is the most likely explanation of action of this agent?
(A) Decreased myocardial perfusion
(B) Decreased preventricular contractions
(C) Decreased myocardial oxygen consumption
(D) Increasing pulmonary arterial blood flow
(E) Venoconstriction

41 A 62-year-old man with a history of myocardial infarction and angina has a prescription for sublingual nitroglycerine but has not taken it. He now complains of erectile dysfunction and is given a prescription for sildenafil 50 mg. He is warned by his physician not to take sildenafil and nitroglycerine because of which of the following possible reactions?
(A) Hypotension
(B) Myocardial infarction
(C) Retinitis pigmentosa
(D) Tinnitus
(E) Vertigo

42 A 58-year-old African American man with hypertension managed with nifedipine presents to his primary care physician for follow-up. His blood pressure is 136/84 mm Hg. Physical examination of the heart, lungs, and abdomen are within normal limits. The most likely effects of this medication to cause blood pressure reduction likely involve
(A) Arterial vasoconstriction
(B) Decrease in smooth muscle vascular tone
(C) Increase in myocardial oxygen consumption
(D) Pronounced improvement in afterload
(E) Synchronized automaticity of the cardiac cycle

43 A 75-year-old man with a history of intermittent angina presents to his primary physician. The anginal attacks are becoming more frequent, and therapy is considered for this reason. His blood pressure is 160/95 mm Hg. Which of the following agents would be least likely to be administered as a first-line agent for this patient?
(A) Diltiazem
(B) Nifedipine
(C) Nitroglycerine
(D) Ranolazine
(E) Verapamil

44 A 56-year-old man with a known history of hypertension treated with a β-blocker presents to his primary care physician for follow-up. His blood pressure usually runs 130/76 mm Hg and today (at 6-month follow-up) is 170/90 mm Hg. What is the most likely explanation for this finding?
(A) Development of cardiac arrhythmia
(B) Development of diabetes mellitus
(C) Lack of patient compliance
(D) Progression of hypertension
(E) Recent stroke

45 A 73-year-old man with a history of coronary disease and angina pectoris is taking aspirin and dipyridamole. The most likely mechanism of action of this agent involves which of the following?
(A) Increased levels of cAMP
(B) Increased levels of cGMP
(C) Increased levels of cGTP
(D) Increased levels of prostacyclin
(E) Increased levels of thrombin

46 A 63-year-old man presents to the emergency department with worsening heart failure following a myocardial infarction 2 weeks previously. The patient complains of shortness of breath. Physical exam reveals +2 pitting edema in his ankles. Past medical history is significant for an allergic reaction following exposure to trimethoprim–sulfamethoxazole. The physician wants to prescribe furosemide as part of this patient's regimen. Which drug should she prescribe him?

(A) Acetazolamide
(B) Ethacrynic acid
(C) Hydrochlorothiazide
(D) Mannitol
(E) The best drug to use in this case is furosemide

47 A 51-year-old man recently started treatment for an arrhythmia. He now presents with what appears to be a sunburn on his face, although he insists he has spent very little time in the sun. Which of the following drugs is he most likely taking?

(A) Amiodarone
(B) Lidocaine
(C) Procainamide
(D) Timolol
(E) Verapamil

48 A 54-year-old man with a history of visual problems presents to the ambulatory surgery center for an outpatient eye surgery. The anesthesiologist gives droperidol for sedation during the procedure. This agent is associated with which of the following risks?

(A) Prolongation of QT interval
(B) Sedation
(C) T wave flattening
(D) T wave inversion
(E) Widening of the QRS interval

49 A 47-year-old man is recovering from a heart attack. He takes a daily baby aspirin to prevent further attacks. He also takes phenelzine for refractory panic disorder. Which of the following characteristics do aspirin and phenelzine share?

(A) Antiplatelet activity
(B) Irreversible inhibition
(C) Inhibit the same enzyme
(D) Should not be taken with tyramine-containing foods
(E) Side effect of hypertension

50 A 41-year-old man who has travelled the world has malaria. He is treated with chloroquine. During follow-up evaluation by the primary care physician, which of the following tests should be ordered?

(A) Echocardiogram
(B) Electrocardiogram
(C) Serum calcium
(D) Serum potassium
(E) Troponin

51 A 28-year-old G3P2 female gives birth to a full-term 7-lb, 6-oz male baby. The neonate's 5-min Apgar score is 8. Physical exam is normal except for a continuous, machine-like murmur on cardiac exam. Which of the following may be necessary for this patient?

(A) Acetaminophen
(B) Dinoprostone
(C) Dopamine
(D) Indomethacin
(E) Propranolol

52 A 64-year-old woman reports to the clinic for her scheduled appointment. She was diagnosed 7 months ago with congestive heart failure. However, the patient refuses to make diet and lifestyle adjustments. She complains her feet are still unable to fit correctly in shoes and her medication has not helped the swelling in her legs and ankles. The doctor decides to increase her level of diuretics after also noting the edematous appearance of her hands. What complication should the doctor be most aware of for this patient?

(A) Diuretic-induced metabolic acidosis
(B) Hepatic encephalopathy
(C) Hypercalcemia
(D) Hyperkalemia
(E) Hypokalemia

53 A 61-year-old man with hypertension develops atrial fibrillation. His medications include simvastatin and metoprolol. His physician prescribes an anticoagulant for clot prophylaxis, which directly inhibits thrombin. Which drug is this?

(A) Aspirin
(B) Dabigatran
(C) Heparin
(D) Ticlopidine
(E) Warfarin

54 A 58-year-old man presents to the emergency department (ED) after experiencing a sudden loss of motor control on his left side accompanied by aphasia. By the time he reached the ED, his symptoms had already resolved. He is given a prescription for a drug that binds platelet ADP receptors to prevent their aggregation. Which drug is this?

(A) Clopidogrel
(B) Enoxaparin
(C) Eptifibatide
(D) Tirofiban
(E) tPA

55 Regarding the interplay between the sympathetic and parasympathetic nervous systems and target organs, most organs receive dual innervation. However, there are some tissues that receive single innervation. Such tissues would include which of the following?
(A) Adrenal cortex
(B) Adrenal medulla
(C) Heart
(D) Ileum
(E) Lungs

56 A 46-year-old Hispanic woman complains of ankle swelling. She has no history of heart failure, and a pregnancy test is negative. Physical exam shows +2 pitting edema on her ankles bilaterally. Current medications include sertraline, amlodipine, sumatriptan, docusate, and montelukast. Which of these medications is most likely causing her edema?
(A) Amlodipine
(B) Docusate
(C) Montelukast
(D) Sertraline
(E) Sumatriptan

57 An IRB-approved animal study involves injection of acetylcholine into the myocardium of a dog to study cardiac changes. Which of the following effects would likely be observed?
(A) Decreased cardiac output
(B) Increased contractility
(C) Increased heart rate
(D) Increased stroke volume
(E) Increased tetanic ability

58 A 19-year-old woman is 24 weeks pregnant. She has received no prenatal care. She presents to the emergency department complaining of an intermittent headache and fatigue during her pregnancy. Her blood pressure has been at least 150/110 mm Hg. What is the most appropriate treatment of this patient?
(A) Hydralazine
(B) Labetalol
(C) Methyldopa
(D) Prazosin
(E) Sodium nitroprusside

59 A 44-year-old man complains of chest palpitations that he has been feeling on and off for months. He denies chest discomfort, shortness of breath, and nausea, and he is not diaphoretic. An ECG reveals premature ventricular contractions but no ST segment changes. He is given acebutolol to abolish the arrhythmia. Which of the following would most likely occur with a very high dose of acebutolol?
(A) Fever
(B) Headache
(C) QT shortening
(D) Tachycardia
(E) Wheezing

60 Drug XY is a potent agent that mimics action of isoproterenol. As a result of this similarity in mechanism of action and function, which of the following properties will this agent exhibit?
(A) Effective when given orally
(B) Low potency
(C) Slow inactivation
(D) Slow CNS penetration

61 Medication AB is an indirect-acting agonist of the adrenergic nervous system. It can block the uptake of norepinephrine and is taken up into the presynaptic neuron. This described which of the following agents?
(A) Cocaine
(B) Epinephrine
(C) Isoproterenol
(D) Norepinephrine
(E) Phenylephrine

62 A 69-year-old man undergoes a five-vessel coronary artery bypass graft procedure. He is currently recovering in the ICU. He is placed on dobutamine to improve cardiac output. He then develops atrial fibrillation. What is the most likely explanation for this finding?
(A) Bundle branch block
(B) Increased AV conduction
(C) Myocardial infarction
(D) Myocardial ischemia
(E) Tolerance

63 A 49-year-old woman with hypertension not controlled well with medication undergoes an abdominal CT scan. Findings reveal a 4-cm adrenal tumor. Urine studies reveal the presence of metanephrines. Prior to surgical removal of the tumor, which of the following interventions should be undertaken?
(A) Epinephrine administration
(B) Fluid restriction
(C) Norepinephrine administration
(D) Phenoxybenzamine administration
(E) Proceed with surgical resection

64 A 65-year-old man with erectile dysfunction is using phentolamine injection to assist with obtaining an erection sufficient for sexual intercourse. Upon administration, which of the following cardiac effects is possible from this medication?
(A) Arrhythmia
(B) Bradycardia
(C) Improved myocardial perfusion
(D) Relief of anginal pain

65 A 72-year-old man with urinary frequency and nocturia presents to his primary care physician for evaluation and treatment. He is found on physical examination to have an enlarged prostate. Treatment with the α-blocker alfuzosin has begun. The patient should be warned about which of the following adverse effects?
(A) Agitation
(B) Headache
(C) Hypertension
(D) Improved energy
(E) Nasal stuffiness

66 A 63-year-old woman with recurrent migraine headaches wishes to take a β-blocker only once a day to control her symptoms. Which of the following agents would allow her to achieve this desired effect?
(A) Albuterol
(B) Esmolol
(C) Labetalol
(D) Nebivolol
(E) Propranolol

67 A 59-year-old man with hypertension presents to his primary care physician with lower extremity edema. Physical examination reveals pitting edema from the ankles to the knees bilaterally. The patient has begun on furosemide. It is important for the physician to be aware of which of the following drug–drug interactions?
(A) Hyperkalemia with corticosteroids
(B) Improves orthostatic hypotension
(C) Ototoxic when combined with thiazide diuretics
(D) Potentiates other antihypertensives

68 A medical student is involved in a summer research project involving the use of varying doses of dopamine on vascular perfusion of various organs. Three doses of dopamine will be used: low, medium, and high. If a high dose of dopamine were infused into an animal model, which of the following effects would be noticed?
(A) Increase in blood pressure
(B) Increase in heart perfusion
(C) Increase in heart stroke volume
(D) Increase in renal blood flow
(E) Increase in urine output

69 A 79-year-old woman with glaucoma has been treated by her primary care physician with timolol eye drops for this condition. At her most recent follow-up appointment, she notes a significant improvement in her symptoms. Which of the following changes has taken placed?
(A) Decreased secretion of aqueous humor
(B) Improved eye focus
(C) Improved pupil size
(D) Improved near vision
(E) Increased intraocular pressure

70 A 62-year-old woman with a history of diabetes mellitus, hypertension, and bilateral lower extremity edema presents to her primary care physician. Physical examination reveals pitting edema of both lower extremities from the ankles to the knees. She was placed on furosemide. The mechanism of action of this agent is in which of the following locations?
(A) Ascending limb of the loop of Henle
(B) Collecting duct
(C) Distal tubule
(D) Proximal tubule

71 A 49-year-old man with a history of hypertension controlled with diet and exercise now has a blood pressure of 160/90 mm Hg. His physician begins treatment with a single agent. However, the patient now complains of tiredness and cannot jog more than 4 miles. In the past, he was able to run a half marathon (13.1 miles). Which one of the following drugs is he most likely to be taking for hypertension?
(A) Albuterol
(B) Atenolol
(C) Ephedrine
(D) Phentolamine
(E) Prazosin

72 A 54-year-old man who is a 50 pack-year smoker (2.5 packs per day for 25 years) complains of chest pain just after he smokes a cigarette. What is the most likely explanation of this finding?
(A) Myocardial infarction
(B) Nicotine-induced vasoconstriction
(C) Pulmonary embolism
(D) Stroke volume change
(E) Tricuspid regurgitation

73 A 32-year-old man who has recently lost his job and found his wife to be having an extramarital affair becomes a cocaine addict. After snorting cocaine, which of the following physiologic effects is likely?
(A) Bradycardia
(B) Hypotension
(C) Pupillary dilation
(D) Vasodilation of peripheral vessels

74 A 48-year-old man with obstructive sleep apnea is planning to undergo a surgical procedure under general anesthesia to relieve his nasal obstruction. Which of the following is a goal of anesthesia for this procedure?

(A) Anxiety
(B) Awareness
(C) Perception of external stimuli
(D) Sedation
(E) Skeletal muscle contraction

75 A 59-year-old man with a long history of untreated hypertension presents to his primary care physician. He is a poor historian. His blood pressure is 160/100 mm Hg. Prior to beginning medical therapy, it is important for the physician to assess for identifiable causes of hypertension that include which of the following?

(A) Acute renal insufficiency
(B) Atrial septal defect
(C) Sleep apnea
(D) Tuberculosis
(E) Viral pneumonia

76 A 54-year-old man with diabetes presents to clinic for a routine checkup. At his prior two visits, he had an elevated blood pressure and has tried lifestyle changes to improve it. Today, his blood pressure is 142/88 mm Hg. His last urinalysis showed a urine microalbumin of 150 mcg. What is the most appropriate initial antihypertensive for this patient?

(A) Doxazosin
(B) Hydrochlorothiazide
(C) Lisinopril
(D) Metoprolol
(E) Nifedipine

77 An 81-year-old female presents to the emergency department with a racing heartbeat. She is subsequently placed on continuous ECG monitor and irregular rhythm is seen. The diagnosis of atrial fibrillation is made. She is started on an amiodarone drip. What side effect should the physician be aware of when starting amiodarone?

(A) Blurry yellow vision
(B) Impotence
(C) Lupus-like syndrome
(D) Prolongation of AV refractory period
(E) Pulmonary fibrosis

78 A 61-year-old female is hospitalized for COPD exacerbation. She is obese and not able to ambulate very far on her own. Upon discharge, the physician wants to send her home on heparin to reduce the risk of deep vein thrombosis. Why would the physician choose a low-molecular-weight heparin (LMWH) instead of unfractionated heparin (UFH)?

(A) LMWH is a better inhibitor of thrombin
(B) LMWH carries no risk of bleeding
(C) LMWH does not cause HIT
(D) LMWH is easier to manage for outpatients
(E) LMWH is more easily reversible

79 A 53-year-old female presents to the emergency department in acute distress from a rapid heart rate and chest pain. She is placed on continuous ECG monitoring and an arrhythmia of supraventricular tachycardia (SVT) is diagnosed. A 6-mg dose of IV adenosine is given and the patient converts back to a normal sinus rhythm. Where does adenosine act on the heart and what is the mechanism of action of adenosine?

(A) AV node, increases efflux of K^+
(B) AV node, increases influx of K^+
(C) SA node, decreases intracellular Ca^{2+}
(D) SA node, increases efflux of K^+
(E) SA node, increases influx of K^+

80 A 52-year-old female presents to the emergency room with swelling over her right calf for the past 3 days. Her right calf is warm, erythematous, and tender to palpation. A duplex is performed and shows a deep vein thrombosis (DVT). This is her first DVT. She is started on warfarin and told that she must continue it for the next 3 months. What effect does warfarin have on the coagulation panel?

(A) Decreases partial thromboplastin time
(B) Decreases prothrombin time
(C) Increases bleeding time
(D) Increases partial thromboplastin time
(E) Increases prothrombin time

81 A 78-year-old man presents to the emergency room with acute-onset left-sided weakness and slurred speech that started 40 min ago. A CT scan of his brain confirms an ischemic stroke. The patient is started on alteplase immediately. What is the mechanism of action of alteplase?

(A) Binds to glycoprotein receptor IIb/IIIa
(B) Blocks ADP receptors
(C) Converts plasminogen to plasmin
(D) Inhibits COX-1 and COX-2
(E) Inhibits thrombin

82 A 24-year-old male with myopia decides to undergo LASIK surgery to correct his vision. Prior to the procedure, the ophthalmologist dilates his pupils with phenylephrine, a sympathomimetic. Which of the following drugs would also cause mydriasis?
(A) Methacholine
(B) Neostigmine
(C) Phentolamine
(D) Scopolamine
(E) Terazosin

83 A 24-year-old man comes to the clinic complaining of vague abdominal pain, headaches, sweating, and unintentional weight loss. Urinalysis reveals elevated levels of vanillylmandelic acid. What substance is likely elevated in this man's serum?
(A) Acetylcholine
(B) Epinephrine
(C) Glutamate
(D) Oxytocin
(E) Serotonin

84 A 74-year-old woman presents to the ophthalmology clinic with progressive vision loss. She has noticed that her peripheral vision is worsening and she often bumps into things. Physical exam and testing confirms the presence of open-angle glaucoma. The physician prescribes a medication that decreases the production of aqueous humor. What medication was most likely prescribed?
(A) Acetazolamide
(B) Brimonidine
(C) Latanoprost
(D) Pilocarpine
(E) Timolol

85 A 45-year-old man is in the operating room under anesthesia when he develops a high fever of 104°F, a heart rate of 126 beats/minute, and a blood pressure of 178/94 mm Hg. Muscle rigidity begins to develop as well. The anesthesiologist suspects malignant hyperthermia and quickly administers a medication. The patient's vital signs and rigidity begin to improve. What is the most likely medication administered?
(A) Bromocriptine
(B) Dantrolene
(C) Diphenhydramine
(D) Nitric oxide
(E) Succinylcholine

86 A 62-year-old man with a herniated lumbar disc at L4 is undergoing spinal surgery to remove the injured disc. During the procedure, propofol is administered intravenously. Which of the following statements about this agent is true?
(A) Increases blood pressure
(B) Myocardial depression
(C) Reduces intracranial pressure
(D) Significant depression of somatosensory-evoked potentials
(E) Systemic vasoconstriction

87 A 56-year-old man presents to his primary care physician complaining of difficulty urinating. Digital rectal exam reveals an enlarged prostate. The patient is started on a trial of terazosin, after which his symptoms improve dramatically. Which of the following side effects is he most likely to experience?
(A) Diarrhea
(B) Dizziness
(C) Flatulence
(D) Headache
(E) Priapism

88 A 7-year-old boy is brought to the emergency department by his parents after being stung by a bee. The parents say he is allergic to bee stings, and the patient is having great difficulty breathing. Epinephrine is administered immediately. His symptoms improve as molecules of epinephrine bind to β_2-receptors in bronchiolar smooth muscle. Which of the following drugs also stimulates these receptors?
(A) Acebutolol
(B) Phenylephrine
(C) Prazosin
(D) Salmeterol
(E) Timolol

89 A 57-year-old man with congestive heart failure presents to the emergency department with shortness of breath. He has +2 pitting edema in his extremities as well. A chest X-ray confirms the presence of pulmonary edema. The patient is given intravenous furosemide to diurese the excess fluid. Where in the nephron does furosemide act?
(A) Collecting tubule
(B) Descending loop of Henle
(C) Distal convoluted tubule
(D) Proximal convoluted tubule
(E) Thick ascending loop of Henle

90 A 62-year-old man with congestive heart failure has been taking a loop diuretic to reduce peripheral edema. His labs today reveal low potassium. Which of the following diuretics would be better to use in this patient?
(A) Acetazolamide
(B) Ethacrynic acid
(C) Hydrochlorothiazide
(D) Methazolamide
(E) Triamterene

91 A 54-year-old woman with severe essential hypertension refractory to treatment switched to a new antihypertensive drug 1 month ago. Her blood pressure is currently well controlled. She now comes complaining of excessive hair growth. What is this drug's mechanism of action?

(A) Blocks calcium channels
(B) Blocks renal Na^+ reabsorption
(C) Increases intracellular cAMP
(D) Increases NO
(E) Inhibits the production of angiotensin II

92 A 32-year-old Caucasian woman experiences chest pain with exertion. She reports having similar episodes in the past. It is determined that she is experiencing stable angina. She is given nitroglycerin to relax her vascular smooth musculature. Which best describes a step on nitroglycerin's mechanism of action?

(A) Activation of adenylate cyclase
(B) Activation of guanylate cyclase
(C) Inhibition of calcium channels
(D) Inhibition of cGMP phosphodiesterase
(E) Preventing calmodulin's activity

93 A medical student is involved in a summer research project involving the administration of subtherapeutic doses of morphine to rats. Cardiovascular effects and parameters are determined approximately 30 min after administration. Which of the following effects is likely?

(A) Bradycardia
(B) Hypertension
(C) Hypotension
(D) No change in heart rate
(E) Tachycardia

94 A 45-year-old man with a family history of hyperlipidemia and heart disease comes to the ER diaphoretic with chest pain radiating to his left arm. An ECG shows ST segment elevation in leads II, III, and aVF. The doctor administers alteplase intravenously. How does alteplase work?

(A) Activates antithrombin III
(B) Activates plasminogen
(C) Activates thrombin
(D) Blocks production of thromboxane A_2
(E) Blocks platelet ADP receptors

95 A 58-year-old man undergoes open heart surgery for a triple coronary artery bypass graft. His surgery goes smoothly, but the next day, he develops chest palpitations. Verapamil is started to keep his supraventricular tachycardia from interfering with ventricular rhythm. Under which Singh–Vaughan Williams class of antiarrhythmics does verapamil fall?

(A) Class Ia
(B) Class Ib
(C) Class Ic
(D) Class II
(E) Class III
(F) Class IV

96 A 63-year-old man with congestive heart failure comes to the cardiologist for a routine visit. He is doing well and has no complaints. He is taking digoxin, metoprolol, and spironolactone. What is the mechanism of action of spironolactone?

(A) Aldosterone receptor antagonist
(B) Carbonic anhydrase inhibitor
(C) Inhibits NaCl reabsorption
(D) Inhibits $Na^+/K^+/2Cl^-$ cotransport
(E) Osmotic diuretic

97 A 57-year-old man with comes to the clinic for a follow-up appointment. For the past two visits, his blood pressure has been 152/88 mm Hg and 150/86 mm Hg. Today, his blood pressure is 150/88 mm Hg. His past medical history is significant for an MI 2 years ago. His physician prescribes fosinopril. Which of the following parameters may change because of fosinopril therapy?

(A) Blood calcium
(B) Blood potassium
(C) Blood lipids
(D) Blood urea nitrogen
(E) White blood cell count

98 A 51-year-old man presents to the urology clinic with difficulty starting and stopping his stream during urination. The symptoms have been worsening over the past year. He also reports that he does not feel he empties his bladder completely. He is started on tamsulosin for benign prostatic hyperplasia. What is a common side effect of tamsulosin?

(A) Cough
(B) Hemorrhagic cystitis
(C) Hypercoagulable state
(D) Impaired blue-green vision
(E) Orthostatic hypotension

99 A 53-year-old woman with a long history of seizure disorder who has failed therapy with other agents is given a trial of pregabalin. She has a history of partial-onset seizures as well as diabetic peripheral neuropathic pain in both extremities. Which of the following statements is correct about this agent?

(A) Drowsiness and blurred vision would be expected
(B) Hepatic excretion will cause jaundice
(C) Her seizures will likely continue
(D) Her neuropathic pain will likely continue
(E) She will likely experience weight loss

100 A 60-year-old Caucasian woman suffers an anterior wall myocardial infarction. She recovers well initially but soon develops left heart failure. Her physician prescribes multiple medications to treat different aspects of heart failure, including digoxin. How does digoxin help in heart failure?

(A) Blocks the activity of angiotensin II at its receptor
(B) Causes excess fluid elimination
(C) Increases cardiac inotropy
(D) Inhibits production of angiotensin II
(E) Reduces preload

101 A 67-year-old man with insulin-dependent diabetes mellitus, hypertension, and congestive heart failure develops exacerbation of heart failure symptoms. Pathophysiology of this condition that relates to potential roles of drug therapy include which of the following?

(A) Peripheral nervous system activity
(B) Loss of cardiac myocytes
(C) Muscle hyperplasia
(D) Muscle inflammatory scar formation
(E) Square geometric configuration of the heart

102 A 61-year-old woman who is a long-term smoker presents to the emergency department with dyspnea and feeling faint. Physical examination reveals bilateral jugular venous distension and significant peripheral edema of both legs up to the knees. Treatment of this condition will be unaffected by which of the following classes of medications?

(A) Antibiotics
(B) β-Blockers
(C) Diuretics
(D) Inhibitors of the renin-angiotensin system
(E) Inotropic agents

103 A 72-year-old man with long-standing heart failure managed with digoxin and a β-blocker suddenly collapses in a shopping mall. Attempts to revive him are unsuccessful. Autopsy is performed. Which of the following changes in his heart would be expected to be noted?

(A) Dilated cardiac chambers
(B) Heart appears small
(C) Heart appears smooth
(D) Increased ability to eject blood
(E) Thinning of the ventricular wall

104 A 67-year-old man with long-standing heart failure managed with digoxin and a β-blocker suddenly collapses in a shopping mall. He has been noncompliant with his medication and now wishes to turn over a new lease on life and care for himself. Which of the following strategies will have the lowest potential of success on improving his health?

(A) Elimination of alcohol
(B) Low dietary intake of sodium (<1500 mg/d)
(C) Judicious use of diuretics
(D) Treatment of his underlying diabetes mellitus
(E) Use of nonsteroidal anti-inflammatory medications

105 A 47-year-old woman with Type-2 diabetes presents to the nephrology clinic for follow-up. She has been doing well other than an increase in her blood sugars lately. She was started on a new medication recently, but she cannot remember the name. All she knows was it affected her kidneys. What is the most likely medication that she started taking?

(A) Acetazolamide
(B) Furosemide
(C) Hydrochlorothiazide
(D) Mannitol
(E) Spironolactone

106 A 57-year-old man with a 40 pack-year history of smoking develops small cell lung cancer. He begins to show signs of hyponatremia, and his urine is highly concentrated. The diagnosis of SIADH is made. Administration of which of the following metal ions may help?

(A) Cobalt
(B) Iron
(C) Lithium
(D) Magnesium
(E) Selenium

107 A 58-year-old man with diabetes has difficulty achieving an erection. He has a history of cardiovascular disease. A friend recommends yohimbine. Which of the following describes yohimbine's likely mechanism of action?

(A) Decreasing parasympathetic tone
(B) Direct vasoconstriction
(C) Direct vasodilation
(D) Increasing sympathetic tone
(E) Stimulation of the pudendal nerve

108 A 55-year-old man complains of poor urinary flow and nocturia. He is found to suffer from benign prostatic hyperplasia. The physician prescribes prazosin to help his symptoms. How does prazosin work?

(A) Antagonizes α_2-adrenergic receptors
(B) Blocks DHT synthesis
(C) Inhibits 5-α-reductase
(D) Inhibits testosterone synthesis
(E) Relaxes prostatic smooth muscle

109 A 53-year-old woman with long-standing hypertension has already been treated with a β-blocker and a calcium channel blocker, which have failed to control her blood pressure. She is now treated with losartan. Which of the following statements is correct regarding its pharmacokinetics?
(A) Converted to an inactive metabolite
(B) Eliminated via skin loss
(C) Extensive first-pass metabolism
(D) Limited binding to plasma proteins
(E) Renal failure is a common complication

110 A 64-year-old man with left heart failure is managed with digoxin and a thiazide diuretic. His primary care physician orders a laboratory panel. Which of the following electrolytes is most likely to be abnormal in this patient?
(A) Calcium
(B) Glucose
(C) Magnesium
(D) Potassium
(E) Sodium

111 Which of the following statements is correct regarding adenosine and its limited role in the treatment of cardiac dysfunction in a 64-year-old man with supraventricular tachycardia?
(A) Decreased conduction velocity
(B) Half-life is 6 h
(C) Improves SA node function
(D) Most efficacious when given intramuscularly
(E) Significant toxicity

112 A 57-year-old retired schoolteacher with a history of Prinzmetal angina presents to his primary care physician for follow-up. He has not had an attack in the last 6 months and wishes to stop preventative medications. Which of the following statements is true?
(A) Continuation of his medications would be helpful
(B) Increased blood flow to the heart worsens symptoms
(C) Symptoms are related to physical activity
(D) Symptoms are worsened with worsening hypertension

113 A 65-year-old man who is an avid golfer has intermittent angina when he plays golf particularly in cold weather. His primary care physician places him on sublingual nitroglycerine to be taken at the onset of symptoms. This patient must be warned of which of the following side effects?
(A) Dry skin
(B) Erectile dysfunction
(C) Headache
(D) Priapism
(E) Slowing of the heart rate

114 A primary care physician is treating several patients with hypertension and chronic angina. Which of the following patient subsets would best benefit from treatment with ranolazine?
(A) A 53-year-old man with acute-onset angina
(B) A 62-year-old man with atrial fibrillation and acute-onset angina
(C) A 65-year-old man with chronic angina who has failed other therapies
(D) A 72-year-old man with acute angina who has just arrived in the emergency department
(E) A 77-year-old man with congestive heart failure and ventricular dysfunction

115 A 72-year-old man who is very athletic and walks half marathons has been successfully treated for exercise-induced angina for several years. He recently has been complaining about being awakened at night with chest pain. Which of the following drugs would be useful in preventing this patient's nocturnal angina?
(A) Amyl nitrite
(B) Esmolol
(C) Hydralazine
(D) Nitroglycerin (sublingual)
(E) Nitroglycerin (transdermal)

116 A 54-year-old man with hypertension presents to his primary care physician for follow-up. His blood pressure is consistently greater than 140/90 mm Hg. The physician urges that the patient begin pharmacotherapy. The patient refuses this suggestion and wants to try lifestyle modifications. Which of the following changes will have the lowest likelihood of blood pressure reduction?
(A) Alcohol intake limited to less than two drinks per day
(B) Diet rich in fruits, vegetables, and low in fat
(C) Reduction of dietary salt to 10 g/d
(D) Regular aerobic activity 30 min/d
(E) Weight management to BMI less than 25

117 A 56-year-old man with male pattern baldness and hypertension is placed on minoxidil. He has had a lack of response to antihypertensive agents with failure to respond to calcium channel blockers and ACE inhibitors. Prolonged use of this agent can be associated with which of the following effects?
(A) Baldness
(B) Fluid retention
(C) Muscular wasting
(D) Thinning of skin on the palms and soles
(E) Uremic pericarditis

118 Five patients with potential need for intravenous sodium nitroprusside are presented as follows. Which patient would best benefit from such an infusion?

(A) A 21-year-old man with pulmonary edema and blood pressure of 180/90 mm Hg
(B) A 43-year-old woman with stroke and blood pressure of 170/100 mm Hg
(C) A 55-year-old man with encephalopathy and blood pressure of 220/160 mm Hg
(D) A 60-year-old man with myocardial infarction and blood pressure of 90/60 mm Hg
(E) A 68-year-old man with pulmonary failure, heart failure, and blood pressure of 80/40 mm Hg

119 Five patient subtypes have hypertension. Which of the following patients would best respond to a calcium channel blocker?

(A) A 40-year-old white woman
(B) A 45-year-old white man
(C) A 50-year-old white man
(D) A 55-year-old white woman
(E) A 60-year-old black man

120 Five pregnant women with hypertension present to the obstetrics clinic for follow-up. Which patient is in need of treatment with an antihypertensive agent?

(A) A 21-year-old woman, 10 weeks pregnant, blood pressure of 130/90 mm Hg
(B) A 24-year-old woman, 20 weeks pregnant, blood pressure of 150/80 mm Hg
(C) A 25-year-old woman, 18 weeks pregnant, blood pressure of 180/110 mm Hg
(D) A 29-year-old woman, 10 weeks pregnant, blood pressure of 120/60 mm Hg
(E) A 35-year-old woman, 10 weeks pregnant, with history of bleeding disorder, blood pressure of 130/90 mm Hg

121 A 57-year-old man presents to his primary care physician for follow-up. He is found to have a blood pressure of 150/100 mm Hg on three successive occasions. He has begun on an antihypertensive agent. After taking the first dose of the medication, he goes out to play golf and collapses on the golf course. Which one of the following drugs may be responsible for his symptoms?

(A) Atenolol
(B) Hydrochlorothiazide
(C) Metoprolol
(D) Prazosin
(E) Verapamil

122 A 57-year-old homeless man with no health insurance has a history of hypertension. He usually takes an antihypertensive agent but has not been able to obtain the medication. He stopped taking the medication yesterday and now is found collapsed in front of a shopping mall. Rescue squad arrives on the scene, and the patient's blood pressure is 190/110 mm Hg. Which one of the following antihypertensive drugs can precipitate a hypertensive crisis following abrupt cessation of therapy?

(A) Clonidine
(B) Diltiazem
(C) Enalapril
(D) Hydrochlorothiazide
(E) Losartan

123 A 72-year-old man is brought to the emergency department with crushing midsternal chest pain. The emergency department believes that he is suffering from a myocardial infarction. Cardiac catheterization is not possible because the cath lab is under renovation. The therapeutic window for myocardial salvage with heparin is which of the following?

(A) 2 to 6 h
(B) 6 to 10 h
(C) 10 to 14 h
(D) Up to 24 h
(E) Up to 48 h

124 A newly built hospital with the latest equipment and medication therapies purports a very high rate of salvage of strokes such that patients have significant recovery of normal function. Alteplase is the first-line agent administered in this facility. For the purported maximum salvage rate following stroke, this agent must be administered in which of the following time intervals?

(A) Within 3 h
(B) Within 6 h
(C) Within 9 h
(D) Within 12 h
(E) Within 24 h

125 A 73-year-old man develops crushing chest pain while walking in a shopping mall. He is brought to the emergency department for evaluation and treatment. He is thought to be having a myocardial infarction. He has immediately begun on streptokinase therapy. Which of the following blood parameters must be carefully monitored during the infusion?

(A) Hemoglobin
(B) Hematocrit
(C) Partial thromboplastin time
(D) Platelet count
(E) Thromboplastin time

126 A 75-year-old man is brought to the emergency department with right calf pain and swelling. Three weeks ago, he underwent a radical cystectomy for invasive bladder cancer. Ultrasound reveals a right pelvic vein deep venous thrombosis. The patient was treated with a bolus of heparin, and a heparin drip was started. One hour later, he was bleeding profusely from the intravenous site. The heparin therapy was suspended, but the bleeding continued. Protamine sulfate was administered intravenously that works in which of the following ways?
(A) Activates the coagulation cascade
(B) Activates tissue plasminogen activator
(C) Degrades the heparin
(D) Inactivates antithrombin
(E) Ionically combines with heparin

127 A 50-year-old man presents to the emergency department with acute-onset left-sided crushing chest pain. An ECG shows ST elevations in II, III, and aVF. He is immediately rushed to the catheterization lab and three stents are placed. Because of the insertion of stents, he has started on ticlopidine. Which of the following is a common side effect of ticlopidine?
(A) Gastric ulcers
(B) Neutropenia
(C) Osteoporosis
(D) Seizures
(E) Tinnitus

128 A 57-year-old man presents with progressively worsening shortness of breath and new-onset hemoptysis. He has a 34 pack-year history of smoking. A chest X-ray reveals a circular lesion in the right upper lobe. He begins taking methotrexate as part of a chemotherapy regimen. Which is a potential complication of methotrexate therapy?
(A) α-Thalassemia
(B) β-Thalassemia
(C) Macrocytic anemia
(D) Microcytic anemia
(E) Normocytic anemia

129 A 78-year-old man with dyspnea is brought to the emergency department for evaluation. Physical examination reveals jugular venous distension and bilateral rales in both lung fields. Chest X-ray reveals pulmonary congestion consistent with fluid overload. What is the best treatment for this patient?
(A) Acetazolamide
(B) Chlorthalidone
(C) Furosemide
(D) Hydrochlorothiazide
(E) Spironolactone

130 A group of medical students is planning to embark on a medical mission to a Third World country where mountain sickness is a possibility for them. Which of the following agents would be an appropriate prophylactic agent to take prior to the trip?
(A) Anticholinergic agent
(B) Carbonic anhydrase inhibitor
(C) Loop diuretic
(D) β-Blocker
(E) Thiazide diuretic

131 A 58-year-old man with diabetes presents to the ambulatory care clinic for follow-up. He has tried to eat better and exercise over the past 6 months. He has lost 10 lb with his new lifestyle. However, his urinalysis shows microalbuminuria. The physician decides to start the patient on captopril. What is a common side effect of captopril?
(A) Acute renal failure
(B) Gynecomastia
(C) Hypertension
(D) Hypokalemia
(E) Ototoxicity

132 A 52-year-old woman presents to the primary care clinic with progressive weakness and muscle aches for the past month. She can still do her daily tasks but can notice a difference in her strength. When she lies down at night, her legs always ache. Her electrolytes are significant for a K^+ of 2.9 mEq/L. She was recently started on a diuretic for peripheral edema. She is pleased that she has not had peripheral edema since starting the diuretic. What is the most appropriate diuretic to treat this patient?
(A) Acetazolamide
(B) Furosemide
(C) Hydrochlorothiazide
(D) Mannitol
(E) Spironolactone

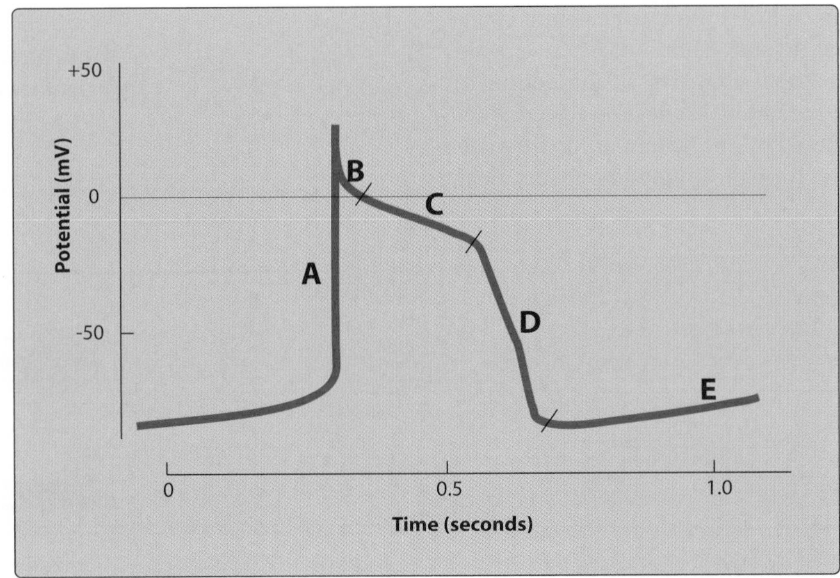

133 The above figure represents the action potential of a Purkinje fiber. At which of the following areas on the succeeding graph do calcium channels close and potassium channels open, resulting in an outward current that leads to membrane repolarization?

(A) Letter A
(B) Letter B
(C) Letter C
(D) Letter D
(E) Letter E

134 A 52-year-old man with chest pain presents to the emergency department for treatment. Three cardiac nitrates are available for treatment. The following is a listing of the agents and their onset and duration of action. Which of the following would be most appropriate for this patient?

(A) Medication A
(B) Medication B
(C) Medication C
(D) Medications B and C

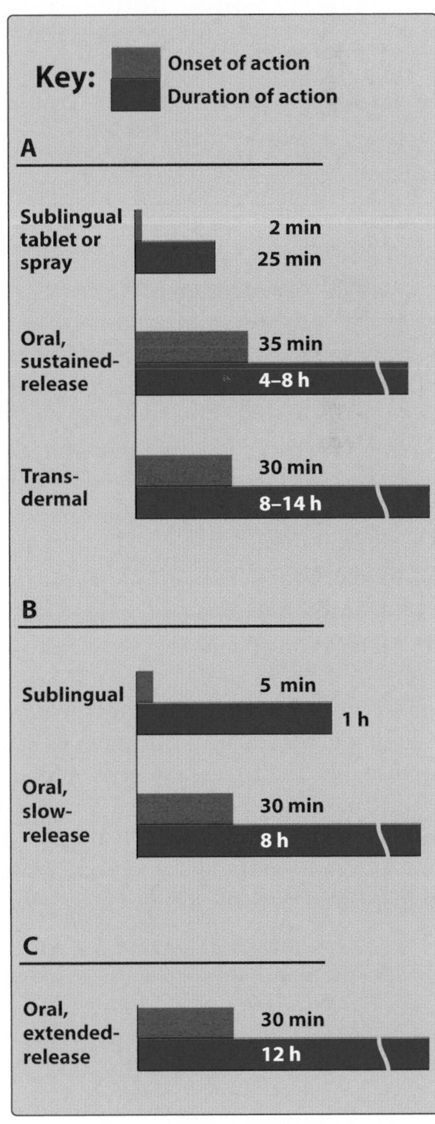

135 A physician is giving consideration to a calcium channel blocker to treat hypertension in a 65-year-old man. He desires an agent that has strong action to dilate coronary arteries and little effect on AV conduction. He is not bothered by the potential for frequent adverse effects. Which of the following agents does this describe?

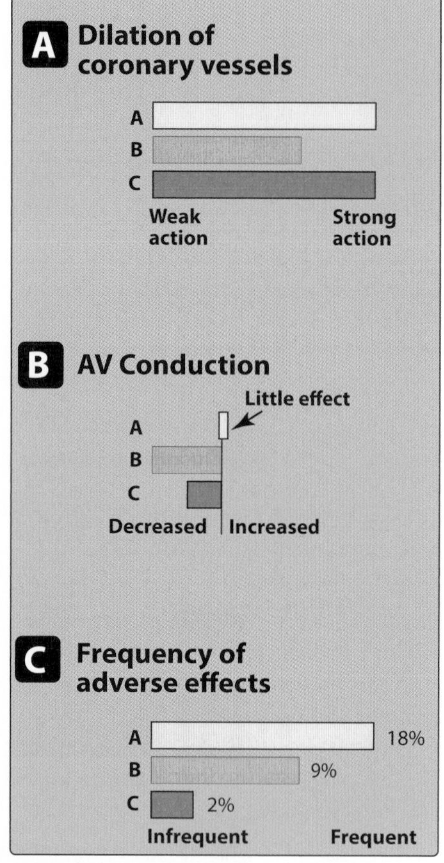

(A) Medication A
(B) Medication B
(C) Medication C
(D) Medications B and C

136 A 59-year-old man with chest pain collapses in a shopping mall. He is brought to the emergency department for treatment. His blood pressure is 210/120 mm Hg. Four medications are available for treatment. The following is a listing of the agents and their onset and duration of action. Which of the following would have the lowest efficacy for this patient?

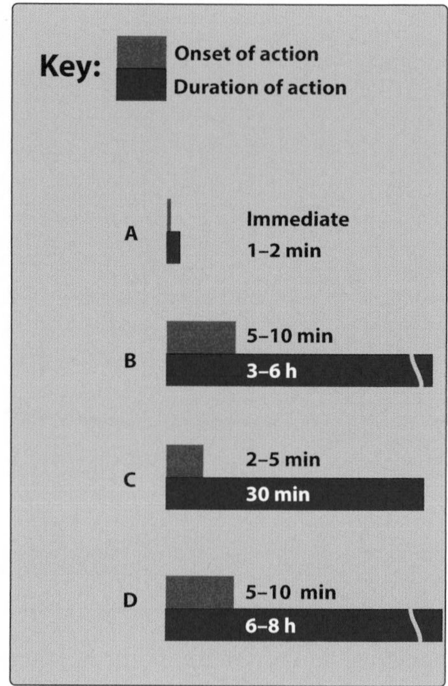

(A) Medication A
(B) Medication B
(C) Medication C
(D) Medication D

137 A 65-year-old man is interested in preventing potential coronary disease through the use of a daily aspirin tablet (81 mg). This agent has a mechanism of action that involves which of the following steps in the succeeding pathway?

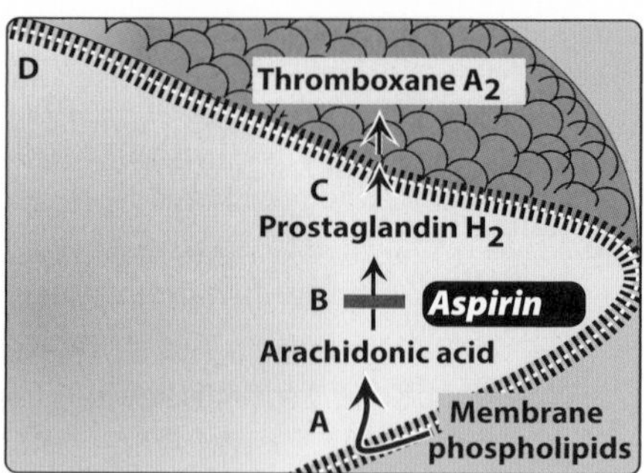

(A) Letter A
(B) Letter B
(C) Letter C
(D) Letter D

138 A 58-year-old man with crushing chest pain is brought to the emergency department for treatment of a suspected myocardial infarction. The following chart presents a comparison of potential thrombolytic enzymes that could be used in the treatment of this patient. Which of the following agents demonstrates high antigenicity, low fibrin specificity, and a half-life of greater than 20 min?

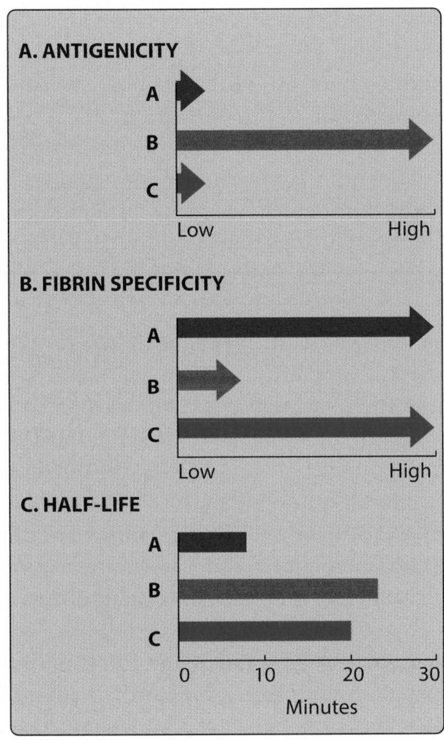

(A) Medication A
(B) Medication B
(C) Medication C
(D) Cannot be determined

139 An 80-year-old woman presents to the emergency department complaining of a right-sided headache and right jaw pain. Physical examination reveals induration of the left temporal artery. Laboratory studies reveal an elevated erythrocyte sedimentation rate, and biopsy of the temporal artery shows granulomatous inflammation. What class of pharmaceuticals is needed to prevent blindness in this patient?

(A) α-Blockers
(B) Anticoagulants
(C) HMG-CoA reductase inhibitors
(D) Steroids
(E) Thrombolytics

140 A 32-year-old pregnant female presents to her obstetrician for a well-baby evaluation. Her blood pressure readings over the past two visits have both been 165/100 mm Hg. The physician suggests that antihypertensive medication is needed in this patient. Chest X-ray is obtained and shows no evidence of infiltrate or effusion. No mass lesions are noted, and the costophrenic angles are sharp. What pharmacologic agent is most effective and safest for this patient?

(A) Furosemide
(B) Hydrochlorothiazide
(C) Lisinopril
(D) Losartan
(E) Methyldopa

141 A 72-year-old man is brought to the emergency department after he passed out at home. Electrocardiography reveals an AV nodal–based arrhythmia. What drug would be most effective at interrupting the AV transmission and breaking the arrhythmic cycle at the AV node?

(A) Adenosine
(B) Flecainide
(C) Lidocaine
(D) Phenytoin
(E) Quinidine

ANSWERS

1 **The answer is D: Pulmonary fibrosis.** Serious cardiac problems may develop, particularly in patients with a history of myocardial infarction. In patients with peripheral vascular disease, a worsening of the vasospasm occurs, and in patients with peptic ulcer, there is a worsening of the ulcer. Because bromocriptine is an ergot derivative, it has the potential to cause pulmonary and retroperitoneal fibrosis. (A) Bromocriptine is not associated with development of adenocarcinoma. (B) Bromocriptine is not associated with development of pneumonia. (C) Bromocriptine is not associated with thromboembolic phenomenon. (E) Bromocriptine is not associated with development of squamous cell carcinoma.

2 **The answer is B: Hyperglycemia.** β_2-Receptor agonists cause hepatic glycogenolysis and muscle glycogenolysis, which will increase serum glucose levels causing hyperglycemia. This can be measured by drawing blood and checking the serum glucose. (A) β_2-Receptor stimulation causes bronchodilation. (C) β_2-Receptor stimulation causes decreased peripheral resistance and decrease in blood pressure. (D) β_2-Receptor stimulation causes uterine relaxation. (E) β_2-Receptor stimulation causes vasodilation.

3 **The answer is D: Insufficient antiplatelet activity because of inadequate platelet cyclooxygenase inhibition.** The two key players here are the eicosanoids thromboxane A_2 (TXA_2), which stimulates aggregation, and prostaglandin I_2 (PGI_2 or prostacyclin), which inhibits platelet aggregation. TXA_2 synthesis occurs in platelets themselves and begins with phospholipase A_2 cleaving membrane phospholipid to release arachidonic acid. This arachidonic acid is converted to prostaglandin H_2 (PGH_2) by platelet cyclooxygenase (COX) enzymes. PGH_2 is then converted to TXA_2 by platelet thromboxane synthase. Prostacyclin is synthesized in endothelial cells. It also starts with arachidonic acid, which is converted to PGH_2 by endothelial COX enzymes. PGH_2 in endothelial cells is then converted to prostacyclin by endothelial prostacyclin synthase. Aspirin and ibuprofen both inhibit COX enzymes in both platelet and endothelial cells, but aspirin inhibition is irreversible, whereas ibuprofen inhibition is reversible. Under chronic aspirin use, endothelial cells can produce new COX enzymes to replace those lost to aspirin's inhibition, but platelets cannot replace deactivated enzymes because they lack a nucleus. Ibuprofen can actually prevent COX deactivation in platelets by aspirin by occupying the active site of the enzyme, so aspirin is unable to enter and modify it. This buys time for the platelet until the aspirin is cleared from the body. Then the reversible inhibition by ibuprofen wears off as ibuprofen is cleared and platelets are left with active COX enzymes to produce TXA_2. (A) Ibuprofen and aspirin do not exhibit synergy with respect to anticoagulation. (B) Ibuprofen's effect on endothelial cells is to prevent formation of prostacyclin by inhibiting COX enzymes, which would favor platelet aggregation. (C) Ibuprofen is not known to increase aspirin's metabolism by cytochrome P450 induction. (E) Ibuprofen would counteract the antiplatelet effect of aspirin.

4 **The answer is A: Impermeability to the blood–brain barrier.** Dopamine is a catecholamine, which is useful in the treatment of shock. It can also be used in the treatment of congestive heart failure and can raise blood pressure. This medication is impermeable to the blood–brain barrier. (B) Dopamine has a short duration of action. (C) Dopamine is administered via intravenous route. (D) Dopamine potentiates hypertension. (E) Dopamine has a rapid onset of action.

5 **The answer is E: Terbutaline.** Terbutaline is used off-label as a uterine relaxant to suppress premature labor. Side effects of β_2-agonists are primarily caused by excessive β_2-receptor activation. One of the most common side effects of these agents is tremor. (A) Albuterol is used in the treatment of asthma. (B) Isoproterenol is used in rare clinical situations. (C) Metaproterenol would not suppress uterine contractions. (D) Metoprolol is an antihypertensive agent.

6 **The answer is D: A 51-year-old man with angina who suffered a heart attack 2 years ago.** Phentolamine-induced reflex cardiac stimulation and tachycardia are mediated by the baroreceptor reflex and by blocking the receptors of the cardiac sympathetic nerves. The drug can also trigger arrhythmias and anginal pain, and phentolamine is contraindicated in patients with decreased coronary perfusion. (A) This is a young patient with no contraindications to phentolamine. (B) Hypertension and renal stones are not contraindications to phentolamine. (C) Parathyroid adenoma and testicular cysts are not contraindications to phentolamine. (E) Hypertension, kidney stones, and renal cysts are not contraindications to phentolamine.

7 **The answer is choice D: Short-term memory loss.** Propranolol has numerous CNS-mediated effects, including depression, dizziness, lethargy, fatigue, weakness, visual disturbances, hallucinations, short-term memory loss, emotional lability, vivid dreams (including nightmares), decreased performance, and depression manifested by insomnia. (A) Visual disturbances can occur as a CNS-mediated effect of propranolol. (B) Insomnia is a CNS-mediated effect of propranolol. (C) Muscle weakness is a CNS-mediated effect of propranolol. (E) Urinary incontinence is not typically seen as a CNS-mediated effect of propranolol.

8 **The answer is C: Improved vascular wall thickening.** Carvedilol is a reversible β-blocker that produces peripheral vasodilation and decreased blood pressure. Additionally, this agent decreases lipid peroxidation and vascular wall thickening, which may be helpful in patients with heart failure. (A) This agent does not alter serum glucose levels. (B) This agent does not alter serum glucose levels. (D) This agent decreases lipid peroxidation. (E) This agent is a vasodilator.

9 **The answer is C: Pindolol.** In general, black patients with hypertension are not well controlled with β-blockers. However, labetalol can be used in those whom increased vascular resistance is undesirable. (A) Labetalol can be used in this patient with efficacy. (B) Methyldopa can be used in this patient with efficacy. (D) Triamterene is a potassium-sparing diuretic with efficacy in black patients. (E) Verapamil is a calcium channel blocker and can be used in black patients.

10 **The answer is D: Nadolol.** Nadolol has a half-life of 12 to 24 h and would be the best agent for β-blockade in a patient who is undergoing a long duration surgical procedure. A single intraoperative dose should suffice the entire case. (A) Acebutolol has a 3- to 4-h half-life. (B) Esmolol has a 10-min half-life. It is the shortest acting β-blocker. (C) Metoprolol has a 3- to 4-h half-life. (E) Pindolol has a 3- to 4-h half-life.

11 **The answer is D: Reserpine.** Reserpine is a plant alkaloid that blocks the Mg^{2+}/ATP-dependent transport of biogenic amines from the cytoplasm into storage vesicles in the adrenergic nerves. This will have an effect on norepinephrine, dopamine, and serotonin concentrations via depletion. This impairs sympathetic function. (A) Atenolol is a β-blocker. (B) Esmolol is a β-blocker. (C) Guanethidine blocks norepinephrine release from storage vesicles. (E) Timolol is a β-blocker.

12 **The answer is A: Dopamine.** Chronic intake of cocaine depletes dopamine. This depletion triggers the vicious cycle of craving for cocaine that temporarily relieves severe depression. In particular, the prolongation of dopaminergic effects in the brain's pleasure system (limbic system) produces the intense euphoria that cocaine initially causes. (B) Epinephrine effects from cocaine will not produce euphoria. (C) Glutamine effects from cocaine will not produce euphoria. (D) Norepinephrine effects from cocaine will not produce euphoria.

13 **The answer is C: Stimulating vascular smooth muscle in arterioles supplying the stomach.** Phenylephrine causes contraction of the dilator muscle by stimulating α_2-receptors to induce mydriasis. The sympathetic nervous system does not always cause smooth muscle contraction in its target organs, however. End-organ effects depend on the receptor type more than on the neurotransmitter, and sympathomimetic drugs have widely varied effects depending on the sympathetic receptors they stimulate. Of the options listed, only stimulating vascular smooth muscle in arterioles supplying the stomach describes an action of the sympathetic nervous system. (A) Contraction of the detrusor muscle of the bladder is mediated acetylcholine (ACh) from the parasympathetic nervous system. (B) Sympathetic stimulation would cause an increase in heart rate (by NE acting on β_1-receptors). Parasympathetic stimulation would cause a decrease in heart rate (by ACh acting on M_2 receptors). (D) NE relaxes vascular smooth muscle in arterioles supplying skeletal muscle by acting on β_2-receptors. (E) NE relaxes bronchiolar smooth muscle by acting on β_2-receptors.

14 **The answer is A: α_1-Adrenergic antagonist.** The -zosin drugs such as terazosin, prazosin, and doxazosin are α_1-adrenergic antagonists. Stimulation of α_1-receptors leads to an increase in intracellular calcium and smooth muscle contraction. Contraction of the smooth muscle of the prostate narrows the prostatic urethra, impeding urine outflow. Terazosin helps with the symptoms of benign prostatic hypertrophy by blocking the contraction of prostatic smooth muscle. (B) Terazosin does not antagonize α_2-receptors. (C) Terazosin is not an anticholinergic agent. (D) Terazosin is not a β_2-adrenergic agonist. (E) Terazosin is not a β_2-adrenergic antagonist.

15 **The answer is A: Amiodarone.** Amiodarone is an antiarrhythmic notorious for its pulmonary side effects including pulmonary fibrosis. Some patients develop fibrosis after a relatively short course, whereas others may take it for much longer and not develop any fibrosis. Amiodarone is indicated in patients with recurring ventricular fibrillation and ventricular tachycardia refractory to other drugs. Amiodarone is a class III antiarrhythmic and also functions as a vasodilator. (B) Digoxin can be used in certain types of arrhythmias but is not known to cause pulmonary fibrosis. (C) Lidocaine is used to treat ventricular tachycardia. It has many side effects, but pulmonary fibrosis is not one of them. (D) Procainamide is used to treat ventricular tachycardia but is not known to cause pulmonary fibrosis. It is better known for being able to cause drug-induced lupus. (E) Verapamil is a calcium channel blocker used for certain types of arrhythmias but not used in ventricular tachycardia. It is also not known to cause pulmonary fibrosis.

16 **The answer is D: Class II.** Metoprolol is a β-adrenergic receptor blocker. Aside from other uses, it can be employed to treat supraventricular tachycardias such as atrial fibrillation and atrial flutter. β-Blockers, as antiarrhythmics, work by slowing signal conduction through the atrioventricular (AV) node. This prevents the spread of arrhythmias from the atria to the ventricles. β-Blockers are categorized as class II antiarrhythmics under the Singh–Vaughan Williams classification. (A) Class Ia contains drugs that block sodium channels with moderate affinity. Class Ia drugs also produce a moderate block on potassium channels. (B) Class Ib contains drugs that block sodium channels with low affinity. They bind best to sodium channels that are more frequently open, providing a use-dependent blockade. (C) Class Ic contains drugs that block sodium channels with high affinity, producing a steady blockade. (E) Class III contains drugs that block potassium channels, slowing repolarization. This increases the refractory period following each action potential making cells less likely to depolarize at inappropriate times. (F) Class IV contains drugs that block calcium channels, slowing conduction through the AV node.

17 The answer is C: Hydrochlorothiazide. Calcium oxalate stones are caused by an increase of calcium, oxalate, or both in the urine. Stone formation can be prevented by lowering the amount of calcium excreted in the urine. Thiazide diuretics, such as hydrochlorothiazide, decrease renal excretion of calcium by an unknown mechanism. (A) Acetazolamide causes diuresis by inhibiting carbonic anhydrase. Acetazolamide actually increases renal excretion of calcium, so it would not be useful in preventing calcium stone formation. (B) Furosemide inhibits sodium, potassium, and chloride resorption in the ascending limb of the loop of Henle. It does not alter calcium handling by the kidney. (D) Mannitol is an osmotic diuretic because it is filtered at the glomerulus but minimally reabsorbed. It does not alter calcium handling by the kidney. (E) Spironolactone is an antagonist of aldosterone. Normally, aldosterone causes resorption of sodium from the distal tubules. It does not alter calcium handling by the kidney.

18 The answer is D: Phase 3. Sotalol is classified as a class III antiarrhythmic, although it also possesses β-blocking (class II) activity. Only its class III effect modifies the cardiac myocyte action potential. Class III antiarrhythmics block the potassium channels in cardiac myocytes, increasing the effective refractory period. Although potassium initially begins to flow out of the cell during phase 1 and 2, phase 3 is dominated by potassium efflux and undergoes the greatest change with sotalol. Prolonging phase 3 is the intended effect of sotalol. (A) Phase 0 corresponds to the influx of sodium ions, depolarizing the cell. Class I antiarrhythmics modify this phase by blocking sodium entry. (B) Phase 1 corresponds to the initial potassium outflow before the phase 2 plateau. Modifying phase 1 is not the intent of sotalol administration. (C) Phase 2 corresponds to an efflux of potassium balancing an influx of calcium, causing a plateau in the action potential. Modifying phase 2 is not the intent of sotalol administration. (E) Phase 4 corresponds to the resting membrane potential dominated by potassium leakage. Modifying phase 4 is not the intent of sotalol administration.

19 The answer is E: Nitroprusside. Lactic acidosis, headache, vertigo, and confusion can be signs of cyanide toxicity. A potential side effect of nitroprusside is cyanide toxicity because nitroprusside is composed of an iron atom bound to five cyanide (CN) ligands and one nitric oxide ligand (NO). The vasodilatory benefit of nitroprusside occurs when the NO molecule is released in the circulation because NO is a potent vasodilator. The CN ligands are also slowly released and can cause toxicity, especially in patients with renal insufficiency. Nitroprusside can still be used in cases of hypertensive crisis, however, because the pharmacologic dose needed for vasodilation does not usually carry enough CN for toxicity. (A) Enalapril is an angiotensin-converting enzyme (ACE) inhibitor. A well-known side effect is to cause a nonproductive cough, thought to be caused in part by accumulation of bradykinin (which is normally degraded by ACE). (B) Labetalol is a mixed α-/β-adrenergic blocker. Common side effects include weakness, drowsiness, and fatigue. (C) Losartan is an angiotensin II receptor blocker (ARB). ARBs and ACE inhibitors have similar effects (both keep angiotensin II from exerting its effects), but ARBs are not associated with cough as ACE inhibitors are. Neither cause the symptoms described in this patient. (D) Nifedipine is a dihydropyridine calcium channel blocker. A common side effect is dizziness from the reduction in blood pressure. It is not associated with the symptoms described in this patient.

20 The answer is C: Minoxidil. This description represents a common scenario of minoxidil use. Minoxidil is used to treat hypertension in patients who have failed therapy of a diuretic plus two other antihypertensives, and a common side effect is hypertrichosis. Minoxidil, in fact, is used to treat alopecia. Its mechanism of action is not entirely understood. The hair growth will regress if minoxidil is discontinued within a month or two. (A) Hydrochlorothiazide is a thiazide diuretic that works on the distal tubule. It also causes resorption of calcium into the blood. It is not known to cause hypertrichosis. (B) Isosorbide dinitrate is converted to nitric oxide (NO) in the body. NO is a potent vasodilator. It is not associated with hypertrichosis. (D) Nifedipine is a dihydropyridine calcium channel blocker. A common side effect is dizziness from the reduction in blood pressure. It is not associated with hypertrichosis. (E) Nitroglycerin is converted to NO in the body. NO is a potent vasodilator. It is not associated with hypertrichosis.

21 **The answer is E: Preventing calmodulin's activity.** Vascular smooth muscle tone is mediated by several factors. Ultimately, phosphorylation of smooth muscle myosin allows its interaction with actin to cause contraction. Myosin is phosphorylated by myosin light chain kinase, which is activated by the calcium-calmodulin complex. Nifedipine is a calcium channel blocker. It prevents calcium from entering the smooth muscle cell, so calmodulin cannot be activated. Other factors include cAMP, which inhibits myosin light chain kinase, and cGMP, which activates myosin phosphatase. Both cAMP and cGMP therefore lead to relaxation. (A) Adenylate cyclase can be activated by epinephrine binding to β_2-receptors. Nifedipine does not activate adenylate cyclase. (B) Guanylate cyclase is activated by nitric oxide (NO). Nifedipine does not activate guanylate cyclase. (C) Increased intracellular NO can be caused by nitrates, leading to activation of guanylate cyclase. Nifedipine does not cause an increase in NO. (D) Sildenafil is an example of a drug that inhibits cGMP phosphodiesterase. This leads to increased cGMP and vasodilation. Nifedipine does not inhibit cGMP phosphodiesterase.

22 **The answer is B: Dry cough.** Angiotensin-converting enzyme (ACE) inhibitors and ARBs both inhibit angiotensin II's ability to cause vasoconstriction and release of aldosterone. ACE inhibitors prevent angiotensin I from being converted to angiotensin II by ACE found in the lungs. ARBs are competitive antagonists for the angiotensin II receptors. ACE also metabolizes bradykinin. Blocking ACE leads to an increase in bradykinin, which is thought to contribute to the development of a dry cough. (A) Dizziness is a possible side effect of both ACE inhibitors and ARBs, although it is more common with high doses of ACE inhibitors. (C) Erectile dysfunction is an uncommon side effect of both ACE inhibitors and ARBs. (D) Hypotension is an uncommon side effect of both ACE inhibitors and ARBs. (E) Tinnitus is not a side effect of ACE inhibitors or ARBs. Tinnitus may be caused by ototoxic drugs such as aminoglycoside antibiotics, vancomycin, and loop diuretics.

23 **The answer is B: Bronchodilation.** Nitrous oxide decreases cerebrovascular resistance, resulting in increased perfusion of the brain. It also causes bronchodilation and decreases both spontaneous minute ventilation (volume of air per unit time moved into or out of the lungs) and hypoxic pulmonary vasoconstriction (increased pulmonary vascular resistance in poorly aerated regions of the lungs, which allows redirection of pulmonary blood flow to regions that are richer in oxygen content). (A) Airway resistance increases at the bases of the lungs. (C) Hypotension will not result from nitrous oxide administration. (D) Blood will be redirected to areas of the lung that have rich oxygen content. (E) Spontaneous minute ventilation decreases.

24 **The answer is E: Patient 5: blood pressure of 80/40 mm Hg, pulse = 60 beats/minute.** Patient 5 is in shock, with hypotension and bradycardia. For inhaled anesthetics, higher CO removes anesthetic from the alveoli faster (because of increased blood flow through the lungs) and thus slows the rate of rise in the alveolar concentration of the gas. It will therefore take longer for the gas to reach equilibrium between the alveoli and the site of action in the brain. Thus, for inhaled anesthetics, higher CO equals slower induction. Again, for inhaled anesthetics, think of the blood as a pharmacologically inactive reservoir. A low CO (shock) speeds the rate of rise of the alveolar concentration of the gas because there is less uptake (removal to peripheral tissues) to oppose input. Blood/gas partition coefficients for some inhalation anesthetics. (A) This patient has neither shock nor bradycardia. (B) This patient has neither shock nor bradycardia. (C) This patient has neither shock nor bradycardia. (D) This patient is hypotensive but is not bradycardic.

25 **The answer is C: D-dimer.** Alteplase is a recombinant form of tissue plasminogen activator (tPA). It falls under the class of drugs called fibrinolytics, meaning it leads to the breakdown of blood clots. The tPA (as its name suggests) activates tissue plasminogen, an endogenous enzyme responsible for cleaving fibrin and fibrinogen. The fibrin split products are called D-dimers, named because they are made up of two D fragments bound together. Dissolving the clot can restore blood flow to the starving myocardium. (A) AST is an enzyme found in many body cells. When these cells are damaged, AST is released into the blood and can be detected. It is not specific to myocardiocytes nor does it result from alteplase administration. (B) CK-MB is an enzyme found in myocardiocytes and skeletal muscle cells. When these cells are damaged, CK-MB is released into the blood and can be detected. It is not specific to myocardiocytes nor does it result from alteplase administration. (D) Myoglobin is a protein found in myocardiocytes and skeletal muscle cells. When these cells are damaged, myoglobin is released into the blood and can be detected. It is not specific to myocardiocytes nor does it result from alteplase administration. (E) Troponin I is a protein found in myocardiocytes. When these cells are damaged, troponin I is released into the blood and can be detected. It is specific to myocardiocytes but does not result from alteplase administration.

26 **The answer is A: Amlodipine.** Calcium channel blockers can be classified as either dihydropyridines or nondihydropyridines. Dihydropyridines are selective for the calcium channels in vascular smooth muscle and have the suffix -dipine. Amlodipine is an example of a dihydropyridine calcium channel blocker. Calcium influx into smooth muscle cells is needed by calmodulin to activate myosin light chain kinase, which phosphorylates myosin to allow interaction with actin leading to muscle contraction. Calcium channel blockers prevent the initial influx of calcium and so prevent smooth muscle contraction. (B) Diltiazem is an example of a nondihydropyridine calcium channel blocker. It affects the calcium channels in heart muscle roughly equally as well as those found in smooth muscle. (C) Losartan is an angiotensin II receptor blocker (ARB), not a calcium channel blocker. It lowers blood pressure by preventing the binding of angiotensin, which is a potent vasoconstrictor. (D) Nitroprusside is not a calcium channel blocker. It works by releasing nitric oxide, which is a potent vasodilator. (E) Verapamil is an example of a nondihydropyridine calcium channel blocker. It works primarily on the calcium channels found in heart muscle and has little effect on those found in smooth muscle.

27 **The answer is C: Blood lipids.** β-Blockers such as metoprolol are known to raise serum triglycerides and lower HDL as well as increase blood glucose. The clinical significance of these changes compared to the benefits on mortality with β-blockers has not been extensively explored, however. It should also be noted that the American Heart Association only recommends β-blockers as a first-line therapy for hypertension in patients with history of MI, heart failure, or angina. (A) β-Blockers do not commonly cause imbalances in blood calcium. Thiazide diuretics are an example of drugs that can cause hypercalcemia. Bisphosphonates are an example of drugs that can cause hypocalcemia. (B) β-Blockers do not commonly cause imbalances in blood potassium. Most diuretics cause hypokalemia, whereas potassium-sparing diuretics such as spironolactone can cause hyperkalemia. (D) β-Blockers do not commonly cause decreased creatinine clearance. Drugs that are nephrotoxic such as aminoglycosides may have this side effect. (E) β-Blockers do not commonly cause leukopenia. Drugs that cause leukopenia include many chemotherapeutics.

28 **The answer is E: Reduces preload.** Heart failure is a complex problem involving many changes to cardiovascular physiology. A decrease in cardiac output (caused by myocardial infarction in this patient's case) will lead to activation of the renin-angiotensin system and increased sympathetic activity. These in turn lead to fluid retention and increased vascular tone. Isosorbide dinitrate is converted to nitric oxide (NO) in the body, which is a potent vasodilator. Vasodilation decreases the preload on the heart. (A) Angiotensin receptor blockers (ARBs) block the activity of angiotensin II at its receptor. Angiotensin II normally causes vasoconstriction and aldosterone secretion. Aldosterone would cause sodium and water retention. (B) Diuretics such as furosemide and hydrochlorothiazide treat heart failure by causing excess fluid to be eliminated. Isosorbide dinitrate does not have a diuretic effect. (C) Cardiac glycosides such as digoxin increase inotropy. Increasing cardiac inotropy leads to an increase in cardiac output. (D) Angiotensin-converting enzyme (ACE) inhibitors block production of angiotensin II. ACE inhibitors and ARBs have a similar effect on heart failure because both interrupt the renin-angiotensin system.

29 **The answer is C: Intracellular vacuolar release of calcium.** Calcium comes from several sources. However, intracellular vacuolar release is not one of those sources. Here are the sources of intracellular calcium: The first is from outside the cell, where opening of voltage-sensitive calcium channels causes an immediate rise in free cytosolic calcium. Calcium may also enter by exchange with sodium. Calcium is also released from the sarcoplasmic reticulum and mitochondria, which further increases the cytosolic level of calcium. (A) Calcium exchange occurs with sodium. (B) Calcium is transported via voltage-sensitive channels. (D) Mitochondrial release of calcium increases cytosolic calcium. (E) Sarcoplasmic reticulum release of calcium increases cytosolic calcium.

30 **The answer is C: Sodium current can be blocked by quinidine in this phase.** During phase 0 (fast upstroke), Na^+ channels open ("fast channels") resulting in a fast inward current. Upstroke ends as Na^+ channels are rapidly inactivated. Sodium current is blocked by antiarrhythmic agents such as quinidine. (A) In phase 0, sodium channels open resulting in a fast inward current. (B) Potassium channels open and rapidly close in phase 1 (partial repolarization). (D) Transient outward current develops in phase 1 (partial repolarization). (E) Phase 1 is called partial repolarization.

31 **The answer is C: Stopping use of nonsteroidal anti-inflammatory agents.** Chronic HF is typically managed by a reduction in physical activity; low dietary intake of sodium (<1500 mg/d); treatment of comorbid conditions; and judicious use of diuretics, inhibitors of the renin-angiotensin system, and inotropic agents. Drugs that may precipitate or exacerbate HF, such as nonsteroidal anti-inflammatory drugs, alcohol, calcium channel blockers, high-dose β-blockers, and some antiarrhythmic drugs, should be avoided if possible. Patients with HF complain of

dyspnea on exertion, orthopnea, paroxysmal nocturnal dyspnea, fatigue, and dependent edema. (A) Vigorous exercise in this deconditioned patient may worsen heart function. (B) Dietary sodium intake should be reduced to 1500 mg/d or less. (D) Use of β-blockers at high doses can worsen heart failure. (E) Use of calcium channel blockers at high doses can worsen heart failure.

32 **The answer is B: Increase in exercise tolerance.** ACE inhibitors and thiazides may improve the clinical signs of heart failure. As such, patients may have some improvement in how they feel and may be able to ambulate without as much exertion. ACE inhibitors decrease vascular resistance, venous tone, and blood pressure. These drugs reduce preload and afterload, resulting in an increased cardiac output. ACE inhibitors also blunt the usual angiotensin II–mediated increase in epinephrine and aldosterone seen in HF. ACE inhibitors improve clinical signs and symptoms in patients also receiving thiazide or loop diuretics and/or digoxin. (A) Blood pressure will decrease in patients taking an ACE inhibitor. (C) Vascular resistance will decrease in patients taking an ACE inhibitor. (D) Venous tone will decrease in patients taking an ACE inhibitor. (E) Jugular venous distension is a clinical sign that may improve with ACE inhibitor therapy.

33 **The answer is D: Potassium.** Digoxin toxicity is one of the most commonly encountered adverse drug reactions. Side effects often can be managed by discontinuing cardiac glycoside therapy, determining serum potassium levels (decreased K^+ increases the potential for cardiotoxicity), and, if indicated, giving potassium supplements. In general, decreased serum levels of potassium predispose a patient to digoxin toxicity. (A) Bicarbonate is less important to follow in this patient than potassium. (B) Chloride levels are usually normal in patients with congestive heart failure and hypertension. (C) Serum glucose levels should be normal in this patient because there is no indication that they have diabetes. (E) Serum sodium levels are less problematic in patients on digoxin.

34 **The answer is B: Atrial conduction arrhythmia.** The common cardiac side effect is arrhythmia, characterized by slowing of AV conduction associated with atrial arrhythmias. A decrease in intracellular potassium is the primary predisposing factor in these effects. Gastrointestinal effects—anorexia, nausea, and vomiting—are commonly encountered adverse effects. (A) Atrial arrhythmias are more common than myocardial problems. (C) Pulmonary embolism is less common than atrial conduction defects. (D) Ventricular septal defect would not be expected in this clinical scenario. (E) Atrial arrhythmias are more common than ventricular tachycardia.

35 **The answer is C: Iatrogenic hyperthyroidism.** Amiodarone contains iodine and is related structurally to thyroxine. It has complex effects, showing class I, II, III, and IV actions. Its dominant effect is prolongation of the action potential duration and the refractory period. Amiodarone has antianginal as well as antiarrhythmic activity. Some of the side effects include interstitial pulmonary fibrosis, gastrointestinal tract intolerance, tremor, ataxia, dizziness, hyperthyroidism or hypothyroidism, liver toxicity, photosensitivity, neuropathy, muscle weakness, and blue skin discoloration caused by iodine accumulation in the skin. (A) This patient does not have hepatitis, although amiodarone is toxic to the liver. (B) This patient does not have hypertrophic cardiomyopathy. (D) This patient has no evidence of skin discoloration as would be seen with iodine toxicity. (E) This patient does not have a systemic lupus-like syndrome. She does not have a malar rash.

36 **The answer is E: Sotalol.** β-Blockers are used for long-term therapy to decrease the rate of sudden death following an acute myocardial infarction. β-Blockers have a modest ability to suppress ectopic beats and to reduce myocardial oxygen demand. They have strong antifibrillatory effects, particularly in the ischemic myocardium. Sotalol was more effective in preventing recurrence of arrhythmia and in decreasing mortality than imipramine, mexiletine, procainamide, propafenone, and quinidine in patients with sustained ventricular tachycardia. (A) Sotalol is a better antiarrhythmic than imipramine to prevent recurrent arrhythmia and decrease mortality. (B) Sotalol is a better antiarrhythmic than mexiletine to prevent recurrent arrhythmia and decrease mortality. (C) Sotalol is a better antiarrhythmic than procainamide to prevent recurrent arrhythmia and decrease mortality. (D) Sotalol is a better antiarrhythmic than propafenone to prevent recurrent arrhythmia and decrease mortality.

37 **The answer is D: Vasodilation.** Erections are mediated by the parasympathetic nervous system causing nitric oxide release from vascular endothelial cells. Nitric oxide diffuses into smooth muscle cells and stimulates guanylate cyclase to produce cGMP. The cGMP activates myosin phosphatase to dephosphorylate myosin, rendering it unable to interact with actin and relaxing the cell. The cGMP is normally broken down by a phosphodiesterase, which sildenafil inhibits to promote smooth muscle relaxation leading to vasodilation. The vasodilation allows more blood to flow into the penis than flows out, leading to erection. (A) Increasing intracellular cAMP in penile vascular smooth muscle would also lead to vasodilation and erection because cAMP inhibits phosphorylation of myosin, but sildenafil does not alter the intracellular cAMP concentrations. (B) Parasympathetic stimulation (of the pelvic nerve) would also lead to erection by

causing nitric oxide production, but sildenafil does not stimulate the parasympathetic nervous system. (C) Sympathetic stimulation is responsible for ejaculation, not erection. Sildenafil does not act on the sympathetic nervous system. (E) Vasoconstriction would inhibit erection by preventing blood from pooling in the penis. Sildenafil does not cause vasoconstriction.

38 **The answer is B: Improved automaticity in the AV node.** Adenosine is a naturally occurring nucleoside, but at high doses, the drug decreases conduction velocity, prolongs the refractory period, and decreases automaticity in the AV node. Intravenous adenosine is the drug of choice for abolishing acute supraventricular tachycardia. It has low toxicity but causes flushing, chest pain, and hypotension. Adenosine has an extremely short duration of action (approximately 15 s). (A) Hypotension is unlikely given that this agent has a duration of action of 15 s. (C) The conduction velocity will decrease. (D) The refractory period will lengthen. (E) The arrhythmia was treated through decrease in automaticity at the AV node.

39 **The answer is D: Unstable angina.** Unstable angina is classified between stable angina and myocardial infarction. In unstable angina, chest pains occur with increased frequency, duration, and intensity and are precipitated by progressively less effort. Any episode of rest angina longer than 20 min, any new onset of angina, any increasing (crescendo) angina, and even sudden development of shortness of breath is suggestive of unstable angina. The symptoms are not relieved by rest or nitroglycerin. (A) Classic angina is the most common form of angina and, therefore, is also called typical angina pectoris. It is characterized by a short-lasting burning, heavy, or squeezing feeling in the chest. (B) This patient does not have symptoms of acid reflux, chest burning, and a relationship of these symptoms to meals. (C) Prinzmetal angina is an uncommon pattern of episodic angina that occurs at rest and is caused by coronary artery spasm.

40 **The answer is C: Decreased myocardial oxygen consumption.** Nitrates inhibit coronary vasoconstriction or spasm, increasing perfusion of the myocardium and thus relieving vasospastic angina. In addition, nitrates relax the veins (venodilation), decreasing preload and myocardial oxygen consumption. Because of this action, nitrates are effective in treating effort-induced angina (classic angina). (A) Nitrates increase myocardial perfusion. (B) Nitrates decrease preload, not preventricular contractions. (D) Nitrates do not increase pulmonary artery blood flow. (E) Nitrates cause venodilation.

41 **The answer is A: Hypotension.** The most common adverse effect of nitroglycerin, as well as of the other nitrates, is headache. From 30% to 60% of patients receiving intermittent nitrate therapy with long-acting agents develop headaches. High doses of organic nitrates can also cause postural hypotension, facial flushing, and tachycardia. Phosphodiesterase V inhibitors such as sildenafil, tardenafil, and vardenafil potentiate the action of the nitrates. To preclude the dangerous hypotension that may occur, this combination is contraindicated. (B) Myocardial infarction would be a rare side effect. Profound hypotension is much more common. (C) Retinitis pigmentosa is a hereditary condition and is not induced by the combination of medications. (D) Tinnitus is unlikely. Headache and hypotension would be expected. (E) Vertigo is unlikely. Headache and hypotension would be expected.

42 **The answer is B: Decrease in smooth muscle vascular tone.** The calcium channel blockers protect the tissue by inhibiting the entrance of calcium into cardiac and smooth muscle cells of the coronary and systemic arterial beds. All calcium channel blockers are, therefore, arteriolar vasodilators that cause a decrease in smooth muscle tone and vascular resistance. At clinical doses, these agents affect primarily the resistance of peripheral and coronary arteriolar smooth muscle. Their use in the treatment of effort-induced angina relies on the reduction in myocardial oxygen consumption resulting from decreased afterload. (A) This agent causes arterial vasodilation. (C) This agent decreases myocardial oxygen consumption because of decreased afterload. (D) This agent reduces afterload. (E) This agent does not function via synchronization of the cardiac cycle.

43 **The answer is D: Ranolazine.** Ranolazine is indicated for the treatment of chronic angina and may be used alone or in combination with other traditional therapies but is most often used as an option in patients with angina who have failed all other antianginal therapies. It is not to be used to treat an acute attack of angina. (A) Diltiazem is a calcium channel blocker and a reasonable choice to be given to this patient. (B) Nifedipine is a calcium channel blocker. It could be given as a first-line agent for this patient. (C) Nitroglycerine would help the angina attacks this patient is currently having problems with. (E) Verapamil is a calcium channel blocker and a reasonable choice to be given to this patient.

44 **The answer is C: Lack of patient compliance.** Lack of patient compliance is the most common reason for failure of antihypertensive therapy. A patient with hypertension is usually asymptomatic and is diagnosed by routine screening before the occurrence of overt end-organ damage. Thus, therapy is generally directed at preventing future disease sequelae rather than relieving the patient's current discomfort. The adverse

effects associated with the hypertensive therapy may influence the patient more than the future benefits. For example, β-blockers can decrease libido and induce erectile dysfunction in males. (A) Patient noncompliance is more common than new-onset development of cardiac arrhythmia. (B) There is no reason to suggest new-onset development of diabetes in this patient. (D) Progression of hypertension is unlikely in this patient. (E) Given the history, there is no reason to suggest stroke in this patient.

45 **The answer is A: Increased levels of cAMP.** Dipyridamole increases intracellular levels of cAMP by inhibiting cyclic nucleotide phosphodiesterase, which results in decreased levels of thromboxane A_2 synthesis. It may also potentiate prostacyclin levels. (B) This agent does not cause a change in cGMP levels. (C) This agent does not cause a change in cGTP levels. (D) This agent may secondarily cause an increase in prostacyclin's ability to antagonize platelet stickiness. (E) This agent does not increase thrombin levels.

46 **The answer is B: Ethacrynic acid.** Diuresis is an important aspect of the treatment of heart failure. Putting a patient with heart failure on a diuretic will help keep excess fluid from accumulating in the lungs and other body tissues. One potential problem with diuretics is that most contain a sulfonamide group, which is the antigen responsible for reactions in patients with a sulfa allergy. Of the diuretics listed, only mannitol and ethacrynic acid do not contain a sulfonamide group. Mannitol should not be used because it is contraindicated in patients with heart failure. Ethacrynic acid is a loop diuretic but is structurally not related to other members of that group. It would be the best option in this patient. (A) Acetazolamide contains a sulfonamide group. No sulfonamide should be used in this patient because of his history of a previous allergic reaction. Further exposure could result in anaphylaxis and death. (C) Hydrochlorothiazide contains a sulfonamide group. (D) Mannitol is an osmotic diuretic. It is contraindicated in patients with heart failure because it initially increases circulatory volume and would likely make his swelling and heart failure worse. (E) Furosemide contains a sulfonamide group.

47 **The answer is A: Amiodarone.** The patient has developed a rash after only a short exposure to sunshine, suggesting photosensitivity because of the medication. There are many drugs that can cause this type of reaction. Of the antiarrhythmics listed, only amiodarone is known to cause photosensitivity. The effect is usually reversible if amiodarone is discontinued. (B) Lidocaine is also used as a local anesthetic. It crosses the blood–brain barrier and is significant for its ability to cause CNS toxicities such as dizziness, light-headedness, and confusion. It is not known to cause photosensitivity. (C) Procainamide's most commonly reported side effects are gastrointestinal, but it is also one of the causes of drug-induced lupus. Procainamide is not known to cause photosensitivity. (D) Timolol is a β-blocker type antiarrhythmic. Usually, it only leads to adverse effects related to its therapeutic action such as bradycardia and hypotension. It is not known to cause photosensitivity. (E) Verapamil is a calcium channel blocker. Its most serious adverse effects are related to its therapeutic action, including bradycardia and heart block. It is not known to cause photosensitivity.

48 **The answer is A: Prolongation of QT interval.** Droperidol is often used during endoscopy and minor surgical procedures as a sedative. It is important to know that this agent can cause prolongation of the QT interval, and it is not as commonly used today. (B) This agent is a sedative, but this would not be considered a risk; it is the therapeutic benefit of this agent. (C) T wave flattening does not occur with this agent. (D) T wave inversion does not occur with this agent. (E) Droperidol does not produce widening of the QRS interval.

49 **The answer is B: Irreversible inhibition.** Phenelzine is an irreversible inhibitor of monoamine oxidase (MAO). Aspirin is an irreversible inhibitor of cyclooxygenase (COX) enzymes. Both aspirin and phenelzine cause an irreversible inhibition of their target enzymes. This property can be a concern because of the potential for additive interactions with other drugs. For example, SNRIs should not be used with MAO inhibitors such as phenelzine, and patients taking aspirin with another antiplatelet drug must be closely monitored. (A) Aspirin irreversibly inhibits COX enzymes found throughout the body, but most cells are able to synthesize new enzymes to replace those inactivated by aspirin. Platelets lack a nucleus and cannot synthesize new COX enzymes, so daily aspirin is particularly effective against platelets. (C) Phenelzine is a monoamine oxidase inhibitor (MAOI), whereas aspirin is a COX inhibitor. These enzymes are not related. (D) This answer refers to phenelzine. Tyramine, found in many foods such as cheeses and beer, causes a release of catecholamines from presynaptic neurons. (E) Without functional MAO to break them down, the catecholamines cause prolonged stimulation of their receptors that can have fatal consequences. Even in the absence of tyramine, MAOIs can lead to hypertension by preventing the natural breakdown of catecholamines.

50 **The answer is B: Electrocardiogram.** Chloroquine should be used cautiously in patients with hepatic dysfunction or severe gastrointestinal problems and in patients with neurologic or blood disorders.

Chloroquine can cause electrocardiographic (ECG) changes because it has a quinidine-like effect. It may also exacerbate dermatitis produced by gold or phenylbutazone therapy. Thus, electrocardiogram should be performed on this patient. (A) Electrocardiogram should be performed to evaluate ECG changes. (C) Serum calcium will likely be normal in this patient. (D) Serum potassium will likely be normal in this patient. (E) Serum troponin would only be elevated in patients with myocardial injury or infarction.

51 **The answer is D: Indomethacin.** This patient's presentation is consistent with a patent ductus arteriosus. In the fetus, the ductus arteriosus is one structure that allows oxygen-rich blood from the right side of the heart to enter systemic circulation. This physiologic shunt must close around birth in order for normal circulation to take place. The ductus patency is maintained by prostaglandin E_2 (PGE_2), so a nonsteroidal anti-inflammatory drug (NSAID) such as indomethacin can be used to block prostaglandin synthesis and allow the ductus to close. (A) Acetaminophen is not an NSAID. It does inhibit cyclooxygenase enzymes but only centrally (not peripherally). Acetaminophen would not block prostaglandin synthesis at the ductus. (B) Dinoprostone is a PGE_2 analog. Administration of dinoprostone would maintain ductus patency, not help it close. (C) Dopamine is a neurotransmitter that can also stimulate β_1-adrenergic receptors at the right concentration. It is not an NSAID and would not decrease prostaglandin synthesis. (E) Propranolol is a β-adrenergic receptor blocker, not an NSAID. It would not decrease prostaglandin synthesis.

52 **The answer is E: Hypokalemia.** Particularly in a patient with cardiac disease, depletion of potassium is an adverse effect that may further compromise function. Hypokalemia can exacerbate underlying arrhythmias and contribute to toxicity. This can usually be avoided by having the patient reduce sodium intake, thus decreasing sodium delivery to the potassium-secreting collecting tubule. Additional KCl supplements or a potassium-sparing diuretic can be effective alternatives as well. (A) Diuretic-induced metabolic alkalosis is a common result of excessive diuretic therapy, not acidosis. (B) Hepatic encephalopathy can result from too much diuretic therapy in a patient suffering from edema associated with liver disease. (C) Hypercalcemia can be a medical emergency when using loop diuretics. If a marked volume contraction occurs, the diuretics become ineffective or counterproductive. Calcium reabsorption in the proximal tube can become markedly enhanced under that circumstance. This is a concern in nonedematous states. (D) Hypokalemia is normally a result of excessive diuretic therapy, not hyperkalemia.

53 **The answer is B: Dabigatran.** Dabigatran is a drug that directly inhibits thrombin. Thrombin, or clotting factor IIa, is formed by the proteolytic cleavage of certain amino acid sites on prothrombin (factor II) by factor Xa. Thrombin, in turn, cleaves certain sites on the soluble fibrinogen molecules to form insoluble fibrin strands that precipitate together, beginning clot formation. By inhibiting thrombin, dabigatran blocks the clotting cascade and prevents thromboembolism. (A) Aspirin is an antiplatelet drug, not an anticoagulant. It inhibits cyclooxygenase activity to block production of thromboxane A_2 (TXA_2), a potent platelet activator. (C) Heparin is a collection of sulfated glycosaminoglycans that activate antithrombin III, which then inactivates thrombin. Heparin does not directly inhibit thrombin. (D) Ticlopidine is an antiplatelet drug, not an anticoagulant. It is an ADP receptor antagonist and prevents platelet adhesion. (E) Warfarin is a vitamin K analog that inhibits vitamin K epoxide reductase. This enzyme is necessary for the γ-carboxylation of factors II, IV, IX, and X and proteins C and S. It does not inhibit thrombin.

54 **The answer is A: Clopidogrel.** This man's presentation is consistent with a transient ischemic attack (TIA), sometimes referred to as a "mini stroke." This occurs when cerebral blood flow is only temporarily disrupted and there is no permanent damage. To prevent a recurrence (which may be more severe), antiplatelet drugs such as aspirin or an ADP inhibitor are given. These decrease the chance of formation of future platelet plugs. Of the medications listed, only clopidogrel binds and inhibits platelet ADP receptors. (B) Enoxaparin is a preparation of low-molecular-weight heparin (LMWH). Heparin is an anticoagulant but is not an antiplatelet drug. (C) Eptifibatide is an antiplatelet drug, but it works by inhibiting Gp IIb/IIIa on platelets. It does not bind platelet ADP receptors. (D) Tirofiban is an antiplatelet drug, but it works by inhibiting Gp IIb/IIIa on platelets. It does not bind platelet ADP receptors. (E) Tissue plasminogen activator (tPA) would be given in the acute phase of ischemia because of clot formation. It does not bind platelet ADP receptors and would not be a good choice for the chemoprophylaxis this patient's needs.

55 **The answer is B: Adrenal medulla.** Although most tissues receive dual innervation, some effector organs, such as the adrenal medulla, kidney, pilomotor muscles, and sweat glands, receive innervation only from the sympathetic nervous system. The control of blood pressure is also mainly a sympathetic activity, with essentially no participation by the parasympathetic nervous system. (A) The adrenal cortex receives both sympathetic and parasympathetic innervation. (C) The heart receives both sympathetic and parasympathetic innervation. (D) The GI tract receives both sympathetic

and parasympathetic innervation. (E) The lungs receive both sympathetic and parasympathetic innervation.

56 **The answer is A: Amlodipine.** Peripheral edema is one of the most common side effects of amlodipine therapy. Amlodipine is a dihydropyridine calcium channel blocker. It works to lower blood pressure by inhibiting contraction of vascular smooth muscle. Unfortunately, this decreased vascular tone also results in tissue edema because the veins become more permeable to fluid. This reaction is dose related, so a lower dose may alleviate the edema. (B) Common side effects of docusate include nausea and diarrhea. It does not commonly cause peripheral edema. (C) A common side effect of montelukast is headache. It does not typically cause peripheral edema. (D) The most common side effects of sertraline are headache, nausea, and diarrhea. It does not commonly cause peripheral edema. (E) A common side effect of sumatriptan is a bad taste in the mouth. It does not commonly cause peripheral edema.

57 **The answer is A: Decreased cardiac output.** Decrease in heart rate and cardiac output: The actions of ACh on the heart mimic the effects of vagal stimulation. For example, if injected intravenously, ACh produces a brief decrease in cardiac rate (negative chronotropy) and stroke volume as a result of a reduction in the rate of firing at the sinoatrial (SA) node. It should be remembered that normal vagal activity regulates the heart by the release of ACh at the SA node. (B) Cardiac contractility will decrease. (C) Heart rate will decrease. (D) Stroke volume will decrease. (E) Tetanic ability will not change.

58 **The answer is A: Hydralazine.** Antihypertensive therapy is indicated if the diastolic blood pressure is repeatedly greater than 110 mm Hg. Hydralazine is the initial antihypertensive of choice and is given in 5 mg increments until blood pressure reduction is achieved. This agent will have no effect on cardiac output or renal blood flow but can cause lethargy, fever, headache, and lupus-like syndrome. (B) Labetalol is associated with a possible decrease in placental perfusion, which can manifest as decreased fetal movements. (C) Methyldopa is a β-blocker and can decrease cardiac output and renal blood flow. (D) Prazosin can increase cardiac output without change in renal blood flow. (E) This agent is a first-line therapy for hypertensive emergencies. It can only be given intravenously and has a very short duration of action.

59 **The answer is E: Wheezing.** Acebutolol is a β_1-selective antagonist, but at high doses, its β-selectivity is diminished and begins to also block β_2-receptors. Stimulation of β_2-receptors in the lungs causes bronchiolar dilation, so high doses of acebutolol could ultimately lead to wheezing because of unopposed bronchoconstriction. The risk of this side effect is greater in patients with a history of reactive airway disease. (A) Chemotherapy drugs are an example of a drug that can cause fever. Acebutolol is not known to cause fever. (B) Headache is a common side effect of many drugs, but acebutolol is not known to cause headaches. (C) QT shortening may be caused by hypercalcemic states as in vitamin D toxicity. Acebutolol does not shorten the QT interval. (D) Acebutolol blocks sympathetic stimulation of β_1-receptors on the heart, allowing unopposed parasympathetic stimulation to decrease heart rate. Bradycardia, not tachycardia, is a possible side effect of acebutolol.

60 **The answer is D: Slow CNS penetration.** Sympathomimetic amines that contain the 3,4-dihydroxybenzene group (such as epinephrine, norepinephrine, isoproterenol, and dopamine) are called catecholamines. These compounds share the following properties. Poor penetration into the CNS: Catecholamines are polar and, therefore, do not readily penetrate into the CNS. Nevertheless, most of these drugs have some clinical effects (anxiety, tremor, and headaches), which are attributable to action on the CNS. (A) Catecholamines have only a brief period of action when given parenterally, and they are ineffective when administered orally because of inactivation. (B) High potency: Drugs that are catechol derivatives (with -OH groups in the three and four positions on the benzene ring) show the highest potency in directly activating or receptors. (C) Rapid inactivation: Not only are the catecholamines metabolized by COMT postsynaptically and by MAO intraneuronally but they are also metabolized in other tissues. For example, COMT is in the gut wall and MAO is in the liver and gut wall.

61 **The answer is A: Cocaine.** Indirect-acting agonists: These agents, which include amphetamine, cocaine, and tyramine, may block the uptake of norepinephrine (uptake blockers) or are taken up into the presynaptic neuron and cause the release of norepinephrine from the cytoplasmic pools or vesicles of the adrenergic neuron. As with neuronal stimulation, the norepinephrine then traverses the synapse and binds to the α- or β-receptors. Examples of uptake blockers and agents that cause norepinephrine release include cocaine and amphetamines, respectively. (B) Epinephrine acts directly on α- or β-receptors, producing effects similar to those that occur following stimulation of sympathetic nerves or release of the hormone epinephrine from the adrenal medulla. (C) Isoproterenol acts directly on α- or β-receptors, producing effects similar to those that occur following stimulation of sympathetic nerves or release of the hormone epinephrine from the adrenal medulla. (D) Norepinephrine is a direct-acting agonist. (E) Phenylephrine is a direct-acting agonist.

62 **The answer is B: Increased AV conduction.** Dobutamine is used to increase cardiac output in acute congestive heart failure as well as for inotropic support after cardiac surgery. The drug increases cardiac output and does not significantly elevate oxygen demands of the myocardium, a major advantage over other sympathomimetic drugs. Dobutamine should be used with caution in atrial fibrillation because the drug increases AV conduction. Other adverse effects are the same as those for epinephrine. Tolerance may develop on prolonged use. (A) Atrial fibrillation results from increase in AV nodal conduction. (C) This patient unlikely is having a myocardial infarction, although it would be important to obtain cardiac enzymes to confirm this. (D) Myocardial ischemia is unlikely to result from this drug toxicity. (E) Although tolerance can develop to dobutamine, it is unlikely to cause cardiac conductivity changes.

63 **The answer is D: Phenoxybenzamine administration.** Phenoxybenzamine is used in the treatment of pheochromocytoma, a catecholamine-secreting tumor of cells derived from the adrenal medulla. Prior to surgical removal of the tumor, patients are treated with phenoxybenzamine to preclude the hypertensive crisis that can result from manipulation of the tissue. This drug is also useful in the chronic management of these tumors, particularly when the catecholamine-secreting cells are diffuse and, therefore, inoperable. (A) Epinephrine administration will worsen the hypertensive crisis that this patient currently has. (B) Fluid restriction is contraindicated. Volume expansion is suggested preoperatively. (C) Norepinephrine administration will worsen the hypertensive crisis that this patient has. (E) Phenoxybenzamine administration is required prior to surgical resection.

64 **The answer is A: Arrhythmia.** Phentolamine produces a competitive block of α_1- and α_2-receptors. This drug's action lasts for approximately 4 h after a single administration. Like phenoxybenzamine, it produces postural hypotension and causes epinephrine reversal. Phentolamine-induced reflex cardiac stimulation and tachycardia are mediated by the baroreceptor reflex and by blocking the α_2-receptors of the cardiac sympathetic nerves. The drug can also trigger arrhythmias and anginal pain, and phentolamine is contraindicated in patients with decreased coronary perfusion. (B) Tachycardia and reflex cardiac stimulation can occur after phentolamine administration. (C) No change should be observed in myocardial perfusion. (D) Anginal pain can worsen with administration of phentolamine.

65 **The answer is B: Headache.** α-Blockers may cause dizziness, lack of energy, nasal congestion, headache, drowsiness, and orthostatic hypotension (although to a lesser degree than that observed with phenoxybenzamine and phentolamine). These agents do not trigger reflex tachycardia to the same extent as the nonselective receptor blockers. (A) Lack of energy and drowsiness are common side effects of α-blockers. (C) Hypotension, not hypertension, can result from administration of α-blockers. (D) Decrease in energy and lethargy can result from administration of α-blockers. (E) Nasal congestion is a common side effect of α-blockers.

66 **The answer is D: Nebivolol.** Nebivolol has a half-life of between 12 and 30 h. β-Blockers are also effective in treating angina, cardiac arrhythmias, myocardial infarction, congestive heart failure, hyperthyroidism, and glaucoma as well as serving in the prophylaxis of migraine headaches. Note: The names of all blockers end in "-olol" except for labetalol and carvedilol. (A) Albuterol has a half-life of 3 to 4 h. (B) Esmolol has a half-life of 10 min. (C) Labetalol has a half-life of 4 to 6 h. (E) Propranolol has a half-life of 4 to 6 h.

67 **The answer is D: Potentiates other antihypertensives.** Furosemide is a loop diuretic with important interactions that treating physicians must be aware of. This agent will potentiate the action of other antihypertensives, and the patient can become hypotensive. (A) Hypokalemia will result when combined with corticosteroids. (B) Orthostatic hypotension is worsened by furosemide. (C) Ototoxicity results when furosemide is combined with aminoglycoside antibiotics.

68 **The answer is A: Increase in blood pressure.** There are several clinical uses of dopamine depending on the dose used. When high-dose dopamine is used, there is an increase in blood pressure, heart rate, and contractility. There is a decrease in renal blood flow. Low-dose dopamine increases renal blood flow only. (B) High-dose dopamine causes an increase in heart rate. (C) High-dose dopamine causes an increase in cardiac contractility. (D) High-dose dopamine causes a decrease in renal blood flow. (E) High-dose dopamine does not change urine output.

69 **The answer is A: Decreased secretion of aqueous humor.** β-Blockers, such as topically applied timolol, betaxolol, or carteolol, are effective in diminishing intraocular pressure in glaucoma. This occurs by decreasing the secretion of aqueous humor by the ciliary body. Many patients with glaucoma have been maintained with these drugs for years. These drugs neither affect the ability of the eye to focus for near vision nor change pupil size, as do the cholinergic drugs. When

administered to the eye, the onset is about 30 min, and the effects last for 12 to 24 h. (B) Cholinergic drugs may improve the eye's ability to focus. (C) Cholinergic drugs may improve pupil size. β-Blockers do not change pupil size. (D) β-Blockers do not improve near vision abilities. (E) β-Blockers will decrease intraocular pressure.

70 **The answer is A: Ascending limb of the loop of Henle.** Furosemide, bumetanide, and ethacrynic acid exert their effects on the ascending limb of the loop of Henle. Osmotic diuretics work mostly on the proximal tubule. Thiazides work mainly on the distal tubule. Spironolactone, amiloride, and triamterene exert their effects on the collecting ducts. (B) Potassium-sparing diuretics act on the collecting ducts. (C) Thiazides work mainly on the distal tubule. (D) Osmotic diuretics work mostly on the proximal tubule.

71 **The answer is B: Atenolol.** Atenolol is a β_1-antagonist and is effective in lowering blood pressure in patients with hypertension. Side effects of blockers include fatigue and exercise intolerance. (A) Albuterol will not change blood pressure in this patient. (C) Ephedrine is not an antihypertensive agent. (D) Phentolamine does not generally cause fatigue in patients. (E) Prazosin is an antagonist that usually does not cause fatigue.

72 **The answer is B: Nicotine-induced vasoconstriction.** Many patients with peripheral vascular disease experience an exacerbation of symptoms with smoking. For example, nicotine-induced vasoconstriction can decrease coronary blood flow, adversely affecting a patient with angina. Stimulation of parasympathetic ganglia also increases motor activity of the bowel. At higher doses, blood pressure falls, and activity ceases in both the gastrointestinal (GI) tract and bladder musculature as a result of a nicotine-induced block of parasympathetic ganglia. (A) There is no indication that this patient has suffered a cardiac event. (C) Pulmonary embolism can occur because of hypercoagulable state, but this is unlikely, given the presentation of this patient. (D) No data is given to suggest stroke volume change. (E) No cardiac findings have been given to suggest valvular dysfunction in this patient.

73 **The answer is C: Pupillary dilation.** Peripherally, cocaine potentiates the action of norepinephrine, and it produces the "fight-or-flight" syndrome characteristic of adrenergic stimulation. This is associated with tachycardia, hypertension, pupillary dilation, and peripheral vasoconstriction. Recent evidence suggests that the ability of baroreceptor reflexes to buffer the hypertensive effect may be impaired. (A) Tachycardia, not bradycardia, will occur as a result of adrenergic stimulation. (B) Hypertension, not hypotension, will occur as a result of adrenergic stimulation. (D) Vasoconstriction of peripheral vasculature will occur.

74 **The answer is D: Sedation.** General anesthesia is a reversible state of central nervous system (CNS) depression, resulting in loss of response to and perception of external stimuli. For patients undergoing surgical and other medical procedures, anesthesia provides these five important benefits: sedation and reduction of anxiety, lack of awareness and amnesia, skeletal muscle relaxation, suppression of undesirable reflexes, and analgesia. (A) General anesthesia should decrease anxiety. (B) General anesthesia should decrease awareness. (C) General anesthesia should suppress perception of external stimuli. (E) General anesthesia should cause skeletal muscle relaxation.

75 **The answer is C: Sleep apnea.** Identifiable causes of hypertension include sleep apnea, drug induced, chronic kidney disease, primary aldosteronism, renovascular disease, pheochromocytoma, and thyroid and parathyroid disease. (A) Acute renal insufficiency is not an identifiable cause of hypertension. (B) Atrial septal defect is not an identifiable cause of hypertension. (D) Tuberculosis is not an identifiable cause of hypertension. (E) Viral pneumonia is not an identifiable cause of hypertension.

76 **The answer is C: Lisinopril.** This patient with diabetes has been diagnosed with hypertension and diabetic nephropathy. Angiotensin-converting enzyme (ACE) inhibitors are the first-choice medications for patients with diabetes and hypertension. This is caused by the combined effect of ACE inhibitors as an antihypertensive and its renal protective effects. (A) Doxazosin is an α_1-selective α-blocker that is used to treat hypertension as well as urinary retention secondary to benign prostatic hyperplasia. (B) Hydrochlorothiazide is a thiazide diuretic that is the most common initial medication for essential hypertension. Because of the patient having diabetes with the initial stages of protein-losing nephropathy, lisinopril is a better choice as the initial antihypertensive. (D) Metoprolol is a β_1-selective blocker that may be used as an initial antihypertensive in patients with compensated CHF or history of coronary artery disease. (E) Nifedipine is a calcium channel blocker that is used commonly to treat isolated systolic hypertension.

77 **The answer is E: Pulmonary fibrosis.** Amiodarone has several well-known side effects, including pulmonary fibrosis, hepatotoxicity, and thyroid imbalances. For this reason, pulmonary function tests, liver function tests, and thyroid function tests should be monitored while taking amiodarone. (A) Blurry yellow vision is

a common side effect of digoxin toxicity, not amiodarone. (B) Impotence is a common side effect of β-blockers, not amiodarone. (C) Lupus-like syndrome is a common side effect of procainamide, not amiodarone. (D) Prolongation of the AV refractory period is a common side effect of class Ic antiarrhythmics, such as flecainide, encainide, and propafenone, not amiodarone.

78 **The answer is D: LMWH is easier to manage for outpatients.** Unfractionated heparin is a collection of sulfated glycosaminoglycans that activate antithrombin III, which then inactivates thrombin and factor Xa. Heparin itself does not directly inhibit any of these. Molecules of heparin smaller than 18 monosaccharide units do not lead to thrombin inhibition, only inhibition of factor X. LMWH has an average size smaller than this, so LMWH inhibits factor X better than it inhibits thrombin. A benefit of LMWH is that it can be used in an outpatient setting, whereas UFH therapy must be followed by laboratory testing. (A) LMWH actually leads to inhibition of factor Xa better than inhibition of thrombin. UFH causes better inhibition of thrombin than LMWH does. (B) LMWH is an anticoagulant and carries a risk of hemorrhage. Even though LMWH is not as strong an inhibitor of thrombin as UFH is, it causes sufficient anticoagulation to carry a risk of bleeding. (C) Heparin-induced thrombocytopenia is caused by platelet-activating antibodies made against the heparin-platelet factor 4 (PF4) complex. LMWH carries a lower risk of HIT than UFH but can cause HIT. (E) LMWH and UFH are made up of large, negatively charged particles. Protamine is strongly positively charged and forms a salt with LMWH and UFH molecules to deactivate them. Protamine works less well against LMWH than it does against UFH.

79 **The answer is A: AV node, increases efflux of K^+.** Adenosine causes a transient (less than 15 sec) heart block at the AV node. This is achieved because adenosine inhibits adenylyl cyclase, which reduces cAMP and causes the efflux of K^+ from cardiac cells. This leads to hyperpolarization and decreased intracellular Ca^{2+}. Adenosine is commonly used to treat supraventricular tachycardia. (B) Adenosine does act at the AV node, but it increases the efflux of K^+, not influx. (C) Adenosine does decrease intracellular Ca^{2+}, but it acts at the AV node, not the SA node. (D) Adenosine does increase the efflux of K^+, but it acts at the AV node, not the SA node. (E) Adenosine does act at the AV node and increases the efflux of K^+.

80 **The answer is E: Increases prothrombin time.** Warfarin inhibits vitamin K metabolism and therefore inactivates vitamin K–dependent clotting factors II, VII, IX, and X. This affects the extrinsic pathway of the clotting cascade and causes an increase in the prothrombin time. (A) Warfarin does not affect the partial thromboplastin time. (B) Warfarin does affect the prothrombin time, but it increases the prothrombin time, not decreases. (C) Warfarin does not affect the bleeding time. (D) Heparin increase the partial thromboplastin time, not warfarin.

81 **The answer is C: Converts plasminogen to plasmin.** Alteplase is a tissue plasminogen activator, which converts plasminogen to plasmin. Plasmin cleaves thrombin and fibrin clots. Alteplase is used in ischemic strokes in an attempt to restore blood flow to the brain. (A) Abciximab is a monoclonal antibody that binds to glycoprotein receptor IIb/IIIa to inhibit platelet aggregation. (B) The mechanism of action of clopidogrel is irreversibly block ADP receptors on platelets to prevent platelet aggregation. (D) The mechanism of action of aspirin is irreversibly inhibiting COX-1 and COX-2. (E) The mechanism of action of lepirudin is the direct inhibition of thrombin.

82 **The answer is D: Scopolamine.** Phenylephrine causes contraction of the dilator muscle by stimulating α_1-receptors to induce mydriasis. Any other drug that stimulates the α_1-adrenergic receptors in the eye will likewise cause mydriasis. Mydriasis would also result from inhibition of the parasympathetic nervous system because the parasympathetic nervous system causes miosis. Of the drugs listed, only scopolamine would block the cholinergic stimulation from the parasympathetic nervous system. (A) Methacholine is a direct cholinergic agonist. It would stimulate cholinergic receptors in the iris and cause miosis, not mydriasis. (B) Neostigmine is an indirect cholinergic agonist. It would lead to stimulation of cholinergic receptors in the iris and cause miosis, not mydriasis. (C) Phentolamine is an α-adrenergic antagonist. It would inhibit adrenergic stimulation of the iris and lead to miosis. (E) Terazosin is an α_1-adrenergic antagonist. It would inhibit adrenergic stimulation of the iris and lead to miosis.

83 **The answer is B: Epinephrine.** Vanillylmandelic acid is the end product of catecholamine metabolism. Three important catecholamines in the body are dopamine, epinephrine, and norepinephrine. Elevated levels of vanillylmandelic acid in this patient's case likely signify an increase in serum epinephrine and norepinephrine. Catecholamine synthesis starts with the amino acid tyrosine. Tyrosine is converted to dihydroxyphenylalanine, or L-dopa, by tyrosine hydroxylase. L-dopa is then converted to dopamine by dopa decarboxylase. Dopamine can be metabolized to homovanillic acid by a two-step process involving monoamine oxidase (MAO) and catechol-*O*-methyltransferase (COMT). Dopamine can also be converted to norepinephrine by dopamine β-hydroxylase. Epinephrine is made from norepinephrine by phenylethanolamine N-methyltransferase (PNMT). Both epinephrine and norepinephrine can be converted to dihydroxymandelic acid by MAO, which is then metabolized to vanillylmandelic acid by COMT. Alternatively, COMT can first convert epinephrine to metanephrine and norepinephrine to normetanephrine. Metanephrine and normetanephrine are then converted to vanillylmandelic acid by MAO. (A) Acetylcholine is the primary neurotransmitter of the peripheral nervous system. Vanillylmandelic acid levels have no connection to levels of acetylcholine. (C) Glutamate is an important CNS stimulatory neurotransmitter. Vanillylmandelic acid levels have no connection to levels of glutamate. (D) Oxytocin is a neuroendocrine peptide hormone that plays an important role in stimulating uterine contractions. Vanillylmandelic acid levels have no connection to levels of oxytocin. (E) Serotonin levels are elevated in carcinoid syndrome, but serotonin is metabolized into 5-hydroxyindoleacetic acid. Vanillylmandelic acid levels have no connection to levels of oxytocin.

84 **The answer is B: Brimonidine.** Brimonidine is an α_2-agonist that decreases the synthesis of aqueous humor. α_2-Agonists inhibit adenylate cyclase, which decreases cAMP and leads to decreased aqueous humor production in the ciliary body. (A) The mechanism of action of acetazolamide is to decrease the secretion of aqueous humor by inhibiting carbonic anhydrase. (C) Latanoprost increases the outflow of aqueous humor; it does not decrease production. (D) Pilocarpine increases the outflow of aqueous humor; it does not decrease production. (E) Timolol is a β-blocker that decreases aqueous humor secretion.

85 **The answer is B: Dantrolene.** Dantrolene is used to treat malignant hyperthermia and neuroleptic malignant syndrome. Dantrolene works by preventing the release of calcium from the sarcoplasmic reticulum in skeletal muscles. (A) Bromocriptine is used for treatment of neuroleptic malignant syndrome but not malignant hyperthermia. (C) Diphenhydramine is used to treat allergy symptoms. It is not used for malignant hyperthermia. (D) Nitric oxide is an inhalation anesthetic that causes malignant hyperthermia and therefore should be stopped when symptoms of malignant hyperthermia develop. (E) Succinylcholine is an inhalation anesthetic that causes malignant hyperthermia and therefore should be stopped when symptoms of malignant hyperthermia develop.

86 **The answer is C: Reduces intracranial pressure.** Although propofol facilitates depression in the CNS, it is occasionally accompanied by excitatory phenomena, such as muscle twitching, spontaneous movement, and hiccups. Propofol decreases blood pressure without depressing the myocardium. It also reduces intracranial pressure mainly because of systemic vasodilation. It has much less of a depressant effect than the volatile anesthetics on CNS-evoked potentials such as somatosensory-evoked potentials. This makes propofol useful for such surgeries as resection of spinal tumors in which somatosensory-evoked potentials are monitored to assess spinal cord functions. (A) Propofol decreases blood pressure. (B) Propofol does not cause myocardial depression. (D) There is limited depression of somatosensory-evoked potentials. (E) This agent causes systemic vasodilation.

87 **The answer is B: Dizziness.** The -zosin drugs such as terazosin, prazosin, and doxazosin are α_1-adrenergic antagonists. Stimulation of α_1-receptors leads to an increase in intracellular calcium and smooth muscle contraction. Contraction of the smooth muscle of the prostate narrows the prostatic urethra, impeding urine outflow. Terazosin helps with the symptoms of benign prostatic hypertrophy by blocking the contraction of prostatic smooth muscle. One of the most common side effects is dizziness because of impaired vasoconstriction. (A) Diarrhea is not commonly associated with terazosin use. As an α_1-blocker, terazosin impairs vasoconstriction and can lead to dizziness. (C) Flatulence is not commonly associated with terazosin use. As an α_1-blocker, terazosin impairs vasoconstriction and can lead to dizziness. (D) Headache has not been shown to be associated with terazosin use. Dizziness, on the other hand, affected up to 19% of patients in some studies. (E) Priapism is not commonly associated with terazosin use. Trazodone is a drug known to be associated with priapism.

88 **The answer is D: Salmeterol.** α- and β-Adrenergic receptors are members of the G protein–coupled receptor (GPCR) class. These receptors are embedded in the cell membrane by a seven-pass transmembrane domain. They also have an extracellular ligand-binding domain and an intracellular domain that exchanges a GTP for a GDP in the associated G protein, activating the G protein to exert its downstream effects. Epinephrine binds to both receptor types, but stimulation of β_2-receptors is responsible for the improvement in his breathing. β-Selective agonists, such as albuterol and salmeterol, are used for this purpose in cases of asthma exacerbation. (A) Acebutolol is a β_1 (cardioselective)-adrenergic antagonist. It does not stimulate β_2-receptors. (B) Phenylephrine is an α_1-adrenergic agonist used as a nasal decongestant, pressor, and pupil dilator. It does not stimulate β_2-receptors. (C) Prazosin is an α_1-adrenergic antagonist used to treat high blood pressure and prostatic hyperplasia. It does not stimulate β_2-receptors. (E) Timolol is a nonselective β-adrenergic receptor blocker used to treat high blood pressure. It does not stimulate β_2-receptors.

89 **The answer is E: Thick ascending loop of Henle.** Furosemide acts on the $Na^+/K^+/2Cl^-$ cotransport in the thick ascending loop of Henle. Furosemide is used in fluid overloaded states, such as congestive heart failure, nephrotic syndrome, and pulmonary edema. (A) Potassium-sparing diuretics, such as spironolactone, act on the collecting tubule. (B) Mannitol, an osmotic diuretic, acts on the descending loop of Henle and the proximal convoluted tubule. (C) Hydrochlorothiazide acts on the distal convoluted tubule. (D) Acetazolamide, a carbonic anhydrase inhibitor, acts on the proximal convoluted tubule.

90 **The answer is E: Triamterene.** Potassium-sparing diuretics such as triamterene or amiloride are commonly used in combination with more potent potassium-wasting diuretics (e.g., loop diuretics) or simply in cases of low serum potassium. Potassium is lost in the urine when high amounts of sodium pass through the distal convoluted tubule (as is the case with potassium-wasting diuretics) because of a sodium-potassium exchange pump on the distal tubule cells. Triamterene and amiloride inhibit this pump, leaving sodium in the urine and potassium in the blood. (A) Acetazolamide is a carbonic anhydrase inhibitor and works in the proximal tubule. It causes mild potassium loss in the urine. (B) Loop diuretics such as ethacrynic acid work by inhibiting the $Na^+/K^+/2Cl^-$ transporter on the ascending limb of the loop of Henle. Loop diuretics are potassium-wasting diuretics. (C) Hydrochlorothiazide inhibits the sodium chloride symporter in the distal tube. It causes calcium retention by an unknown mechanism but does not cause potassium retention. (D) Methazolamide is a carbonic anhydrase inhibitor and works in the proximal tubule. It causes mild potassium loss in the urine.

91 **The answer is C: Increases intracellular cAMP.** This description represents a common scenario of minoxidil use. Minoxidil is used to treat hypertension in patients that have failed therapy of a diuretic plus two other antihypertensives, and a common side effect is hypertrichosis. Minoxidil, in fact, is used to treat alopecia. Its mechanism of action is not entirely understood. The hair growth will regress if minoxidil is discontinued within a month or two. It is a direct vasodilator that appears to work at least in part by inhibiting cAMP breakdown in arterial smooth muscle. (A) Dihydropyridine calcium channel blockers such as nifedipine and amlodipine decrease blood pressure by impairing contraction of vascular smooth muscle. Minoxidil does not block calcium channels. (B) Hydrochlorothiazide is a diuretic that blocks Na^+ reabsorption in the renal distal tubule. Minoxidil does not lower blood pressure through diuresis. (D) Nitroglycerin is converted to nitric oxide (NO) in the body, which is a potent vasodilator. Minoxidil does not work by increasing NO. (E) Angiotensin-converting enzyme (ACE) inhibitors such as lisinopril block production of angiotensin II. Minoxidil does not inhibit angiotensin production.

92 **The answer is B: Activation of guanylate cyclase.** Vascular smooth muscle tone is mediated by several factors. Ultimately, phosphorylation of smooth muscle myosin allows its interaction with actin to cause contraction. Myosin is phosphorylated by myosin light chain kinase, which is activated by the calcium-calmodulin complex. Other factors include cAMP, which inhibits myosin light chain kinase, and cGMP, which activates myosin phosphatase. Both cAMP and cGMP therefore lead to relaxation. Nitroglycerin causes an increase in intracellular NO, which leads to activation of guanylate cyclase. (A) Adenylate cyclase can be activated by epinephrine binding to β_2-receptors. Nitroglycerin does not activate adenylate cyclase. (C) Nifedipine is a calcium channel blocker. It prevents calcium from entering the smooth muscle cell, so calmodulin cannot be activated. (D) Sildenafil is an example of a drug that inhibits cGMP phosphodiesterase. This leads to increased cGMP and vasodilation. Nitroglycerin does not inhibit cGMP phosphodiesterase. (E) Nifedipine is a calcium channel blocker. It prevents calcium from entering the smooth muscle cell, so calmodulin cannot be activated.

93 **The answer is D: No change in heart rate.** Morphine has no major effects on the blood pressure or heart rate except at large doses at which hypotension and bradycardia may occur. Because of respiratory depression and carbon dioxide retention, cerebral vessels dilate and increase cerebrospinal fluid (CSF) pressure. Therefore, morphine is usually contraindicated in individuals with head or severe brain injury. (A) Morphine has no major effects on the blood pressure or heart rate except at large doses. (B) This animal will have normal blood pressure. (C) This animal will have normal blood pressure. (E) This animal will have normal heart rate.

94 **The answer is B: Activates plasminogen.** Alteplase is a recombinant form of tissue plasminogen activator (tPA). It falls under the class of drugs called fibrinolytics, meaning it leads to the breakdown of blood clots. The tPA (as its name suggests) activates tissue plasminogen, an endogenous enzyme responsible for cleaving fibrin and fibrinogen. The fibrin split products are called D-dimers, named because they are made up of two D fragments bound together. Dissolving the clot can restore blood flow to the

oxygen-starved myocardium. (A) Antithrombin III is activated by heparin and inhibits thrombin to stop further clot formation. Alteplase does not activate antithrombin III. (C) Thrombin is the enzyme responsible for cleaving fibrinogen into fibrin to form a clot. Activating thrombin would not be beneficial to this patient. Alteplase does not activate thrombin. (D) Aspirin is a drug with antiplatelet properties because it inhibits platelet production of procoagulating thromboxane A_2 (TXA_2). Alteplase does not inhibit TXA_2 production. (E) Clopidogrel is an antiplatelet drug that inhibits platelet activation by blocking ADP receptors. Alteplase does not block ADP receptors.

95 **The answer is F: Class IV.** Verapamil is a calcium channel blocker. It can be employed to treat supraventricular tachycardias such as atrial fibrillation and atrial flutter. Verapamil works by slowing signal conduction through the atrioventricular (AV) node. This prevents the spread of arrhythmias from the atria to the ventricles. Calcium channel blockers are categorized as class IV antiarrhythmics under the Singh–Vaughan Williams classification. (A) Class Ia contains drugs that block sodium channels with moderate affinity. Class Ia drugs also produce a moderate block on potassium channels. (B) Class Ib contains drugs that block sodium channels with low affinity. They bind best to sodium channels that are more frequently open, providing a use-dependent blockade. (C) Class Ic contains drugs that block sodium channels with high affinity, producing a steady blockade. (D) Class II contains β-adrenergic blockers such as metoprolol. β-Blockers as antiarrhythmic drugs act by slowing conduction through the AV node, similar to calcium channel blockers. (E) Class III contains drugs that block potassium channels, slowing repolarization. This increases the refractory period following each action potential making cells less likely to depolarize at inappropriate times.

96 **The answer is A: Aldosterone receptor antagonist.** The mechanism of action of spironolactone is as an aldosterone receptor antagonist. The aldosterone receptors are found in the cortical collecting tubule of the nephron. It is commonly used because of its potassium-sparing characteristics. (B) The mechanism of action of acetazolamide is the inhibition of carbonic anhydrase. (C) The mechanism of action of hydrochlorothiazide is inhibiting NaCl reabsorption in the distal tubule. (D) The mechanism of action of furosemide is the inhibition of the $Na^+/K^+/2Cl^-$ cotransport. (E) The mechanism of action of mannitol is through osmotic diuresis in the proximal tubule.

97 **The answer is D: Blood urea nitrogen.** Fosinopril is an angiotensin-converting enzyme (ACE) inhibitor. ACE normally converts angiotensinogen into angiotensin II (ATII), which is a potent vasoconstrictor. Fosinopril lowers blood pressure by decreasing the amount of circulating ATII. In patients with heart failure, chronic kidney disease, or bilateral renal artery stenosis, ACE inhibitors can precipitate a reduction in GFR and rise in BUN. This patient's history of myocardial infarction places him at increased risk for a rise in BUN following fosinopril use. (A) ACE inhibitors do not commonly cause imbalances in blood calcium. Thiazide diuretics are an example of drugs that can cause hypercalcemia. Bisphosphonates are an example of drugs that can cause hypocalcemia. (B) ACE inhibitors do not commonly cause imbalances in blood potassium. Most diuretics cause hypokalemia, whereas potassium-sparing diuretics such as spironolactone can cause hyperkalemia. (C) ACE inhibitors are not known to disrupt a patient's lipid profile. β-Blockers may raise triglycerides and lower HDL. (E) ACE inhibitors do not commonly cause leukopenia. Drugs that cause leukopenia include many chemotherapeutics.

98 **The answer is E: Orthostatic hypotension.** Tamsulosin is an α_1-receptor antagonist used to treat benign prostatic hyperplasia because of its ability to relax smooth muscle. Although it is selective for prostatic α-receptors, and not vascular, orthostatic hypotension has still been reported. (A) A common side effect of ACE inhibitors is cough. (B) Hemorrhagic cystitis is seen with cyclophosphamide, not tamsulosin. (C) Oral contraceptive pills have been known to cause a hypercoagulable state. (D) Sildenafil, not tamsulosin, can cause impaired blue-green vision.

99 **The answer is A: Drowsiness and blurred vision would be expected.** Pregabalin binds to the secondary site, an auxiliary subunit of voltage-gated calcium channels in the CNS, inhibiting excitatory neurotransmitter release. The exact role this plays in treatment is not known, but the drug has proven effects on partial-onset seizures, neuropathic pain associated with diabetic peripheral neuropathy, postherpetic neuralgia, and fibromyalgia. More than 90% of pregabalin is eliminated renally, with no indication of CYP involvement. Drowsiness, blurred vision, weight gain, and peripheral edema have been reported. (B) This medication is excreted renally. (C) She will likely have improvement in seizures and neuropathic pain. (D) Her neuropathic pain will likely improve with this agent. (E) She will likely experience weight gain.

100 **The answer is C: Increases cardiac inotropy.** Heart failure is a complex problem involving many changes to cardiovascular physiology. A decrease in cardiac output (caused by myocardial infarction in this patient's case) will lead to activation of the renin-angiotensin system and increased sympathetic activity. These in

turn lead to fluid retention and increased vascular tone. Cardiac glycosides such as digoxin increase inotropy, which leads to an increase in cardiac output. (A) Angiotensin receptor blockers (ARBs) block the activity of angiotensin II at its receptor. Angiotensin II normally causes vasoconstriction and aldosterone secretion. Aldosterone would cause sodium and water retention. (B) Diuretics such as furosemide and hydrochlorothiazide treat heart failure by causing excess fluid to be eliminated. Digoxin does not have a diuretic effect. (D) Angiotensin-converting enzyme (ACE) inhibitors block production of angiotensin II. ACE inhibitors and ARBs have a similar effect on heart failure because both interrupt the renin-angiotensin system. (E) Isosorbide dinitrate is converted to nitric oxide (NO) in the body, which is a potent vasodilator. Vasodilation decreases the preload on the heart. Digoxin does not work by reducing preload.

101 The answer is B: Loss of cardiac myocytes. Chronic activation of the sympathetic nervous system and the renin-angiotensin-aldosterone axis is associated with remodeling of cardiac tissue, characterized by loss of myocytes, hypertrophy, and fibrosis. This prompts additional neurohumoral activation, creating a vicious cycle that, if left untreated, leads to death. (A) Chronic activation of the sympathetic nervous system occurs in heart failure. (C) Cardiac muscle hypertrophy occurs with heart failure. (D) Cardiac muscle fibrosis occurs with heart failure. (E) The geometry of the heart becomes less elliptical and more spherical, interfering with its ability to efficiently function as a pump.

102 The answer is A: Antibiotics. The goals of treatment of heart failure are to alleviate symptoms, slow disease progression, and improve survival. Accordingly, six classes of drugs have been shown to be effective: (1) inhibitors of the renin-angiotensin system, (2) β-adrenoreceptor blockers, (3) diuretics, (4) direct vasodilators, (5) inotropic agents, and (6) aldosterone antagonists. Antibiotics will not likely help this patient's symptoms. (B) β-Blockers will improve symptoms in this patient. (C) Diuretics will improve symptoms in this patient. (D) Inhibitors of the renin-angiotensin system will improve symptoms in this patient. (E) Inotropic agents are going to be important in treating this patient.

103 The answer is A: Dilated cardiac chambers. The heart increases in size, and the chambers dilate and become more globular. Initially, stretching of the heart muscle leads to a stronger contraction of the heart. However, excessive elongation of the fibers results in weaker contractions, and the geometry diminishes the ability to eject blood. This type of failure is termed "systolic failure" and is the result of a ventricle being unable to pump effectively. Less commonly, patients with HF may have "diastolic dysfunction," a term applied when the ability of the ventricles to relax and accept blood is impaired by structural changes such as hypertrophy. The thickening of the ventricular wall and subsequent decrease in ventricular volume decrease the ability of heart muscle to relax. In this case, the ventricle does not fill adequately, and the inadequacy of cardiac output is termed "diastolic HF." (B) The heart will have increased in size and became more globular. (C) The heart will have stretching of the muscles. (D) The heart would have decreased ability to eject blood. (E) The ventricular wall becomes thickened.

104 The answer is E: Use of nonsteroidal anti-inflammatory medications. Chronic heart failure is typically managed by a reduction in physical activity; low dietary intake of sodium (<1500 mg/d); treatment of comorbid conditions; and judicious use of diuretics, inhibitors of the renin-angiotensin system, and inotropic agents. Drugs that may precipitate or exacerbate HF, such as nonsteroidal anti-inflammatory drugs, alcohol, calcium channel blockers, high-dose β-blockers, and some antiarrhythmic drugs, should be avoided if possible. (A) Elimination of alcohol would help in improving this patient's overall health. (B) Low-sodium diet may improve blood pressure and fluid balance. (C) Judicious use of diuretics will help blood pressure control. (D) Treatment of this patient's underlying diabetes mellitus will help in his overall health.

105 The answer is C: Hydrochlorothiazide. A side effect of hydrochlorothiazide is hyperglycemia. The exact mechanism of the cause of hyperglycemia is unknown; however, it is believed to be through decreased insulin secretion. (A) Acetazolamide can lead to hyperchloremic metabolic acidosis but not commonly hyperglycemia. (B) Furosemide may lead to ototoxicity or hypokalemia but not commonly hyperglycemia. (D) Mannitol may lead to pulmonary edema but not commonly hyperglycemia. (E) Spironolactone may lead to gynecomastia or hyperkalemia but not commonly hyperglycemia.

106 The answer is C: Lithium. Antidiuretic hormone (ADH) is normally only secreted in response to hypovolemia and increased serum osmolarity. When ADH is inappropriately secreted (as in ADH secretion by cancer cells), serum sodium concentration is diminished because the kidneys retain too much free water. This is known as the syndrome of inappropriate ADH secretion (SIADH). Demeclocycline (a tetracycline antibiotic) and lithium correct this by blocking ADH's effects on the kidney's collecting ducts. (A) Cobalt is an essential nutrient as part of vitamin B_{12}, also known as cobalamin. It has no role in the treatment of SIADH. (B) Iron is the metal ion found in many important mammalian proteins and enzymes such as hemoglobin and cytochromes. It would not be useful to treat SIADH. (D) Magnesium is important in hundreds of human enzyme-catalyzed reactions, including all enzymes involved in ATP synthesis. It would not be useful to treat SIADH. (E) Selenium is an antioxidant that functions as a cofactor for glutathione peroxidase—the enzyme that catalyzes the reaction that uses glutathione to break down hydrogen peroxide. It would not be useful to treat SIADH.

107 **The answer is D: Increasing sympathetic tone.** Normally, erections are mediated by the parasympathetic nervous system causing nitric oxide release from vascular endothelial cells. Nitric oxide diffuses into smooth muscle cells and stimulates guanylate cyclase to produce cGMP, which activates myosin phosphatase to dephosphorylate myosin, rendering it unable to interact with actin and relaxing the cell. This relaxation leads to vasodilation, allowing more blood to flow into the penis than flows out that causes an erection. Yohimbine is thought to bypass the parasympathetic pathway and cause an increase in penile blood flow by blocking α_2-adrenergic receptors (negative feedback receptors) centrally. This increases sympathetic tone to increase penile blood flow. (A) Normally, parasympathetic tone directly causes erection. Decreasing parasympathetic tone would not result in an erection nor is this yohimbine's mechanism of action. (B) Vasoconstriction would impair this patient's ability to achieve erection. Yohimbine causes increased blood flow, not vasoconstriction. (C) Vasodilation would help this patient achieve an erection and is likely part of yohimbine's mechanism of action, although yohimbine indirectly causes vasodilation. Sildenafil is a drug that causes direct vasodilation. (E) Stimulation of the pudendal nerve would lead to erection, but this is not yohimbine's mechanism of action. Yohimbine likely works by blocking α_2-adrenergic receptors in order to increase sympathetic tone and ultimately penile blood flow.

108 **The answer is E: Relaxes prostatic smooth muscle.** Prazosin and terazosin are examples of α_1-antagonists. These are used to treat BPH because by blocking α_1-receptors, they lead to relaxation of prostatic smooth muscle. This makes it easier for urine to flow through the prostate. Prazosin and terazosin can also be used to treat hypertension because antagonizing α_1-receptors they decrease vascular tone. (A) α_2-Receptors are negative feedback receptors; antagonizing these receptors would increase norepinephrine release. This would ultimately increase prostatic smooth muscle contraction and worsen this patient's symptoms. (B) Prazosin works by inhibiting α_1-receptors to cause prostatic smooth muscle relaxation. Finasteride is a drug that blocks synthesis of DHT. (C) Finasteride is a drug that inhibits the enzyme 5-α-reductase. This enzyme is responsible for DHT production, which is a hormone that drives prostate enlargement. Prazosin does not block 5-α-reductase. (D) Ketoconazole is a drug that can be used to inhibit testosterone synthesis (useful in polycystic ovarian syndrome). Prazosin does not inhibit testosterone synthesis.

109 **The answer is C: Extensive first-pass metabolism.** Losartan, the first approved member of the class, differs from the others in that it undergoes extensive first-pass hepatic metabolism, including conversion to its active metabolite. The other drugs have inactive metabolites. Elimination of metabolites and parent compounds occurs in urine and feces. The proportion is dependent on the individual drug. All are highly plasma protein bound (greater than 90%). (A) Losartan is converted to an active metabolite. (B) Losartan is eliminated via urine and feces. (D) Losartan has extensive binding to plasma proteins. (E) Losartan is not commonly associated with development of renal failure.

110 **The answer is D: Potassium.** Digoxin can cause electrolyte abnormalities. Hypokalemia can precipitate serious arrhythmia. Reduction of serum potassium levels is most frequently observed in patients receiving thiazide or loop diuretics, which can usually be prevented by use of a potassium-sparing diuretic or supplementation with potassium chloride. Hypercalcemia and hypomagnesemia also predispose to digoxin toxicity. (A) Calcium abnormalities are less common than potassium abnormalities. (B) Glucose abnormalities are unlikely unless the patient has diabetes. (C) Magnesium abnormalities are less common than potassium abnormalities. (E) Sodium abnormalities are unlikely in this patient.

111 **The answer is A: Decreased conduction velocity.** Adenosine is a naturally occurring nucleoside, but at high doses, the drug decreases conduction velocity, prolongs the refractory period, and decreases automaticity in the AV node. Intravenous adenosine is the drug of choice for abolishing acute supraventricular tachycardia. It has low toxicity but causes flushing, chest pain, and hypotension. Adenosine has an extremely short duration of action (approximately 15 s). (B) The half-life of adenosine is 15 min. (C) This medication decreases automaticity at the AV node. (D) This agent works best when given intravenously. (E) This agent has low toxicity.

112 **The answer is A: Continuation of his medications would be helpful.** Prinzmetal angina is an uncommon pattern of episodic angina that occurs at rest and is caused by coronary artery spasm. Symptoms are

caused by decreased blood flow to the heart muscle from the spasm of the coronary artery. Although individuals with this form of angina may have significant coronary atherosclerosis, the angina attacks are unrelated to physical activity, heart rate, or blood pressure. Prinzmetal angina generally responds promptly to coronary vasodilators, such as nitroglycerin and calcium channel blockers. (B) Decrease in blood flow causes coronary artery spasm. (C) Symptoms are unrelated to physical activity. (D) Symptoms are not worsened with changes in heart rate or blood pressure.

113 **The answer is C: Headache.** The most common adverse effect of nitroglycerin, as well as of the other nitrates, is headache. From 30% to 60% of patients receiving intermittent nitrate therapy with long-acting agents develop headaches. High doses of organic nitrates can also cause postural hypotension, facial flushing, and tachycardia. Phosphodiesterase V inhibitors such as sildenafil, tardenafil, and vardenafil potentiate the action of the nitrates. To preclude the dangerous hypotension that may occur, this combination is contraindicated. (A) Sweating is more likely to occur than dry skin associated with the use of nitrates. (B) Organic nitrates do not cause erectile dysfunction. (D) Organic nitrates are not associated with priapism. (E) Organic nitrates can cause tachycardia and flushing.

114 **The answer is C: A 65-year-old man with chronic angina who has failed other therapies.** Ranolazine inhibits the late phase of the sodium current (late INa) improving the oxygen supply-and-demand equation. Inhibition of late INa reduces intracellular sodium and calcium overload, thereby improving diastolic function. Ranolazine is indicated for the treatment of chronic angina and may be used alone or in combination with other traditional therapies but is most often used as an option in patients with angina who have failed all other antianginal therapies. It is not to be used to treat an acute attack of angina. (A) Ranolazine is not indicated in the treatment of acute angina. (B) Ranolazine is not indicated in the treatment of acute angina. (D) This agent is not effective in the management of acute coronary events. (E) This patient does not have evidence of chronic angina. This patient has congestive failure and outflow obstruction.

115 **The answer is E: Nitroglycerin (transdermal).** Transdermal nitroglycerin can sustain blood levels for as long as 24 h. Because tolerance occurs, however, it is recommended that the patch be removed after 10 to 12 h to allow recovery of sensitivity. (A) This agent has a short duration of action. (B) This agent has a short duration of action. (C) Hydralazine may actually precipitate an angina attack. (D) Transdermal nitroglycerin is a better selection than sublingual nitroglycerin.

116 **The answer is C: Reduction of dietary salt to 10 g/d.** Lifestyle modifications to improve blood pressure include the following: weight—maintain normal body weight (BMI 18.5 to 24.9); DASH diet—rich in fruits, vegetables, grains, low-fat dairy products; and low in fat, cholesterol, and sodium; salt—reduce dietary sodium to no more than 2.4 g/d of sodium or 6 g/d of NaCl; exercise—regular aerobic activity such as walking (30 min/d on most days); and alcohol—limit to no more than two drinks per day for men and one drink per day for women. (A) This is a useful modification that may improve blood pressure. (B) This is a useful modification that may improve blood pressure. (D) This is a useful modification that may improve blood pressure. (E) This is a useful modification that may improve blood pressure.

117 **The answer is B: Fluid retention.** This drug causes dilation of resistance vessels (arterioles) but not of capacitance vessels (venules). Minoxidil is administered orally for treatment of severe to malignant hypertension that is refractory to other drugs. Reflex tachycardia and fluid retention may be severe and require the concomitant use of a loop diuretic and a β-blocker. Minoxidil causes serious sodium and water retention, leading to volume overload, edema, and congestive heart failure. Minoxidil treatment also causes hypertrichosis (the growth of body hair). This drug is used topically to treat male pattern baldness. (A) This agent is used to treat male pattern baldness. (C) This agent is not associated with muscle wasting. (D) This agent does not cause thinning of the skin on the palms or soles. (E) This agent does not cause uremic pericarditis.

118 **The answer is C:A 55-year-old man with encephalopathy and blood pressure of 220/160 mm Hg.** Hypertensive emergency is a rare but life-threatening situation in which the diastolic blood pressure is either greater than 150 mm Hg (with systolic blood pressure greater than 210 mm Hg) in an otherwise healthy person or greater than 130 mm Hg in an individual with preexisting complications, such as encephalopathy, cerebral hemorrhage, left ventricular failure, or aortic stenosis. The therapeutic goal is to rapidly reduce blood pressure. (A) This patient does not have a hypertensive emergency. (B) This patient does not have a hypertensive emergency. (D) This patient is hypotensive. Administration of sodium nitroprusside will worsen hypotension. (E) This patient is hypotensive and has two systems in failure. Administration of sodium nitroprusside will worsen hypotension.

119 **The answer is E: A 60-year-old black man.** There are some predictable differences in the response to antihypertensive drugs among patient groups, which can be summarized by the AB/CD guidelines: α (A) or β (B).

For older (and black) patients, consider starting on a calcium channel blocker (C) or diuretic (D). The best choice antihypertensive agent for a 60-year-old black man would be a calcium channel blocker. (A) This patient may respond nicely to a β-blocker. (B) This patient may respond nicely to a β-blocker. (C) This patient may respond nicely to a β-blocker. (D) This patient would best respond to a calcium-channel blocker.

120 **The answer is C: A 25-year-old woman, 18 weeks pregnant, with blood pressure of 180/110 mm Hg.** Mild hypertension associated with preeclampsia typically does not warrant treatment. Severe hypertension (systolic pressures ≥150 mm Hg and diastolic blood pressures ≥100 mm Hg) is treated acutely with labetalol to prevent maternal cerebrovascular complications. Avoid ACE inhibitors, ARBs, and aliskiren because these drugs may cause fetal injury or death. Nitroprusside is contraindicated in the later stages of pregnancy because of possible fetal cyanide poisoning if used for more than 4 h. (A) This pregnant woman does not have preeclampsia. (B) This pregnant woman does not have preeclampsia. (D) This pregnant woman does not have preeclampsia. (E) This pregnant woman does not have preeclampsia.

121 **The answer is D: Prazosin.** Prazosin produces first-dose hypotension, presumably by blocking α_1-receptors. This effect is minimized by initially giving the drug in small, divided doses. (A) Atenolol does not cause first-dose hypotension. (B) Hydrochlorothiazide does not cause first-dose hypotension. (C) Metoprolol does not cause first-dose hypotension. (E) Verapamil does not cause first-dose hypotension.

122 **The answer is A: Clonidine.** Increased sympathetic nervous system activity occurs if clonidine therapy is abruptly stopped after prolonged administration. Uncontrolled elevation in blood pressure can occur. Patients should be slowly weaned from clonidine while other antihypertensive medications are initiated. (B) Diltiazem does not cause increased sympathetic activity after abrupt discontinuation. (C) Enalapril does not cause increased sympathetic activity after abrupt discontinuation. (D) Hydrochlorothiazide does not cause increased sympathetic activity after abrupt discontinuation. (E) Losartan does not cause increased sympathetic activity after abrupt discontinuation.

123 **The answer is A: 2 to 6 h.** For myocardial infarction, intracoronary delivery of the drugs is the most reliable in terms of achieving recanalization. However, cardiac catheterization may not be possible in the 2- to 6-h "therapeutic window," beyond which significant myocardial salvage becomes less likely. Thus, thrombolytic agents are usually administered intravenously, because this route is rapid, inexpensive, and does not have the risks of catheterization. (B) The therapeutic window for antithrombotics to be effective in cardiac vessel recanalization is 2 to 6 h. (C) This window is too long and recanalization of the damaged cardiac vessels will not occur. (D) The therapeutic window for antithrombotics to be effective in cardiac vessel recanalization is 2 to 6 h. (E) This window is too long and recanalization of the damaged cardiac vessels will not occur.

124 **The answer is A: Within 3 h.** Alteplase is approved for the treatment of myocardial infarction, massive pulmonary embolism, and acute ischemic stroke. Alteplase seems to be superior to streptokinase in dissolving older clots and, ultimately, may be approved for other applications. Alteplase administered within 3 h of the onset of ischemic stroke significantly improves clinical outcome, that is, the patient's ability to perform activities of daily living. Reteplase is similar to alteplase and can be used as an alternative. (B) Alteplase must be administered within 3 h of the onset of stroke for maximal effectiveness. (C) Alteplase must be administered within 3 h of the onset of stroke for maximal effectiveness. (D) Alteplase must be administered within 3 h of the onset of stroke for maximal effectiveness. (E) Alteplase must be administered within 3 h of the onset of stroke for maximal effectiveness.

125 **The answer is E: Thromboplastin time.** Streptokinase therapy is instituted within 4 h of a myocardial infarction and is infused for 1 h. Its half-life is less than half an hour. Thromboplastin time is monitored and maintained at twofold to fivefold the control value. On discontinuation of treatment, either heparin or oral anticoagulants may be administered. (A) Hemoglobin will be unchanged following streptokinase infusion. (B) Hematocrit should not change during streptokinase infusion. (C) Partial thromboplastin time should not change during streptokinase infusion. (D) Platelet count should not change during streptokinase infusion.

126 **The answer is E: Ionically combines with heparin.** Excessive bleeding may be managed by ceasing administration of the drug or by treating with protamine sulfate. Infused slowly, protamine sulfate combines ionically with heparin to form a stable, inactive complex. The other effects listed are not those of protamine sulfate. (A) Protamine does not activate the coagulation cascade. (B) Protamine does not activate the tissue plasminogen activator. (C) Protamine does not degrade heparin. (D) Protamine does not inactivate antithrombin.

127 **The answer is B: Neutropenia.** Ticlopidine irreversibly blocks ADP receptors on platelets, which inhibits

their aggregation. Side effects of ticlopidine are neutropenia and thrombotic thrombocytopenic purpura. It is rarely used anymore because of clopidogrel having less side effects. (A) Gastric ulcers are more commonly seen with aspirin, not ticlopidine. (C) Osteoporosis is more commonly seen with steroids or heparin, not ticlopidine. (D) Seizures are more commonly seen with bupropion, not ticlopidine. (E) Tinnitus is more commonly seen with aspirin, not ticlopidine.

128 **The answer is C: Macrocytic anemia.** Methotrexate is a folate antimetabolite. It inhibits the enzyme dihydrofolate reductase, which is necessary for recycling folate from its oxidized form to its usable, reduced form, tetrahydrofolate. Without tetrahydrofolate, cells cannot replicate DNA. This not only makes methotrexate useful against the rapidly dividing cells of cancer but may also significantly impair DNA synthesis in normal cells with prolonged use. In particular, extended use of methotrexate can disrupt mitosis of hematopoietic cells and lead to megaloblastic anemia, a form of macrocytic anemia. (A) α-Thalassemia is a genetic anemia caused by the loss of function of one or more α-globin genes. Methotrexate does not cause α-thalassemia. (B) β-Thalassemia is a genetic anemia caused by the loss of function of one or more β-globin genes. Methotrexate does not cause β-thalassemia. (D) Microcytic anemia occurs when hematopoietic cell growth is slowed but the rate of DNA synthesis is unchanged. Methotrexate impairs DNA synthesis, so would not result in microcytic anemia. (E) Normocytic anemia means a decrease in total hemoglobin but with normal-sized erythrocytes, as would occur following the loss of a large amount of blood. Methotrexate would instead cause a macrocytic anemia because it creates a condition in which hematopoietic cells grow at the normal rate but are unable to divide as often because of impaired DNA synthesis.

129 **The answer is C: Furosemide.** This is a potentially fatal situation. It is important to administer a diuretic that will reduce fluid accumulation in the lungs and thus improve oxygenation and heart function. The loop diuretics are most effective in removing large fluid volumes from the body and are the treatment of choice in this situation. Furosemide is usually administered intravenously. (A) Acetazolamide is not an appropriate consideration to treat pulmonary edema. (B) Chlorthalidone is an outpatient treatment for hypertension. (D) Hydrochlorothiazide is not an appropriate treatment consideration for pulmonary edema. (E) Spironolactone is a potassium-sparing diuretic used to treat hypertension.

130 **The answer is B: Carbonic anhydrase inhibitor.** Acetazolamide is used prophylactically for several days before an ascent above 10,000 feet. This treatment prevents the cerebral and pulmonary problems associated with the syndrome as well as other difficulties, such as nausea. (A) Anticholinergic agents will have no effect on cerebral or circulatory problems, although they may have some benefit for overactive bowel or bladder. (C) Loop diuretics may improve symptoms of pulmonary edema but would be otherwise not helpful in prevention of mountain sickness. (D) β-Blockers will not improve pulmonary or cerebral symptoms of mountain sickness. (E) Thiazide diuretics are used in the outpatient management of hypertension.

131 **The answer is A: Acute renal failure.** Captopril is used to protect the kidneys against diabetic nephropathy once proteinuria develops. A side effect of captopril is reversible acute renal failure as evident by an increase in creatinine. The exact reason for renal failure is unknown, but it is believed to be related to the decrease in glomerular filtration rate from decreased angiotensin II. (B) Gynecomastia is more commonly associated with spironolactone, not captopril. (C) Hypotension is more commonly seen with captopril. (D) Hyperkalemia is more commonly seen with captopril. (E) Ototoxicity is more commonly associated with furosemide, not captopril.

132 **The answer is E: Spironolactone.** Spironolactone is a potassium-sparing diuretic that can be used for diuresis. Spironolactone competitively inhibits aldosterone receptors in the collecting tubules. It decreases the secretion of potassium in the urine. (A) Acetazolamide causes the excretion of potassium leading to hypokalemia. (B) Furosemide causes the excretion of potassium leading to hypokalemia. (C) Hydrochlorothiazide causes the excretion of potassium leading to hypokalemia. (D) Mannitol causes the excretion of potassium leading to hypokalemia.

133 **The answer is D: Letter D.** Letter D represents phase 3 repolarization. In this phase, calcium channels close. Potassium channels open resulting in an outward current that leads to membrane repolarization. The net result of the action potential to this point is a net gain of sodium and loss of potassium. (A) Letter A represents the fast phase 0 upstroke. (B) Letter B represents the phase 1 partial repolarization. (C) Letter C represents the phase 2 plateau. (E) Letter E represents the phase 4 forward current.

134 **The answer is A: Medication A.** Medication A is nitroglycerin and is the agent of choice in acute chest pain. The sublingual dose has an onset of action in 2 min and a duration of 25 min. (B) Medication B is isosorbide dinitrate, which has an onset of action of 5 min. (C) Medication C is isosorbide mononitrate and only

has an extended-release formulation and is not suitable in this patient. (D) Combination nitrate therapy is not indicated in this patient.

135 **The answer is A: Medication A.** Nifedipine is represented by medication A. This agent has strong action to dilate coronary arteries with little effect on AV conduction. Side effects are common at approximately 18%. (B) Medication B is verapamil with a less strong action on dilation of coronary vessels. (C) Medication C is diltiazem, which has strong action on dilation of coronary vessels and a limited side effect profile. (D) Combination therapy is not suggested in this patient.

136 **The answer is D: Medication D.** Medication D is nicardipine. This agent has an onset of action of 5 to 10 min and a duration of action of 6 to 8 h. It is not useful in this patient who has a hypertensive emergency. The medication of choice is medication A, which is sodium nitroprusside. (A) Medication A is sodium nitroprusside and is the medication of choice for this patient. (B) Medication B is labetalol, which has an onset of action of 5 to 10 min. (C) Medication C is fenoldopam, which has an onset of action of 2 to 5 min.

137 **The answer is B: Letter B.** Aspirin blocks the conversion of arachidonic acid to prostaglandin H_2. This causes a decrease in cyclooxygenase 1 (COX-1). This will inhibit aggregation of platelets. (A) Aspirin inhibits COX-1. (C) Aspirin inhibits formation of prostaglandin H_2 and COX-1. (D) Letter D is not part of the cyclooxygenase pathway.

138 **The answer is B: Medication B.** Streptokinase demonstrates high antigenicity, low fibrin specificity, and a half-life of approximately 22 min. It is an agent of choice as a thrombolytic agent. (A) This medication is alteplase, which has low antigenicity, high fibrin specificity, and a short half-life. (C) This medication is urokinase, which has low antigenicity, high fibrin specificity, and a 20-min half-life. (D) This information describes streptokinase.

139 **The answer is D: Steroids.** This patient is presenting with temporal arteritis or giant cell arteritis, which typically affects branches of the carotid artery. If left untreated, this patient may develop occlusion of the ophthalmic artery resulting in permanent blindness. The only medications shown to slow or stop the granulomatous occlusion of these arteries are steroids. (A) α-Blockers such as phenoxybenzamine and prazosin would decrease systemic blood pressure and decrease constriction of blood vessels but would not stop the progression of the granulomatous process. (B) Anticoagulants such as heparin and warfarin would not be effective because this is not the result of platelet coagulation. (C) HMG-CoA reductase inhibitors such as lovastatin decrease the long-term occlusion of vessels by reducing the deposition of cholesterol found in atherosclerotic plaques and would not decrease the formation of granulomas. (E) Thrombolytics such as tPA and streptokinase would not be effective because the occlusion of the ophthalmic artery is not a result of clot formation.

140 **The answer is E: Methyldopa.** Methyldopa, a centrally acting α_2-agonist similar to clonidine, is the first choice for pregnant women with hypertension and results in a decreased sympathetic output reducing blood pressure. Methyldopa has shown no threatening side effects and no teratogenic effects on the fetus. (A) Loop diuretics such as furosemide are generally avoided because of the electrolyte imbalances and the possibility for dehydration resulting in compromised blood flow to the fetus. (B) Hydrochlorthiazide is not recommended in pregnancy. (C) Angiotensin-converting enzyme (ACE) inhibitors (lisinopril) are contraindicated in the pregnant women. (D) Angiotensin II receptor antagonists such as losartan are contraindicated in the pregnant women.

141 **The answer is A: Adenosine.** The arrhythmia described involves dysfunction of the AV node, which has led to syncope in this patient. A treatment is required to act fast and block the AV node in order to reset the heart's normal innate automaticity. Adenosine is the best choice because of its ability to block AV node function rapidly and transiently (for only 15 to 20 s). (B) Flecainide is a very dangerous antiarrhythmic and has also been shown to actually induce arrhythmias in some cases. It is still occasionally used to treat recalcitrant ventricular arrhythmias. (C) Lidocaine is both a local anesthetic and a class Ib antiarrhythmic for ventricular arrhythmias. Generally, lidocaine is used post-MI because it prevents the formation of arrhythmias in the infarcted tissue while increasing blood supply as well. (D) Phenytoin is both an epileptic drug and a treatment for a special drug-induced arrhythmia. Phenytoin's usage as a treatment for arrhythmia is generally limited to digitalis toxicity. (E) Quinidine is a class Ia antiarrhythmic that is used as a long-term treatment for atrial and ventricular arrhythmias. This would not have a fast enough onset for this patient.

Chapter 4

Endocrine Pharmacology

QUESTIONS

Select the single best answer.

1 A 67-year-old man injures his shoulder in an ATV accident. Over-the-counter ibuprofen is unable to control the pain satisfactorily. The patient asks about glucocorticoid injections, so his doctor begins to explain the myriad effects of glucocorticoids in the body. Which of the following glucocorticoid actions would be most desirable in this patient?

(A) Antiemetic
(B) Decreasing synthesis of HGF, a growth factor
(C) Decreasing translocation of GLUT4 receptors to the cell membrane
(D) Increasing synthesis of IκB
(E) Stimulating gluconeogenesis

2 A 37-year-old kidney transplant recipient presents to her primary care physician for follow-up. Among other immunosuppressant drugs, she has been taking daily prednisone for the past 2 months since her transplant. With only a few doses of prednisone left, she gets snowed into her house and cannot refill her prescription (but she has enough of the other medications to last a few more weeks). If she runs out of prednisone and cannot get it refilled, what is she most at risk for developing?

(A) Cardiovascular collapse (adrenal crisis)
(B) Osteoporosis
(C) Increased risk of infection
(D) Insomnia (short-term oral/parenteral)
(E) Nausea/vomiting (short-term oral/parenteral)

3 A 72-year-old woman with myasthenia gravis is brought to the emergency department with decreased responsiveness. She has a history of diabetes, hypertension, Alzheimer's disease, and stroke. Physical examination reveals significant abdominal tenderness with guarding and peritoneal signs. Which of the following is a medication that should be discontinued immediately in this patient?

(A) Insulin
(B) Neostigmine
(C) Nifedipine
(D) Rivastigmine
(E) Tacrine

4 A 58-year-old man with depression who takes a monoamine oxidase inhibitor has a love for aged cheese and wine. His depression is well controlled in this regimen. He must be alert to which of the following significant events?

(A) Diarrhea
(B) Hypertensive headaches
(C) Lacrimation
(D) Sweating
(E) Tremors

5 Five patients with sexual dysfunction present to their primary care physician for evaluation and treatment. Which of the following would most likely benefit from treatment with this medication yohimbine?

(A) A 19-year-old man with sexual arousal difficulties
(B) A 29-year-old man with erectile and ejaculatory dysfunction
(C) A 47-year-old man with erectile dysfunction and hypertension
(D) A 57-year-old man with erectile dysfunction and diabetes mellitus
(E) A 80-year-old man with erectile dysfunction and myocardial infarction

6 A 29-year-old man with a family history of heart disease presents to his primary care physician for a routine checkup. A lipid profile on a blood draw reveals high LDL and low HDL. One way to decrease the amount of LDL in the blood is to hinder the liver's ability for de novo cholesterol synthesis. Which of the following drugs blocks de novo cholesterol synthesis in hepatocytes?

(A) Cholestyramine
(B) Colesevelam
(C) Colestipol
(D) Ezetimibe
(E) Rosuvastatin

7 A 37-year-old woman with hyperlipidemia is taking a drug to lower her triglyceride and blood cholesterol levels. She is considering stopping her therapy, however, because of a red, itchy rash on her face and neck that occurs following some doses. Which drug is she taking?

(A) Atorvastatin
(B) Fenofibrate
(C) Gemfibrozil
(D) Nicotinic acid
(E) Omacor

8 A 41-year-old man with end-stage HIV disease has lost approximately 50 lb from his baseline weight of 160 lb. He now weighs in the fifth percentile for his age group. He is given dronabinol to achieve a change in this area. The most plausible mechanism of action for this medication is

(A) Appetite stimulant
(B) Induction of chemotactic centers of the brain
(C) Stimulation of epidermal growth factor
(D) Stimulation of keratinocyte growth factor
(E) Stimulation of growth hormone

9 A 63-year-old woman falls at home and fractures her wrist. She has a 40 pack-year history of smoking. Her doctor recommends a DXA scan, which reveals a very low bone density and prescribes alendronate. How will alendronate help this patient?

(A) Enhancing GI calcium absorption
(B) Inhibiting calcium excretion in the kidneys
(C) Inhibiting osteoclasts
(D) Providing the starting material for bone mineralization
(E) Stimulating osteoblasts

10 A 33-year-old woman presents to her primary care physician with tachycardia, heat intolerance, tremor, and unintentional weight loss. A thyroid scan shows multiple regions of thyroid taking up excess iodine. She is prescribed with a drug that will decrease synthesis of thyroid hormones and decrease the peripheral conversion of T_4 to T_3. Which drug is this?

(A) Lanreotide
(B) Levothyroxine
(C) Methimazole
(D) Octreotide
(E) Propylthiouracil

11 A 27-year-old man was recently diagnosed with Type-2 diabetes mellitus and placed on a medication. As he was drinking with his friends, he became violently ill. What medication is he most likely taking?

(A) Acarbose
(B) Glyburide
(C) Metformin
(D) Pioglitazone
(E) Tolbutamide

12 A 43-year-old woman with Type-2 diabetes has been taking insulin with meals as well as metformin. Her blood glucose remains poorly controlled. Her doctor prescribes an additional drug, which is an analog of an endogenous peptide that inhibits glucagon secretion. What is the most likely medication this patient is taking?

(A) Exenatide
(B) Glipizide
(C) Miglitol
(D) Pramlintide
(E) Rosiglitazone

13 A 57-year-old man with a 40 pack-year history of smoking develops small cell lung cancer. His serum sodium is 121 mEq/L and his urine has a specific gravity of 1.030. Which of the following is a tetracycline antibiotic that can also be used in the treatment of SIADH?

(A) Demeclocycline
(B) Doxycycline
(C) Minocycline
(D) Tetracycline
(E) Tigecycline

14 A young married couple has been unable to conceive after 3 years of unprotected intercourse. The husband's sperm count is normal. They both agree that they would like the wife to undergo fertility treatment. Which of the following drugs has the ability to either stimulate or inhibit ovulation depending only on the dosing schedule?

(A) Bromocriptine
(B) Clomiphene
(C) Estrone sulfate
(D) hCG
(E) Leuprolide

15 A 59-year-old man with long-standing hypertension presents to his primary care physician for a follow-up visit and guidance. His blood pressure is 160/80 mm Hg. His current medications include a calcium channel blocker. He is now switched to losartan. Which of the following properties of this medication can limit its efficacy for this patient?

(A) Extensive hepatic first-pass metabolism
(B) Drug interaction with antacids
(C) Oral administration
(D) Renal excretion
(E) Requirement to be taken on a full stomach

16 A 72-year-old man with congestive heart failure is hospitalized because of worsening pulmonary and peripheral edema. He is given intravenous furosemide. This agent will likely improve hemodynamics in which of the following ways?
(A) Decrease venous return to the heart
(B) Increase blood pressure
(C) Increase circulatory volume
(D) Increase heart rate
(E) Increase plasma volume

17 A 46-year-old man with hypertension presents to his primary care physician for follow-up. He has a good blood pressure control as evidenced by normal levels on his home blood pressure machine. He currently takes hydrochlorothiazide. Which of the following laboratory studies should be undertaken in this patient?
(A) Complete blood count
(B) Electrolytes
(C) Hemoglobin electrophoresis
(D) Hematocrit
(E) Plasma protein levels

18 A 65-year-old man with long-standing hypertension on enalapril presents to his primary care physician complaining of a chronic cough. The cough began when he started this medication. The most likely explanation for this finding is
(A) Bradykinin stimulation
(B) Bronchiolar congestion
(C) Pulmonary embolism
(D) Pulmonary exudate
(E) Restrictive cardiomyopathy

19 A 29-year-old man is found to have primary pulmonary hypertension while undergoing a workup for shortness of breath and fatigue. A defect in his BMPR2 gene is discovered. This gene product normally inhibits smooth muscle proliferation. Which of the following drugs would best help this patient?
(A) Bosentan
(B) Captopril
(C) Furosemide
(D) Labetalol
(E) Valsartan

20 A 52-year-old man is prescribed with furosemide by his physician to help treat his hypertension. His physician further advises him to avoid NSAIDs for pain because they may antagonize the effects of furosemide. Which of the following describes how NSAIDs may interfere with the effects of furosemide?
(A) Afferent arteriole vasoconstriction
(B) Efferent arteriole vasoconstriction
(C) Increase tubular sodium reabsorption
(D) Stimulation of the ADH receptor
(E) The physician is mistaken; pain management with NSAIDs has no bearing on furosemide use

21 A 21-year-old woman plans to spend a semester high in the Andes. She shares a concern with her doctor about the elevation because 1 year ago, she went on a ski trip to Colorado and developed altitude sickness. Her doctor prescribes a diuretic that can help her if she begins to have symptoms of altitude sickness. Which diuretic did her doctor likely prescribe?
(A) Acetazolamide
(B) Furosemide
(C) Hydrochlorothiazide
(D) Mannitol
(E) Spironolactone

22 A 19-year-old woman presents to her primary care physician for evaluation of elevated triglycerides. Her mother, father, sister, and brother all have the same problem. Her serum cholesterol and triglyceride levels are normal. What is the most appropriate initial treatment for this patient?
(A) Dietary modification to include increased protein and fats
(B) Exercise regimen approximately 5 d/wk
(C) HMG-CoA reductase inhibitor 5 d/wk
(D) Introduction of a statin drug 5 d/wk
(E) Watchful waiting and follow-up in 1 year

23 A 56-year-old man with a known history of hyperlipidemia and coronary artery disease on simvastatin develops chest pain while golfing (usually 4 d/wk). His weight is 75 kg. He is brought to the emergency department, is found to be asystolic, and dies. His most recent serum cholesterol level was in the normal range. Which of the following statements is true?
(A) His exercise regimen was inadequate
(B) His dietary modifications were inadequate
(C) His weight was above normal
(D) Lowering cholesterol does not reduce cardiac mortality completely
(E) Lowering cholesterol directly caused his mortality

24 A 45-year-old man has high serum LDL and low serum HDL. He presents to his primary care physician for treatment guidance. In addition to exercise and diet modification, which of the following agents would provide him with the most efficacious improvement of serum LDL and HDL levels?
(A) Cholestyramine
(B) Fluvastatin
(C) Lovastatin
(D) Simvastatin

25 A 76-year-old man with a history of falls, hypertension, and kidney stones presents to his primary care physician for follow-up. His blood pressure is 140/100 mm Hg. He is placed on hydrochlorothiazide. This agent may be helpful in prevention of renal stones through which of the following mechanisms?
(A) Binding to urine calcium
(B) Binding to urine sodium
(C) Causing resorption of calcium in the renal tubules
(D) Increasing calcium excretion in the renal tubules
(E) Increasing sodium resorption in the renal tubules

26 A 79-year-old woman with diabetes mellitus, hypertension, and visual disturbances presents to her ophthalmologist for management of her eye condition. She is found to have open-angle glaucoma. Prescription for acetazolamide is given to produce which of the following responses?
(A) Decrease production of aqueous humor
(B) Increasing intraocular pressure
(C) Inhibition of sodium-calcium transport
(D) Stimulating carbonic anhydrase
(E) Stimulating ciliary body function in acute glaucoma

27 A 45-year-old man with insulin-dependent diabetes mellitus on insulin injection decides that he wants to "drink" the insulin instead of taking the injection form. He is tired of the pain he gets during the injections. Which of the following is the most likely sequelae of this action?
(A) Diarrhea
(B) Nausea
(C) Persistent hyperglycemia
(D) Transient ischemic attack
(E) Uremia

28 A 39-year-old man with insulin-dependent diabetes mellitus is brought to the emergency department after collapsing in a shopping mall. His blood sugar is 589 mg/dL. Which of the following preparations would have the least minimal effect on his blood sugar levels?
(A) Insulin aspart
(B) Insulin glargine
(C) Insulin lispro
(D) Regular insulin

29 A 56-year-old male with insulin-dependent diabetes and with poorly controlled blood sugar is on regular insulin. His primary care physician adds pramlintide in an effort to further reduce his blood sugar levels. An important condition to rule out in this patient would be which of the following?
(A) Gastric retention
(B) Acute-angle glaucoma
(C) Wide-angle glaucoma
(D) Pneumonia
(E) Urinary retention

30 A 65-year-old man with non–insulin-dependent diabetes mellitus presents to his primary care physician for follow-up. He is currently managed with glyburide. His weight has increased from a baseline of 195 lb to 230 lb during the past year. He walks approximately 30 min every other day throughout the year and eats three balanced meals per day. What is the most likely explanation for these findings?
(A) Lack of physical exercise
(B) Lack of proper diet
(C) Medication side effect
(D) Underlying hyperthyroidism
(E) Underlying malignancy

31 A 42-year-old man with a history of diabetes mellitus on metformin is going to have a CT scan of the abdomen with contrast to evaluate his chronic right lower quadrant pain. Which of the following statements about his metformin and this radiographic study is correct?
(A) He can continue taking metformin prior to and after the CT scan
(B) He can continue taking metformin and should increase the dose prior to the CT scan
(C) He can continue taking metformin and should stop the medicine just prior to the CT scan
(D) He should be hospitalized and given Benadryl and continue taking metformin at the usual dosage

32 A 62-year-old female with diabetes presents to her primary care physician for follow-up. She takes pioglitazone daily and her blood sugar ranges approximately from 100 to 180 mg/dL. Which of the following indicators would likely have minimal or no change from baseline values with this therapy?
(A) Glucose
(B) Hemoglobin A_{1c}
(C) Insulin
(D) Low-density lipoprotein
(E) Triglycerides

33 A 56-year-old man with Type-2 diabetes mellitus managed with acarbose presents to his primary care physician for a follow-up evaluation. His most recent laboratory studies indicate normal serum glucose levels and low serum amylase. What is the most likely explanation for this finding?

(A) Drug toxicity
(B) Inhibition of pancreatic amylase
(C) Pancreatitis
(D) Pancreatic carcinoma
(E) Subtherapeutic pharmacologic effect

34 A 58-year-old female with diabetes on sitagliptin presents to her primary care physician because of recurrent sinusitis and sore throat. Her blood sugar is 130 mg/dL. What is the most likely explanation for this finding?

(A) Allergic phenomenon to dander
(B) Gastroesophageal reflux
(C) Treatment-related side effect
(D) Underlying nasopharyngeal obstruction
(E) Viral infection

35 A 65-year-old woman with postmenopausal atrophy and hot flashes is prescribed with estrogen therapy by her primary care physician. She has a family history of endometrial cancer and is concerned about her risk for this condition. Which of the following statements is true?

(A) Breast cancer is unlikely
(B) Postmenopausal bleeding is unlikely
(C) The risk can be offset by adding a proestrogen product
(D) Thromboembolic events are unlikely

36 A 20-year-old woman becomes pregnant out of wedlock and wants to terminate the pregnancy with an oral abortifacient. The use of mifepristone (RU-486) as an oral abortifacient is based on which of the following characteristics?

(A) Anticoagulant properties
(B) Interference with progesterone
(C) Potent mineralocorticoid activity
(D) Teratogenicity
(E) Uremic encephalopathy development

37 A 22-year-old woman is using a vaginal ring as a contraceptive agent. She has no other medical problems. She is concerned about device failure and becoming pregnant. What is the most likely reason for this failure to occur?

(A) Having 1 of every 4 weeks vaginal ring free
(B) Insertion into the vagina for 3 weeks
(C) Low levels of ethinyl estradiol and etonogestrel
(D) Slippage of the ring from the vaginal vault

38 A 19-year-old woman who was intoxicated at a party finds that she had nonconsenting sexual intercourse after awakening without clothes on the following morning. She presents to the ambulatory care clinic and is administered with postcoital contraception. She is still very concerned that she may become pregnant. An estimation of the risk of pregnancy in this scenario is approximately

(A) 0%
(B) 1% to 3%
(C) 5%
(D) 15%
(E) 30%

39 A 38-year-old woman on oral contraceptives for 18 years thinks that this preparation may prove to be not only beneficial in preventing pregnancy but also beneficial in reduction of cancer risk. Which of the following cancers may show a decreased incidence because of her prolonged use of oral contraceptives?

(A) Breast cancer
(B) Cervical cancer
(C) Lung cancer
(D) Ovarian cancer
(E) Thyroid cancer

40 A 32-year-old woman with endometriosis of the uterus, pelvic sidewall, and bladder has chronic unrelenting pelvic pain. She is prescribed with danazol. Over the next few weeks, she experiences a 40% improvement in her symptoms. What physiologic changes are likely to be found in this patient as a result of this medication?

(A) Decreased aromatase
(B) Decreased hair growth
(C) Decreased libido
(D) Decreased FSH
(E) Decreased testosterone

41 An 18-year-old male high school baseball player is interested in improving his hitting ability. He receives twice weekly injections of anabolic steroids. Over the next year, which of the following effects would be likely observed in this patient?

(A) Depression
(B) Hepatic hemangioma
(C) Premature epiphyseal long bone closing
(D) Testicular hyperplasia
(E) Tubercle development

42 A 44-year-old woman with systemic lupus erythematosus presents to her primary care physician for follow-up. She is currently being managed with an oral glucocorticoid agent. The most likely mechanism of action of this medication involves which of the following?

(A) Inhibition of erythrocytes
(B) Inhibition of macrophages
(C) Stimulation of cyclooxygenase 2 synthesis
(D) Stimulation of phospholipase A_2
(E) Stimulation of T cells

43 A 66-year-old woman with a history of Cushing's disease treated with oral glucocorticoids presents to her primary care physician for follow-up. She was recently hospitalized for a hip fracture following a fall. What is the most likely mechanism for hip fracture in this patient?
(A) Increased intestinal calcium absorption
(B) Increased sex hormone synthesis
(C) Inhibition of bone formation
(D) Osteoarthritis
(E) Osteochondroma

44 A 49-year-old woman with a history of hypertension is treated with spironolactone. She has good blood pressure control and in the last 6 months has shown an improvement in her hirsutism. What is the most likely explanation for these findings?
(A) Androgen receptor inhibition of the hair follicle
(B) Drug toxicity
(C) Hypoaldosteronism
(D) Testosterone levels are elevated
(E) Idiopathic effect

45 A 34-year-old man who is obese has been unable to lose weight by diet management and exercise. He also has hypertension and prediabetes. His physician prescribes orlistat to cut down on the amount of calories he takes in. Which of the following describes the mechanism of orlistat?
(A) Binding bile salts
(B) Inhibition of α-glucosidase
(C) Inhibition of chylomicron formation
(D) Inhibition of lipase
(E) Inhibition of trypsin

46 A 23-year-old male college graduate student with a history of asthma presents to the ambulatory care clinic for follow-up. He uses a β_2-agonist via inhaler when he has an attack. The treating physician should be alert to which of the following possible findings on examination and laboratory studies?
(A) Bradycardia
(B) Hyperglycemia
(C) Hyperkalemia
(D) Hypermagnesemia
(E) Hypertension

47 A 78-year-old woman with known osteoporosis presents to her primary care physician for follow-up. She is managed with alendronate. Physical examination reveals a woman with a height of 5 ft 3 in and weight of 143 lb. The most likely effects on bone would be which of the following?
(A) Increased osteoblastic bone resorption
(B) Inhibition of cholesterol biosynthesis
(C) Inhibition of osteoclastic apoptosis
(D) Inhibition of osteocyte activation
(E) Inhibition of osteocyte formation

48 A 78-year-old woman who is still an active tennis player has osteoporosis. She has been treated with calcium supplementation and now begins therapy with teriparatide. This unique agent is a recombinant segment of which of the following hormones?
(A) Follicle-stimulating hormone
(B) Growth hormone
(C) Luteinizing hormone
(D) Parathyroid hormone
(E) Thyroid hormone

49 A 17-year-old woman presents to her primary care physician with polydipsia and polyuria. She is found to have high amounts of amino acids, phosphates, bicarbonate, and glucose in her urine. She reports that after complaining to a friend about her acne, her friend gave her some old acne medication that she had in her medicine cabinet. Which medication did she likely use?
(A) Benzoyl peroxide
(B) Clindamycin
(C) Erythromycin
(D) Isotretinoin
(E) Tetracycline

50 A 37-year-old woman who is obese with hyperglycemia complains of polyuria and polydipsia. Her physician prescribes glipizide to help control her blood sugar. After a few days of taking glipizide, she develops a pruritic rash. The physician prescribes a different drug. In light of her rash and in the absence of other contraindications, which of the following drugs would be safe for her to take?
(A) Celecoxib
(B) Hydrochlorothiazide
(C) Losartan
(D) Sulfamethoxazole
(E) Sulfasalazine

51 A 45-year-old man who is obese presents with increasing agitation and anxiety. He has many medical problems, and his list of drugs include metformin, verapamil, hydrochlorothiazide, venlafaxine, and atorvastatin. Which of the following drugs is most likely causing his anxiety and agitation?

(A) Atorvastatin
(B) Hydrochlorothiazide
(C) Metformin
(D) Venlafaxine
(E) Verapamil

52 A 48-year-old postmenopausal woman undergoes a hysterectomy prophylactically because of a strong family history of endometrial cancer. After her procedure, she complained of difficulty moving her bowels. Physical exam revealed decreased bowel sounds in all four quadrants. A white blood cell count showed 9,000 cells per microliter. The physician gives her a drug to stimulate her intestines until normal function resumes. Which of the following is most likely the drug given?

(A) Benztropine
(B) Bethanechol
(C) Epinephrine
(D) Methscopolamine
(E) Oxybutynin

53 A son brings his 72-year-old father into his scheduled follow-up after being placed on a new pharmacotherapy for his chronic hypertension. The patient also suffers from renal failure, and his son is his primary caretaker. Although the patient was on the maximum dose of hydralazine in addition to an ACE inhibitor and diuretic, the therapy has not effectively managing his severe hypertension. If the doctor replaces the hydralazine in the patient's drug regime, what medication is most likely to be chosen as a replacement?

(A) Calcium channel blockers
(B) Diazoxide
(C) Fenoldopam
(D) Minoxidil
(E) Sodium nitroprusside

54 A 76-year-old man with stage 5 chronic kidney disease who has been on hemodialysis for 2 years presents with muscle cramping. His serum phosphate is markedly elevated. His physician prescribes sevelamer. How will sevelamer help this patient?

(A) Decrease phosphate resorption from bone
(B) Increased excretion in the feces
(C) Increased excretion in the sweat
(D) Increased excretion in the urine
(E) Sevelamer does not affect phosphate handling; it is a muscle relaxant that will ease his cramps

55 Regarding the release of ACTH from the anterior pituitary in a 24-year-old man who is a marathon runner, which of the following is the next step in the process?

(A) Activation of protein S
(B) Increase of cGMP
(C) Stimulation of conversion of cholesterol to pregnenolone
(D) Release of adrenocorticosteroids
(E) Synthesis of pulmonary ACTH

56 Regarding the normal function of triiodothyronine and thyroxine in a 19-year-old female who has just finished menses, which of the following statements is true?

(A) Food administration decreases absorption of T_3
(B) Hormones are metabolized through the microsomal P450 system
(C) Phenytoin slows metabolism of thyroid hormones
(D) Rifampin slows metabolism of thyroid hormones
(E) T_3 is absorbed after subcutaneous administration

57 A 34-year-old man with a history of thyroid problems is brought to the emergency department with tachycardia, chest pressure, and sweating. He is thought to have thyroid storm. Which of the following treatment strategies is important in the management of this patient?

(A) Intravenous administration of medication is most efficacious
(B) Medications used are given at lower doses than hyperthyroidism
(C) Medications used are given at QD frequencies
(D) Use of an angiotensin-converting enzyme inhibitor would be useful for symptoms of heart failure

58 A 36-year-old man who is obese with a history of mildly elevated serum glucose levels (range from 110 to 118 mg/dL) presents to his primary care physician for follow-up. Physical examination of the heart, lungs, and abdomen are within normal limits. Which of the following strategies will cause the lowest improvement in serum glucose in this patient?

(A) Corrective glasses
(B) Diet modification
(C) Exercise
(D) Weight loss

59 A 45-year-old man with diabetes mellitus has begun on intensive therapy with insulin (dosed approximately three to five times per day). His blood glucose levels run in the range of 120 to 160 mg/dL. The long-term use of this treatment regimen will have the least significant clinical effect for

(A) Macrovascular disease
(B) Nephropathy
(C) Neuropathy
(D) Retinopathy
(E) Serum glucose normalization

60 A 56-year-old woman with diabetes who takes metformin is scheduled to undergo a CT scan of the abdomen and pelvis with IV contrast. Her last dose of metformin was this morning. She presents to the imaging center ready for the test. When she tells the technician that she takes metformin, her CT scan is cancelled despite her serum creatinine being 1 mg/dL. What is the reason for cancellation of the test?

(A) Allergic reaction potential
(B) Lactic acidosis development
(C) Nephrotoxic effects of the contrast
(D) Neurotoxic effects of the contrast
(E) Uremic potential of the contrast

61 A 16-year-old girl with primary dysmenorrhea, abnormal menses, and pelvic pain presents to her primary care physician for treatment. She has a history of asthma and allergic rhinitis. Her physician begins therapy with oral estradiol. Which of the following is the most common adverse effect for this patient to be aware of?

(A) Blood clotting
(B) Breast discharge
(C) Diarrhea
(D) Nausea
(E) Vomiting

62 A 37-year-old woman with diabetes is brought to the emergency department unresponsive by her husband. She recently started taking a new medication to control her blood sugar, but her husband could not remember the name of it. Her blood sugar is 45 mg/dL. Which of the following diabetes medications is most likely for her condition?

(A) Acarbose
(B) Glipizide
(C) Metformin
(D) Pramlintide
(E) Sitagliptin

63 A cell within the body that secretes a chemical that acts locally on cells in their immediate environment and does not enter the blood stream describes which of the following?

(A) Epinephrine
(B) Histamine
(C) Norepinephrine
(D) Thyroxine
(E) Testosterone

64 A 28-year-old man who is obese is found to have a hemoglobin A_{1c} of 9.5%. He has been unable to adequately control his blood sugar with diet and exercise alone. His physician wishes to prescribe an insulin product to help control his blood sugar level. Which of the following is the longest acting to provide this patient a low, baseline insulin dose that will last throughout the day?

(A) Insulin aspart
(B) Insulin glargine
(C) Insulin lispro
(D) Lente insulin
(E) NPH insulin

65 A 44-year-old black man is brought to the emergency department by a friend with 6 h of worsening lethargy and confusion. Past medical history is significant for easy bruising, 3 months of bone pain, and frequent pneumococcal infections. Labs were ordered, revealing a serum calcium of 17 mg/dL (normal: 9 to 10.5 mg/dL). Which of the following may be used to rapidly lower his serum calcium?

(A) Calcitonin
(B) Colesevelam
(C) Hydrochlorothiazide
(D) Teriparatide
(E) Vitamin D

66 A 16-year-old girl plans to become sexually active. She does not want a pregnancy, so she requests an oral contraceptive pill from her primary care physician. The physician prescribes a pill that contains both an estrogen analog and a progesterone analog. What is an effect of the progesterone analog?

(A) Hirsutism
(B) Milk production
(C) Peripheral muscle wasting
(D) Sodium retention
(E) Thickened cervical mucus

67 A 51-year-old premenopausal woman requests an estrogen-containing contraceptive from her primary care physician. Her social history is significant for being sexually active, smoking one pack per day of cigarettes, and consuming one to two alcoholic drinks per week. She has no personal or family history of breast, ovarian, or endometrial cancer. Why might be the physician will choose to avoid an estrogen-containing contraceptive?

(A) The patient is at high risk for developing cancer
(B) The physician fears a disulfiram-like reaction
(C) The physician fears that estrogen will disrupt the patient's lipid profile and increase her risk of cardiovascular disease
(D) The physician has no reason to avoid an estrogen-containing contraceptive
(E) This patient has a high risk of thromboembolism

68 A 67-year-old man injures his shoulder in an ATV accident. Over-the-counter and prescription ibuprofen are unable to control the pain and swelling satisfactorily. The patient asks about glucocorticoid injections, so his doctor begins to explain the myriad effects of glucocorticoids in the body. How might glucocorticoids help this patient?

(A) Enhance the immune system to protect against possible underlying infection
(B) Decrease activity of phospholipase A_2
(C) Improve healing by enhanced collagen production
(D) Increase blood flow by vasodilation
(E) Stabilize the joint by causing skeletal muscle hypertrophy

69 A 48-year-old woman has a history of urinary retention and progressive neuromuscular weakness. CT scan does not reveal any abnormalities of the head and neck. Consideration for an edrophonium test is being undertaken by the treating physician. Which of the following statements is correct?
(A) Diagnosis of thymic aplasia is possible
(B) Edrophonium is a tertiary amine
(C) Edrophonium binds irreversibly to acetylcholine
(D) Renal excretion takes approximately 24 h
(E) This agent is rapidly absorbed with a short duration of action

70 A 37-year-old woman who is a kidney transplant recipient has been taking daily prednisone for the past 2 months since her transplant. With only a few doses of prednisone left, she gets snowed in to her house and cannot refill her prescription (but she has enough of the other medications to last a few more weeks). Which of the following classes do steroids belong to?
(A) Biogenic amine
(B) Catecholamine
(C) Ion
(D) Lipid
(E) Peptide

71 A 26-year-old woman with infertility and her 23-year-old husband with a history of bilateral undescended testicles desires to start a family. She is currently taking a fertility medication but is troubled by some unusual and troubling side effects. She experiences heat and cold intolerance and mood swings. She complains of visual changes, and this makes her depressed. Which of the following medications is she most likely taking?
(A) Clomiphene citrate
(B) Danocrine
(C) Human chorionic gonadotropin
(D) Pulsatile GnRH
(E) Pergonal (human gonadotropins)

72 A 43-year-old man with dyslipidemia comes to the clinic for a routine checkup. He currently takes atorvastatin but is not achieving his target lipid profile. The physician prescribes colesevelam to help. Which of the following changes is expected as a result of this new therapy?
(A) Decreased HDL
(B) Decreased triglycerides
(C) Hyperglycemia
(D) Increased LDL
(E) Increased triglycerides

73 A 43-year-old man with a history of low libido and erectile dysfunction presents to his primary care physician for treatment. Physical examination reveals normal testicular size. Serum testosterone is 200 mg/dL. He is on treatment with testosterone 1% gel. Which of the following adverse effects is possible as a result of this preparation?
(A) Breast pain
(B) Hypotension
(C) Prostate inflammation
(D) Stomatitis
(E) Virilization in adults

74 A 33-year-old woman has difficulties with redness of her eyes especially after swimming. She takes oxymetazoline eye drops, which gives her relief. However, this medication can get into the systemic circulation and cause which of the following adverse effects?
(A) Calming
(B) Diarrhea
(C) Fatigue
(D) Headache
(E) Sleepiness

75 A 59-year-old man with hypertension is taking a β-blocker (acebutolol). His most recent blood pressure is 120/78 mm Hg. This agent is likely to alter which of the following laboratory values?
(A) Chylomicrons
(B) HDL
(C) LDL
(D) VLDL
(E) Lipid metabolism remains unchanged

76 A week-old newborn male presents to clinic for a routine checkup. His birth history and delivery were uncomplicated. He is being breastfed and has had no difficulty feeding. The parents are concerned because he does not seem to have male genital characteristics. Physical examination reveals female external genitalia seen without a scrotum or descended testicles. What androgen is the patient lacking that is the cause of his condition?
(A) Androstenedione
(B) Androsterone
(C) Dehydroepiandrosterone (DHEA)
(D) Dihydrotestosterone (DHT)
(E) Testosterone

77 A 42-year-old man is a habitual coffee drinker of caffeinated products. Chronic use of this product has led to his addiction. What is the most likely mechanism of action of caffeine?
(A) Increase in adenosine diphosphate
(B) Increase in cyclic guanosine monophosphate
(C) Inhibition of guanosine receptors
(D) Inhibition of thymine receptors
(E) Inhibition of uracil receptors

78 A 67-year-old woman with diabetes presents to clinic for an annual visit. She has been doing well over the past, and her hemoglobin A_{1c} is 6.9%. Her fasting cholesterol showed a total cholesterol of 152 mg/dL, LDL of 68 mg/dL, and HDL of 31 mg/dL. Which medication is shown to have the greatest increase in HDL?
(A) Cholestyramine
(B) Ezetimibe
(C) Gemfibrozil
(D) Lovastatin
(E) Niacin

79 A 55-year-old man with hypertension presents for an annual visit. He admits to exercising less and eating fast food more often over the past year. His fasting cholesterol panel shows a total cholesterol of 266 mg/dL, LDL of 178 mg/dL, and HDL of 43 mg/dL. The physician would like to start him on lovastatin. What lab tests should the physician order prior to starting lovastatin?
(A) BUN/creatinine
(B) Complete blood count
(C) Fasting blood glucose
(D) Liver function tests
(E) Uric acid level

80 A 42-year-old woman presents to clinic with fatigue for the past 2 weeks. She has a history of diabetes, hypothyroidism, lupus, hypertension, and GERD. She currently takes metformin, levothyroxine, prednisone, hydrochlorothiazide, and cimetidine. She reports that her blood sugar has been well controlled. Her TSH and free T_4 are both within normal limits. She has not had a recent lupus flare. The physician is unsure of the cause of her fatigue and gathers some blood work. The complete blood count is significant for a white blood cell count of 16.1. What medication may be responsible for her elevated white blood cell count?
(A) Cimetidine
(B) Hydrochlorothiazide
(C) Levothyroxine
(D) Metformin
(E) Prednisone

81 A 78-year-old postmenopausal woman has been steadily losing weight over the past 6 months. She has no family history of breast or endometrial cancer. Which steroid hormone could she be given to increase her appetite?
(A) Drospirenone
(B) Ethinyl estradiol
(C) Medroxyprogesterone
(D) Megestrol
(E) Norgestrel

82 A 47-year-old woman presents to the clinic for her annual visit. Her last fasting blood glucose on her last visit showed she has borderline diabetes. She tried to make lifestyle changes to improve her blood sugars. However, her fasting blood glucose is 215 mg/dL this year. She is started on metformin and encouraged to live a healthier lifestyle. What is a side effect associated with metformin?
(A) Disulfiram-like reaction
(B) Hypoglycemia
(C) Lactic acidosis
(D) Pancreatitis
(E) Weight gain

83 A 63-year-old female presents to clinic for a diabetes follow-up. She has been taking metformin for 3 years now, but her blood sugars have not been well controlled over the past year. Her average morning fasting blood sugar is 165 mg/dL, and her 2-h postprandial is 205 mg/dL. Glimepiride is added to her regimen. What is the mechanism of action of glimepiride?
(A) Decreased glucagon release
(B) Increased insulin release
(C) Increased insulin sensitivity in peripheral tissues
(D) Inhibits hepatic gluconeogenesis
(E) Inhibits intestinal brush border enzymes

84 An 18-year-old female with diabetes presents to the clinic for her annual visit. Over the past year, she has experienced daily nausea and occasional vomiting. She has learned that eating small amounts of food at a time helps to decrease the frequency of vomiting. She is diagnosed with diabetic gastroparesis and started on metoclopramide. What is a side effect of metoclopramide?
(A) Dry mouth
(B) Gynecomastia
(C) Headache
(D) Increased risk of abortion
(E) Tardive dyskinesia

85 A 29-year-old man with a family history of heart disease comes to your office for a routine checkup. A lipid profile on a blood draw reveals high LDL and low HDL. One way to decrease the amount of LDL in the blood is to hinder intestinal absorption of cholesterol. Which of the following drugs blocks brush border enzymes to inhibit intestinal absorption of cholesterol?
(A) Cholestyramine
(B) Colesevelam
(C) Colestipol
(D) Ezetimibe
(E) Rosuvastatin

86 A 37-year-old woman patient with hyperlipidemia is taking a drug to lower her triglyceride and blood cholesterol levels. She is considering stopping her therapy, however, because of a red, itchy rash on her face and neck that occurs following some doses. What could she use to avoid this side effect?

(A) Aspirin
(B) Calamine lotion
(C) Cimetidine
(D) Diphenhydramine
(E) This reaction is unavoidable

87 A 35-year-old man presents to the emergency department complaining of a cough and runny nose of 1-week duration. While being evaluated, it is discovered that his blood pressure is 230/120 mm Hg. An antihypertensive is immediately administered. Later, he develops lactic acidosis, headache, vertigo, and confusion. Which of the following initial therapies would best treat his new symptoms?

(A) Activated charcoal
(B) Methylene blue
(C) Nothing; these symptoms are temporary and result from a rapid decrease in blood pressure
(D) Penicillamine
(E) Sodium nitrite

88 A 27-year-old woman presents to clinic with infertility over the past 2 years. Her husband had a normal sperm analysis. She has also had weight gain and increased facial hair. Her labs show an increase in both her LH and FSH, with a ratio of LH:FSH of 2:1. What is the most appropriate medication to help her with her infertility?

(A) Clomiphene
(B) Combined estrogen–progestin pill
(C) Dinoprostone
(D) Estrogen
(E) Mifepristone

89 A 62-year-old man has developed worsening hypertension in spite of therapy. His physician wants to prescribe an additional medication that will dilate his blood vessels to help lower his blood pressure. Which of the following is a calcium channel blocker that affects vascular smooth muscle and cardiac muscle equally well?

(A) Amlodipine
(B) Diltiazem
(C) Losartan
(D) Nitroprusside
(E) Verapamil

90 A 33-year-old woman presents with tachycardia, heat intolerance, tremor, and unintentional weight loss. Her TSH level is markedly elevated. Her physician prescribes a drug that will block TSH release. Which drug is this?

(A) Levothyroxine
(B) Methimazole
(C) Octreotide
(D) Potassium iodide
(E) Propylthiouracil

91 A 57-year-old man was recently diagnosed with Type-2 diabetes mellitus and placed on a medication. He began having myalgias and feeling sick and later developed respiratory distress, so he went to the hospital. His pH was 7.2, and he had elevated blood lactate levels. Which drug is likely causing his problem?

(A) Acarbose
(B) Glyburide
(C) Metformin
(D) Pioglitazone
(E) Tolbutamide

92 A 76-year-old man presents to the clinic for follow-up of his benign prostatic hyperplasia. He has been doing well with his symptoms since starting finasteride. He no longer has as much difficulty starting his stream and feels that he empties his bladder completely. What is the mechanism of action of finasteride?

(A) 5α-Reductase inhibitor
(B) α_1-Antagonist
(C) GnRH agonist
(D) GnRH antagonist
(E) Nonsteroidal competitive inhibitor at the testosterone receptor

93 A 43-year-old woman with Type-2 diabetes has been taking insulin with meals as well as metformin. Her blood glucose remains poorly controlled. Her doctor prescribes an additional drug, which is an analog of an endogenous peptide that enhances insulin secretion. What drug is this?

(A) Exenatide
(B) Glipizide
(C) Miglitol
(D) Pramlintide
(E) Rosiglitazone

94 A 64-year-old woman presents to her primary care physician for follow-up. She is being treated for a ventricular arrhythmia. She is placed on a new medication and now complains of feeling tired. She also has diarrhea and weight loss. She also feels very anxious and nervous. Laboratory studies indicate low thyroxin and elevated thyroid-stimulating hormone levels. Which of the following antiarrhythmic drugs is the likely cause of these signs and symptoms?

(A) Amiodarone
(B) Procainamide
(C) Propranolol
(D) Quinidine
(E) Verapamil

95 A 52-year-old overweight woman presents to the clinic for a diabetes management. She had not been doing well controlling her blood sugars with metformin. Her last hemoglobin A_{1c} was 13.4%, despite her taking her medication every day. The physician decides to start her on a long-acting insulin that is injected only once a day for better glucose control. Also, he wants the insulin to have a minimal risk of hypoglycemia. What is the most likely medication given to this patient?

(A) Insulin aspart
(B) Insulin glargine
(C) Insulin lispro
(D) NPH insulin
(E) Regular insulin

96 A 23-year-old woman presents to her primary care physician with an enlarging neck mass and weight loss. The large mass is seen in the midline of the neck. She has lost 15 lb over the past month, feels like her heart is racing, and is always hot. The patient is diagnosed with Graves' disease and started on propylthiouracil. Which of the following is a side effect of propylthiouracil?

(A) Agranulocytosis
(B) Arrhythmias
(C) Diabetes
(D) Hypertension
(E) Tachycardia

97 A 34-year-old man presents to his primary care physician because of an enlarging jaw and hands over the past 6 months. He has noticed enlargement of most his facial features, including his jaw, forehead, nose, and tongue. His hands have gotten bigger as well. He is diagnosed with acromegaly. What is the most appropriate treatment for this patient?

(A) Desmopressin
(B) Growth hormone
(C) Octreotide
(D) Oxytocin
(E) Propylthiouracil

98 A 42-year-old man with hypertriglyceridemia comes from a family with the same abnormality as his brother, sister, father, and father's brother. He presents to a primary care physician in a new city. Which of the following is the most cost-effective treatment of this condition?

(A) Diet
(B) Niacin
(C) Riboflavin
(D) Statin therapy
(E) Watchful waiting

99 Five patients with elevated cholesterol present to the ambulatory care clinic for treatment of abnormalities of cholesterol. Which of the following patients would best benefit from treatment with an HMG-CoA reductase inhibitor?

(A) Total cholesterol = 180 mg/dL, HDL = 100 mg/dL
(B) Total cholesterol = 180 mg/dL, LDL = 100 mg/dL
(C) Total cholesterol = 180 mg/dL, HDL = 60 mg/dL
(D) Total cholesterol = 220 mg/dL, HDL= 100 mg/dL
(E) LDL = 60 mg/dL, HDL = 100 mg/dL

100 A 54-year-old man with elevated cholesterol levels is treated with niacin. Within 2 weeks of starting therapy, he develops an uncomfortable feeling of warmth and itchiness. Which of the following is the most appropriate next step in the management of this patient?

(A) Administer aspirin prior to niacin
(B) Administer prednisone orally and continue niacin
(C) Administer prednisone orally and discontinue niacin
(D) Consider a twice-daily dosage of niacin
(E) Transfer patient to an emergency department for intravenous prednisone

101 A 48-year-old female who is obese with elevated cholesterol is treated with fenofibrate for elevated cholesterol levels. She complains of acute onset of right upper quadrant pain, nausea, and vomiting after eating a fatty meal. She is brought to the emergency department for further evaluation. Which of the following is the most likely explanation for these findings?

(A) Drug overdose
(B) Gallstone formation
(C) Iatrogenic effect
(D) Myositis
(E) Inflammatory pancreatitis

102 A 57-year-old woman with elevated triglycerides and cholesterol takes a medication that binds bile acids in the intestine, thus preventing their return to the liver via the enterohepatic circulation. This description suggests that the patient is taking which of the following medications?

(A) Cholestyramine
(B) Fenofibrate
(C) Fluvastatin
(D) Lovastatin
(E) Niacin

103 A 37-year-old man is found to have hypercholesterolemia during a routine checkup. The physician prescribes lovastatin and counsels the patient to make healthy dietary and lifestyle changes to keep his cholesterol under control. Two months later, he returns for a follow-up visit, and the physician discovers his LDL level remains virtually unchanged. He insists that he is taking the medication exactly as prescribed. The physician knows lovastatin is metabolized by the cytochrome P450 3A4. What else may he be using that would explain his condition?

(A) Cimetidine
(B) Diltiazem
(C) Ketoconazole
(D) Ritonavir
(E) St. John's wort supplement

104 A young married couple complains of being unable to conceive after 9 months of unprotected sex. The wife has normal TSH and FSH levels and a normal pelvic exam. They agree to a trial of letrozole to see if they can increase their fecundity. How does letrozole work?

(A) Blocks E_2 receptors on the hypothalamus
(B) Increases sperm production
(C) Inhibits aromatase
(D) Stimulates follicular development
(E) Suppresses prolactin secretion

105 A 45-year-old woman with diabetes and hypertension presents to the primary care clinic with a cough. The nonproductive cough started about 2 weeks ago. She has not had a fever, congestion, or been around any sick contacts. However, she was recently started on lisinopril. The physician decides to switch her to losartan, and the patient reports that her cough has ceased. What is the mechanism of action of losartan?

(A) Activates angiotensin I receptor
(B) Activates angiotensin II receptor
(C) Inhibits angiotensin-converting enzyme
(D) Inhibits angiotensin I receptor
(E) Inhibits angiotensin II receptor

106 An 18-year-old woman presents to the primary care clinic for a routine visit. She has been feeling well over the past year. She tells the physician she is in a long-term relationship with a boyfriend and has been sexually active. She would like to start using oral contraceptive pills. The physician should inform the patient about what possible side effect?

(A) Headaches
(B) Increased menstrual bleeding
(C) Increased risk of ovarian cancer
(D) Venous thromboembolism
(E) Weight gain

107 A 54-year-old woman presents to the primary care clinic with hot flashes and irregular menstrual cycles. These symptoms started about 3 months ago and have worsened recently. She has always had regular menstrual cycles until 3 months ago. She would like to start hormone replacement therapy but estrogen only. What is a common side effect of unopposed estrogen replacement therapy?

(A) Depression
(B) Increased risk of endometrial cancer
(C) Osteoporosis
(D) Rash
(E) Vaginal atrophy

108 A 44-year-old woman with a long history of diarrhea, sweating, and weight loss is thought to have hyperthyroidism. This condition can be worsened with which of the following treatments?

(A) Iodide
(B) Methimazole
(C) Propylthiouracil
(D) Surgical removal of the thyroid gland
(E) Triiodothyronine

109 A 57-year-old man with hyperlipidemia presents to the emergency department with severe pain in his first right toe. The pain is a 10/10 and worse with any contact. The toe is erythematous, inflamed, and warm to touch. Joint aspiration confirms gout. He had an episode of gout about 10 years ago. What medication used to treat his hyperlipidemia may have led to his gout flare?

(A) Cholestyramine
(B) Ezetimibe
(C) Gemfibrozil
(D) Lovastatin
(E) Niacin

110 A 43-year-old woman presents to the primary care clinic for follow-up. During her last visit, her fasting lipid panel showed a triglyceride level of 315 mg/dL. She tried to eat healthier and increase her exercise regimen. Her lipid panel was rechecked and showed a total cholesterol of 189 mg/dL, LDL of 88 mg/dL, HDL of 52 mg/dL, and triglycerides of 286 mg/dL. What medication will lower the triglyceride level the most?

(A) Colestipol
(B) Ezetimibe
(C) Gemfibrozil
(D) Niacin
(E) Rosuvastatin

111 A 38-year-old woman with hyperlipidemia presents to the primary care clinic with worsening muscle aches. Her total cholesterol was 268 mg/dL, her LDL was 167 mg/dL, her HDL was 42 mg/dL, and her triglycerides was 254 mg/dL during her last visit. The decision was made to add another lipid-lowering medication to her simvastatin. She never had muscle aches before and is wondering if the new medication is causing her new pain. What medication was most likely added to her simvastatin?

(A) Cholestyramine
(B) Colestipol
(C) Ezetimibe
(D) Gemfibrozil
(E) Niacin

112 A 23-year-old healthy man receives an infusion of 100 mL of glucose solution. Which of the following curves would represent his plasma insulin concentration at 2 min after infusion?

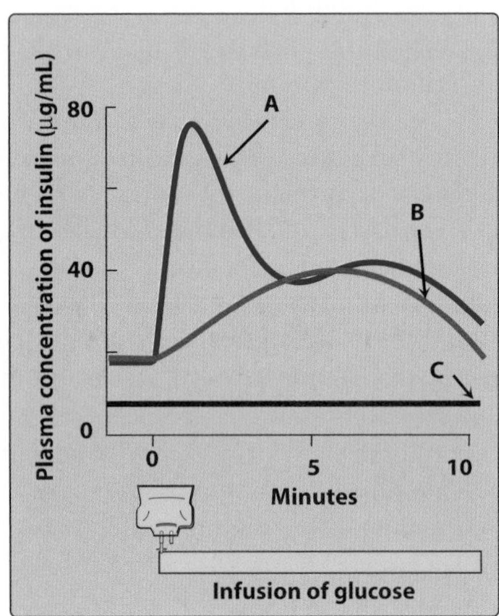

(A) Letter A
(B) Letter B
(C) Letter C
(D) Cannot be determined

113 A 57-year-old man with Type-2 diabetes presents to the primary care clinic for follow-up. He has been taking metformin and has had good control of his sugars. He denies any hypoglycemic episodes or peripheral neuropathy. His hemoglobin A_{1c} is 8.3%, which is increased from 7.9% previously. The physician decides to add miglitol to his regimen. What is the mechanism of action of miglitol?

(A) Decreased glucagon release
(B) Increased insulin release
(C) Increased insulin sensitivity in peripheral tissues
(D) Inhibits hepatic gluconeogenesis
(E) Inhibits intestinal brush border enzymes

114 A 72-year-old man with Type-2 diabetes and hypertension presents to the emergency department after feeling dizzy and falling. In the emergency department, he becomes confused and does not know where he is. His blood pressure is 134/76 mm Hg. His blood sugar is 34 mg/dL. He is given dextrose, and as his blood sugar improves, so does his mental status. What medication most likely caused this patient's hypoglycemia?

(A) Acarbose
(B) Exenatide
(C) Glyburide
(D) Metformin
(E) Pioglitazone

115 A 44-year-old man with Type-2 diabetes presents to the ambulatory care clinic for follow-up. He was diagnosed with diabetes 6 months ago and was started on oral medication then. His blood sugar has been under good control with a hemoglobin A_{1c} of 6.7%. He has not had any hypoglycemic episodes. His only complaint is that despite daily exercise and eating healthier, he has gained 12 lb in the last 6 months. What medication is most likely to cause his weight gain?

(A) Acarbose
(B) Exenatide
(C) Glyburide
(D) Metformin
(E) Pioglitazone

116 A 75-year-old man with metastatic prostate cancer is placed on leuprolide administered monthly in an intramuscular injection. This agent will act at which of the following areas on the succeeding diagram?

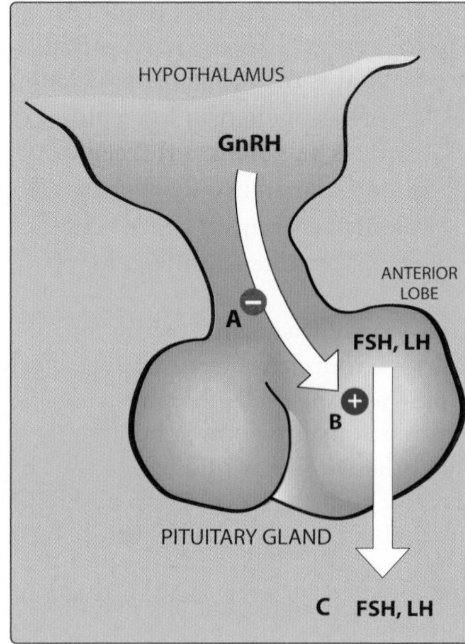

(A) Letter A
(B) Letter B
(C) Letter C
(D) Cannot be determined

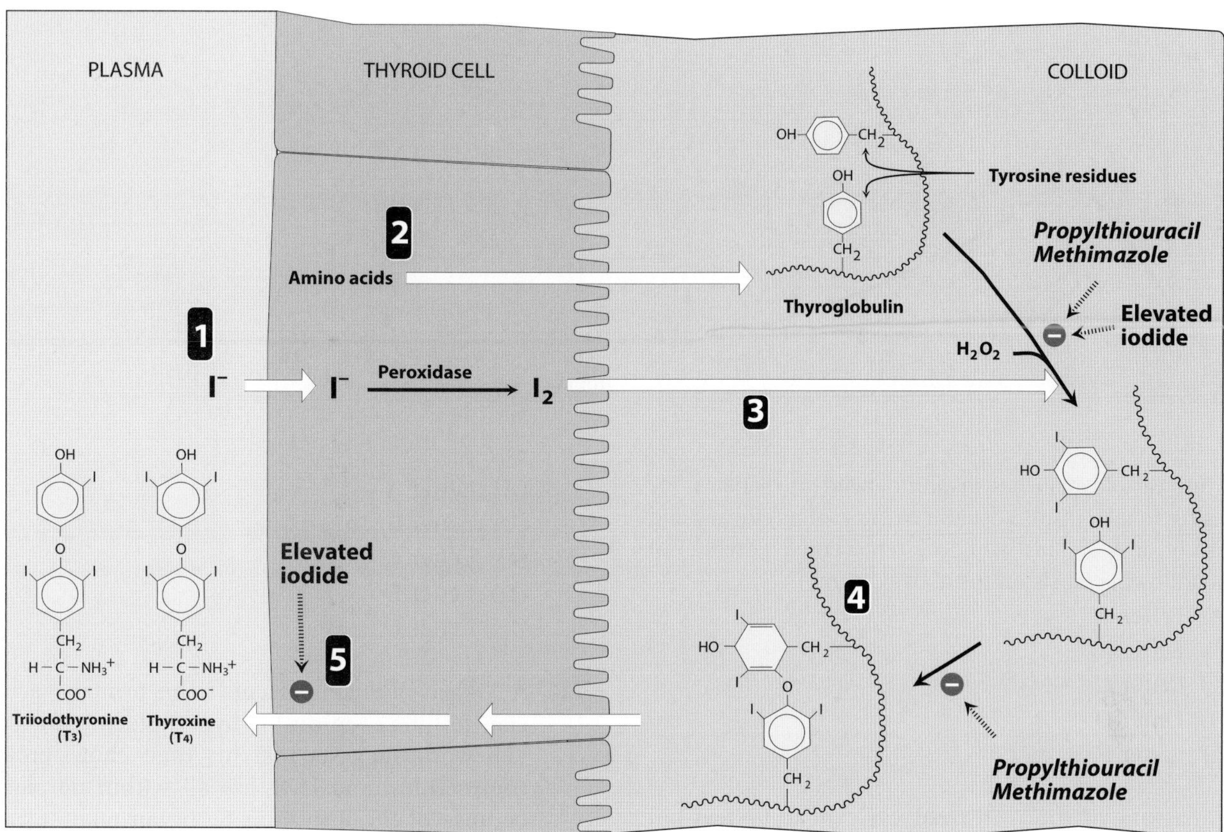

117 Regarding the biosynthesis of thyroid hormones, if a novel medication was developed to block the proteolytic release of hormones, this medication would act at which of the following sites?

(A) Location 1
(B) Location 2
(C) Location 3
(D) Location 4
(E) Location 5

118 In the following figure, five patients (A through E) have various stages of diabetes mellitus. Which of the following patients would best benefit from therapy with diet and exercise alone?

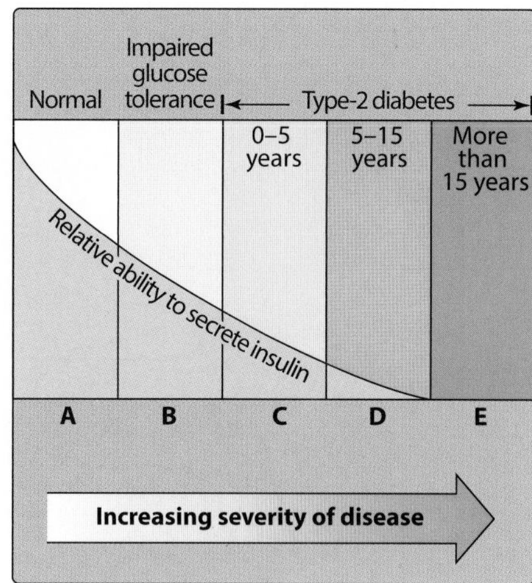

(A) Patient A
(B) Patient B
(C) Patient C
(D) Patient D
(E) Patient E

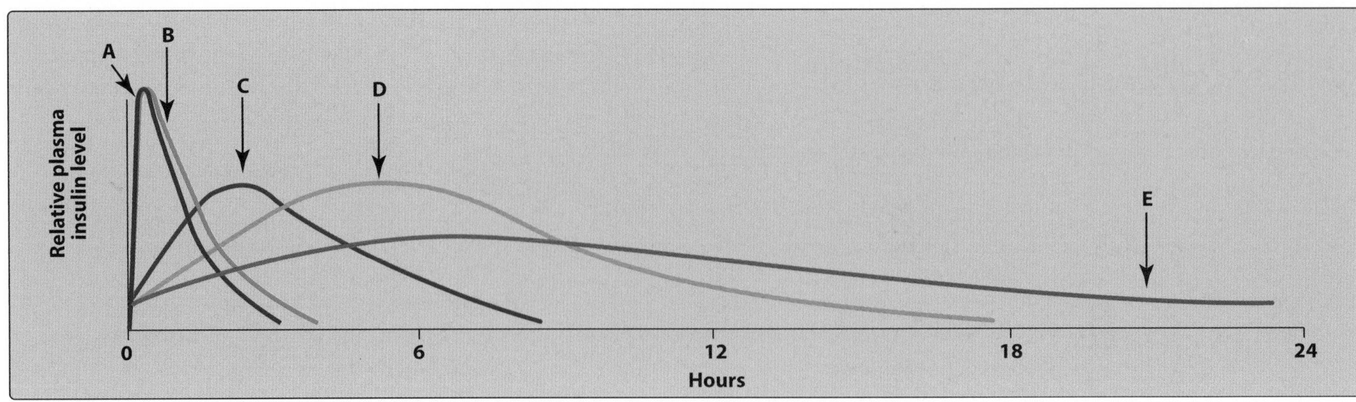

119 A 54-year-old man has insulin-dependent diabetes. He desires to take insulin detemir because of its efficacy and ease of dosing. This would be represented as which of the following labels on the above diagram?

(A) Letter A
(B) Letter B
(C) Letter C
(D) Letter D
(E) Letter E

120 A diagram of the menstrual cycle in a 19-year-old woman who complains of dysmenorrhea is shown as follows. Which of the following points represents the highest level of estradiol?

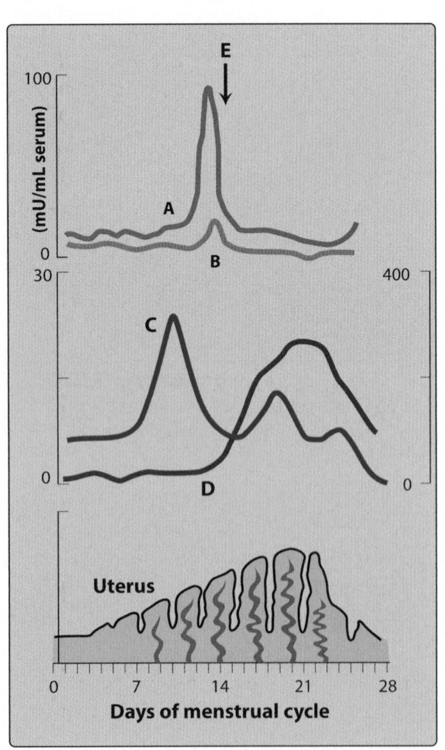

(A) Letter A
(B) Letter B
(C) Letter C
(D) Letter D
(E) Letter E

121 A 55-year-old man presents to his primary care physician to follow up on his hyperlipidemia medication. Lab work suggests that his total cholesterol, LDL, triglycerides, and HDL are all within normal limits because of the lovastatin he began taking 2 months ago. He has not visited the office since being prescribed this medication. Which of the following lab tests should be obtained at the present office visit?

(A) Electrocardiogram
(B) Hemoglobin A_{1c} levels
(C) Liver function tests
(D) Pulmonary function tests
(E) Potassium levels

ANSWERS

1 **The answer is D: Increasing synthesis of IκB.** Glucocorticoids affect many cell types in the body. In this case, the patient would benefit most from inhibiting inflammation. All the responses listed are known glucocorticoid effects, but only increasing synthesis of IκB would decrease inflammation. IκB inhibits NF-κB, which is a transcription factor for enzymes that make inflammatory cytokines. (A) Exogenous dexamethasone given along with ondansetron to patients with low cortisol levels before chemotherapy had less nausea than those given ondansetron alone. This effect would not be as useful as inhibiting inflammation in this patient. (B) Glucocorticoid suppression of growth factors leading to decrease proliferation would not be as useful as inhibiting inflammation in this patient. (C) Glucocorticoids raise blood glucose levels by several mechanisms, two of which are to decrease GLUT4 receptors in the cell membrane and to stimulate gluconeogenesis. (E) Increased blood glucose is an unfortunate side effect and would not be useful in this patient.

2 **The answer is A: Cardiovascular collapse (adrenal crisis).** Chronic use of glucocorticoids (such as prednisone) will lead to adrenal atrophy because the exogenous steroid suppresses the hypothalamic-pituitary-adrenal (HPA) axis. If the exogenous steroid is abruptly withdrawn, the atrophied adrenal gland is unable to compensate by producing endogenous steroids quickly enough. The sudden loss of adrenal steroids is termed "adrenal crisis" and can result in cardiovascular collapse and death. (B) Osteoporosis is a possible result of continued chronic glucocorticoid therapy, not abrupt cessation. (C) Increased risk of infection is a result of continued chronic glucocorticoid therapy, not abrupt cessation. (D) Insomnia is a possible side effect from short-term oral or parenteral glucocorticoid therapy. (E) Nausea/vomiting are possible side effects from short-term oral or parenteral glucocorticoid therapy.

3 **The answer is B: Neostigmine.** This patient has evidence of peritonitis based on the physical examination findings of guarding and rebound tenderness. Neostigmine is contraindicated when intestinal or urinary bladder obstruction is present. It should not be used for patients who have peritonitis or inflammatory bowel disease. (A) This patient has diabetes and should have her insulin continued as scheduled. (C) Nifedipine should be continued in this patient as scheduled. (D) Rivastigmine should be continued in this patient as scheduled. (E) Tacrine should be continued in this patient as scheduled.

4 **The answer is B: Hypertensive headaches.** Tyramine is not a clinically useful drug, but it is important because it is found in fermented foods, such as aged cheese and Chianti wine. It is a normal byproduct of tyrosine metabolism. Normally, it is oxidized by MAO in the gastrointestinal tract, but, if the patient is taking MAOIs, it can precipitate serious vasopressor epinephrine. Like amphetamines, tyramine can enter the nerve terminal and displace stored norepinephrine. The released catecholamine then acts on adrenoceptors. (A) Tyramine is unlikely to cause diarrhea. (C) Tyramine is unlikely to cause increase in tear formation and release. (D) Tyramine is unlikely to cause sweating. (E) Tremors are unlikely to be a result of catecholamine surge.

5 **The answer is A: A 19-year-old man with sexual arousal difficulties.** Yohimbine is a selective competitive α_2-blocker. It is found as a component of the bark of the yohimbe tree and is sometimes used as a sexual stimulant. The efficacy of yohimbine for the treatment of impotence has never been clearly demonstrated. Yohimbine works at the level of the CNS to increase sympathetic outflow to the periphery. (B) This patient would benefit from a medication to treat erectile dysfunction such as sildenafil, tadalafil, or vardenafil. (C) This patient would benefit from a medication to treat erectile dysfunction such as sildenafil, tadalafil, or vardenafil. (D) This patient would benefit from an erectogenic agent similar to the previous patient description. (E) This patient probably should be treated with an erectogenic agent because he has cardiac problems.

6 **The answer is E: Rosuvastatin.** Cholesterol in the body has two sources: diet and de novo synthesis in hepatocytes. All "statin" drugs (including rosuvastatin) inhibit the rate-limiting enzyme in cholesterol synthesis—HMG-CoA reductase. Hepatocytes use cholesterol to make bile. When they cannot synthesize sufficient cholesterol de novo, they upregulate LDL receptors on their surfaces to increase uptake of cholesterol in LDL from the blood. This, in turn, lowers blood LDL levels. (A) Cholestyramine binds up bile salts in the intestine, preventing their reabsorption and recycling. This means hepatocytes must make much more bile salts than normal to replace those that are lost in the feces. (B) Colesevelam prevents bile salt reabsorption in the intestine. The high demand on hepatocytes to make more bile salts translates into a large increase in need for cholesterol. (C) Colestipol binds up bile salts in the intestine. It increases de novo synthesis of cholesterol and increased uptake of LDL in the blood result. (D) Ezetimibe works by inhibiting dietary uptake of cholesterol at the intestinal brush border. Ezetimibe is synergistic with the statins but ineffective when used alone because of a compensatory increase in de novo synthesis of cholesterol.

7 **The answer is D: Nicotinic acid.** Nicotinic acid and niacin are both names for vitamin B_3. Niacin in large doses is effective for preventing lipolysis, increasing HDL levels, and decreasing LDL levels. Its primary adverse effect is flushing, which may be itchy and occurs usually on the head, neck, and chest. The mechanism for niacin's beneficial effects on lipids is unknown, but the flushing appears to be caused largely by niacin-induced release of prostaglandin D_2 from mast cells (which causes vasodilation). (A) Atorvastatin is an HMG-CoA reductase inhibitor blocking de novo cholesterol synthesis. HMG-CoA reductase inhibitors are known for their potential to cause rhabdomyolysis. (B) Fenofibrate is not known to cause flushing. (C) Gemfibrozil is not known to cause flushing. (E) Omacor is omega-3 fatty acids and is not known to cause flushing.

8 **The answer is A: Appetite stimulant.** Dronabinol is indicated as an appetite stimulant for patients with acquired immunodeficiency syndrome who are losing weight. Dronabinol is administered orally and has a peak effect in 2 to 4 h. Its psychoactive effects can last up to 6 h, but its appetite-stimulant effects may persist for 24 h. It is also sometimes given for the severe emesis caused by some cancer chemotherapeutic agents. (B) This agent does not stimulate chemotactic centers of the brain. (C) This agent does not stimulate epidermal growth factor. (D) This agent does not stimulate keratinocyte growth factor. (E) This agent does not stimulate growth hormone.

9 **The answer is C: Inhibiting osteoclasts.** Osteoporosis develops as the result of an imbalance between bone formation and breakdown. Osteoblasts stimulate bone formation by secreting organic osteoid, which is then mineralized by incorporating calcium and phosphate. Osteoclasts secrete enzymes to break down the organic component of bone and acid to dissolve the inorganic component. Bone formation and bone breakdown are constant and normally balanced. Decreased serum calcium, increased osteoclast activity, or decreased osteoblast activity can all lead to osteoporosis. Alendronate works primarily by inhibiting osteoclast activity. (A) Vitamin D increases intestinal absorption of calcium. Alendronate's primary mechanism of action is to inhibit osteoclasts. (B) Thiazide diuretics are an example of drugs that decrease renal calcium excretion. Vitamin D also decreases renal calcium excretion. Alendronate's primary mechanism of action is to inhibit osteoclasts. (D) Alendronate does not provide starting materials for bone mineralization. Alendronate's primary mechanism of action is to inhibit osteoclasts. (E) Alendronate does not stimulate osteoblasts. Alendronate's primary mechanism of action is to inhibit osteoclasts.

10 **The answer is E: Propylthiouracil.** Methimazole and propylthiouracil both decrease the synthesis of thyroid hormone, but only propylthiouracil decreases the peripheral conversion of T_4 to T_3. These drugs both inhibit thyroid peroxidase, which is the enzyme responsible for oxidation and organification of iodide for its incorporation into T_3 and T_4. Because it also inhibits peripheral conversion to T_3, propylthiouracil may be preferred in severe hyperthyroidism. (A) Lanreotide is a somatostatin analog used in secondary hyperthyroidism because somatostatin normally inhibits TSH secretion. (B) Levothyroxine is a synthetic T_4. It is used to treat hypothyroidism and would worsen this patient's condition. (C) Methimazole does decrease the synthesis of thyroid hormone but does not decrease the peripheral conversion of T_4 to T_3. (D) Octreotide is a somatostatin analog used in secondary hyperthyroidism because somatostatin normally inhibits TSH secretion.

11 **The answer is E: Tolbutamide.** This scenario describes a disulfiram-like effect of his medication. Disulfiram inhibits the enzyme acetaldehyde dehydrogenase. When alcohol is consumed, it is metabolized to acetaldehyde (a toxic metabolite) by alcohol dehydrogenase, and then acetaldehyde is metabolized to harmless acetic acid by acetaldehyde dehydrogenase. When acetaldehyde dehydrogenase is inhibited, acetaldehyde reaches high levels and causes nausea, vomiting, and headache. First-generation sulfonylureas such as tolbutamide are known to produce a disulfiram-like effect. (A) Acarbose inhibits intestinal brush border enzymes to decrease the amount of carbohydrate absorption after a meal and can cause GI discomfort. It is not known to cause a disulfiram-like reaction. (B) Glyburide is a second-generation sulfonylurea. Second-generation sulfonylureas work the same way as first-generation sulfonylureas but do not have the disulfiram-like side effect. (C) Metformin's most severe adverse reaction is lactic acidosis, but this is rare. It is not known to cause a disulfiram-like reaction. (D) Pioglitazone adverse effects include hepatotoxicity and weight gain. It is not known to cause a disulfiram-like reaction.

12 **The answer is D: Pramlintide.** Glucagon is inhibited by two endogenous peptides: insulin and amylin. Pramlintide is an analog of amylin. Pramlintide also diminishes the postprandial blood glucose spike by slowing gastric emptying and suppressing the appetite. Currently, pramlintide is indicated only in patients with diabetes taking insulin with meals. (A) Exenatide mimics incretin secretion, which increases glucose-dependent insulin secretion. It does not inhibit secretion. (B) Glipizide is a second-generation sulfonylurea. These drugs enhance insulin secretion but do not block glucagon secretion.

(C) Miglitol inhibits intestinal brush border α-glucosidase. This enzyme is needed for the final steps in carbohydrate breakdown before absorption, so miglitol decreases the amount of dietary carbohydrate absorbed. (E) Rosiglitazone lowers blood glucose by increasing insulin sensitivity in peripheral tissues. It does not inhibit glucagon secretion.

13 **The answer is A: Demeclocycline.** Antidiuretic hormone (ADH) is normally only secreted in response to hypovolemia and increased serum osmolarity. When ADH is inappropriately secreted (as in ADH secretion by cancer cells), serum sodium concentration is diminished because the kidneys retain too much free water. This is known as the syndrome of inappropriate ADH secretion (SIADH). Demeclocycline corrects this by blocking ADH effects on the kidneys' collecting ducts. (B) Doxycycline is a tetracycline antibiotic and has no effect on the kidneys' response to ADH. (C) Minocycline is a tetracycline antibiotic and has no effect on the kidneys' response to ADH. (D) Tetracycline has no effect on the kidneys' response to ADH. (E) Tigecycline is a derivative of minocycline but belongs to a newer class of antibiotics called the glycylcyclines.

14 **The answer is E: Leuprolide.** Female infertility may be caused simply by decreased oocyte production by the ovaries. If this is the case, stimulating the ovaries with gonadotropins could easily restore fertility. Gonadotropins are released from the anterior pituitary when it is stimulated by gonadotropin-releasing hormone (GnRH). GnRH secretion is normally pulsatile; constant exposure of the anterior pituitary to GnRH results in inhibition of gonadotropin release. Leuprolide is a GnRH analog. As such, constant administration of leuprolide will suppress gonadotropin release and ovulation, whereas pulsatile administration will stimulate gonadotropin release and ovulation. (A) Bromocriptine allows gonadotropin release by inhibiting prolactin secretion. It may also directly stimulate some gonadotropin release. Its effect does not alternate between inhibitory and stimulatory based on its dosing schedule. (B) Clomiphene acts directly on the hypothalamus to cause GnRH secretion. Its effect does not alternate between inhibitory and stimulatory based on its dosing schedule. (C) Estrone sulfate (as well as other estrogens) enhances fertility by offsetting the thickened cervical mucus that can be caused by clomiphene therapy. Its effect does not alternate between inhibitory and stimulatory based on its dosing schedule. (D) Human chorionic gonadotropin (hCG) mimics the activity of luteinizing hormone, the gonadotropin responsible for ovulation. Its effect does not alternate between inhibitory and stimulatory based on its dosing schedule.

15 **The answer is A: Extensive hepatic first-pass metabolism.** Losartan, the first approved member of the class, differs from the others in that it undergoes extensive first-pass hepatic metabolism, including conversion to its active metabolite. The other drugs have inactive metabolites. Elimination of metabolites and parent compounds occurs in urine and feces. The proportion depends on the individual drug. (B) This patient is not taking antacids, so this should not be a problem for him. (C) The route of administration should not pose a problem for this patient. (D) Renal excretion of losartan should not compromise efficacy. (E) This medication is not required to be taken with a full stomach.

16 **The answer is A: Decrease venous return to the heart.** Diuretics relieve pulmonary congestion and peripheral edema. These agents are also useful in reducing the symptoms of volume overload, including orthopnea and paroxysmal nocturnal dyspnea. Diuretics decrease plasma volume and, subsequently, decrease venous return to the heart (preload). This decreases the cardiac workload and the oxygen demand. Diuretics may also decrease afterload by reducing plasma volume, thereby decreasing blood pressure. (B) Diuretics will decrease blood pressure. (C) Diuretics will decrease circulatory volume. (D) Diuretics do not act as inotropes and will not change heart rate. (E) Diuretics will decrease plasma volume, which will reduce afterload.

17 **The answer is B: Electrolytes.** Thiazide diuretics induce hypokalemia and hyperuricemia in 70% of patients and hyperglycemia in 10% of patients. Thus, serum electrolytes should be monitored periodically in these patients. Acute gout attacks may be triggered. Hypomagnesemia may also occur. Serum potassium levels should be monitored closely in patients who are predisposed to cardiac arrhythmias (particularly individuals with left ventricular hypertrophy, ischemic heart disease, or chronic heart failure) and those who are concurrently being treated with both thiazide diuretics and digoxin. (A) Serum electrolytes are more likely to be abnormal than hemoglobin and white blood cell count. (C) There is no reason to suggest a hemoglobinopathy in this patient. (D) Hematocrit is likely to be normal in this patient. (E) Plasma proteins are likely to be normal in this patient.

18 **The answer is A: Bradykinin stimulation.** Common side effects include dry cough, rash, fever, altered taste, hypotension (in hypovolemic states), and hyperkalemia. The dry cough, which occurs in about 10% of patients, is thought to be caused by increased levels of bradykinin in the pulmonary tree. It occurs more frequently in women and nonsmokers and with longer acting ACE inhibitors. (B) Bradykinin stimulation causes chronic cough, not an inflammatory process. (C) Pulmonary embolism is highly unlikely in this patient. (D) This is not an infectious process. It is an inflammatory process mediated by bradykinin. (E) This patient does not have a restrictive cardiomyopathy.

19 **The answer is A: Bosentan.** Primary pulmonary hypertension is a rare form of pulmonary hypertension that can be caused by a mutation in the BMPR2 gene. The BMPR2 gene product normally inhibits excessive smooth muscle proliferation. In the absence of functional BMPR2, pulmonary vascular smooth muscle proliferates more than normal, leading to a decrease in the compliance of pulmonary arteries and an increase in pressure. Bosentan is an endothelin receptor antagonist that is useful in blocking this proliferation. Bosentan would be the best choice of drug to help this patient's pulmonary hypertension. (B) Captopril is an angiotensin-converting enzyme inhibitor. It is used in the treatment of systemic hypertension. It would not be the best choice because it would not affect the underlying cause of hypertension in this patient's case. (C) Furosemide is a loop diuretic. It is used in the treatment of systemic hypertension to reduce fluid load. It would not be the best choice in this patient's case. (D) Labetalol is a β-adrenergic receptor blocker that can be used to treat systemic hypertension. It would not be the best choice because it would not affect the underlying cause of hypertension in this patient's case. (E) Valsartan is an angiotensin II receptor blocker. It is used to treat systemic hypertension. Because it would not affect the underlying cause of hypertension in this patient, it would not be the best choice.

20 **The answer is A: Afferent arteriole vasoconstriction.** Furosemide is a loop diuretic. It works by inhibiting ion (and therefore water) uptake in the ascending limb of the loop of Henle. NSAIDs combat pain by inhibition of cyclooxygenase enzymes. These enzymes are key in the production of prostaglandins. Prostaglandins have many effects, including pain sensitization and stimulation of inflammation. In the kidneys, prostaglandins are important for causing vasodilation of the afferent arteriole. NSAIDs use will inhibit prostaglandin synthesis, therefore causing afferent arteriole vasoconstriction. This in turn leads to decreased renal perfusion and decreased glomerular filtration rate (GFR), attenuating the effects of furosemide. (B) NSAIDs do not significantly affect the tone of the efferent arteriole. If they did lead to efferent arteriole vasoconstriction, this would actually increase the GFR because more fluid would be forced into the glomerular capsule. (C) Aldosterone is an endogenous hormone that increases sodium reabsorption in the distal tubule. NSAIDs do not interfere with aldosterone signaling. (D) Antidiuretic hormone (ADH), also known as vasopressin, is the endogenous hormone that stimulates the ADH receptor. Desmopressin is a synthetic analog. NSAIDs do not impact ADH signaling. (E) Although using NSAIDs while on furosemide is not contraindicated, the physician is correct to warn his patient of the decreased efficacy of furosemide because of NSAID use.

21 **The answer is A: Acetazolamide.** A principal issue at high altitude is the low partial pressure of oxygen. The low amount of oxygen stimulates the body to breath faster and deeper, leading to a respiratory alkalosis because too much carbon dioxide is breathed off. Acetazolamide reverses this alkalosis by inhibiting carbonic anhydrase in the kidneys, causing bicarbonate to be excreted in the urine. Administration of acetazolamide in many patients leads to resolution of the symptoms of altitude sickness. (B) Furosemide is a loop diuretic. Loop diuretics produce the greatest amount of diuresis of any type of diuretic and so are useful for fluid overload states (as in heart failure). Furosemide would not be useful in treating altitude sickness. (C) Hydrochlorothiazide is a diuretic that also increases calcium reabsorption. In addition to its diuretic properties, it may be used in patients with calcium-containing kidney stones (to keep calcium out of the urine) and in patients who could use more calcium (as in patients with osteoporosis). Hydrochlorothiazide would not be useful in treating altitude sickness. (D) Mannitol is an osmotic diuretic. It (along with acetazolamide) can also be used to treat glaucoma. Mannitol would not be useful in treating altitude sickness. (E) Spironolactone is a potassium-sparing diuretic. Potassium-sparing diuretics are useful in patients with (or at risk of) hypokalemia who need diuresis.

22 **The answer is B: Exercise regimen approximately 5 d/wk.** Elevated triacylglycerol (triglyceride) levels are independently associated with increased risk of CHD. Diet and exercise are the primary modes of treating hypertriacylglycerolemia. If indicated, niacin and fibric acid derivatives are the most efficacious in lowering triacylglycerol levels. Triacylglycerol reduction is a secondary benefit of the statin drugs (the primary benefit being LDL cholesterol reduction). (A) Dietary modification should include a low-fat diet. (C) HMG-CoA reductase inhibitor therapy is considered a second-line therapy. (D) Statin therapy will lower LDL cholesterol levels. (E) This patient should receive some treatment regimen, which initially should include diet modification and exercise.

23 **The answer is D: Lowering cholesterol does not reduce cardiac mortality completely.** It should be noted that, in spite of the protection afforded by cholesterol lowering, about one-fourth of the patients treated with these drugs still present with coronary events. Thus, additional strategies, such as diet, exercise, and additional agents, may be warranted. (A) This patient appeared to

have a good exercise regimen. (B) This patient appeared to have a good dietary plan. (C) This patient had a reasonably normal body weight. (E) Lowering cholesterol did not directly cause his mortality; his underlying cardiac disease played a major role.

24 **The answer is D: Simvastatin.** Simvastatin will reduce serum LDL cholesterol by 41% and increase serum HDL cholesterol by 12%. Thus, of the choices presented, this agent will serve both problems of this patient rather well. (A) Cholestyramine will decrease serum LDL and have lesser effects on raising serum HDL levels. (B) Fluvastatin will decrease serum LDL by 24% and raise serum HDL by 8%. (C) Lovastatin will decrease serum LDL by 34% and raise serum HDL by 9%.

25 **The answer is C: Causing resorption of calcium in the renal tubules.** Thiazide diuretics decrease the Ca^{2+} content of urine by promoting the resorption of Ca^{2+}. This effect contrasts with the loop diuretics, which increase the Ca^{2+} concentration of the urine. There is evidence from epidemiologic studies that use of thiazides preserves bone mineral density at the hip and spine and that the risk for hip fracture is reduced by a third. (A) This agent does not bind to urine calcium. (B) This agent does not bind to urine sodium. (D) This agent does not increase calcium excretion in the renal tubules. This best described the mechanism of action of furosemide. (E) This agent does not increase sodium resorption in the renal tubules.

26 **The answer is A: Decrease production of aqueous humor.** The most common use of acetazolamide is to reduce the elevated intraocular pressure of open-angle glaucoma. Acetazolamide decreases the production of aqueous humor, probably by blocking carbonic anhydrase in the ciliary body of the eye. It is useful in the chronic treatment of glaucoma but should not be used for an acute attack. (B) This agent will decrease intraocular pressure. (C) The mechanism of action of acetazolamide does not involve the sodium-calcium transport system. (D) Acetazolamide inhibits carbonic anhydrase. (E) Acetazolamide should not be used for acute glaucoma treatment. Better results are noted for treatment of chronic glaucoma.

27 **The answer is C: Persistent hyperglycemia.** This patient will likely have persistent hyperglycemia. Because insulin is a polypeptide, it is degraded in the gastrointestinal tract if taken orally. Therefore, it is generally administered by subcutaneous injection. In a hyperglycemic emergency, regular insulin is injected intravenously. Continuous subcutaneous insulin infusion (insulin pump) has become popular because it does not require multiple daily injections. (A) Diarrhea is an unlikely sequelae of this process. (B) Nausea is an unlikely sequelae of this process. (D) Transient ischemic attacks are unlikely to occur following administration of oral insulin. (E) Uremia is unlikely because there is no evidence of infection or renal obstructive process in this patient.

28 **The answer is B: Insulin glargine.** Insulin lispro is usually administered 15 min prior to a meal or immediately following a meal, whereas glulisine can be taken either 15 min before a meal or within 20 min after starting a meal. Insulin aspart should be administered just prior to the meal or up to 15 min following the meal. Insulin glargine has a long onset of action and could take 12 to 24 h for the most significant glucose lowering effects to be noted. (A) Insulin aspart has a rapid onset of action and could be useful in this patient to lower blood sugar levels. (C) Insulin lispro also has a rapid onset of action and would be useful in treating this patient. (D) Regular insulin has an important treatment role in this patient. It is the best choice agent to use.

29 **The answer is A: Gastric retention.** Pramlintide may not be mixed in the same syringe with any insulin preparation. Adverse effects are mainly gastrointestinal and consist of nausea, anorexia, and vomiting. Pramlintide should not be given to patients with diabetic gastroparesis (delayed stomach emptying), cresol hypersensitivity, or a history of hypoglycemic unawareness. (B) Pramlintide can be given to patients with acute-angle glaucoma. (C) Pramlintide can be given to patients with wide-angle glaucoma. (D) Pramlintide is not contraindicated in patients with pneumonia. (E) Caution should be exercised when giving pramlintide to patients with urinary retention. Gastric retention is a much more common and problematic condition to be concerned about.

30 **The answer is C: Medication side effect.** Shortcomings of the sulfonylureas are their propensity to cause weight gain, hyperinsulinemia, and hypoglycemia. These drugs should be used with caution in patients with hepatic or renal insufficiency because delayed excretion of the drug and resulting accumulation may cause hypoglycemia. Renal impairment is a particular problem in the case of those agents that are metabolized to active compounds such as glyburide. (A) This patient walks 30 min every other day as stated in the question stem. (B) This patient eats three balanced meals as stated in the question stem. (D) This patient does not have signs of hyperthyroidism because weight loss would be expected, not weight gain. (E) This patient has no evidence of underlying malignancy.

31 **The answer is C: He can continue taking metformin and should stop the medicine just prior to the CT scan.** Metformin should be used with caution in patients older than age 80 years and in those with a history of

congestive heart failure or alcohol abuse. Metformin should be temporarily discontinued in patients undergoing diagnosis requiring IV radiographic contrast agents. Rarely, potentially fatal lactic acidosis may occur. Long-term use may interfere with vitamin B absorption. (A) Metformin and radiographic contrast can produce nephrotoxicity, and thus, metformin should be stopped prior to the CT scan. (B) Metformin doses should never be increased before a contrast CT scan. (D) There is no reason to hospitalize this patient. The metformin and contrast reaction is not an allergic reaction. It is a nephrotoxic potentiation reaction.

32 **The answer is D: Low-density lipoprotein.** Hyperglycemia, hyperinsulinemia, hypertriglyceridemia, and elevated HbA_{1c} levels are improved. Interestingly, LDL levels are neither affected by pioglitazone monotherapy nor when the drug is used in combination with other agents, whereas LDL levels have increased with rosiglitazone. (A) Serum glucose levels will decrease with pioglitazone therapy. (B) Hemoglobin A_{1c} levels will decrease with pioglitazone therapy. (C) Serum insulin levels will decrease with pioglitazone therapy. (E) Serum triglyceride levels will decrease with pioglitazone therapy.

33 **The answer is B: Inhibition of pancreatic amylase.** Acarbose is used in the treatment of Type-2 diabetes. Acarbose also inhibits pancreatic amylase, thereby interfering with the breakdown of starch to oligosaccharides. Consequently, the postprandial rise of blood glucose is blunted. Unlike other oral glucose-lowering agents, these drugs neither stimulate insulin release nor increase insulin action in target tissues. Thus, as monotherapy, they do not cause hypoglycemia. (A) This is a therapeutic effect of acarbose, not a toxic effect. (C) This patient does not have any physical signs or symptoms of pancreatitis. (D) It is unlikely that this patient has pancreatic carcinoma. (E) This patient likely has therapeutic levels of acarbose because his blood sugar is normal.

34 **The answer is C: Treatment-related side effect.** This patient is taking sitagliptin. In general, this medicine is well tolerated, with the most common adverse effects being nasopharyngitis and headache. Rates of hypoglycemia are comparable to those with placebo when these agents are used as monotherapy or in combination with metformin or pioglitazone. (A) This patient does not have an allergy to dander. This is an adverse drug reaction. (B) Although this patient can have underlying gastroesophageal reflux, the nasopharyngitis is a treatment-related side effect. (D) There is no evidence to suggest nasopharyngeal obstruction. (E) There is no evidence to suggest a viral infection in this patient.

35 **The answer is C: The risk can be offset by adding a proestrogen product.** Nausea and breast tenderness are among the most common adverse effects of estrogen therapy. Postmenopausal uterine bleeding can occur. In addition, the risk of thromboembolic events, myocardial infarction, and breast and endometrial cancer is increased with use of estrogen therapy. The increased risk of endometrial cancer can be offset by including a progesterone along with the estrogen therapy. (A) Estrogens can be associated with an increased risk of breast cancer. (B) Postmenopausal bleeding is possible with estrogen preparations. (D) Thromboembolic events are possible with estrogen preparations.

36 **The answer is B: Interference with progesterone.** Mifepristone (also designated as RU-486) is a progesterone antagonist with partial agonist activity. Mifepristone also has potent antiglucocorticoid activity. Administration of this drug to females early in pregnancy usually results in abortion of the fetus because of interference with the progesterone needed to maintain pregnancy. (A) This agent interferes with progesterone. (C) This agent has potent antiglucocorticoid activity. (D) This agent is an abortifacient, not a teratogen. (E) Uremic encephalopathy is unlikely with this agent.

37 **The answer is D: Slippage of the ring from the vaginal vault.** An additional contraceptive option is a vaginal ring containing ethinyl estradiol and etonogestrel. The ring is inserted into the vagina and is left in place for 3 weeks. Week 4 is ring free, and withdrawal bleeding occurs. The contraceptive vaginal ring has efficacy, contraindications, and adverse effects similar to those of oral contraceptives. One caveat with the vaginal ring is that it may occasionally slip or be expelled accidentally. (A) The ring is placed for 3 weeks, and the fourth week is ring free for withdrawal bleeding to occur. (B) The ring is inserted into the vagina for 3 weeks. (C) The ring contains ethinyl estradiol and etonogestrel.

38 **The answer is B: 1% to 3%.** Postcoital or emergency contraception reduces the probability of pregnancy to between 0.2% and 3.0%. Emergency contraception uses high doses of progestin (e.g., 0.75 mg of levonorgestrel) or high doses of estrogen (100 μg of ethinyl estradiol) plus progestin (0.5 mg of levonorgestrel) administered within 72 h of unprotected intercourse (the "morning-after pill"). For these regimens, a second dose of emergency contraception should be taken 12 h after the first dose. (A) Abstinence would make the pregnancy rate 0%. (C) The pregnancy rate is 1% to 3%. (D) Unprotected sex 3 days prior to ovulation results in a pregnancy rate of 15%. (E) Unprotected sex 1 to 2 days prior to ovulation results in a pregnancy rate of 30%.

39 **The answer is D: Ovarian cancer.** Oral contraceptives have been shown to decrease the incidence of endometrial and ovarian cancer. The incidence of cervical cancer may be increased with oral contraceptives because women are less likely to use additional barrier methods of contraception that reduce exposure to human papilloma virus (the primary risk factor for cervical cancer). The ability of oral contraceptives to induce other neoplasms is controversial. The production of benign tumors in the liver that may rupture, and hemorrhage is rare. (A) Breast cancer incidence does not change with oral contraceptives. (B) Cervical cancer incidence may increase with oral contraceptives. (C) Lung cancer incidence does not change with oral contraceptives. (E) Thyroid cancer incidence is unchanged following prolonged use of oral contraceptives.

40 **The answer is D: Decreased FSH.** Danazol, a mild androgen, is used in the treatment of endometriosis (ectopic growth of the endometrium) and fibrocystic breast disease. Danazol also possess antiestrogenic activity. It inhibits release of FSH and LH but has no effect on the aromatase. Weight gain, acne, decreased breast size, deepening voice, increased libido, and increased hair growth are among the adverse effects. Danazol has been reported occasionally to suppress adrenal function. (A) Danazol will have no change on aromatase levels. (B) This patient will have an increase in hair growth. (C) This patient will have an increase in libido. (E) Testosterone levels will be unchanged or slightly decrease in this patient.

41 **The answer is C: Premature epiphyseal long bone closing.** Use of anabolic steroids, (e.g., DHEA) by athletes can cause premature closing of the epiphysis of the long bones, which stunts growth and interrupts development. High doses taken by young athletes may result in reduction of testicular size, hepatic abnormalities, increased aggression ("roid rage"), major mood disorders, and other adverse effects described earlier. (A) Mood disorders such as mania are common in steroid abuse. (B) Hepatic abnormalities such as hepatitis and hepatocellular carcinoma are possible in this patient. (D) Testicular atrophy, not testicular hyperplasia, can occur in this patient. (E) Tubercle development is not likely following steroid abuse.

42 **The answer is B: Inhibition of macrophages.** The most important therapeutic property of the glucocorticoids is their ability to dramatically reduce the inflammatory response and to suppress immunity. The exact mechanism is complex and incompletely understood. However, the lowering and inhibition of peripheral lymphocytes and macrophages is known to play a role. Also involved is the indirect inhibition of phospholipase A_2 (because of the steroid-mediated elevation of lipocortin), which blocks the release of arachidonic acid (the precursor of the prostaglandins and leukotrienes) from membrane-bound phospholipid. Cyclooxygenase 2 synthesis in inflammatory cells is further reduced. (A) Glucocorticoids do not stimulate erythrocytosis. (C) Glucocorticoids inhibit cyclooxygenase 2 synthesis. (D) Glucocorticoids inhibit phospholipase A_2. (E) Glucocorticoids may inhibit T-cell function.

43 **The answer is C: Inhibition of bone formation.** Osteoporosis is the most common adverse effect because of the ability of glucocorticoids to suppress intestinal Ca^{2+} absorption, inhibit bone formation, and decrease sex hormone synthesis. Alternate-day dosing does not prevent osteoporosis. Patients are advised to take calcium and vitamin D supplements. Drugs that are effective in treating osteoporosis may also be beneficial. (A) Glucocorticoid use decreases intestinal calcium absorption. (B) Glucocorticoid use decreases sex hormone synthesis. (D) Osteoporosis is associated with glucocorticoid use. (E) Osteochondroma is uncommon in this presentation.

44 **The answer is A: Androgen receptor inhibition of the hair follicle.** Spironolactone is an antihypertensive drug that competes for the mineralocorticoid receptor and, thus, inhibits sodium resorption in the kidney. It can also antagonize aldosterone and testosterone synthesis. It is effective against hyperaldosteronism. Spironolactone is also useful in the treatment of hirsutism in women, probably because of interference at the androgen receptor of the hair follicle. Adverse effects include hyperkalemia, gynecomastia, menstrual irregularities, and skin rashes. (B) This is not a drug toxicity effect. (C) Hyperaldosteronism is treated with spironolactone. (D) Gynecomastia and menstrual abnormalities are common in patients who are taking spironolactone. (E) This is not an idiopathic effect.

45 **The answer is D: Inhibition of lipase.** Orlistat inhibits lipase to block digestion of dietary fats. The intended result is a negative energy balance leading to weight loss. An obvious side effect is fat in the stool (steatorrhea) because a lot of dietary fat is not digested. Because it works on enzymes in the GI lumen, orlistat does not need to be absorbed to work. (A) Cholestyramine is a drug that binds bile salts. It also impairs fat digestion and absorption, but its primary purpose is to decrease blood cholesterol. It does this by blocking recycling of bile salts to cause the liver to increase LDL uptake from the bloodstream. Orlistat does not work by binding bile salts. (B) α-Glucosidase is a brush border enzyme and the rate-limiting enzyme for carbohydrate digestion. It is inhibited by acarbose, not by orlistat. (C) Chylomicrons are lipid-carrying particles produced by enterocytes.

Their function is not impaired by orlistat. (E) Trypsin is an enzyme important for protein digestion. An endogenous trypsin inhibitor, α_1-antitrypsin, prevents trypsin produced by neutrophils from destroying elastin in the lungs, but trypsin is not inhibited by orlistat.

46 **The answer is B: Hyperglycemia.** The β_2-agonists are not catecholamines and thus are not inactivated by catechol-*O*-methyltransferase. Adverse effects, such as tachycardia, hyperglycemia, hypokalemia, and hypomagnesemia, are minimized with delivery via inhalation versus systemic routes. Although tolerance to the effects of β_2-agonists on nonairway tissues occurs, it is uncommon with normal dosages. These agents can cause β_2-mediated skeletal muscle tremors. (A) Tachycardia is an adverse effect of β_2-agonist therapy. (C) Hypokalemia is an adverse effect of β_2-agonist therapy. (D) Hypomagnesemia is an adverse effect of β_2-agonist therapy. (E) β_2-Agonist therapy should not produce any change in blood pressure.

47 **The answer is B: Inhibition of cholesterol biosynthesis.** The bisphosphonates decrease osteoclastic bone resorption via several mechanisms including inhibition of cholesterol biosynthesis pathway, which is important for osteoclast function. There is also a small gain in bone mass in this patient. (A) Osteoclastic bone resorption is decreased by alendronate. (C) Increased osteoclastic apoptosis, programmed cell death, occurs with alendronate. (D) Osteoclast activation is inhibited by alendronate. (E) Osteoclast formation is inhibited by alendronate.

48 **The answer is D: Parathyroid hormone.** Teriparatide is a recombinant segment of human parathyroid hormone that is administered subcutaneously for the treatment of osteoporosis. This causes dissolution of bone but can more commonly cause bone formation. In can increase spinal bone density. (A) Follicle-stimulating hormone has no effect on development of osteoporosis. (B) Levels of growth hormone are unrelated to the pathogenesis of osteoporosis. (C) Luteinizing hormone levels do not play a role in the development of osteoporosis. (E) It is possible that low levels of thyroid hormone may contribute to decrease in bone density associated with osteoporosis.

49 **The answer is E: Tetracycline.** This patient's presentation is consistent with Fanconi syndrome, a defect in proximal renal tubule function. The proximal tubule is responsible for reabsorbing the phosphate, bicarbonate, amino acids, and glucose filtered that would otherwise be lost in the urine. Fanconi syndrome can be inherited or, as in this patient's case, acquired. One of the causes of acquired Fanconi syndrome is expired tetracycline antibiotics. (A) Benzoyl peroxide produces reactive oxygen species that damage and kill bacteria. It is used topically and is not known to cause Fanconi syndrome. (B) Clindamycin binds the 50S subunit of bacterial ribosomes to inhibit protein synthesis. It is not known to cause Fanconi syndrome. (C) Erythromycin is a macrolide antibiotic that also inhibits the 50S subunit of bacterial ribosomes. It is not known to cause Fanconi syndrome. (D) Isotretinoin is a vitamin A derivative. It is a potent teratogen but is not known to cause Fanconi syndrome.

50 **The answer is C: Losartan.** Glipizide is a sulfonylurea. Sulfonylureas stimulate pancreatic β-islet cells to secrete insulin. Sulfonylureas contain a sulfonamide group, which is the likely cause behind this patient's apparent allergic reaction to glipizide. Further exposure to drugs containing a sulfonamide group may lead to a severe, life-threatening allergic reaction and should be avoided. Of the drugs listed, only losartan has no sulfonamide group. (A) Celecoxib is a selective COX-2 inhibitor. It contains a sulfonamide group and should not be given to this patient. (B) Hydrochlorothiazide is a thiazide diuretic. It contains a sulfonamide group and should not be given to this patient. (D) Sulfamethoxazole is an antibiotic usually coadministered with trimethoprim. It contains a sulfonamide group and should not be given to this patient. (E) Sulfasalazine is metabolized by colonic bacteria to sulfapyridine and mesalamine—two drugs used to treat Crohn's disease. Sulfasalazine contains a sulfonamide group and should not be given to this patient.

51 **The answer is D: Venlafaxine.** Venlafaxine is an antidepressant of the serotonin-norepinephrine reuptake inhibitor class. Venlafaxine can also be used to treat anxiety disorders and panic disorders. Ironically, venlafaxine can cause anxiety, agitation, and worsening of depression. Of the medications listed, venlafaxine is the most likely cause of this patient's agitation and anxiety. (A) Atorvastatin is known to cause myalgia and rhabdomyolysis. It is not known to cause agitation or anxiety. (B) Hydrochlorothiazide may cause constipation and hypercalcemia. It is not known to cause agitation or anxiety. (C) Metformin has been known to cause a possibly life-threatening metabolic acidosis, although this is rare. It is not known to cause agitation or anxiety. (E) Verapamil may cause sinus bradycardia and AV block. It is not known to cause agitation or anxiety.

52 **The answer is B: Bethanechol.** Surgical anesthesia may cause a temporary postoperative ileus. To prevent complications, a cholinergic drug may be administered that will stimulate the gastrointestinal (GI) tract. Of the drugs listed, only bethanechol is a cholinergic agonist. Bethanechol binds to muscarinic acetylcholine receptors on smooth muscle cells of the GI tract to increase motility, mimicking acetylcholine.

(A) Benztropine is a muscarinic antagonist. Administration of benztropine would further inhibit gut motility in this patient. (C) Epinephrine binds to β_2-adrenergic receptors in the gut. β_2-Receptors cause smooth muscle relaxation and would lead to decreased gut motility. (D) Methscopolamine is a muscarinic antagonist. Administration of methscopolamine would further inhibit gut motility in this patient. (E) Oxybutynin is a muscarinic antagonist. Administration of oxybutynin would further inhibit gut motility in this patient.

53 **The answer is D: Minoxidil.** Minoxidil is a very effective vasodilator. Like hydralazine, the medication dilates only arterioles, not veins. The active metabolite, minoxidil sulfate, causes the potassium channels in smooth muscle membranes to open, which reduces the likelihood of contraction. Because of its potency and adverse side effects, minoxidil should be used only when maximal doses of hydralazine are ineffective or in patients with renal failure and severe hypertension who do not respond well to hydralazine. (A) Calcium channel blockers are effective at reducing peripheral resistance and blood pressure in addition to their antianginal and antiarrhythmic effects. Some epidemiologic studies reported an increased risk of mortality in patients receiving short-acting nifedipine for hypertension. Specific calcium channel blockers with longer half-lives or are administered through sustained release are more appropriate for the treatment of hypertension. (B) Diazoxide is a long-acting arteriolar dilator that is occasionally used to treat hypertensive emergencies. (C) Fenoldopam is a peripheral arteriolar dilator used for hypertensive emergencies and postoperative hypertension. (E) Sodium nitroprusside is a powerful vasodilator used in treating hypertensive emergencies as well as severe heart failure. It affects both arterioles and veins.

54 **The answer is B: Increased excretion in the feces.** The primary source of phosphate in hyperphosphatemia is dietary. Normally, excess dietary phosphate is excreted by the kidneys. In patients with kidney disease, phosphate cannot be renally excreted. Phosphate levels build and the excess phosphate precipitates with calcium, which leads to many of the symptoms of hyperphosphatemia. Sevelamer is a phosphate binder and retains phosphate in the gut lumen to be excreted in the feces. (A) Sevelamer does not interfere with bone metabolism. It decreases serum phosphate by inhibiting dietary phosphate absorption. (C) Sweat is not an important vehicle for phosphate excretion. Sevelamer decreases serum phosphate by inhibiting dietary phosphate absorption. (D) This patient has hyperphosphatemia because his kidneys can no longer excrete phosphate. Sevelamer does not work on the kidneys; even if it did, it would not be useful in this patient. (E) Sevelamer is not a muscle relaxant. Sevelamer decreases serum phosphate by inhibiting dietary phosphate absorption.

55 **The answer is C: Stimulation of conversion of cholesterol to pregnenolone.** The target organ of ACTH is the adrenal cortex, where it binds to specific receptors on the cell surfaces. The occupied receptors activate G protein–coupled processes to increase cyclic adenosine monophosphate (cAMP), which in turn stimulates the rate-limiting step in the adrenocorticosteroid synthetic pathway (cholesterol to pregnenolone). This pathway ends with the synthesis and release of the adrenocorticosteroids and the adrenal androgens. (A) The occupied receptors activate G protein–coupled processes. (B) The activated G protein complex increases cyclic AMP. (D) Release of adrenocorticosteroids occurs after they are synthesized. (E) Pulmonary ACTH is produced in disease states such as oat cell carcinoma.

56 **The answer is B: Hormones are metabolized through the microsomal P450 system.** Both T_4 and T_3 are absorbed after oral administration. Food, calcium preparations, and aluminum-containing antacids can decrease the absorption of T_4 but not of T_3. T_4 is converted to T_3 by one of two distinct deiodinases, depending on the tissue. The hormones are metabolized through the microsomal P450 system. Drugs that induce the P450 enzymes, such as phenytoin, rifampin, and phenobarbital, accelerate metabolism of the thyroid hormones. Enzyme induction can increase the metabolism of the thyroid hormones. T_3 = triiodothyronine; T_4 = thyroxine. (A) Food administration decreases absorption of T_4 but not T_3. (C) Phenytoin accelerates metabolism of thyroid hormones. (D) Rifampin accelerates metabolism of thyroid hormones. (E) T_3 and T_4 are absorbed after oral administration.

57 **The answer is A: Intravenous administration of medication is most efficacious.** Thyroid storm presents with extreme symptoms of hyperthyroidism. The therapeutic options for thyroid storm are the same as those for hyperthyroidism, except that the drugs are given in higher doses and more frequently. β-Blockers that lack sympathomimetic activity, such as propranolol, are effective in blunting the widespread sympathetic stimulation that occurs in hyperthyroidism. Intravenous administration is effective in treating thyroid storm. An alternative in patients suffering from severe heart failure or asthma is the calcium channel blocker diltiazem. Time is required for patients with Graves hyperthyroidism to become euthyroid with normal serum T_4 and T_3 concentrations. (B) Medications are given at higher dosing than that for patients with hyperthyroidism. (C) Medications are given at higher dosing

frequencies than that for patients with hyperthyroidism. (D) Use of calcium channel blockers are useful for patients with thyroid storm and severe heart failure.

58 **The answer is A: Corrective glasses.** The goal in treating Type-2 diabetes is to maintain blood glucose concentrations within normal limits and to prevent the development of long-term complications of the disease. Weight reduction, exercise, and dietary modification decrease insulin resistance and correct the hyperglycemia of Type-2 diabetes in some patients. However, most patients depend on pharmacologic intervention with oral glucose-lowering agents. (B) Diet modification can lower serum glucose levels and is effective in this patient. (C) Exercise will lower serum glucose and can prevent development of diabetes mellitus. (D) Weight loss is important for this patient because it can maintain blood glucose levels within normal limits.

59 **The answer is A: Macrovascular disease.** Patients on intensive therapy show a significant reduction in such long-term complications of diabetes as retinopathy, nephropathy, and neuropathy compared to patients receiving standard care. Intensive therapy should generally not be recommended for patients with long-standing diabetes, significant microvascular complications, advanced age, and those with hypoglycemic unawareness. Intensive therapy has not been shown to significantly reduce the macrovascular complications of diabetes. (B) This patient will have a significant risk reduction of developing diabetic nephropathy. (C) This patient will have a significant risk reduction of developing diabetic neuropathy. (D) This patient will have a significant risk reduction of developing diabetic retinopathy. (E) Serum glucose should be in the normal range in this patient who is receiving intensive insulin therapy.

60 **The answer is B: Lactic acidosis development.** Metformin should be temporarily discontinued in patients undergoing diagnosis requiring IV radiographic contrast agents. Rarely, potentially fatal lactic acidosis may occur. Long-term use may interfere with vitamin B absorption. (A) Metformin can react with IV contrast to cause lactic acidosis. (C) IV contrast can be nephrotoxic when patients have renal insufficiency. This patient has normal renal function. (D) The combination of metformin and IV contrast should not create a neurotoxic effect. (E) Uremia could be possible if this patient had renal insufficiency or failure and was given an IV contrast.

61 **The answer is D: Nausea.** Nausea and breast tenderness are among the most common adverse effects of estrogen therapy. Postmenopausal uterine bleeding can occur. In addition, the risk of thromboembolic events, myocardial infarction, and breast and endometrial cancer is increased with use of estrogen therapy. The increased risk of endometrial cancer can be offset by including a progestogen along with the estrogen therapy. (A) Thromboembolism is a possible but less common effect of estrogen therapy. (B) Breast tenderness, not breast discharge, is a common side effect of estrogen therapy. (C) Nausea, not diarrhea, is a common side effect of estrogen therapy. (E) Vomiting is not a common side effect of estrogen therapy.

62 **The answer is B: Glipizide.** The negative consequences of diabetes occur only because of elevated blood sugar levels. Pharmacotherapy of diabetes, therefore, relies on keeping sugar levels within the normal range. Because of their mechanism of action, some of these drugs can cause hypoglycemia (as in this patient's case). Sulfonylureas such as glipizide are an example of drugs that can cause hypoglycemia. (A) Acarbose blocks the brush border glucosidases necessary for the final stage of carbohydrate metabolism. It is not associated with hypoglycemia. (C) Metformin works by inhibiting gluconeogenesis and intestinal carbohydrate absorption. It is known to cause hypoglycemia but much less commonly than sulfonylureas. (D) Pramlintide is an amylin analog and works by slowing gastric emptying, impairs glucagon secretion, and suppresses the appetite. Alone, it is not known to cause hypoglycemia. (E) Sitagliptin mimics incretins, which increase insulin secretion following a meal. Sitagliptin does not increase insulin secretion when blood glucose drops below about 90 mg/dL and does not produce significantly more hypoglycemia than placebo.

63 **The answer is B: Histamine.** Histamine is an example of a local mediator. Most cells in the body secrete chemicals that act locally, that is, on cells in their immediate environment. Because these chemical signals are rapidly destroyed or removed, they do not enter the blood and are not distributed throughout the body. (A) Epinephrine is a hormone. A hormone travels throughout the bloodstream, exerting effects on broadly distributed target cells in the body. (C) Norepinephrine is a hormone. A hormone travels throughout the bloodstream, exerting effects on broadly distributed target cells in the body. (D) Thyroxine is a hormone. A hormone travels throughout the bloodstream, exerting effects on broadly distributed target cells in the body. (E) Testosterone is a hormone. A hormone travels throughout the bloodstream, exerting effects on broadly distributed target cells in the body.

64 **The answer is B: Insulin glargine.** Insulin and its analogs act to lower blood sugar by causing the cells of the body to pull glucose from the blood into their

cytoplasm. The different formulations of insulin are used to produce different effects on the body. Short-acting insulin preparations such as insulin aspart and insulin lispro peak rapidly and can be used at meal times. Long-acting insulin preparations such as insulin glargine produce a much lower peak and provide a low, baseline insulin level throughout the day and night. (A) Insulin aspart is a rapid-acting insulin preparation. It would not provide a long-lasting baseline insulin level. (C) Insulin lispro is a rapid-acting insulin preparation. It would not provide a long-lasting baseline insulin level. (D) Lente insulin is an intermediate-acting insulin preparation. It would not provide as good baseline insulin coverage as insulin glargine. (E) NPH insulin is an intermediate-acting insulin preparation. It would not provide as good baseline insulin coverage as insulin glargine.

65 **The answer is A: Calcitonin.** Of the medications listed, only calcitonin would cause a decrease in this patient's serum calcium level. The physiologic role of calcitonin is unclear, but high doses are known to decrease serum calcium. This effect, however, is short lived, so calcitonin should be combined with bisphosphonates, which work longer but have a slower onset. (B) Colesevelam is used to lower cholesterol by binding bile salts in the gut lumen to inhibit their resorption. This forces the liver to use cholesterol to synthesize new bile salts. Colesevelam would not be an effective measure to lower this patient's calcium level. (C) Hydrochlorothiazide is a diuretic that causes calcium retention. It is used in patients with recurrent kidney stones because it decreases urinary calcium, but it increases serum calcium. (D) Teriparatide is a recombinant form of parathyroid hormone. Administration of this drug would cause an increase in this patient's serum calcium level. (E) Vitamin D increases serum calcium by various mechanisms. It would not be useful in lowering this patient's calcium.

66 **The answer is E: Thickened cervical mucus.** Both estrogen and progesterone have contraceptive effects therapeutically. When used in combination, they also provide better menstrual cycle control than when used alone. Both help prevent the LH surge necessary for ovulation. Additionally, estrogen stabilizes the endometrium to prevent breakthrough bleeding. Progesterone also causes the cervical mucus to thicken, preventing sperm entry. (A) Androgens such as DHE and androstenedione can cause hirsutism. Neither estrogen nor progesterone analogs cause hirsutism. (B) Prolactin from the anterior pituitary causes milk production. Progesterone actually inhibits milk production. (C) Glucocortecoids can produce peripheral muscle wasting and trunchal obesity. Progesterone does not cause peripheral muscle wasting. (D) Aldosterone, a mineralocorticoid, causes sodium retention. Progesterone does not cause sodium retention.

67 **The answer is E: This patient has a high risk of thromboembolism.** Estrogen is known to increase the risk of thromboembolism. This patient has two additional risk factors: being older than 35 years old and smoking. These three risk factors combined would present a serious risk for thromboembolism in this patient. The physician's best choice would be to prescribe a progesterone-only contraceptive. (A) This patient has no personal or family history of breast or endometrial cancer. Her cancer risk is not significantly higher than the baseline. (B) Disulfiram causes extreme nausea and headaches in patients who drink alcohol because disulfiram blocks the metabolism of acetaldehyde. Some other drugs have a disulfiram-like effect, but estrogens do not. (C) Estrogen has a favorable effect on lipid profiles. This patient's only risk for cardiovascular disease is her smoking habit. (D) Adding estrogen therapy to this patient's two existing risk factors for thromboembolism would present a serious health concern. The physician's best choice in this case would be to prescribe a progesterone-only contraceptive.

68 **The answer is B: Decrease activity of phospholipase A_2.** Glucocorticoids affect many cell types in the body. In this case, the patient would benefit most from inhibiting inflammation. Inflammation is mediated in large part by prostaglandins produced from arachidonic acid. Arachidonic acid, in turn, is released from cell membrane phospholipids by the action of phospholipase A_2. Glucocorticoids stimulate the production molecules that inhibit phospholipase A_2 to decrease inflammation. (A) Glucocorticoids cause a moderate but transient rise in circulating neutrophils, but their overall effect on the immune system is immunosuppression. Care should be taken when administering glucocorticoids because they can mask the signs of infection. (C) Glucocorticoids decrease collagen deposition in tissues. Prolonged exposure (as in Cushing's syndrome) can lead to skin weakening and striae. (D) Prostaglandins lead to inflammation in part by causing vasodilation. By blocking prostaglandin synthesis, glucocorticoids lead to a decrease in vasodilation and inflammation. (E) Androgens are catabolic and cause skeletal muscle hypertrophy, but glucocorticoids are anabolic and cause muscle wasting. Prolonged exposure (as in Cushing's syndrome) leads to peripheral muscle wasting.

69 **The answer is E: This agent is rapidly absorbed with a short duration of action.** Edrophonium is the prototype short-acting AChE inhibitor. Edrophonium binds reversibly to the active center of AChE, preventing hydrolysis of ACh. It is rapidly absorbed and has

a short duration of action of 10 to 20 minutes because of rapid renal elimination. Edrophonium is a quaternary amine, and its actions are limited to the periphery. It is used in the diagnosis of myasthenia gravis, which is an autoimmune disease caused by antibodies to the nicotinic receptor at NMJs. This causes their degradation, making fewer receptors available for interaction with the neurotransmitter. Intravenous injection of edrophonium leads to a rapid increase in muscle strength. (A) Diagnosis of myasthenia gravis is possible with the edrophonium test. (B) Edrophonium is a quaternary amine with peripheral actions. (C) Edrophonium binds reversibly to the active center of acetylcholinesterase. (D) Renal excretion and elimination of edrophonium is rapid.

70 **The answer is D: Lipid.** Steroids are built on a cholesterol backbone and are highly lipophilic. This makes it possible for them to easily diffuse across cellular membranes. This means that their receptors need not be found on the cell surface, although some are. Steroid hormone receptors can also be found in the nucleus, but most are found in the cytoplasm. Because of their lipid nature, steroids can diffuse across the membrane to interact with cytoplasmic receptors without the need of any transport mechanism. (A) Biogenic amines are substances made from chemically modified amino acids rather than chains of amino acids (as in peptides). This group includes histamine, tyramine, serotonin, and the catecholamines. Steroids are not biogenic amines. (B) Catecholamines are a subset of biogenic amines made from tyrosine. These include dopamine, norepinephrine, and epinephrine. Steroids are not biogenic amines. (C) Ions are molecules that carry a charge. Common signaling ions include sodium, calcium, and glutamate. Lipophilic molecules such as steroids are uncharged. (E) Peptides are molecules made from chains of amino acids attached with a peptide bond. Oxytocin, vasopressin, and insulin are peptide hormones.

71 **The answer is A: Clomiphene citrate.** Clomid is an antiestrogen, and so its side effects appropriately remind one of those associated with menopause or decreased circulating estrogen: hot flashes, emotional lability, changes in vision, and depression. It also has multiple gestational pregnancies as a side effect in 8% of patients. (B) Danocrine is an androgen-derived substance used to treat endometriosis because it decreases FSH and LH. (C) Human chorionic gonadotropin (hCG) structurally resembles LH and induces ovulation. (D) Lutrepulse is a GnRH agonist and would not have these side effects. (E) Pergonal is purified FSH and LH distilled from postmenopausal women's urine. This drug has multiple gestational pregnancy as a side effect 20% of the time.

72 **The answer is E: Increased triglycerides.** Atorvastatin and colesevelam both work to decrease LDL levels, although by different mechanisms. Colesevelam is a bile acid–binding resin. It sequesters bile acids in the gut lumen to prevent their reuptake and recycling, which forces the liver to synthesize new bile acids by pulling LDL cholesterol from the bloodstream. Colesevelam has the unfortunate side effect of increasing triglycerides. It also lowers blood glucose and hemoglobin A_{1c} levels by an unknown mechanism. (A) Colesevelam's primary action is to decrease the blood LDL level. It will also cause an increase in the HDL level. (B) Fibric acid derivatives such as fenofibrate and clofibrate are effective at lowering triglycerides. Colesevelam has the unfortunate side effect of increasing triglycerides. (C) Hyperglycemia is a side effect of many drugs but not of colesevelam. Colesevelam actually lowers blood glucose and hemoglobin A_{1c} levels by an unknown mechanism. (D) Colesevelam decreases blood LDL. It is a bile acid–binding resin that sequesters bile acids in the gut lumen to prevent their reuptake and recycling, which forces the liver to synthesize new bile acids by pulling LDL cholesterol from the bloodstream.

73 **The answer is A: Breast pain.** Adverse reactions associated with topical testosterone therapy include local reactions at the skin level, gynecomastia, breast pain, edema, virilization in children, and nervousness. (B) Hypertension can result from topical testosterone therapy. (C) Prostate inflammation is a rare adverse effect of testosterone therapy. (D) Stomatitis is unlikely following topical therapies. (E) Virilization in children is possible after testosterone administration.

74 **The answer is D: Headache.** Oxymetazoline is found in many over-the-counter short-term nasal spray decongestant products (applied every 12 h) as well as in ophthalmic drops for the relief of redness of the eyes associated with swimming, colds, and contact lenses. The mechanism of action of oxymetazoline is direct stimulation of receptors on blood vessels supplying the nasal mucosa and the conjunctiva to reduce blood flow and decrease congestion. Oxymetazoline is absorbed in the systemic circulation regardless of the route of administration and may produce nervousness, headaches, and trouble sleeping. (A) Oxymetazoline will likely cause nervousness and agitation. (B) Oxymetazoline does not usually cause diarrhea. (C). Oxymetazoline may cause headaches but not usually fatigue. (E) Oxymetazoline may cause trouble sleeping.

75 **The answer is E: Lipid metabolism remains unchanged.** Blockers with ISA minimize the disturbances of lipid and carbohydrate metabolism that are seen with other blockers. For example, these agents do not decrease plasma HDL levels. (A) Chylomicron level is unchanged with acebutolol. (B) HDL levels remain unchanged with acebutolol. (C) LDL levels remain unchanged with acebutolol. (D) VLDL levels remain unchanged with acebutolol.

76 **The answer is D: Dihydrotestosterone (DHT).** Dihydrotestosterone is responsible for the formation of the penis, scrotum, and prostate during embryology. Without dihydrotestosterone, a female genitalia will be present. Testosterone is converted to dihydrotestosterone by 5α-reductase. (A) Androstenedione is a precursor of testosterone and has been used by athletes and body builders to increase muscle mass. (B) Androsterone is a by-product of androgen breakdown. Although not very potent, it does have a masculinizing effect. (C) Dehydroepiandrosterone is produced by the adrenal cortex and a precursor to testosterone. It has been proposed to play a role in the immune system. (E) Testosterone functions in embryology to differentiate the epididymis, vas deferens, and seminal vesicles. It is not responsible for the formation of the external genitalia.

77 **The answer is B: Increase in cyclic guanosine monophosphate.** Several mechanisms have been proposed for the actions of methylxanthines including translocation of extracellular calcium, increase in cyclic adenosine monophosphate and cyclic guanosine monophosphate caused by inhibition of phosphodiesterase, and blockade of adenosine receptors. (A) Caffeine causes an increase in cyclic adenosine monophosphate. (C) Caffeine causes blockade of adenosine receptors. (D) Caffeine causes blockade of adenosine receptors. (E) Caffeine causes blockade of adenosine receptors.

78 **The answer is E: Niacin.** Niacin has been shown to increase HDL the most of any of the listed medications; however, it is most likely to cause side effects. The mechanism of action of niacin is inhibiting lipolysis in adipose tissue. (A) Cholestyramine decreases LDL, increases HDL, and increases triglycerides. However, it does not increase HDL as much as niacin. (B) Ezetimibe decreases LDL and has no effect on HDL or triglycerides. (C) Gemfibrozil has its greatest effect on decreasing triglyceride. It also decreases LDL and increases HDL. However, it does not increase HDL as much as niacin. (D) Lovastatin has its greatest effect on decreasing LDL. It increases HDL and decreases triglycerides. However, it does not increase HDL as much as niacin.

79 **The answer is D: Liver function tests.** Lovastatins and other HMG-CoA reductase inhibitors are known to cause hepatotoxicity and rhabdomyolysis. The hepatotoxicity should be monitored by following liver function tests, and baseline values are needed. The rhabdomyolysis commonly presents with muscle aches. (A) BUN/creatinine are monitored for nephrotoxic medications, for example, amphotericin B and ACE inhibitors. (B) Complete blood counts do not need to be monitored when starting lovastatin. Complete blood counts should be monitored with medications, such as chloramphenicol, which causes aplastic anemia. (C) A baseline fasting blood glucose could be ordered for a patient starting niacin, which can cause hyperglycemia. Lovastatin does not commonly cause hyperglycemia. (E) Uric acid levels should be monitored in patients starting niacin, which can cause hyperuricemia. Lovastatin does not commonly cause hyperuricemia.

80 **The answer is E: Prednisone.** Prednisone is a glucocorticoid used in the treatment of lupus. Patients on steroids may have a rise in their neutrophil count. Other side effects of steroids are Cushing's syndrome, osteoporosis, and thin skin. (A) Cimetidine has antiandrogenic properties that may cause decreased libido or gynecomastia in men but not an increased white blood cell count. (B) Hydrochlorothiazide may cause hypokalemia, hyperuricemia, hyperlipidemia, or hypercalcemia but not an increased white blood cell count. (C) Levothyroxine may cause symptoms of hyperthyroidism, such as tachycardia and heat intolerance, but not an increased white blood cell count. (D) Metformin may cause GI upset or lactic acidosis but not an increased white blood cell count.

81 **The answer is D: Megestrol.** Decreased appetite is more common in the elderly than in other patient populations and may cause significant morbidity and even mortality from malnourishment. A variety of drugs exist that can stimulate the appetite; one of the best drugs for this is a progestin called megestrol. The mechanism by which it suppresses the appetite may be caused by interference with cachexia. It has also demonstrated antineoplastic activity against endometrial cancer. (A) Drospirenone is a synthetic progestin that also possesses antimineralocorticoid activity. It is used in combination with an estrogen to treat atrophic vaginitis in postmenopausal women. It does not stimulate the appetite. (B) Ethinyl estradiol is a synthetic estrogen often used in combination with a progestin to treat atrophic vaginitis in postmenopausal women. It does not stimulate the appetite. (C) Medroxyprogesterone is a synthetic progestin that is used in contraceptives to inhibit gonadotropin secretion. It does not stimulate the appetite as much as megestrol. (E) Norgestrel is a synthetic progestin that is used in contraceptives to inhibit gonadotropin secretion. It does not stimulate the appetite as much as megestrol.

82 **The answer is C: Lactic acidosis.** Lactic acidosis is one of the most dangerous side effects of metformin.

Metformin inhibits hepatic gluconeogenesis, which uses lactate. This allows for the accumulation of lactate. The most common side effect of metformin is GI upset, particularly diarrhea. (A) Disulfiram-like reaction can be seen with first-generation sulfonylureas, such as tolbutamide or chlorpropamide. (B) Hypoglycemia is a common side effect of insulin, glyburide, and pramlintide. (D) Pancreatitis is more commonly seen as a side effect of exenatide, not metformin. (E) Weight gain is more commonly seen with pioglitazone and rosiglitazone. Some reports show metformin may actually cause weight loss.

83 **The answer is B: Increased insulin release.** Glimepiride is a second-generation sulfonylurea that works by increasing insulin release. This is achieved by binding to and inhibiting K^+ channels on β-cell membranes causing depolarization and the influx of Ca^{2+}. This leads to the release of insulin from the pancreatic β-cells. (A) Decreased glucagon release is seen with pramlintide and exenatide. (C) The mechanism of action of pioglitazone and rosiglitazone is increased insulin sensitivity in peripheral tissues. (D) The mechanism of action of metformin is inhibiting hepatic gluconeogenesis. (E) The mechanism of action of acarbose and miglitol is inhibiting the intestinal brush border α-glucosidases.

84 **The answer is E: Tardive dyskinesia.** Metoclopramide is a D_2-receptor antagonist. Because of the inhibition of dopamine, Parkinson-like symptoms can occur, such as tardive dyskinesia. Tardive dyskinesia is most common in young adults who are on metoclopramide for more than 3 months. (A) Dry mouth is a more common side effect of muscarinic antagonists, such as pirenzepine and propantheline, not metoclopramide. (B) Gynecomastia is a more common side effect of cimetidine because of its antiandrogenic properties. (C) Headache is more common side effect of ondansetron, not metoclopramide. (D) Misoprostol, a prostaglandin E_1 analog, is contraindicated in pregnancy because of the increased risk of abortion.

85 **The answer is D: Ezetimibe.** Cholesterol in the body has two sources: diet and de novo synthesis in hepatocytes. All "statin" drugs (including rosuvastatin) inhibit the rate-limiting enzyme in cholesterol synthesis—HMG-CoA reductase. Hepatocytes use cholesterol to make bile. When they cannot synthesize sufficient cholesterol de novo, they upregulate LDL receptors on their surfaces to increase uptake of cholesterol in LDL from the blood. This, in turn, lowers blood LDL levels. Ezetimibe works by inhibiting dietary uptake of cholesterol at the intestinal brush border. Ezetimibe is synergistic with the statins but ineffective when used alone because of a compensatory increase in de novo synthesis of cholesterol. (A) Cholestyramine is a cholesterol-binding resin that binds up bile salts in the intestine, preventing their resorption and recycling. This means that hepatocytes must make much more bile salts than normal to replace those that are lost in the feces. The high demand on hepatocytes to make more bile salts translates into a large increase in need for cholesterol. Both increased de novo synthesis of cholesterol and increased uptake of LDL in the blood result. (B) Colesevelam is another cholesterol-binding resin. It does not inhibit brush border enzymes. (C) Colestipol is another cholesterol-binding resin. It does not inhibit brush border enzymes. (E) Rosuvastatin is an HMG-CoA reductase inhibitor. It works by blocking de novo synthesis of cholesterol.

86 **The answer is D: Diphenhydramine.** Nicotinic acid and niacin are both names for vitamin B_3. Niacin in large doses is effective for preventing lipolysis, increasing HDL levels, and decreasing LDL levels. Its primary adverse effect is flushing, which may be itchy and occurs usually on the head, neck, and chest. The mechanism for niacin's beneficial effects on lipids is unknown, but the flushing appears to be caused largely by niacin-induced release of prostaglandin D_2 from mast cells (which causes vasodilation). Diphenhydramine is an H_1-receptor blocker useful for treating allergic reactions. The niacin flush has been shown to work independent of histamine. (A) Taking aspirin or another NSAID has been shown to relieve the symptoms. (B) Calamine lotion is an antipruritic preparation commonly used for insect bites and poison ivy exposure. It would not be expected to improve this patient's flushing as aspirin would. (C) Cimetidine is an H_2-receptor blocker. H_2 receptors are found in the stomach, not in the skin, and the niacin flush has been shown not to involve histamine anyway. (E) This reaction is avoidable. An NSAID such as aspirin can significantly reduce the amount of flushing caused by niacin.

87 **The answer is E: Sodium nitrite.** Lactic acidosis, headache, vertigo, and confusion can be signs of cyanide toxicity. A potential side effect of nitroprusside is cyanide toxicity because nitroprusside is composed of an iron atom bound to five cyanide (CN) ligands and one nitric oxide ligand (NO). The vasodilatory benefit of nitroprusside occurs when the NO molecule is released in the circulation because NO is a potent vasodilator. The CN ligands are also slowly released and can cause toxicity when CN ligands bind to cytochrome oxidase and disrupt oxidative phosphorylation. Cyanide toxicity can be mitigated by administration of a nitrite such as sodium nitrite, which converts hemoglobin into methemoglobin. Methemoglobin has a high affinity for CN and decreases the amount of CN that binds cytochrome oxidase. Nitrite therapy would be followed by

methylene blue (to regenerate hemoglobin) and sodium thiosulfate (to convert the cyanomethemoglobin into thiocyanate, which can be excreted in urine). (A) Activated charcoal, administered orally, is useful for absorbing toxins from the GI tract before they can be absorbed. Activated charcoal would not be useful in this case because the toxin, cyanide, is already in the patient's bloodstream. (B) Methylene blue would be given to this patient only after receiving sodium nitrite. Sodium nitrite helps the body get rid of cyanide but in the process produces methemoglobin. Methylene blue then converts methemoglobin back to hemoglobin. (C) If the cyanide toxicity is mild, oxygen administration until the liver can dispose of the cyanide may be adequate. In more severe cases, sodium nitrite may help avoid excessive damage from hypoxia. Doing nothing will likely result in morbidity or mortality. (D) Penicillamine is a chelator that is used to treat toxicity from copper and arsenic. It would not be helpful in this patient whose symptoms are caused by cyanide toxicity.

88 **The answer is A: Clomiphene.** This patient most likely has polycystic ovarian syndrome, which is the cause of her infertility. Clomiphene induces ovulation by being a partial agonist of estrogen receptors in the hypothalamus. This leads to an increase in the release of LH and FSH from the pituitary because of a disruption of normal feedback inhibition on the hypothalamus. (B) The combined estrogen–progestin pill is an oral contraceptive used to prevent pregnancy. (C) Dinoprostone is a prostaglandin E_2 analog used to induce labor. (D) Estrogen is most commonly used for hormone replacement in women who are postmenopausal, not to induce ovulation. (E) Mifepristone is used to terminate pregnancy, not induce ovulation.

89 **The answer is B: Diltiazem.** Calcium channel blockers (CCBs) can be classified as either dihydropyridines or nondihydropyridines. Dihydropyridines are selective for the calcium channels in vascular smooth muscle and have the suffix -dipine such as amlodipine. Diltiazem and verapamil are nondihydropyridine CCBs. Verapamil is selective for cardiac muscle cells, whereas diltiazem affects the calcium channels in heart muscle roughly equally as well as those found in smooth muscle. Calcium influx into smooth muscle cells is needed by calmodulin to activate myosin light chain kinase, which phosphorylates myosin to allow interaction with actin leading to muscle contraction. CCBs such as the dihydropyridines and diltiazem prevent the initial influx of calcium and so prevent smooth muscle contraction. (A) Amlodipine is a dihydropyridine CCB. It affects principally those calcium channels in vascular smooth muscle. (C) Losartan is an angiotensin II receptor blocker (ARB), not a calcium channel blocker. It lowers blood pressure by preventing the binding of angiotensin, which is a potent vasoconstrictor. (D) Nitroprusside is not a calcium channel blocker. It works by releasing nitric oxide, which is a potent vasodilator. (E) Verapamil is an example of a nondihydropyridine calcium channel blocker. It works primarily on the calcium channels found in heart muscle and has little effect on those found in smooth muscle.

90 **The answer is C: Octreotide.** This patient's presentation of hyperthyroidism with an elevated thyroid-stimulating hormone (TSH) level is consistent with a pituitary thyrotropinoma. Her hyperthyroidism is secondary to increased TSH release from the anterior pituitary gland. Somatostatin is an endogenous hormone that inhibits TSH release, so administration of a somatostatin analog such as octreotide would block TSH release in this patient. (A) Levothyroxine is synthetic T_4. It is used to treat hypothyroidism and would worsen this patient's condition. (B) Methimazole does decrease the synthesis of thyroid hormone but does not decrease TSH release. Octreotide is the only drug listed that would decrease TSH secretion. (D) Potassium iodide is used to treat acute thyrotoxic crises. The effect is rapid, but this drug will usually not work indefinitely. (E) Propylthiouracil does decrease the synthesis of thyroid hormone but does not decrease TSH release. Octreotide is the only drug listed that would decrease TSH secretion.

91 **The answer is C: Metformin.** This scenario describes a case of lactic acidosis. Lactic acidosis is a rare but serious potential side effect of metformin. The first symptoms are often vague, such as the malaise and myalgias experienced by this patient. Mortality from this lactic acidosis approaches 50%. Although this is a serious complication, it appears to occur only in patients with comorbid conditions that also predispose to lactic acidosis. (A) Acarbose inhibits intestinal brush border enzymes to decrease the amount of carbohydrate absorption after a meal and can cause GI discomfort. It is not known to cause lactic acidosis. (B) Glyburide is a second-generation sulfonylurea. Sulfonylureas may cause hypoglycemia but are not known to cause lactic acidosis. (D) Pioglitazone adverse effects include hepatotoxicity and weight gain. It is not known to cause lactic acidosis. (E) Tolbutamide is a first-generation sulfonylurea. First-generation sulfonylureas may cause a disulfiram-like reaction when used with alcohol but are not known to cause lactic acidosis.

92 **The answer is A: 5α-Reductase inhibitor.** Finasteride is a 5α-reductase inhibitor used for the treatment of benign prostatic hyperplasia. 5α-Reductase is an enzyme used to convert testosterone to dihydrotestosterone. Without dihydrotestosterone, the prostate

volume decreases, relieving urinary symptoms. (B) The mechanism of action of tamsulosin is as an α_1-antagonist. (C) Leuprolide when used in pulsatile dosing is a GnRH agonist used to treat infertility. (D) Leuprolide when used in continuous dosing is a GnRH antagonist used in the treatment of prostate cancer. (E) The mechanism of action of flutamide is as a nonsteroidal competitive inhibitor of androgens at the testosterone receptor. It is used in the treatment of prostate cancer.

93 **The answer is A: Exenatide.** Insulin release is stimulated primarily by elevated levels of blood glucose. Insulin secretion is also stimulated by endogenous hormones called incretins. The two known human incretins are GLP-1 and GIP. These molecules cause insulin release following oral glucose intake even before blood glucose levels are elevated. Additionally, they appear to slow gastric emptying and reduce food intake. Exenatide is a GLP-1 analog found in Gila monsters' venom. (B) Glipizide is a second-generation sulfonylurea. These drugs enhance insulin secretion, but they are not analogs of an endogenous peptide. (C) Miglitol inhibits intestinal brush border α-glucosidase. This enzyme is needed for the final steps in carbohydrate breakdown before absorption, so miglitol decreases the amount of dietary carbohydrate absorbed. It is not a peptide analog. (D) Pramlintide is an analog of amylin, which is cosecreted with insulin in response to a rise in glucose but does not enhance insulin secretion. Along with insulin, it inhibits glucagon secretion. (E) Rosiglitazone lowers blood glucose by increasing insulin sensitivity in peripheral tissues. It does not inhibit glucagon secretion.

94 **The answer is A: Amiodarone.** The patient is exhibiting symptoms of hypothyroidism, which is often associated with amiodarone therapy. It has complex effects, showing class I, II, III, and IV actions. Its dominant effect is prolongation of the action potential duration and the refractory period. Amiodarone has antianginal as well as antiarrhythmic activity. (B) Procainamide can cause lupus-like syndrome. (C) Propranolol could slow the heart but would not produce the changes in thyroid function. (D) Quinidine does not cause changes in thyroid function. (E) Verapamil does not cause changes in thyroid function.

95 **The answer is B: Insulin glargine.** Insulin glargine is a long-acting insulin that has a duration of action of 18 to 26 h. It reaches its peak quickly and remains stable over the course of a day for steady control. Because of its steady state, the risk of hypoglycemia is lower than with other insulins. (A) Insulin aspart is a fast-acting insulin that starts to work in 15 min, peaks around an hour, and lasts 3 to 5 h. (C) Insulin lispro is a fast-acting insulin that starts to work in 15 min, peaks around an hour, and lasts 3 to 5 h. (D) NPH insulin is an intermediate-acting insulin that starts to work in 1 to 2 h, peaks in 4 to 10 h, and lasts 18 to 24 h. It is associated with a higher risk of hypoglycemia compared to insulin glargine. (E) Regular insulin is a short-acting insulin that starts to work in 30 to 60 min, peaks in 2 to 4 h, and lasts 6 to 10 h.

96 **The answer is A: Agranulocytosis.** Propylthiouracil is used to treat hyperthyroidism and can be used in Graves' disease. A side effect is agranulocytosis. Patients should be watched for the risk of increased infections. (B) Arrhythmias would be a more common side effect of levothyroxine. (C) Diabetes would be a more common side effect of steroids. (D) Hypertension would be a more common side effect of sibutramine. (E) Tachycardia would be a more common side effect of levothyroxine.

97 **The answer is C: Octreotide.** The most appropriate medical treatment for acromegaly is octreotide, which is a somatostatin analog. It is an inhibitor of growth hormone, which is overproduced in acromegaly. (A) Desmopressin is used in the treatment of central diabetes insipidus, not acromegaly. (B) Growth hormone is used in the treatment of growth hormone deficiency. There is an excess of growth hormone in acromegaly. (D) Oxytocin is used to induce labor by causing uterine contractions, not to acromegaly. (E) Propylthiouracil is used in the treatment of hyperthyroidism, not acromegaly.

98 **The answer is A: Diet.** In type V familial mixed hypertriglyceridemia, serum VLDL and chylomicrons are elevated. LDL is normal or decreased. This results in elevated cholesterol and greatly elevated TG levels. The cause is either increased production or decreased clearance of VLDL and chylomicrons. Usually, it is a genetic defect. It occurs most commonly in adults who are obese and/or with diabetes. The treatment is diet. If necessary, drug therapy includes niacin, and/or fenofibrate, or a statin. (B) Diet is the most cost-effective therapy of familial mixed hypertriglyceridemia. (C) Riboflavin is ineffective for this condition. (D) Statin therapy is effective but involves a monthly medication cost. (E) Watchful waiting will not change serum medication levels.

99 **The answer is D: Total cholesterol = 220 mg/dL, HDL = 100 mg/dL.** Treatment with an HMG-CoA reductase inhibitor will best benefit the patient with elevated total cholesterol. This patient has elevated total cholesterol with normal levels of HDL cholesterol. (A) This patient has normal total cholesterol and HDL cholesterol. (B) This patient has normal total cholesterol and

LDL cholesterol. (C) This patient has normal total cholesterol and borderline/desirable HDL cholesterol. (E) This patient has normal LDL cholesterol and normal HDL cholesterol.

100 **The answer is A: Administer aspirin prior to niacin.** The most common side effects of niacin therapy are an intense cutaneous flush (accompanied by an uncomfortable feeling of warmth) and pruritus. Administration of aspirin prior to taking niacin decreases the flush, which is prostaglandin mediated. The sustained-release formulation of niacin, which is taken once daily at bedtime, reduces bothersome initial adverse effects. (B) This patient does not require treatment with prednisone. (C) This patient does not require treatment with prednisone. (D) This patient would benefit from treatment with a sustained-release formulation of niacin. (E) This patient needs basic treatment with aspirin prior to administration of niacin.

101 **The answer is B: Gallstone formation.** Fenofibrate and gemfibrozil are derivatives of fibric acid that lower serum triacylglycerols and increase HDL levels. Both have the same mechanism of action. However, fenofibrate is more effective than gemfibrozil in lowering plasma LDL cholesterol and triglyceride levels. Because these drugs increase biliary cholesterol excretion, there is a predisposition to the formation of gallstones. (A) This is not a drug overdose case. Cholestasis and increased biliary cholesterol excretion are the most likely causes. (C) This is not an unexplained effect. (D) Although myositis is also an adverse effect of this medication, it does not explain the cholelithiasis. (E) Inflammatory pancreatitis is unlikely; gallstone pancreatitis would be more likely.

102 **The answer is A: Cholestyramine.** Cholestyramine is an anion-exchange resin that binds negatively charged bile acids and bile salts in the small intestine. The resin/bile acid complex is excreted in the feces, thus preventing the bile acids from returning to the liver by the enterohepatic circulation. (B) Fenofibrate does not bind intestinal bile acids. (C) Fluvastatin does not bind intestinal bile acids. (D) Lovastatin inhibits HMG-CoA reductase. (E) Niacin does not bind intestinal bile acids.

103 **The answer is E: St. John's wort supplement.** Lovastatin (and many other -statin drugs) is metabolized by the cytochrome P450 3A4 (CYP3A4) enzyme in the liver. This enzyme is the site of many drug interactions. It metabolizes dozens of drugs but can also be induced or inhibited by others. Cimetidine, diltiazem, ketoconazole, and ritonavir are all CYP3A4 inhibitors. Given with lovastatin, these would cause an increase in lovastatin's concentration because they inhibit the enzyme responsible for breaking lovastatin down. St. John's wort, a herbal supplement, is a CYP3A4 inducer. It would cause a decrease in lovastatin's concentration, making it appear that he has been taking less than prescribed. (A) Cimetidine is a CYP3A4 inhibitor. Taking it together with lovastatin would cause an increase in lovastatin's concentration. (B) Diltiazem is a CYP3A4 inhibitor. Taking it together with lovastatin would cause an increase in lovastatin's concentration. (C) Ketoconazole is a CYP3A4 inhibitor. Taking it together with lovastatin would cause an increase in lovastatin's concentration. (D) Ritonavir is a CYP3A4 inhibitor. Taking it together with lovastatin would cause an increase in lovastatin's concentration.

104 **The answer is C: Inhibits aromatase.** Although infertility can only be diagnosed following 1 year of unprotected sex, 75% of couples are able to conceive after 9 months. This couple appears to have a decreased fecundity (ability to conceive), but no abnormalities were immediately seen in the wife. It is not yet known whether the problem lies in the husband or the wife, so a trial of letrozole is started with the wife. Letrozole is an aromatase inhibitor, which blocks the peripheral conversion of endogenous androgens to estrogens. By reducing the wife's overall estrogen load, letrozole may increase her fertility through decreasing the negative feedback from estrogen on the hypothalamus. Letrozole is a good choice for an early try to increase fertility because it is generally well tolerated with a mild side effect profile. (A) Clomiphene works by blocking estrogen receptors on the hypothalamus in order to allow GnRH release. Letrozole does not block estrogen receptors. (B) Letrozole works in the female partner to reduce her overall estrogen load in order to permit more GnRH release from the hypothalamus. It does not increase sperm production. (D) Follitropin is a recombinant form of FSH (r-FSH). It acts like endogenous FSH to directly stimulate the development of ovarian follicles. Letrozole does not work in this manner. (E) Bromocriptine is a dopamine receptor agonist that suppresses prolactin secretion. High levels of prolactin suppress GnRH and FSH to decrease fertility. Letrozole does not interfere with prolactin secretion.

105 **The answer is E: Inhibits angiotensin II receptor.** Losartan is an angiotensin II receptor inhibitor. It does not increase the level of bradykinin, like angiotensin-converting enzyme inhibitors, and therefore does not cause a cough. It is often the substitute used when a cough develops on angiotensin-converting enzyme inhibitors. (A) Losartan does not affect the angiotensin I receptor. (B) Losartan inhibits, not activates, the angiotensin II receptor. (C) Lisinopril is an angiotensin-converting enzyme inhibitor, not losartan. (D) Losartan does not affect the angiotensin I receptor.

106 **The answer is D: Venous thromboembolism.** Oral contraceptive pills lead to increased risk of venous thrombosis, and patients should be counseled about the signs and symptoms. The risk is increased more with smoking and older age. In patients older than age 35 years, smoking is a contraindication to using oral contraceptive pills. (A) Headaches are more common side effect with nitroglycerin and sildenafil, not oral contraceptive pills. (B) Oral contraceptive pills lead to a decrease menstrual bleeding. (C) Oral contraceptive pills lead to a decreased risk of endometrial and ovarian cancer. (E) Recent studies have confirmed that oral contraceptive pills do not lead to significant weight gain.

107 **The answer is B: Increased risk of endometrial cancer.** Estrogen-only replacement therapy increases the risk of endometrial cancer and therefore is usually reserved for patients who had total hysterectomies. Progesterone is added to the estrogen as a protective effect for the endometrial lining. Hormone replacement therapy is usually used for no more than 5 years. (A) Estrogen replacement therapy will usually improve the mood of perimenopausal patients. (C) Estrogen replacement therapy decreases the risk of osteoporosis. (D) Estrogen replacement therapy does not commonly cause a rash. A rash would be more commonly seen as an allergic reaction to antibiotics. (E) Estrogen replacement therapy maintains the vaginal lining to prevent atrophy.

108 **The answer is E: Triiodothyronine.** Triiodothyronine is a thyroid hormone that is overproduced in hyperthyroidism. The other choices are hyperthyroidism treatments. (A) Iodine is a treatment for hyperthyroidism. (B) Methimazole is a treatment for hyperthyroidism. (C) Propylthiouracil is a treatment for hyperthyroidism. (D) Surgical removal of the thyroid gland is a treatment for hyperthyroidism.

109 **The answer is E: Niacin.** A side effect of niacin is causing increased levels of uric acid, which can cause gout flares. It is thought to occur because niacin competes with uric acid for excretion in the kidneys. It usually only occurs when high doses of niacin are used. (A) Cholestyramine may cause gallstones but not hyperuricemia. (B) Ezetimibe may cause an elevation of liver enzymes but not hyperuricemia. (C) Gemfibrozil may cause gallstones but not hyperuricemia. (D) Lovastatin may cause hepatotoxicity or muscle aches but not hyperuricemia.

110 **The answer is C: Gemfibrozil.** Gemfibrozil is used to significantly lower triglyceride levels; however, it has little effect on LDL and HDL. Gemfibrozil increases the synthesis of lipoprotein lipase, which increases the clearance of triglycerides. (A) Colestipol has been shown to minimally increase triglyceride levels. (B) Ezetimibe has very little effect on triglyceride levels. (D) Niacin will decrease triglyceride levels but not as much as gemfibrozil. (E) Rosuvastatin will decrease triglyceride levels but not as much as gemfibrozil.

111 **The answer is D: Gemfibrozil.** Gemfibrozil interacts with the statin class of cholesterol medications to cause an increased risk of muscle aches and rhabdomyolysis. Because of the increased risk and limited benefits seen with the combination of gemfibrozil and statins, it is not recommended. (A) It is generally safe to add cholestyramine to statins for better cholesterol control. (B) It is generally safe to add colestipol to statins for better cholesterol control. (C) It is generally safe to add ezetimibe to statins for better cholesterol control. (E) Niacin is usually poorly tolerated because of GI side effects, but it is generally safe to add to statins.

112 **The answer is A: Letter A.** Letter A represents the insulin response in a normal individual to a glucose load. Pancreatic function is normal in this patient. (B) Letter B represents the insulin response in a patient with Type-2 diabetes. (C) Letter C represents the insulin response in a patient with Type-1 diabetes. (D) This information can be determined from the curves presented.

113 **The answer is E: Inhibits intestinal brush border enzymes.** Miglitol inhibits the intestinal brush border enzyme, α-glucosidase. The enzyme breaks down complex sugars into monosaccharides that are absorbed in the intestinal tract. It can be poorly tolerated because of GI upset. (A) Decreased glucagon release is seen with pramlintide and exenatide. (B) Sulfonylureas, such as glyburide, increase the release of insulin. (C) The mechanism of action of pioglitazone and rosiglitazones is increased insulin sensitivity in peripheral tissues. (D) The mechanism of action of metformin is inhibiting hepatic gluconeogenesis.

114 **The answer is C: Glyburide.** A side effect of glyburide is that it can cause hypoglycemia. Glyburide is a second-generation sulfonylurea that increases the release of insulin. The dose has to be closely monitored to ensure that the patient does not become hypoglycemic. (A) Acarbose does not usually cause hypoglycemia. If hypoglycemia would occur, the patient must ingest monosaccharides because polysaccharides will not be broken down. (B) Exenatide can cause GI upset and pancreatitis but does not usually cause hypoglycemia. (D) Metformin is effective at lowering hemoglobin A_{1c} but does not usually cause hypoglycemia. (E) Pioglitazone can cause weight gain and hepatotoxicity but does not usually cause hypoglycemia.

115 **The answer is E: Pioglitazone.** Weight gain is commonly seen with pioglitazone. The weight gain is caused by an increase in subcutaneous adipose tissue. Other side effects of pioglitazone include edema and hepatotoxicity. (A) A common side effect of acarbose is GI upset, not weight gain. (B) A common side effect of exenatide is pancreatitis, not weight gain. (C) Hypoglycemia is a common side effect of glyburide. (D) Lactic acidosis is one of the most dangerous side effects of metformin.

116 **The answer is A: Letter A.** Leuprolide is an inhibitor of GnRH in a negative fashion. This agent will decrease production of LH, which will lower serum testosterone levels. Testosterone causes prostate cancer to grow. Thus, inhibition may cause cancer regression. (B) Letter B is the pituitary gland. (C) Letter C is the target organs such as the testes. (D) This information can be determined from the figure.

117 **The answer is E: Location 5.** Location 5 is the site of proteolytic release of hormones. T_3 and T_4 levels will subsequently increase as a result of this function. (A) Location 1 is the update of iodide ion. (B) Location 2 is the synthesis of thyroglobulin. (C) Location 3 is the site of iodination. (D) Location 4 is the site of condensation.

118 **The answer is B: Patient B.** Patient B has mild impairment of glucose tolerance but has reasonable ability to secrete insulin. This patient can be treated with dietary modification and exercise. Medical therapy is not required for this patient. (A) Patient A does not require treatment for diabetes mellitus. (C) Patient C required therapy with metformin and dietary modifications. (D) Patient D requires combination therapy for diabetes mellitus. (E) Patient E requires injections of insulin to treat diabetes mellitus.

119 **The answer is E: Letter E.** Insulin detemir is represented by letter E. This agent can be given daily and has activity for 12 to 24 h. (A) Letter A represents insulin glulisine. (B) Letter B represents insulin aspart. (C) Letter C represents regular insulin. (D) Letter D represents NPH insulin.

120 **The answer is C: Letter C.** Letter C represents the relative concentrations of estradiol. This hormone has peak levels at approximately days 7 to 10 of the menstrual cycle. (A) Letter A represents LH. (B) Letter B represents FSH. (D) Letter D represents progesterone. (E) Letter E represents ovulation.

121 **The answer is C: Liver function tests.** There are two main concerns when starting any patient on a statin: myopathy and hepatotoxicity. However, because the statins are such effective medications at lowering LDL and triglyceride levels, physicians still prescribe these medications and follow closely liver function tests and creatine kinase levels to ensure proper liver and muscle function, respectively. (A) Although an electrocardiogram may be warranted, it is clearly not as important as looking for toxic manifestations of the lovastatin. (B) Hemoglobin A_{1c} would be an important monitoring test to follow a diabetic's sugar control over the last 3 months. However, we have no indication of diabetes in this patient, and a hemoglobin A_{1c} would not be used to diagnose diabetes. (D) Pulmonary function tests are often monitored in drugs that lead to pulmonary fibrosis. Those drugs include bleomycin, amiodarone, and busulfan; but no statins are thought to have any pulmonary complications. (E) Potassium levels are often associated with various diuretics; urine potassium levels increase with all diuretic classes except potassium-sparing diuretics. Statins are not associated with any changes in potassium levels.

Chapter 5

Drugs Affecting Other Systems (Including GI and Pulmonary)

QUESTIONS

Select the single best answer.

1 A 28-year-old woman is hospitalized (hospital day 3) on the maternity floor after cesarean section delivery of her first child. The child was born at term by C-section because of failure of labor to progress. The patient has been unable to void normally since the procedure. Which of the following is the most appropriate treatment for this patient?

(A) Bethanechol
(B) Carbachol
(C) Physostigmine
(D) Pilocarpine
(E) Tacrine

2 A 45-year-old male who is obese presents to his primary care physician complaining of postprandial epigastric pain. The pain does not appear after every meal. He has noticed the pain especially after eating spicy foods and oatmeal. He is not currently taking any medications. Which of the following drugs prevents acid secretion by antagonizing a receptor?

(A) Aluminum hydroxide
(B) Fexofenadine
(C) Misoprostol
(D) Omeprazole
(E) Ranitidine

3 A 52-year-old man with glaucoma is seen by a new ophthalmologist who prescribes latanoprost for his glaucoma that is refractory to medical treatments. The physician must warn the patient about which of the following possible adverse effects of this medication?

(A) Decreased iris pigmentation
(B) Diarrhea
(C) Hair growth of eyelashes
(D) Nausea
(E) Transient myopia

4 A 47-year-old immigrant from Japan with a long history of untreated gastric ulcers develops stomach cancer. One drug in his initial treatment regimen is 5-fluorouracil (5-FU) as well as ondansetron to control nausea. While receiving this drug, the patient develops redness and numbness on the palms of his hands and soles of his feet. How can this reaction be avoided?

(A) Do not coadminister ondansetron with 5-fluorouracil
(B) Give 5-FU by bolus rather than continuous infusion
(C) Give 5-FU by continuous infusion rather than bolus
(D) Give with leucovorin
(E) This is a rare, bizarre side effect of 5-FU and cannot be avoided

5 A 62-year-old man with congestive heart failure has been taking a loop diuretic to reduce peripheral edema. His labs reveal a serum potassium of 3.1 mEq/L, so a potassium-sparing diuretic, triamterene, is added to his regimen. Which of the following is the site of action of this agent?

(A) Ascending limb of loop of Henle
(B) Collecting tubule
(C) Descending limb of loop of Henle
(D) Distal convoluted tubule
(E) Proximal convoluted tubule

6 A 43-year-old man presents to his primary care physician for evaluation of urinary urgency, frequency, and dysuria. Urinalysis reveals nitrates, leukocytes, and red blood cells. His serum creatinine is 1.5 mg/dL. He is given a prescription for ciprofloxacin to take for 10 days. Because of his renal insufficiency, he will likely have compensatory drug excretion via

(A) Breath
(B) Liver
(C) Salivary gland
(D) Skin
(E) Spleen

7 A medical student is involved in a summer research project that involves evaluating the effect of inhalational halothane tagged with a carbon-labeled radiotracer. Rats (2 kg in weight) are being studied and then sacrificed according to institutional protocol. Which of the following organs or systems would have the least amount of halothane carbon-labeled radiotracer picked up?

(A) Brain
(B) Heart
(C) Liver
(D) Pancreas
(E) Thoracic wall muscle

8 A first-year anesthesiology resident reaches for isoflurane as the induction agent for a patient who is about to receive general anesthesia. When the attending faculty sees this, he quickly takes the syringe away from the resident because this agent can cause which of the following effects when used for induction?

(A) Coughing
(B) Dry mouth
(C) Hypertension
(D) Laryngeal relaxation
(E) Muscle relaxation

9 Five patients will undergo surgery for a hip replacement. Which of the following patients is at greatest risk for the anesthetic agents entering the cerebral blood flow?

(A) A 19-year-old man with blood pressure of 120/80 mm Hg and pulse of 80 beats/minute
(B) A 41-year old man with sinusitis and hypertension
(C) A 62-year-old man with a history of four-vessel coronary artery bypass
(D) A 71-year-old man who has run four marathons

10 A 49-year-old woman with a deviated septum is going to undergo repair under anesthesia. Induction with intravenous propofol will first be given prior to placement of a laryngeal mask airway. Advantages of this agent include which of the following?

(A) Administered orally
(B) Half-life up to 4 h
(C) Low perfusion to the brain
(D) Plasma levels maintained for several hours
(E) Use allowed in moderate renal failure

11 A 12-year-old boy with obsessive-compulsive disorder and depression desires to be managed with a single pharmacologic agent. Which of the following agents would be best used in this patient?

(A) Bupropion
(B) Fluoxetine
(C) Fluvoxamine
(D) Mirtazapine
(E) Sertraline

12 A 39-year-old man with schizophrenia presents to his primary care physician for follow-up. He is currently taking thioridazine. Which of the following statements regarding his recovery is true?

(A) Complete normalization of behavior is expected
(B) Delusions typically persist despite therapy
(C) Hallucinations typically improve with therapy
(D) Thought processing remains dysfunctional despite therapy
(E) Withdrawal from social situations is markedly improved

13 A 45-year-old woman complains of intractable hiccups. She has no prior medical or surgical history. Physical examination and direct laryngoscopy fails to reveal any anatomic defects. What is the most appropriate treatment for this patient?

(A) Chlorpromazine
(B) Pimozide
(C) Promethazine
(D) Tetracycline
(E) Thioridazine

14 A 52-year-old man with a history of chronic low back pain caused by herniated L5 disk and depression is currently taking fluoxetine and tramadol. He presents to his primary care physician for follow-up. The combination of these two agents should raise the treating physician's concern for which of the following reactions?

(A) Encephalitis
(B) Meningitis
(C) Parkinson disease
(D) Seizures
(E) Stroke

15 A 55-year-old man complains of poor urinary flow and nocturia. He is found to suffer from benign prostatic hyperplasia. The physician prescribes finasteride to help his symptoms. What is the mechanism of action of this agent?

(A) Antagonizes α_1-adrenergic receptors
(B) Blocks DHT receptors
(C) Inhibits 5-α-reductase
(D) Inhibits testosterone synthesis
(E) Relaxes prostatic smooth muscle

16 A 56-year-old man presents to his primary care physician for a follow-up examination. He is known to have hypertension. Physical examination of the heart, lungs, and abdomen are within normal limits. Which of the following concomitant conditions is he most likely to suffer from?

(A) Angina
(B) Asthma
(C) Diabetes
(D) Prior myocardial infarction
(E) Renal impairment

17 A 38-year-old businessman is on a trip to Mexico when he develops diarrhea. He has to give a presentation in a few hours and needs rapid relief. He takes an antidiarrheal preparation containing loperamide. Which of the following is a property of loperamide that makes it useful in treating diarrhea?

(A) Anticholinergic
(B) Broad-spectrum antibiotic
(C) Gram-negative antibiotic
(D) Inhibitor of myenteric plexus activity
(E) Sympathetic nervous system stimulant

18 A 37-year-old man complains of chest pain after meals. He says this pain has gone on for a few months and gets only minimal relief from antacid tablets. The physician prescribes a drug that will decrease the amount of acid secreted by binding to and inhibiting an ATPase on the lumenal surface of parietal cells. Which of the following drugs works by this mechanism?

(A) Atropine
(B) Cimetidine
(C) Misoprostol
(D) Octreotide
(E) Omeprazole

19 A 56-year-old man who is a chronic alcoholic is brought to the emergency department because of altered mental status. Blood tests reveal normal creatinine but indicate hyperammonemia. The patient is given lactulose after which his blood ammonia soon drops to a more suitable level. Which of the following organs is lactulose's site of action?

(A) Brain
(B) Colon
(C) Kidney
(D) Liver
(E) Spleen

20 A 3-year-old girl is brought to the pediatrics clinic by her parents. They say that their daughter has had a runny nose for a few days and recently began complaining of ear pain. The parents also say that she has been treated for ear infections in the past but once broke out in a rash while taking an antibiotic. The physician is worried about an allergic reaction but knows that some antibiotics can cause a nonallergic rash and that she may not be allergic to this class of antibiotics. Which of the following antibiotics is known for causing a nonallergic rash?

(A) Amoxicillin
(B) Ceftriaxone
(C) Erythromycin
(D) Gentamicin
(E) Vancomycin

21 A 74-year-old man with a history of transient ischemic attacks takes a baby aspirin (81 mg) per day at the suggestion of his cardiologist to prevent heart disease. One day, he accidentally takes six baby aspirins. Which of the following sequelae is most likely to occur?

(A) Cholecystitis
(B) Gastrointestinal bleeding
(C) Pancreatitis
(D) Splenic infarct
(E) Transient ischemic attack

22 A 32-year-old man presents to his primary care physician for evaluation of elevated triglycerides. His mother, father, sister, and brother all have the same problem. His serum cholesterol and triglyceride levels are normal. What is the most likely explanation for these findings?

(A) Diabetes insipidus
(B) Diabetes mellitus
(C) Increased production of triglycerides
(D) Increased clearance of VLDL

23 A 69-year-old man with a history of hypertension on a thiazide diuretic once daily is planning to have hip replacement. He sees the anesthesiologist preoperatively and is found to have a serum potassium of 2.9 mEq/L on routine laboratory studies. His blood pressure is 110/86 mm Hg. What is the best course of action for this patient at this time?
(A) Begin exercise regimen immediately
(B) Cardiac enzyme evaluation for possible myocardial infarction
(C) Discontinue thiazide diuretic and begin ACE inhibitor therapy
(D) Increase thiazide diuretic dose to be administered twice daily
(E) Supplement potassium by increasing intake of fruits and bananas

24 A 67-year-old man with long-standing hypertension presents to his primary care physician for follow-up. He is managed with spironolactone. Physical examination reveals bilateral gynecomastia. He states that he has recently underwent an endoscopy, which revealed gastric ulcers. What is the most likely explanation for these findings?
(A) Chronic stress
(B) Drug toxicity
(C) Pituitary tumor
(D) Thyroid disease
(E) Thyroid storm

25 A 47-year-old man presents to the ambulatory care center with symptoms of hypoglycemia and is found to have an insulinoma. His medical history is significant for occasional asthma, which he treats using an albuterol inhaler, and an MI for which he takes daily low-dose aspirin. Because he takes aspirin, he is not able to immediately undergo surgery. The physician prescribes diazoxide for therapy until the tumor can be removed. Diazoxide stimulates potassium channels leading to inhibition of insulin release. Which of the following is most likely to occur in this patient as a result of diazoxide therapy?
(A) Bronchoconstriction
(B) Hypertension
(C) Hypoglycemia
(D) Hypotension
(E) Seizures

26 A 27-year-old man complains of occasional heartburn. His physician makes a few suggestions of diet and lifestyle changes he could make as well as some medications he can take for symptom management. The patient decides to try a magnesium hydroxide (MgOH) preparation. Which of the following is a side effect of MgOH that the physician should warn him about?
(A) Constipation
(B) Diarrhea
(C) Headache
(D) Impotence
(E) Seizures

27 A 42-year-old woman with a history of asthma has an attack and is brought to the emergency department for evaluation and treatment. She is wheezing and is short of breath. What is the most likely pathophysiology of this condition?
(A) Bronchodilation
(B) Increased secretion of mucus
(C) Inflammation of the bronchial serosa
(D) Relaxation of bronchial smooth muscle

28 A 57-year-old man with chronic gastroesophageal reflux disease on cimetidine presents to a new primary care physician. He states that he has been doing well and has been taking this medication for about 15 years. Which of the following statements is true about therapy with this agent?
(A) Dose adjustment is required in hepatic failure
(B) Has a long half-life
(C) 70% inactivated in the liver
(D) 30% excreted in the urine

29 A 37-year-old man with gastroesophageal reflux takes over-the-counter cimetidine. He has no health care insurance and thus does not go to see a physician. This patient must be aware of which of the following side effects of this medication?
(A) Confusion
(B) Constipation
(C) Hallucinations
(D) Headache
(E) Muscular pain

30 A 55-year-old woman with end-stage ovarian cancer with extensive carcinomatosis has chronic nausea and vomiting. She inquires about a marijuana derivative to help. She realizes that this is not considered an approved therapy. Should she elect to pursue this agent, she should be concerned about which of the following effects?
(A) Disorientation
(B) Euphoria
(C) Excitation
(D) Vomiting
(E) Uremic pericarditis

31 A 42-year-old woman with irritable bowel syndrome with diarrhea predominance presents to her primary care physician for treatment. The physician suggests an exercise regimen, dietary modifications, and a bulk laxative. The likely mechanism of action of this agent would involve which of the following?

(A) Gel formation in the intestine
(B) Neuromodulation of the S3 nerve root
(C) Nonabsorbable salt
(D) Osmotic laxative
(E) Stimulation of the cholinergic nervous system

32 A 37-year-old man who is morbidly obese (weight is 375 lb) is referred for weight-reducing surgery via gastric bypass. After hearing the risks of the surgery, the patient decides on a medical approach to treatment. He begins therapy with phentermine. Which of the following is the most important for both the patient and the family to know about this medication?

(A) Abuse potential
(B) Cardiovascular toxicities
(C) Hypertension
(D) Risk of stroke
(E) Seizures

33 A 49-year-old man with a history of peptic ulcer disease and gastroesophageal reflux disorder is being treated with cimetidine for approximately 20 years. He now complains of breast swelling and breast discharge. What is the most likely explanation for these findings?

(A) Abscess
(B) Antiandrogenic effect
(C) Inflammatory response
(D) Neoplastic process
(E) Overwhelming edema

34 A 67-year-old woman with known peptic ulcer disease found at endoscopy to be on maintenance treatment with misoprostol at 125% of the recommended dose. The rationale behind this dose is to maximize which of the following?

(A) Decrease in gastric acid secretion
(B) Improve bicarbonate balance
(C) Improve gastric emptying
(D) Improve sphincter tone of the lower esophagus
(E) Lower gastric luminal pressures

35 A 78-year-old woman with osteoporosis and occasional gastroesophageal reflux presents to her primary care physician for follow-up. Physical examination of the heart, lungs, and abdomen are unremarkable. Which of the following agents would be best to treat both of her underlying conditions?

(A) Aluminum hydroxide
(B) Calcium carbonate
(C) Magnesium hydroxide
(D) Sodium bicarbonate
(E) Warm milk

36 A 47-year-old man with a history of NSAID-induced ulcers has been placed on sucralfate. He has been on the medicine for 1 year and does complain of intermittent chest pressure after meals. Upper endoscopy is performed. Which of the following findings is most likely to occur?

(A) Duodenitis
(B) Duodenal perforation
(C) Gastric ulcers that appear unhealed
(D) Normal gastric epithelium
(E) Normal lower esophageal epithelium

37 A 23-year-old man with mild erectile dysfunction presents to his primary care physician. He has no other medical problems. He does have an anxiety disorder. Physical examination of the abdomen and genitalia are within normal limits. Which of the following is the best agent for treatment of this patient?

(A) Penile prosthesis
(B) Sildenafil
(C) Tadalafil
(D) Vardenafil
(E) Vacuum erection device

38 A 53-year-old man who is a 40 pack-year smoker presents to his primary care physician with a productive cough, fever, and chills. He sits in an office all day and recently began using an air conditioner as the weather has warmed. No organisms were visible with a gram stain of sputum, but a silver stain reveals rods. His medical history includes myocardial infarction, for which he takes ticlopidine; hyperglycemia, for which he takes metformin; and a congenital QT segment prolongation. For which of the following reasons would the physician be hesitant to prescribe erythromycin to treat his legionellosis?

(A) Drug interaction with metformin
(B) Drug interaction with ticlopidine
(C) History of hyperglycemia
(D) History of myocardial infarction
(E) QT prolongation

39 A 63-year-old woman is hospitalized in the intensive care unit with overwhelming sepsis. She is on multiple intravenous medications and is now begun on imipenem/cilastatin. The treating physician must be concerned about which of the following side effects of this therapy?

(A) Cardiotoxicity
(B) Gastrointestinal ischemia
(C) Pulmonary fibrosis
(D) Renal failure
(E) Seizures

40 A 59-year-old man with multiple organ system failure and sepsis is treated with multiple medications, including gentamicin. Unfortunately, because of an error in the pharmacy, the patient is given a dose of daptomycin. Over the next few hours, the patient becomes tachypneic and develops a fever of 103°F. What is the most likely rationale for this response?
(A) Atrial fibrillation
(B) Cardiac arrest
(C) Inactivation of surfactant
(D) Pulmonary embolus
(E) Pulmonary infarct

41 A 23-year-old woman with a history of an MRSA skin boil is treated with telavancin. During therapy, she does complain of some foamy urine and nausea. The most important complication to warn this patient of is which of the following?
(A) Pregnancy complications
(B) Pulmonary embolism
(C) QT interval prolongation
(D) T wave inversion
(E) Uremic pericarditis

42 A 36-year-old man with multiple medical problems including diabetes, hypertension, and morbid obesity is hospitalized for treatment of a vancomycin-resistant *Enterobacter* infection. Recent blood cultures are positive. He is given quinupristin/dalfopristin intravenously through the antecubital vein. Which of the following sequelae is most likely?
(A) Arthritis
(B) Hepatic dysfunction
(C) Muscle fatigue
(D) Renal failure
(E) Venous irritation

43 A 55-year-old man with multidrug-resistant methicillin-resistant *Staphylococcus aureus* is treated with intravenous linezolid for 40 days. He is currently hospitalized in the intensive care unit. Which of the following consultations should be ordered in this patient at this time?
(A) Gastroenterology
(B) Ophthalmology
(C) Podiatry
(D) Pulmonary medicine
(E) Urology

44 A 43-year-old woman with recurrent urinary tract infections who is usually sensitive to ciprofloxacin now has three consecutive UTIs in a 4-month period. Each time, the culture and sensitivity reveal resistance to ciprofloxacin. What is the most likely source of resistance?
(A) DNA gyrase
(B) DNA polymerase
(C) DNA topoisomerase I
(D) DNA topoisomerase II
(E) DNA topoisomerase III

45 A 35-year-old G1P0 woman presents to her primary care physician at 35 weeks gestation with headaches. Her blood pressure is 164/90 mm Hg, although 6 months ago it was 124/74 mm Hg. She has no proteinuria and no edema. Which of the following antihypertensive would be best for this patient?
(A) Atenolol
(B) Lisinopril
(C) Losartan
(D) Methyldopa
(E) Nifedipine

46 It is well established that the use of fluoroquinolones is associated with a risk of rupture of the Achilles tendon. Five patients with infections are considered for therapy with a quinolone antibiotic. Which of the following patient profile is at the lowest risk for Achilles tendon rupture or tendon inflammation?
(A) A 30-year-old man with a history of diabetes mellitus
(B) A 35-year-old woman with rheumatoid arthritis who takes prednisone
(C) A 40-year-old man with liver and renal failure awaiting transplantation
(D) A 60-year-old man who received a renal transplant 3 years ago
(E) A 65-year-old man with a history of hypertension and sleep apnea

47 A 52-year-old woman with a long history or recurrent urinary tract infections now has another one. Review of culture results reveal that the organism is resistant to sulfa drugs. What is the most likely mechanism of resistance to this medication?
(A) Enhanced production of PABA
(B) Increased cellular permeability
(C) Increased tetrahydrofolate reductase
(D) Increased tetrahydrofolate synthase

48 A 21-year-old woman presents to her primary care physician with worsening alogia as well as harboring the delusion that an ex-boyfriend (who now lives in a different state) is spying on her through her computer. Her physician prescribes chlorpromazine, a low-potency antipsychotic. The physician warns her of possible anticholinergic side effects. Which of the following is an anticholinergic effect?

(A) Bradycardia
(B) Diarrhea
(C) Lacrimation
(D) Miosis
(E) Urinary retention

49 A 51-year-old man with systemic candidemia is hospitalized in the intensive care unit. He has failed treatment with outpatient oral medications. He has begun on intravenous amphotericin. Approximately 1 h after administration of amphotericin, the patient develops fever and chills. What is the most appropriate course of action to take?

(A) Continue infusion; premedicate with antipyretic for next doses
(B) Discontinue the infusion
(C) Intravenous prednisone and discontinue amphotericin
(D) Intravenous tetracycline and discontinue amphotericin
(E) Transfusion of one unit of packed red blood cells

50 A 58-year-old man with systemic candidemia is hospitalized in the intensive care unit. He has failed treatment with outpatient oral medications. He also has a history of prostate cancer that was treated with external beam radiotherapy. He has begun on intravenous amphotericin and flucytosine. Which of the following is an important side effect for the treating physician to be aware of?

(A) Bone marrow depression
(B) Necrotizing enterocolitis
(C) Neutrophilia
(D) Transient hepatitis
(E) Thrombocytosis

51 A 49-year-old man with a fungal infection is hospitalized and is being treated with oral ketoconazole. To help with intestinal absorption of this agent, which of the following agents should be given to this patient?

(A) Calcium carbonate
(B) Calcium citrate
(C) Cimetidine
(D) Coca-Cola
(E) Sodium bicarbonate

52 A 42-year-old man with HIV disease is hospitalized for refractory fungemia. He has begun on a course of caspofungin. After administration of the first intravenous dose, the patient develops flushing and sweats. What is the most likely mechanism of action for this finding?

(A) Histamine release from mast cells
(B) Pancreatic pseudocyst
(C) Parathyroid adenoma
(D) Parathyroid hyperplasia
(E) Pheochromocytoma

53 A 39-year-old man with recurrent fungal infections is seen by his primary care physician. Consideration is given to prescribing terbinafine for this patient. Although the medication can be given without regard to meals, a possible problem with this medication can be which of the following?

(A) Accumulation in tissues
(B) Nephrotoxicity
(C) Neuromuscular blockade
(D) Ototoxicity
(E) Uremia

54 A 22-year-old man is transferred to a tertiary care center for the management of trypanosomal infection. He has a significant history of travel abroad in Africa. When melarsoprol is used in the treatment of trypanosomal infections, which of the following serious side effects must the treating physician be concerned with?

(A) Cardiac arrest
(B) Encephalopathy
(C) Pulmonary embolism
(D) Tetany
(E) Uremia

55 A 32-year-old man with HIV disease is hospitalized in the intensive care unit. He is receiving intravenous pentamidine for suspected *Pneumocystis* pneumonia. After 3 days of therapy, his serum glucose level is 250 mg/dL. He is not known to be a diabetic. What is the most likely explanation for this finding?

(A) Hypertension
(B) Pancreatitis
(C) Pancreatic carcinoma
(D) Pheochromocytoma
(E) Toxicity of pancreatic cells

56 A 6-year-old boy returns home from his last day of school before thanksgiving break. Over the break, he develops a cough, stuffy nose, headache, and fever. His mother administers a cough syrup containing guaifenesin. Which of the following effects is likely caused by guaifenesin?

(A) Cough becomes more productive
(B) Cough stops altogether
(C) Fever diminishes
(D) Headache resolves
(E) Headache worsens

57 A 16-year-old boy with cystic fibrosis undergoes many types of treatments intended to loosen and thin the mucus obstructing his airways in order for him to expel it. He also takes an oral pancreatic enzyme because his pancreas is unable to secrete sufficient amounts because of mucus obstruction. Which of the following medications thins cystic fibrosis mucus by cleaving extracellular DNA?

(A) Acetylcysteine
(B) Bromhexine
(C) Dornase alfa
(D) Guaifenesin
(E) Ipratropium

58 A 17-year-old female with cystic fibrosis began taking a new medication to help loosen the mucus in her respiratory tract. The patient has not been adherent to her regimen of this drug, complaining that its smell makes her sick. Which is the most likely drug?

(A) Acetylcysteine
(B) Bromhexine
(C) Calfactant
(D) Dornase alfa
(E) Guaifenesin

59 A 33-year-old man with a history of HIV disease presents to the ambulatory care clinic complaining of right-sided flank pain. His current medications include indinavir. He has right CVA tenderness. Ultrasound of the abdomen reveals right-sided hydronephrosis. What is the most likely diagnosis?

(A) Hepatitis
(B) Gallstone pancreatitis
(C) Renal stone
(D) Small bowel obstruction
(E) Transverse colon colitis

60 A 35-year-old man with nonseminomatous germ cell tumor of the testis and bulky lymphadenopathy undergoes orchiectomy followed by multiagent chemotherapy with high-dose methotrexate. His serum creatinine rises from 1.10 mg/dL at baseline to 3.50 mg/dL after 4 weeks of therapy. What is the most likely explanation for this finding?

(A) Collecting duct extravasation
(B) Crystallization in the renal tubules
(C) Distal tubular cell necrosis
(D) Glomerular necrosis
(E) Proximal tubular cell necrosis

61 A 33-year-old man with advanced Crohn disease is treated with multiagent therapy including 6-mercaptopurine. On his most recent CT scan, there is evidence of disease progression to include the entire ileum and right colon. What is the most likely explanation for these findings?

(A) Ability to transform 6-MP to a nucleotide
(B) Decreased metabolism to other metabolites
(C) Decreased metabolism to thiouric acid
(D) Increased dephosphorylation
(E) Increased levels of HGPRT

62 A 57-year-old man who has chronic leukemia with brain metastasis has begun on high-dose intrathecal cytarabine. The treating physician must be aware of which of the following significant adverse effects?

(A) Myocardial infarction
(B) Paralysis
(C) Pulmonary embolism
(D) Renal cast formation
(E) Uremic pericarditis

63 A 37-year-old woman presents to the plastic surgery group for the second round of treatment to address her wrinkles. She complains that her right eyelid and forehead are “too droopy” and has a persistent headache since her first Botox treatment 5 days ago. What is the mechanism of action for this treatment?

(A) Binds α-receptors preventing activation
(B) Binds muscarinic receptors preventing activation
(C) Blocks uptake of choline into nerve terminals
(D) Prevents release of cholinergic vesicles
(E) Prevents storage of cholinergic vesicles

64 A 24-year-old Caucasian woman with dysplastic nevus syndrome presents to her annual checkup with a suspicious-looking mole. The physician decides to remove it. To prepare the site, she injects a lidocaine preparation. The surrounding tissue blanches. What is most likely present with the lidocaine that causes the blanching?

(A) Epinephrine
(B) Levothyroxine
(C) Nifedipine
(D) Nothing—lidocaine is thick and white itself and only appears to cause blanching
(E) Sodium bicarbonate

65 A 43-year-old man with a history of peptic ulcer disease has developed hypersensitivity to H_2 blockers. He now complains of worsening of his dyspepsia. Physical examination reveals mild tenderness on the midepigastric region. If misoprostol is prescribed to this patient, which of the following mechanisms of action would be most plausible for this agent?
(A) Enhance mucosal resistance
(B) Inhibition of gastrin secretion
(C) Inhibition of proton pump secretion
(D) Inhibition of somatostatin release
(E) Inhibition of uric acid secretion

66 A 39-year-old man with recurrent migraine headaches presents to his primary care physician for evaluation and treatment. Physical examination of the head and neck is unremarkable. Treatment with zolmitriptan has begun. This agent acts on which of the following receptors in the brain?
(A) Acetylcholine
(B) Choline
(C) Dopamine
(D) Epinephrine
(E) Serotonin

67 The parents of an 8-year-old boy complain of his inability to concentrate and focus and his impulsiveness. Following multiple visits and tests, he is given a diagnosis and prescribed a mixture of amphetamine salts. The parents are initially pleased with the results but soon remark that they find him excessively preoccupied with tasks and "zombielike." How can the physician best address this concern?
(A) Apologize for making a hasty and incorrect diagnosis
(B) Change to another drug of this class
(C) Decrease the dose
(D) Explain that this is an unfortunate but inevitable side effect
(E) Increase the dose

68 A 27-year-old woman complains of a 3-year history of depressed mood, loss of interest in her hobbies, and low energy levels following a job change and a move to a new city. Her physician prescribes fluoxetine to help improve her mood. After 2 weeks, she returns stating that she feels no better. What is the physician's best response?
(A) Add sertraline
(B) Do nothing
(C) Increase the dose
(D) Stop the drug
(E) Switch to another drug

69 An 83-year-old woman nursing home resident complains of trouble falling asleep at night. Her daughter also mentions that her mother's mood appears depressed, and the nursing home staff state that she is not eating well. Which of the following medications could best help this patient?
(A) Amitriptyline
(B) Buspirone
(C) Mirtazapine
(D) Olanzapine
(E) Venlafaxine

70 A 34-year-old construction worker injured his right leg while on the job. His medical history includes poorly controlled Type-2 diabetes mellitus. He now presents with cellulitis in his right leg, for which he is given empiric IV vancomycin. He also complains of nausea, for which he is given an antiemetic. Which of the following antiemetics is also an antihistamine?
(A) Droperidol
(B) Famotidine
(C) Loratadine
(D) Ondansetron
(E) Promethazine

71 A 24-year-old man complains of recurring episodes of bloody diarrhea and abdominal pain. A flexible sigmoidoscopy reveals pseudopolyps and erythematous, friable mucosa. One of the drugs given to this patient is diphenoxylate. How could diphenoxylate help this patient?
(A) Antimicrobial effects
(B) Blocks TNF-α signaling
(C) Inhibition of dihydrofolate reductase
(D) Inhibition of phospholipase A_2
(E) Slows peristalsis

72 A 33-year-old woman who is obese complains of postprandial, burning chest pain. Her physician prescribes pantoprazole. Pantoprazole may impair absorption of which of the following nutrients?
(A) Calcium
(B) Carbohydrates
(C) Fatty acids
(D) Vitamin A
(E) Vitamin D

73 A 64-year-old woman is hospitalized for COPD exacerbation. While in the hospital, she becomes constipated. She also takes metoprolol for hypertension and mirtazapine for depression. The physician gives her docusate. Which of the following adverse reactions is most likely to occur as a result of docusate administration in this patient?
(A) Cardiac arrhythmia
(B) Diarrhea
(C) Hypertension
(D) Rash
(E) Worsening depression

74 A 58-year-old male is hospitalized for COPD exacerbation. While in the hospital, he becomes constipated. He has a history of hyperlipidemia and gout. The physician gives him docusate. How does docusate work to relieve constipation?
(A) Binds water in the lumen
(B) Increases chloride secretion into the gut lumen
(C) Increases water absorption by the stool
(D) Irritation of the bowel mucosa to stimulate peristalsis
(E) Stimulation of the myenteric plexus

75 A 53-year-old postmenopausal woman presents with urinary urge incontinence. Medical history is significant for hypertension, which is controlled with losartan. She is not a surgical candidate so pharmacological therapy is chosen to treat her condition, and she begins treatment with solifenacin. Which of the following side effects is most likely to occur in this patient?
(A) Diarrhea
(B) Hypertension
(C) Photosensitivity
(D) Restless leg syndrome
(E) Xerostomia

76 A researcher is creating a novel medication to act at M_1 receptors. This agent will likely have which of the following augmentative effects on target organs?
(A) Cardiac muscle contractility
(B) Constipation
(C) Diarrhea
(D) Gastric acid secretion
(E) Stroke volume

77 A 34-year-old man with a sacral spinal cord injury has neurogenic bowel. He is on a bowel regimen that involves periodic bowel cleansing with soapsuds enemas. He is given a trial of bethanechol for this condition. Which of the following adverse events must his treating physician be aware of?
(A) Bronchodilation
(B) Diarrhea
(C) Dry mouth
(D) Dry skin
(E) Sigmoid colonic stasis

78 A 69-year-old man with a history of squamous cell carcinoma of the larynx underwent treatment with surgical resection and postoperative radiation therapy. He currently has significant xerostomia. Which of the following would be the best course of treatment for this patient?
(A) Bethanechol
(B) Carbachol
(C) Oral liquid intake
(D) Resection of the parotid gland
(E) Pilocarpine

79 A 78-year-old woman with a long history of chronic open-angle glaucoma has failed numerous treatments with oral and topical agents. She has begun on a treatment regimen with an ophthalmic solution of echothiophate. Which of the following effects must the treating physician be aware of?
(A) Cataracts
(B) Narrow-angle glaucoma
(C) Open-angle glaucoma
(D) Venous nicking of the retina
(E) Uremia

80 The use of atropine drops to the eye of a 37-year-old man who is a stockbroker would produce which of the following effects?
(A) Cycloplegia
(B) Decreased intraocular pressure
(C) Miosis
(D) Responsiveness to light

81 A 53-year-old man with a history of cataracts and retinal disease is going to undergo a 6- to 10-h procedure that will require mydriasis to complete the procedure. Which of the following ophthalmic agents would be most useful for this situation?

(A) Atropine
(B) Cyclopentolate
(C) Nicotine
(D) Tropicamide

82 A 38-year-old man with third-degree burns on 40% of his body undergoes a debridement procedure in the operating room. Succinylcholine is used at supratherapeutic dose. On postoperative day 1, the patient's serum potassium is 7.3 mEq/L. What is the most likely source of this problem?

(A) Iatrogenic overdose of intravenous fluids
(B) Medication reaction between H_2 blocker and burn eschar
(C) Potassium release from intracellular stores
(D) Succinylcholine overdose

83 A 75-year-old man with a 40-pack-year history of smoking and known chronic obstructive pulmonary disease complains of intermittent cough. Physical examination reveals wheezing, which is suggestive of bronchospasm. Which of the following is the most appropriate treatment for this patient?

(A) Ipratropium aerosol
(B) Mecamylamine
(C) Nicotine
(D) Oxygen
(E) Scopolamine

84 A 52-year-old woman complains of dizziness when she looks up or rapidly changes the position of her head. These dizzy spells are often accompanied by nausea and vomiting. She complains that these episodes severely limit her ability to work and function normally. Which of the following medications would best help control her symptoms?

(A) Amlodipine
(B) Meclizine
(C) Midodrine
(D) Mirtazapine
(E) Ondansetron

85 A researcher is developing a medication that selectively stimulates β_2-receptors without affecting any other receptors. As a result of such stimulation, which of the following effects is possible?

(A) Bronchoconstriction
(B) Glucagon release
(C) Renin release
(D) Uterine smooth muscle contraction
(E) Vasoconstriction

86 A 19-year-old man cuts his hand while slicing a bagel. He sustains a 4-cm laceration of the palmar aspect of his hand. The wound will be sutured with absorbable sutures. Prior to beginning the procedure, the wound is injected with lidocaine containing 1:100,000 parts epinephrine. The rationale behind the use of epinephrine is which of the following?

(A) Augment pain sensation
(B) Increase bleeding to improve toxin release from the wound
(C) Slow anesthetic metabolism from tissue
(D) Vasodilation at the side of administration

87 A 23-year-old man with erectile dysfunction refuses to see a physician for his problem. Instead, he purchases an over-the-counter product that contains yohimbine. He claims that he now has improved sexual function with improved quality of his erections. What is the most likely explanation for this finding?

(A) Cavernosal artery stimulation
(B) Cavernosal nerve stimulation
(C) Development of hypertension
(D) Development of priapism
(E) Improved sympathetic outflow to the periphery

88 A 45-year-old man who is obese complains of postprandial epigastric pain. The pain does not appear after every meal. He has noticed the pain especially after eating spicy foods. He is not currently taking any medications. You suspect gastroesophageal reflux disease (GERD) and want to try a drug that will lower the amount of acid in his stomach. Which of the following drugs chemically elevates the pH?

(A) Aluminum hydroxide
(B) Fexofenadine
(C) Misoprostol
(D) Omeprazole
(E) Ranitidine

89 A group of teenage boys present to the emergency department after ingesting a plant they heard would make them high. One member of the group still had some plant parts in his pocket, which you use to identify deadly nightshade. They present with xerostomia, dry eyes, flushed skin, blurry vision, and tachycardia. Which substance is likely causing their symptoms?

(A) Atropine
(B) Bethanechol
(C) Physostigmine
(D) Strychnine
(E) Tyramine

90 A 9-year-old boy with chronic otitis media infections is scheduled to undergo bilateral ear tube placement under inhalational anesthesia. Which of the following will occur as a result of administration of this agent?

(A) Bronchoconstriction
(B) Decrease in cerebrovascular resistance
(C) Decrease in brain perfusion
(D) Decrease in pulmonary vascular resistance
(E) Pulmonary vasodilation

91 A 19-year-old male presents to the emergency room with a broken ankle after a fall. He is given hydrocodone for the pain and, soon after, his stomach becomes upset. He has vomited once. The patient is given ondansetron to treat his nausea. What is the mechanism of action of ondansetron?

(A) 5-HT_3 antagonist
(B) D_2-receptor antagonist
(C) H_2-receptor inhibitor
(D) Serotonin-norepinephrine reuptake inhibitor
(E) Substance P antagonist

92 A 37-year-old female with mild arthritis presents to the clinic for follow-up. She states that she is doing much better because of doubling her dose of ibuprofen. Some days, she even triples her dose throughout the day. The physician warns the patient about peptic ulcers and bleeding from taking too much ibuprofen. She is offered alternatives, but the patient refuses because the ibuprofen works so well. What is the most appropriate therapy for this patient to prevent peptic ulcers?

(A) Bismuth
(B) Famotidine
(C) Lansoprazole
(D) Misoprostol
(E) Pirenzepine

93 A 48-year-old male presents to the emergency department with chest pain for the past 2 days. The pain is nonradiating and burning in nature. An ECG is normal, and serial troponins are negative. The physician makes the diagnosis of GERD. What is the most potent therapy for the prevention of GERD?

(A) Bismuth
(B) Famotidine
(C) Misoprostol
(D) Omeprazole
(E) Pirenzepine

94 A 21-year-old man presents to his primary care physician with 6 weeks of painful, bloody stools. Flexible sigmoidoscopy reveals erythema and friability with pseudopolyps. Which drug used for ulcerative colitis is made of two identical smaller molecules linked together with an azo bond?

(A) Azathioprine
(B) Cyclosporine
(C) Sulfasalazine
(D) Mesalamine
(E) Olsalazine

95 A 26-year-old G2P1001 woman at 33 weeks gestation presents to the emergency department with pain and swelling in her right calf. On physical examination, Homans sign is positive. A duplex of the right calf confirms the presence of a deep vein thrombosis (DVT). What is the most appropriate treatment for the rest of her pregnancy?

(A) Abciximab
(B) Aspirin
(C) Heparin
(D) Streptokinase
(E) Warfarin

96 A 33-year-old pregnant woman begins taking a new drug, Drug X, for morning sickness. Drug X has been found to have adverse fetal effects in animal models, but no adequate human studies have been done. Under which FDA pregnancy category would Drug X fall?

(A) Category A
(B) Category B
(C) Category C
(D) Category D
(E) Category X

97 A 37-year-old man with a history of inguinal hernia undergoes elective surgical repair. The anesthesiologist is concerned about potential adverse effects of the inhalational agent chosen—halothane. The initial symptom of halothane's adverse reaction is which of the following?

(A) Anorexia
(B) Fever
(C) Hepatitis
(D) Nausea
(E) Vomiting

98 Isoflurane is used as the induction agent in a 9-year-old girl who is undergoing tonsillectomy and adenoidectomy. She has a history of obstructive sleep apnea and has developmental delay. Which of the following characteristics of this agent is correct?
(A) Can induce cardiac arrhythmia
(B) Causes peripheral vasoconstriction
(C) Fruity smelling gaseous agent
(D) Produces dose-dependent hypotension
(E) Undergoes significant metabolism

99 A 58-year-old man with a long history of depression is evaluated for treatment by his primary care physician. The physician begins treatment with sertraline. The patient is concerned about the possibility of sexual dysfunction. Which of the following changes is possible?
(A) Altered penile sensation
(B) Delayed ejaculation
(C) Normal libido
(D) Normal orgasm
(E) Rust-colored ejaculate

100 A 23-year-old woman presents to the emergency department with a headache. Her headaches began on the right frontal side and radiated to the back of the right side of her head. She has vomited twice. She has photophobia and phonophobia. She usually takes sumatriptan as her headache begins, but she has none left. What is the mechanism of action of sumatriptan?
(A) 5-HT_{1A} agonist
(B) 5-HT_{1A} antagonist
(C) 5-$HT_{1B/1D}$ agonist
(D) 5-HT_{1B} antagonist
(E) 5-HT_3 agonist

101 A 5-year-old boy is brought to the clinic by his parents who say that he often has trouble catching his breath when he has been playing hard outside. He is allergic to peanuts. At the moment, he is breathing fine. Which of the following drugs would dilate his bronchioles in an acute asthma attack?
(A) Albuterol
(B) Methacholine
(C) Neostigmine
(D) Nicotine
(E) Pilocarpine

102 A 45-year-old man with a history of depression presents to the emergency department with priapism. He has had an erection for the past 2 h, and it is extremely painful. He is given pseudoephedrine and the erection subsides. What medication is the most likely cause of his priapism?
(A) Bupropion
(B) Fluoxetine
(C) Maprotiline
(D) Trazodone
(E) Venlafaxine

103 A 27-year-old woman complains of right flank pain and hematuria. She has passed calcium oxalate stones in the past and likely has another stone. After treating her for her stone, which of the following diuretics should she avoid to prevent future calcium oxalate stones?
(A) Amiloride
(B) Furosemide
(C) Hydrochlorothiazide
(D) Mannitol
(E) Spironolactone

104 A 65-year-old man with long-standing schizophrenia has been taking an antipsychotic agent since his diagnosis of schizophrenia at age 19 years. He has been in and out of psychiatric hospitals for most of his adult life. Long-term adverse effects of these agents may include which of the following?
(A) Hypertension
(B) Myocardial infarction
(C) Poikilothermia
(D) Pulmonary edema
(E) Pulmonary embolism

105 A 39-year-old man with chronic back pain from a spinal cord injury has a pain medication pump placed in his body. Unfortunately, meperidine was placed in the pump instead of the usual medication—morphine. Which of the following effects is possible as a result of this mistake?
(A) Cough
(B) Diarrhea
(C) Neurotoxicity
(D) Pain relief
(E) Urinary retention

106 A 44-year-old woman with a history of refractory seizure disorder has been treated with numerous antiepileptic agents, which have failed to control her seizures. She has begun on therapy with rufinamide. This agent is contraindicated in which of the following situations?

(A) Egg allergy
(B) Familial short QT syndrome
(C) Milk allergy
(D) Women with birth control ring
(E) Women with tubal ligation

107 A 23-year-old woman with a history of seizure disorder is planning to become pregnant. She realizes that being on this medication during pregnancy can have fetal effects of mental retardation. Which of the following agents would likely produce a newborn with the lowest intelligence quotient (IQ)?

(A) Carbamezapine
(B) Lamotrigine
(C) Phenytoin
(D) Valproic acid

108 A 48-year-old woman with epilepsy refractory to medical therapy is hospitalized for deep brain stimulation. This new modality uses a pacemaker-like device to stimulate which of the following structures?

(A) Cerebrum
(B) Cerebellum
(C) Hypothalamus
(D) Muscles of the lower extremities
(E) Thalamus

109 A 23-year-old woman with lifelong epilepsy controlled with medication has just found out that she is pregnant. She has seizures once a month but seem to be controlled at present. Which of the following statements about epilepsy in pregnancy is true?

(A) Barbiturates should be considered
(B) Divalproex is considered a drug of choice
(C) Maintenance medication doses should be increased
(D) She should be taking high doses of folic acid
(E) She will likely have no change in seizure activity during pregnancy

110 A 54-year-old woman with diabetes presents to the clinic for follow-up. On her last two visits, her blood pressure was elevated. She measured her blood pressure at home daily and it was elevated. The physician decides to start her on enalapril. She returns in 1 week with a persistent cough. What causes the cough associated with enalapril?

(A) Decrease in aldosterone
(B) Decrease in angiotensin II
(C) Increase in angiotensin I
(D) Increase in bradykinins
(E) Increase in renin

111 A 17-year-old man is brought to the emergency department with severe right lower quadrant pain that he first felt around his umbilicus. His white blood cell count is 12,000/μL of blood. He is taken to the OR for emergent appendectomy. About an hour into the surgery, his body temperature spikes and CO_2 production rises uncontrollably. What was done differently in this patient's procedure to lead to this outcome?

(A) Anesthesia used is an outdated drug
(B) He is experiencing an allergic reaction to an anesthetic
(C) Nothing was done differently—this outcome is caused by a genetic defect
(D) Surgery was excessively prolonged and his appendix ruptured
(E) This is a reaction between the anesthetic and one of his prescriptions from home

112 A 74-year-old man with bladder cancer and refractory depression is tried on a new agent to help his depression. Tranylcypromine is begun by his primary care physician. Which of the following adverse reactions may be expected in this patient?

(A) Anxiety
(B) Hepatitis
(C) Normalization of blood glucose levels
(D) Salivation
(E) Tachypnea

113 A 21-year-old woman presents to the emergency department (ED) after she intentionally took 20 alprazolam 15 min ago in a suicide attempt. She has never been on benzodiazepines before in the past. The ED physician wants to reverse the effects of the alprazolam immediately. What is the most appropriate treatment?

(A) Ammonium chloride
(B) Flumazenil
(C) N-acetylcysteine
(D) Naloxone
(E) Sodium bicarbonate

114 A 34-year-old man who recently had a renal transplant presents to clinic for follow-up. He has been feeling well and has no specific complaints. His laboratory test results look normal other than an elevated blood glucose of 197 mg/dL. The physician believes the elevated blood glucose may be caused by a medication. What is the most likely medication to cause hyperglycemia?

(A) Azathioprine
(B) Cyclosporine
(C) Muromonab
(D) Sirolimus
(E) Tacrolimus

115 A 34-year-old woman with long-standing hypertension is taking an ACE inhibitor. She is now newly married. Which of the following potential adverse effects is most applicable to her at this time?

(A) Angioedema
(B) Hyperkalemia
(C) Persistent cough
(D) Renal insufficiency
(E) Toxicity to fetus

116 Which of the following patient presentations would best benefit from therapy with digoxin?

(A) A 52-year-old man with right-sided heart failure
(B) A 55-year-old man with diastolic heart failure
(C) A 65-year-old man with heart failure and atrial fibrillation
(D) A 72-year-old man with mild dyspnea on exertion because of pulmonary edema
(E) A 77-year-old man with Alzheimer dementia and minimal angina

117 A 62-year-old man presents to his primary care physician for follow-up. He has a history of an atrial arrhythmia. He takes multiple medications but does not know the names of them. He now complains of headache, dizziness, and tinnitus. Which one of the following antiarrhythmic drugs is the most likely cause?

(A) Amiodarone
(B) Procainamide
(C) Propranolol
(D) Quinidine
(E) Verapamil

118 A 31-year-old woman presents to the clinic for follow-up of her abdominal pain. The pain has been occurring for a couple of years but has worsened recently. She is often constipated and then will have periods of diarrhea. Her pain does usually improve after a bowel movement. After multiple negative tests, the diagnosis of constipation-predominant irritable bowel syndrome is made. Which of the following is an appropriate treatment for this patient?

(A) Infliximab
(B) Metoclopramide
(C) Ondansetron
(D) Sulfasalazine
(E) Tegaserod

119 A 58-year-old man with a history of occasional GERD presents to the clinic with diarrhea for the past 3 months. He has not been sick and feeling quite well otherwise. Further history uncovers that 3 months ago, he switched the type of antacid he uses for reflux. He stopped the antacid and calls back 1 month later, saying he has not had diarrhea since then. Which of the following antacids was most likely causing the patient's diarrhea?

(A) Aluminum hydroxide
(B) Bismuth
(C) Calcium carbonate
(D) Magnesium hydroxide
(E) Sodium bicarbonate

120 A 58-year-old man who is a smoker with chronic obstructive pulmonary disease (COPD) presents to the emergency department (ED) with shortness of breath and a productive cough. This is the fourth time this year he has come to the ED because of COPD exacerbation. After this hospital stay, his primary care physician prescribes roflumilast in hopes of decreasing his ED visits for COPD exacerbation. What is roflumilast's mechanism of action?

(A) Blocks arachidonic acid production
(B) Bronchodilation
(C) Inhibition of leukocyte chemotaxis by interfering with microtubules
(D) PDE4 inhibitor
(E) Thins and loosens mucus

121 A newlywed 23-year-old woman presents to the urgent care center with 24 h of burning and pain with urination. She also feels a constant need to urinate but produces only small amounts of urine at a time. She is given trimethoprim–sulfamethoxazole to treat her urinary tract infection. Three days into her regimen, she develops fever and a sore throat. Physical exam reveals ulcerations in her throat. Which of the following is a potential complication if her treatment is continued?

(A) Anaphylaxis
(B) Lactic acidosis
(C) Rhabdomyolysis
(D) She will recover more rapidly with continued antibiotics because these are signs of infection
(E) Toxic epidermal necrolysis

122 A 38-year-old businessman is on a trip to Mexico when he develops diarrhea. He has to give a presentation in a few hours and needs rapid relief. He takes an antidiarrheal preparation containing diphenoxylate. Which of the following describes diphenoxyate's mechanism of action?

(A) Anticholinergic
(B) Broad-spectrum antibiotic
(C) Gram-negative antibiotic
(D) Inhibitor of myenteric plexus activity
(E) Sympathetic nervous system stimulant

123 A 26-year-old man presents to an urgent care clinic with a dry cough for the past week. The cough was associated with a fever and chills for 2 days, but he has since been afebrile. He has no other symptoms. What opioid is most appropriate to treat this patients' cough?

(A) Butorphanol
(B) Dextromethorphan
(C) Diphenoxylate
(D) Guaifenesin
(E) Loperamide

124 A 72-year-old woman presents to her primary care physician with vision loss over the past year. She has noticed painless loss of her peripheral vision. Her peripheral vision has become darker. She is diagnosed with open-angle glaucoma and started on medication. She returns in 1 month and says her vision has improved, but now her blue eyes turned brown. What was the most likely medication given to treat her glaucoma?

(A) Acetazolamide
(B) Epinephrine
(C) Latanoprost
(D) Pilocarpine
(E) Physostigmine

125 A 34-year-old man with a seizure disorder presents to the emergency department with severe left-sided flank pain. The pain began suddenly this morning and has not improved. His urinalysis shows microscopic hematuria, and a KUB confirms a kidney stone. Which pain medication should be avoided in this patient?

(A) Acetaminophen
(B) Butorphanol
(C) Fentanyl
(D) Morphine
(E) Tramadol

126 A 37-year-old man complains of chest pain after meals. He says this pain has gone on for a few months, and he gets only minimal relief from antacid tablets. The physician prescribes a drug that will decrease the amount of acid secreted by blocking a histamine receptor. Which of the following drugs works by this mechanism?

(A) Atropine
(B) Cimetidine
(C) Misoprostol
(D) Octreotide
(E) Omeprazole

127 An 8-year-old boy is brought to the pediatrician because of his continued bedwetting despite many treatment attempts. He has tried a bed alarm and desmopressin but still wets the bed at least twice a week for the past 2 months. He has been healthy otherwise and does not have urinary accidents other than at night. Which of the following antidepressants is the most appropriate treatment?

(A) Citalopram
(B) Imipramine
(C) Mirtazapine
(D) Trazodone
(E) Venlafaxine

128 A 7-year-old boy is brought to the ambulatory care clinic by his mother because of acting out in class and at home. In class, he often talks out of turn and does not stay focused on tasks. At home, his mother cannot get him to do his chores, and he never sits still. What is the most appropriate treatment for this patient?

(A) Clomipramine
(B) Fluoxetine
(C) Lithium
(D) Methylphenidate
(E) Venlafaxine

129 A 68-year-old man with congestive heart failure presents to the emergency department with shortness of breath. He has +2 pitting edema in his extremities as well. A chest X-ray confirms the presence of pulmonary edema. The patient is given ethacrynic acid to diurese the excess fluid. Where in the nephron does ethacrynic acid act?

(A) Collecting tubule
(B) Descending loop of Henle
(C) Distal convoluted tubule
(D) Proximal convoluted tubule
(E) Thick ascending loop of Henle

130 A 39-year-old woman with chronic migraine headaches manages her condition with ibuprofen 200 mg. Most days, she does well with 200 to 400 mg. Adverse reactions to this therapy include which of the following?

(A) Gastrointestinal upset
(B) Hives
(C) Seizure disorder
(D) Teratogenicity
(E) Throat tightness

131 A 48-year-old woman with a history of chronic migraine headaches has failed therapy with conservative measures and ibuprofen. Her primary care physician begins treatment with ergotamine. Important adverse reactions to be aware of include which of the following?

(A) Cold extremities
(B) Diarrhea
(C) Improved muscle strength
(D) Skin dryness
(E) Tachycardia

132 A 54-year-old woman with a history of migraine headaches has begun on therapy with Topamax as prophylaxis. She is poorly communicative and a poor historian. Which of the following would be important coexisting conditions to know about?

(A) Depression
(B) Kidney stones
(C) Nearsightedness
(D) Pulmonary deficits
(E) Tinnitus

133 An 11-year-old boy with tonsillar hypertrophy is going to undergo elective tonsillectomy. He will be intubated for the procedure. A 2% aqueous lidocaine jelly is administered topically. Which of the following adverse reactions is possible?

(A) Bradycardia
(B) Erythema
(C) Hypertension
(D) Temperature change
(E) Tinnitus

134 A 22-year-old woman recently began medical treatment for a seizure disorder. She presents with dysuria; and a urine dipstick shows microhematuria but no leukocytes and no nitrites. A KUB X-ray shows calcifications in the renal pelvis, although she has neither personal nor family history of kidney stones. Which seizure medicine is she likely taking?

(A) Ethosuximide
(B) Phenobarbital
(C) Phenytoin
(D) Topiramate
(E) Valproic acid

135 A 54-year-old man with hypertension, alcoholic cirrhosis, and HIV disease is hospitalized for abdominal pain, fatigue, and weakness. His ascites and edema are markedly worse. Physical examination reveals a palpable abdominal fluid wave. Which of the following treatments may be beneficial for this patient?

(A) Acetazolamide
(B) Chlorthalidone
(C) Furosemide
(D) Hydrochlorothiazide
(E) Spironolactone

136 A 59-year-old man with a history of recurrent bilateral kidney stones is placed on a medication to decrease calcium excretion. Unfortunately, 3 months after beginning this medication, he develops gout in his right great toe. The most likely explanation of these findings relates to which of the following medications?

(A) Furosemide
(B) Hydrochlorothiazide
(C) Spironolactone
(D) Triamterene
(E) This is not a medication effect

137 A 24-year-old G1P1 woman presents to the emergency department days after giving birth to her first child. She lost a large amount of blood during birth. Her hemoglobin level is 12.5 g/dL (normal is 12.1 to 15.1 g/dL). Her gynecologist prescribes ferrous sulfate to help raise her hemoglobin levels. Which of the following is a common side effect of this medication?

(A) Constipation
(B) Diarrhea
(C) Hypercoagulability
(D) Hypotension
(E) Seizures

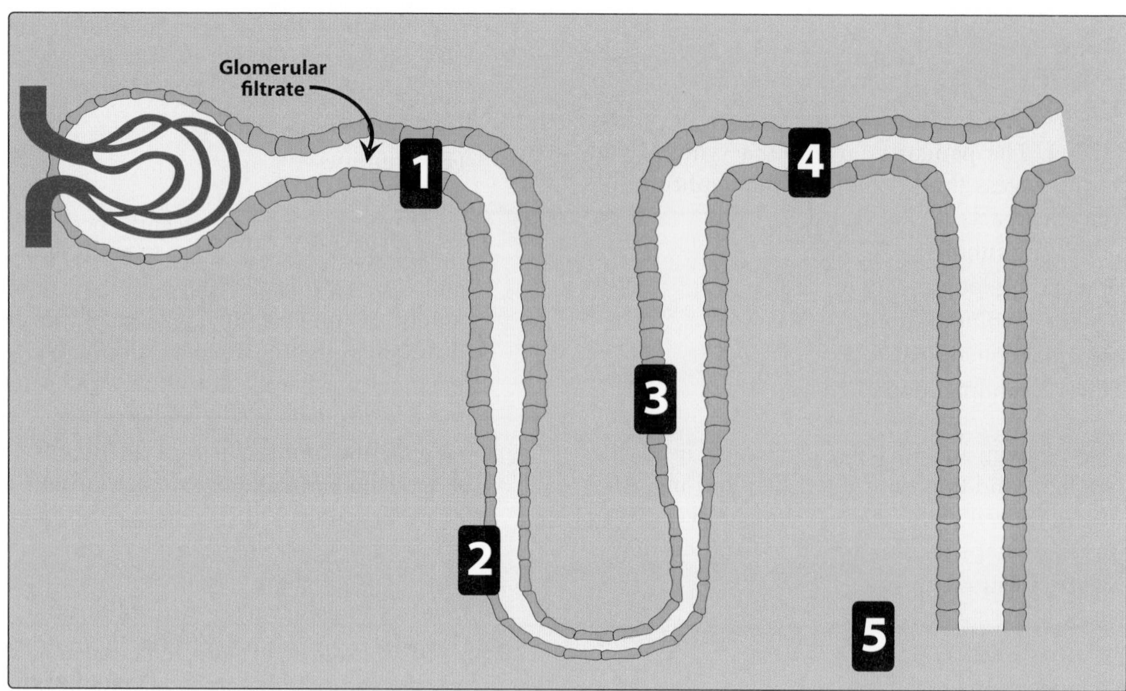

138 A 44-year-old man with multiple medical problems is placed on a carbonic anhydrase inhibitor which inhibits bicarbonate reabsorption and acts as a weak diuretic. This agent works at which of the following areas in the above diagram?

(A) Location 1
(B) Location 2
(C) Location 3
(D) Location 4
(E) Location 5

139 A 46-year-old woman is undergoing a laparoscopic supracervical hysterectomy for menometrorrhagia secondary to extensive leiomyomas. She is anesthetized with general anesthetic. The surgeon begins once she has lost her eyelash reflex and her breathing pattern became regular. Under which stage of anesthesia does this fall?

(A) Stage I
(B) Stage II
(C) Stage III
(D) Stage IV
(E) Stage V

140 A 34-year-old man presents to the emergency department with fever and right upper quadrant pain for the past 8 days since returning from Thailand. His fever is 102.4°F and his pain is a 9/10 in the Numeric Pain Rating Scale, sharp, constant ache. He also has associated jaundice of his hands and face. While in Thailand, he enjoyed the local cuisine including many meals of raw sushi. The physician wants to treat the patient right away to prevent the development of cholangiocarcinoma. What is the most appropriate treatment for this patient?

(A) Diethylcarbamazine
(B) Ivermectin
(C) Praziquantel
(D) Pyrantel pamoate
(E) Sodium stibogluconate

141 A 32-year-old man who traveled to Brazil 1 week ago presents to the emergency department with swelling of his right eye. He has decreased vision in his right eye because of the swelling. His left eye is unaffected. A peripheral blood smear shows the presence of a parasite. The patient does remember being warned of reduviid bugs and that their bites are painless. What is the most appropriate treatment for this patient?

(A) Chloroquine
(B) Melarsoprol
(C) Nifurtimox
(D) Sodium stibogluconate
(E) Suramin

142 A 42-year-old woman presents to the emergency department with fevers and headaches for the past 3 days. The fevers are off and on but are usually at least 102.5°F. Her headaches usually occur at the same time as the fevers. Splenomegaly is noted on examination. Peripheral blood smear confirms the presence of *Plasmodium vivax*. What is the most appropriate treatment for the dormant form of the parasite in the liver?

(A) Chloroquine
(B) Clindamycin
(C) Metronidazole
(D) Primaquine
(E) Sodium stibogluconate

143 A 33-year-old woman patient needs to be anesthetized before a dilation and curettage for abnormal uterine bleeding. Her anesthesia is induced initially with an inhaled, nonflammable anesthetic that contains no halogenated carbons. Of the following, which agent best fits this description?

(A) Enflurane
(B) Diethyl ether
(C) Halothane
(D) Nitrous oxide
(E) Propofol

144 An 18-year-old man is brought to the emergency department by a friend after smoking crack cocaine because he was "acting funny." His temperature is 38°C (100.4°F), pulse is 110 beats/minute, and he appears agitated. What is the action of cocaine on sympathetic nerves?

(A) Increase norepinephrine synthesis
(B) Inhibition of catechol-*O*-methyltransferase (COMT)
(C) Inhibition of monoamine oxidase (MAO)
(D) Inhibition of norepinephrine reuptake
(E) Stimulation of nicotinic receptors in postganglionic autonomic neurons

145 The potency of inhaled anesthetics is defined as the minimum alveolar concentration. Five anesthetic gases are infused into 2-kg rats denoted as gas A through gas E with the MACs noted. Which of the following gases would likely be nitrous oxide?

(A) Gas A MAC 0.75%
(B) Gas B MAC 1.2%
(C) Gas C MAC 2%
(D) Gas D MAC 6%
(E) Gas E MAC 105%

146 The replacement of the normal lung gases with the inspired anesthetic mixture defines which of the following terms?

(A) Anesthetic uptake
(B) Alveolar wash-in
(C) Minimum alveolar concentration
(D) Solubility

147 A 44-year-old man with depression is currently being managed with paroxetine. He presents to his primary care physician complaining of loss of libido, delayed ejaculation, and occasional inability to ejaculate. Which of the following is the best course of action for this patient?

(A) Continue medication at current dose
(B) Dose frequency of medication at every other day
(C) Referral for outpatient psychotherapy
(D) Referral for outpatient sexual therapy
(E) Stop paroxetine and begin bupropion

148 A 27-year-old man was prescribed with an antidepressant for his insomnia. He now presents to the emergency department with priapism of 3 h duration. Which antidepressant was he likely taking?

(A) Bupropion
(B) Duloxetine
(C) Imipramine
(D) Sertraline
(E) Trazodone

149 A 73-year-old man presents to the primary care clinic with increasing shortness of breath. He has had shortness of breath for many years, but it has been progressively worsening. It is associated with peripheral edema and dry cough. A transthoracic echocardiogram shows pulmonary hypertension. What is the most appropriate treatment for this patient?

(A) Albuterol
(B) Bosentan
(C) Guaifenesin
(D) *N*-acetylcysteine
(E) Theophylline

ANSWERS

1 **The answer is A: Bethanechol.** Bethanechol is used to stimulate the atonic bladder, particularly in postpartum urinary retention as well as in nonobstructive urinary retention. This agent can also be used to treat neurogenic atony and megacolon. (B) Carbachol is an anticholinergic agent with muscarinic and nicotinic properties. (C) Physostigmine is used to treat intestinal atony. It is a second-line agent to treat bladder atony. (D) Pilocarpine is an anticholinergic agent used in ophthalmology. (E) Tacrine is an anticholinergic agent that may have promise in the treatment of Alzheimer disease.

2 **The answer is E: Ranitidine.** Multiple factors contribute to acid secretion by parietal cells in gastric mucosa. Gastrin from G cells, histamine from enterochromaffin-like (ECL) cells (acting on H_2 receptors), and acetylcholine from parasympathetic neurons all act directly on parietal cells to induce acid secretion. Prostaglandins from surface mucous cells and somatostatin from D cells directly inhibit acid secretion. Ranitidine is an H_2-receptor antagonist, meaning it blocks the proacid effect of endogenous histamine. (A) Aluminum hydroxide does not bind a receptor. It is a base that decreases acid by a simple chemical reaction: $H^+ + OH^- \rightarrow H_2O$. (B) Fexofenadine is a second-generation H_1 antagonist. It would not be expected to significantly bind H_2 receptors. (C) Misoprostol is a prostaglandin agonist, not antagonist. It decreases acid by mimicking the inhibitory effect of endogenous prostaglandins. (D) Omeprazole does not bind a receptor. It decreases acid secretion by blocking the proton pump on the luminal surface of parietal cells.

3 **The answer is C: Hair growth of eyelashes.** Latanoprost is a prostaglandin-like topical medication used to treat glaucoma. This agent has few important side effects to be aware of including red eye and excessive hair growth of eyelashes. Its mechanism of action involves an increase in aqueous humor outflow. (A) Increased iris pigmentation can be seen with this agent. (B) Diarrhea can be seen with the carbonic anhydrase inhibitors. (D) Nausea can be seen with the carbonic anhydrase inhibitors. (E) Transient myopia can be seen with the carbonic anhydrase inhibitors.

4 **The answer is B: Give 5-FU by bolus rather than continuous infusion.** Palmar–plantar erythrodysesthesia, or hand–foot syndrome, is a common reaction with many chemotherapy drugs such as 5-FU. The exact mechanism is unclear, but excessive friction (as with walking and working with hands) and high temperatures seem to make it worse. Hand–foot syndrome is more commonly associated with continuous infusion of 5-FU than with bolus administration, so giving the drug by bolus helps to avoid it. (A) Ondansetron and 5-FU are not known to interactions adversely. (C) Giving 5-FU by continuous infusion increases the likelihood that the patient will develop hand–foot syndrome. (D) Leucovorin, or folinic acid, can perform the same role as folic acid in DNA synthesis. Leucovorin is used to decrease toxicity of methotrexate, which inhibits folic acid recycling. Leucovorin is not known to protect against hand–foot syndrome caused by 5-FU. (E) Hand–foot syndrome is a common side effect of 5-FU administration, with some reports describing 50% of treated patients being affected. The likelihood of developing hand–foot syndrome can be lessened by giving 5-FU as a bolus rather than continuous infusion.

5 **The answer is D: Distal convoluted tubule.** Potassium-sparing diuretics such as triamterene or amiloride are commonly used in combination with more potent potassium-wasting diuretics (e.g., loop diuretics) to offset their effects on serum potassium. Potassium is lost in the urine when high amounts of sodium pass through the distal convoluted tubule (as is the case with potassium-wasting diuretics) because of a sodium-potassium exchange pump on the distal tubule cells. Triamterene and amiloride inhibit this pump, leaving sodium in the urine and potassium in the blood. (A) Loop diuretics such as furosemide work by inhibiting the $Na^+/K^+/Cl^{-2}$ transporter on the ascending limb of the loop of Henle. (B) Antidiuretic hormone (ADH) works on the collecting tubule by causing preformed aquaporins to be inserted on the apical membrane of the tubular cells, allowing water to leave the urine back into the blood. (C) There is currently no diuretic in use that works on the descending limb of the loop of Henle. (E) Carbonic anhydrase inhibitors work in the proximal tubule.

6 **The answer is B: Liver.** Ciprofloxacin is eliminated primarily by renal excretion. However, this drug is also metabolized through the biliary system of the liver and through the intestine. These alternative pathways of drug elimination compensate for the reduced renal excretion. (A) Ciprofloxacin is not excreted via the breath. (C) Ciprofloxacin is not excreted via the salivary gland. (D) Ciprofloxacin is not excreted via the skin. (E) Ciprofloxacin is not excreted via the spleen.

7 **The answer is E: Thoracic wall muscle.** Brain, heart, liver, kidney, and endocrine glands—these highly perfused tissues rapidly attain a steady state with the partial pressure of anesthetic in the blood. Skeletal muscles are poorly perfused during anesthesia. This, and the fact that they have a large volume, prolongs the time required to achieve steady state. Thus, thoracic wall muscle will not pick up very much halothane carbon-labeled radiotracer. (A) Brain is highly perfused and will attain good levels of halothane.

(B) Heart is also highly perfused and will attain good levels of halothane. (C) Liver is well perfused and will attain good levels of halothane. (D) Pancreas and other endocrine glands are well perfused and will attain good levels of halothane.

8 **The answer is A: Coughing.** Isoflurane does not induce cardiac arrhythmias and does not sensitize the heart to the action of catecholamines. However, like the other halogenated gases, it produces dose-dependent hypotension because of peripheral vasodilation. It has a pungent odor and stimulates respiratory reflexes (e.g., breath-holding, salivation, coughing, and laryngospasm) and is, therefore, not used for inhalation induction. (B) Isoflurane induces salivation. (C) Isoflurane induces dose-dependent hypotension. (D) Isoflurane induces laryngeal spasm. (E) Isoflurane stimulates respiratory reflexes.

9 **The answer is C: A 62-year-old man with a history of four-vessel coronary artery bypass.** The patient with a history of cardiac disease is at greatest risk of anesthetic agents entering the cerebral blood circulation. In circumstances in which CO is reduced (e.g., in patients in shock, the elderly, cardiac disease, etc.), the body compensates by diverting an increased proportion of the CO to the cerebral circulation to preserve cerebral blood flow. A greater proportion of any given drug will enter the cerebral circulation under these circumstances. As a result, the dose of induction drug must be reduced. (A) This patient is not at increased risk of anesthetic agent entering the brain. (B) Hypotension would put the patient at risk of anesthetic agent entering the brain. (D) In general, elderly patients are at increased risk of the anesthetic agent entering the brain. However, this patient is a healthy marathon runner and is likely not at increased risk.

10 **The answer is E: Use allowed in moderate renal failure.** Following an IV bolus, there is rapid equilibration between the plasma and the highly perfused tissue of the brain, as described earlier. Plasma levels decline rapidly as a result of redistribution, followed by a more prolonged period of hepatic metabolism and renal clearance. The initial redistribution half-life is between 2 and 4 min. The pharmacokinetics of propofol are not altered by moderate hepatic or renal failure. (A) This agent is administered intravenously. (B) The half-life is between 2 and 4 min. (C) There is rapid equilibration to the brain because of perfusion. (D) Plasma levels of propofol are maintained for several minutes.

11 **The answer is B: Fluoxetine.** Fluoxetine is the best choice to treat both depression and OCD. Antidepressants should be used cautiously in children and teenagers because about 1 out of 50 children report suicidal ideation as a result of SSRI treatment. Pediatric patients should be observed for worsening depression and suicidal thinking whenever any antidepressant is started or its dose is increased or decreased. Fluoxetine, sertraline, and fluvoxamine are U.S. Food and Drug Administration (FDA)–approved for use in children to treat obsessive-compulsive disorder, and fluoxetine is approved to treat childhood depression. (A) Bupropion would only treat depression in this patient. (C) Fluvoxamine would only treat obsessive-compulsive disorder in this patient. (D) Mirtazapine would only treat depression in this patient. (E) Sertraline would only treat obsessive-compulsive disorder in this patient.

12 **The answer is C: Hallucinations typically improve with therapy.** Hallucinations are positive symptoms of schizophrenia and improve with therapy. The antipsychotics are considered to be the only efficacious treatment for schizophrenia. Not all patients respond, and complete normalization of behavior is seldom achieved. The first-generation antipsychotics are most effective in treating positive symptoms of schizophrenia (delusions, hallucinations, thought processing, and agitation). The newer agents with 5-HT_{2A} receptor–blocking activity may be effective in many patients who are resistant to the traditional agents, especially in treating the negative symptoms of schizophrenia (social withdrawal, blunted emotions, ambivalence, and reduced ability to relate to people). (A) Complete normalization of behavior does not always occur. (B) Delusions typically improve with therapy. (D) Thought processing typically improves with therapy. (E) Withdrawal from social situations is a negative symptom of schizophrenia and does not usually improve with first-line therapy.

13 **The answer is A: Chlorpromazine.** The antipsychotic drugs can be used as tranquilizers to manage agitated and disruptive behavior secondary to other disorders. Antipsychotics are used in combination with narcotic analgesics for treatment of chronic pain with severe anxiety. Chlorpromazine is used to treat intractable hiccups. (B) Pimozide is primarily indicated for treatment of the motor and phonic tics of Tourette disorder. (C) Although promethazine is not an effective antipsychotic drug, this agent is used in treating pruritus because of its antihistaminic properties. (D) Tetracycline is an antibiotic and is not used to treat hiccups. (E) Thioridazine would be effective in the treatment of schizophrenia.

14 **The answer is D: Seizures.** Tramadol is a centrally acting analgesic that binds to the μ-opioid receptor. Toxicity through drug–drug interactions with medications, such as selective serotonin reuptake inhibitors

and tricyclic antidepressants, or in overdose, leads to CNS excitation and seizures. Tramadol should also be avoided in patients taking MAOIs. (A) This patient is not at risk for an inflammatory process such as encephalitis. (B) This patient is not at risk for an inflammatory process such as meningitis. (C) This combination of medication is not likely to produce extrapyramidal effects. (E) Development of thromboembolism is unlikely given this combination of medications.

15 **The answer is C: Inhibits 5-α-reductase.** Benign prostatic hyperplasia (BPH) is an enlargement of the prostate gland that can impinge on the urethra as it travels through the prostate. This impingement leads to the symptoms of BPH—decreased force of stream, hesitancy, urinary retention, and nocturia—by slowing or blocking the flow of urine through the prostate. The prostate enlarges under the influence of dihydrotestosterone (DHT). Finasteride improves BPH symptoms and reduces the volume of the prostate by inhibiting 5-α-reductase's ability to convert testosterone to DHT. (A) Prazosin is used to treat BPH because, by blocking α_1-receptors, they lead to relaxation of prostatic smooth muscle, making it easier for urine to flow through the prostate. (B) Finasteride works by inhibiting synthesis of DHT, not by blocking its receptors. (D) Ketoconazole is a drug that can be used to inhibit testosterone synthesis (useful in polycystic ovarian syndrome). Finasteride does not inhibit testosterone synthesis. (E) Terazosin is used to treat BPH because, by blocking α_1-receptors, they lead to relaxation of prostatic smooth muscle, making it easier for urine to flow through the prostate.

16 **The answer is A: Angina.** Angina coexists with hypertension in approximately 15% of patients. This is important for physicians to know about because one might consider dual therapy in the treatment of such patients. Of the choices listed, angina is the most common condition to coexist with hypertension. (B) Asthma is the least common coexisting condition with hypertension. The incidence of coexistence is 5%. (C) Diabetes coexists with hypertension in approximately 13% of patients. (D) Prior myocardial infarction coexists with hypertension in approximately 9% of patients. (E) Renal impairment coexists with hypertension in approximately 7% of patients.

17 **The answer is D: Inhibitor of myenteric plexus activity.** Loperamide is an opioid-receptor agonist but does not affect the central nervous system. It binds to μ-receptors on the myenteric plexus and, like other opioids, decreases myenteric plexus activity. By inhibiting the myenteric plexus, GI smooth muscle activity is decreased. Stool transit time is increased, and it is thought that this allows more time for water absorption from the feces to decrease diarrhea. (A) Atropine is an example of an anticholinergic that can be used to treat diarrhea. Loperamide does not influence signaling with acetylcholine. (B) Many antidiarrheals (including loperamide) have no antibiotic capability. They simply increase transit time in the bowels to allow for more water reabsorption. (C) This agent is not an antibiotic. (E) Clonidine is an example of a sympathetic nervous system stimulant that can be used for diarrhea. Data are limited as to its efficacy in treating diarrhea, and it is usually only used in refractory cases. Loperamide does not treat diarrhea by modulating sympathetic nervous system activity.

18 **The answer is E: Omeprazole.** The ATPase on the lumenal surface of parietal cells described in the question stem is known as the "proton pump." It uses energy from ATP cleavage to force hydrogen ions out of the cell and potassium ions in. The proton pump inhibitors generally have the *-prazole* suffix, as in omeprazole. These drugs bind to and inhibit the function of the H^+/K^+ ATPase to significantly reduce acid secretion. (A) Atropine decreases gastric acid secretion by blocking acetylcholine signaling from the vagus nerve to parietal cells. It is not commonly used to treat GERD because of its systemic anticholinergic side effects. (B) Cimetidine decreases gastric acid secretion by blocking histamine signaling from ECL cells to parietal cells. It blocks the H_2 receptor. (C) Misoprostol is a prostaglandin analog. Prostaglandins inhibit acid secretion by binding GI receptors, which lead to a decrease in intracellular cAMP and in turn to decreased H^+/K^+ ATPase activity. They do not bind directly to the proton pump. (D) Octreotide is a somatostatin analog. Although it would decrease gastric acid production, it is not used to treat GERD because of its systemic side effects.

19 **The answer is B: Colon.** This patient's altered mental status was caused by high levels of ammonia in his blood. Normally, the liver converts excess ammonia into water-soluble urea to be excreted by the kidneys; but in patients with impaired liver function, this may not happen. When ammonia cannot be converted to urea, it will build up in the body to toxic and deadly levels unless it can be removed some other way. Lactulose is a synthetic molecule that cannot be digested by human enzymes. Once it arrives in the colon, however, it is converted to various organic acids, which lower the pH of the colonic lumen. Ammonia that diffuses into the colon is converted to ammonium ion (NH_4+) that cannot diffuse back out. In this way, lactulose works in the colon to ion trap excess ammonia for excretion. (A) Lactulose cannot be broken down or absorbed by the human body. It does not reach the brain. (C) This patient's kidneys appear to be functioning normally, judging by his creatinine level. Normal kidneys will have no problem

excreting urea. This patient's problem is that he cannot make urea. Lactulose does not work in the kidneys. (D) This man's liver is not able to metabolize ammonia rapidly enough to prevent its accumulation. Lactulose does not work in the liver and has no effect on the speed at which his liver can produce urea from ammonia. (E) The spleen serves no function in the excretion of ammonia. Lactulose does not work on the spleen.

20 **The answer is A: Amoxicillin.** The aminopenicillins, amoxicillin and ampicillin, are known for causing a nonallergic type skin rash. It is important to distinguish between this type of rash and an allergic type skin rash because a patient allergic to an aminopenicillin will likely have an allergic reaction to any other penicillin derivative. A small portion of people allergic to penicillins will also have an allergic reaction to the cephalosporins. This type of nonallergic reaction is not an absolute contraindication to aminopenicillin use but can be serious and must be considered before reexposure. (B) Ceftriaxone is not known for its ability to cause a nonallergic rash. It is known for its ability to cause biliary sludging, which is usually benign but may lead to jaundice. (C) Erythromycin is not known for its ability to cause a nonallergic rash. It is known to increase the QT interval on ECGs, which may precipitate torsades de pointes. (D) Gentamicin is not known for its ability to cause a nonallergic rash. It (as well as the other aminoglycoside antibiotics) is known for its nephrotoxicity and ototoxicity. (E) Vancomycin is not known for its ability to cause a nonallergic rash. It can cause a condition known as "red man syndrome," a skin flushing related to rapid infusion.

21 **The answer is B: Gastrointestinal bleeding.** "Baby aspirin" or an 81-mg aspirin is most commonly used in the United States. Bleeding time is prolonged by aspirin treatment, causing complications that include an increased incidence of hemorrhagic stroke as well as gastrointestinal (GI) bleeding, especially at higher doses of the drug. Aspirin is frequently used in combination with other drugs having anticlotting properties, such as heparin or clopidogrel. Acetylation of cyclooxygenase 1 by aspirin. (A) Cholecystitis is unlikely to occur with an increased dose of aspirin. (C) Pancreatitis is unlikely to occur with an increased dose of aspirin. (D) Splenic infarct is unlikely to occur with an increased dose of aspirin. (E) Hemorrhagic stroke is a possible complication of increased dose of aspirin.

22 **The answer is C: Increased production of triglycerides.** This patient has type V familial mixed hypertriglyceridemia. Serum VLDL and chylomicrons are elevated. LDL is normal or decreased. This results in elevated cholesterol and greatly elevated TG levels. The cause is either increased production or decreased clearance of VLDL and chylomicrons. Usually, it is a genetic defect. It occurs most commonly in adults who are obese and/or has diabetes. The treatment is diet. If necessary, drug therapy includes niacin and/or fenofibrate or a statin. (A) Diabetes mellitus is an associated finding in these patients. (B) These patients are often adults who are obese and/or has diabetes. (D) These patients can have increased production or decreased clearance of chylomicrons or VLDL.

23 **The answer is E: Supplement potassium by increasing intake of fruits and bananas.** Hypokalemia is the most frequent problem encountered with the thiazide diuretics, and it can predispose patients who are taking digoxin to ventricular arrhythmias. Often, K^+ can be supplemented by diet alone such as by increasing the intake of citrus fruits, bananas, and prunes. In some cases, K^+ salt supplementation may be necessary. (A) This patient must have his hypokalemia managed immediately. (B) There is no indication that this patient is having a myocardial infarction. (C) This patient has good blood pressure control on the thiazide diuretic. (D) The thiazide is working nicely on a daily dose regimen. Blood pressure is well controlled.

24 **The answer is B: Drug toxicity.** Spironolactone frequently causes gastritis and can cause peptic ulcers. Because it chemically resembles some of the sex steroids, spironolactone may act at receptors in other organs to induce gynecomastia in male patients and menstrual irregularities in female patients. Therefore, the drug should not be given at high doses on a chronic basis. (A) Chronic stress can produce gastric ulcers but not gynecomastia. (C) Pituitary tumor would not be likely to produce gynecomastia and gastric ulcers. (D) Thyroid disease does not usually produce gynecomastia. (E) This patient has no clinical findings to suggest thyroid storm.

25 **The answer is D: Hypotension.** By stimulating potassium channels, diazoxide hyperpolarizes cells. Hyperpolarized smooth muscle cells are less likely to contract, whereas hyperpolarized β-pancreatic islet cells are less likely to release insulin. It is used to inhibit insulin release in cases of inoperable insulinomas and in cases of hypertensive emergencies to lower blood pressure. Common side effects, therefore, are hypotension and hyperglycemia. (A) Hyperpolarization of smooth muscle cells would lead to bronchodilation rather than bronchoconstriction. Diazoxide is not known to cause bronchoconstriction. (B) Diazoxide is used to treat hypertension because it hyperpolarizes cells. A hyperpolarized cell is less likely to constrict. (C) Diazoxide is used to treat cases of hypoglycemia caused by excess insulin secretion. The hyperpolarization produced by diazoxide inhibits insulin release.

(E) Seizures represent a hyperexcitable state, opposite the hyperpolarization created by diazoxide. It is not known to cause seizures.

26 **The answer is B: Diarrhea.** Magnesium hydroxide is a base that neutralizes gastric acid. The reaction produces magnesium and chloride ions. The magnesium is not absorbed by the intestine and acts as an osmolyte to retain water in the lumen. This results in increased volume and gut motility that can lead to diarrhea. (A) Magnesium hydroxide is also used to treat constipation because magnesium stays in the gut lumen as an osmolyte. Aluminum hydroxide is a drug used to treat heartburn that can cause constipation. (C) Cimetidine is a drug used to treat heartburn that causes headache in about 3% of people. It is an H_2 blocker usually used to treat more severe cases of heartburn than in this patient. Magnesium hydroxide is not known to cause headaches. (D) Some of the H_2 blockers, including cimetidine and ranitidine, can cause impotence. Magnesium hydroxide is not known to cause impotence. (E) Seizure is a rare complication of both famotidine and lansoprazole. Magnesium hydroxide is not known to cause seizures.

27 **The answer is B: Increased secretion of mucus.** Airflow obstruction in asthma is caused by bronchoconstriction that results from contraction of bronchial smooth muscle, inflammation of the bronchial wall, and increased secretion of mucus. Asthmatic attacks may be related to recent exposure to allergens or inhaled irritants, leading to bronchial hyperactivity and inflammation of the airway mucosa. The symptoms of asthma may be effectively treated by several drugs, but no agent provides a cure. (A) Bronchoconstriction results in asthma, a reactive airway disease. (C) Asthma causes inflammation of the bronchial wall. (D) Asthma causes bronchial smooth muscle contraction.

28 **The answer is A: Dose adjustment is required in hepatic failure.** Cimetidine and the other H_2 antagonists are given orally, distribute widely throughout the body (including into breast milk and across the placenta), and are excreted mainly in urine. Cimetidine normally has a short serum half-life, which is increased in renal failure. Approximately 30% of a dose of cimetidine is slowly inactivated by the liver's microsomal mixed-function oxygenase system (see p. 14) and can interfere in the metabolism of many other drugs. The other 70% is excreted unchanged in urine. The dosage of all these drugs must be decreased in patients with hepatic or renal failure. (B) Cimetidine has a short half-life. (C) Thirty percent of a dose of cimetidine is slowly inactivated in the liver. (D) Seventy percent of a dose of cimetidine is excreted unchanged in the urine.

29 **The answer is E: Muscular pain.** The adverse effects of cimetidine are usually minor and are associated mainly with reduced gastric acid production, the major pharmacologic activity of the drug. Side effects occur only in a small number of patients and generally do not require discontinuation of the drug. The most common side effects are headache, dizziness, diarrhea, and muscular pain. Other central nervous system effects (such as confusion and hallucinations) occur primarily in elderly patients and after intravenous administration. (A) Confusion is common in elderly patients after IV infusion of cimetidine. (B) Diarrhea is a common side effect of cimetidine. (C) Hallucinations are common in elderly patients after IV infusion of cimetidine. (D) Headache is a common side effect of nearly all medications.

30 **The answer is A: Disorientation.** Marijuana derivatives are effective as an antiemetic agent. This is not approved for use by the FDA. Disorientation, dysphoria, and hallucinations can occur with this product. The antiemetic properties do not involve the brain. (B) Dysphoria would be expected with marijuana use. (C) Sedation, not excitation, would be expected with marijuana use. (D) Marijuana is an antiemetic agent and would inhibit vomiting. (E) Uremic pericarditis is not a known side effect of marijuana use.

31 **The answer is A: Gel formation in the intestine.** Bulk laxatives include hydrophilic colloids. They form gels in the large intestine that cause water retention and intestinal distension, which increases peristalsis. This agent should be used with caution because of the potential for intestinal obstruction. (B) Sacral nerve stimulation is a surgical procedure that stimulates the S3 nerve root. (C) Magnesium citrate is a nonabsorbable salt. (D) Lactulose is a semisynthetic sugar that also acts as an osmotic diuretic. (E) Cholinomimetic agents stimulate the cholinergic nervous system.

32 **The answer is A: Abuse potential.** Phentermine is an appetite suppressant. This is a schedule IV controlled agent because of the potential of dependence or abuse. Other common effects include dry mouth, sedation, headache, insomnia, and constipation. (B) Cardiovascular toxicities are uncommon with phentermine. (C) Hypertension is uncommon with phentermine. (D) Risk of stroke is low with phentermine. (E) Risk of seizures is low with phentermine.

33 **The answer is B: Antiandrogenic effect.** Cimetidine can also have endocrine effects because it acts as a nonsteroidal antiandrogen. These effects include gynecomastia and galactorrhea (continuous release/discharge of milk). Drugs such as ketoconazole, which depend on an acidic medium for gastric absorption, may not be efficiently absorbed if taken with one of these H_2 receptor

antagonists. (A) Cimetidine is associated with endocrine effects such as breast swelling and tenderness. This is not caused by an abscess. (C) This process is not inflammatory in nature. This process is an endocrine side effect of cimetidine. (D) This patient has no evidence by history of examination to suggest breast cancer. (E) This is an overgrowth of breast tissue, not a buildup of interstitial fluid in the chest.

34 **The answer is A: Decrease in gastric acid secretion.** Misoprostol, a stable analog of prostaglandin E_1, as well as some PPIs, are approved for the prevention of gastric ulcers induced by NSAIDs. It is less effective than H_2 antagonists and the PPIs for acute treatment of peptic ulcers. Although misoprostol has cytoprotective actions, it is clinically effective only at higher doses that diminish gastric acid secretion. (B) Misoprostol is an analog of prostaglandin E_1 and does not affect bicarbonate balance. (C) Misoprostol does not improve gastric muscular tone. (D) Misoprostol does not alter lower esophageal sphincter tone. (E) Misoprostol does not change gastric luminal pressures.

35 **The answer is B: Calcium carbonate.** Aluminum- and magnesium-containing antacids are used for symptomatic relief of peptic ulcer disease and GERD, and they may also promote healing of duodenal ulcers. However, they are used as last-line therapy for acute gastric ulcers because the evidence for efficacy is less compelling. Calcium carbonate preparations are also used as calcium supplements for the treatment of osteoporosis. (A) Aluminum hydroxide will help with the GERD symptoms but not the osteoporosis. (C) Magnesium hydroxide will help with the GERD symptoms but will not improve bone mineralization as needed in osteoporosis. (D) Sodium bicarbonate is an effective antacid but is not of benefit in the treatment of osteoporosis. (E) Warm milk may worsen gastroesophageal reflux and will have limited benefit for osteoporosis.

36 **The answer is C: Gastric ulcers that appear unhealed.** Sucralfate should not be administered with PPIs, H_2 antagonists, or antacids. Little of the drug is absorbed systemically. It is very well tolerated, but it can interfere with the absorption of other drugs by binding to them. This agent does not prevent NSAID-induced ulcers, and it does not heal gastric ulcers. (A) NSAID-induced ulcers are typically gastric and less likely to be duodenal. (B) Duodenal perforation would present with peritoneal signs and significant abdominal pain. (D) Normal gastric epithelium is unlikely to be present because active ulceration would be expected. (E) The lower esophagus likely has inflammatory changes.

37 **The answer is C: Tadalafil.** Tadalafil has a slower onset of action than sildenafil and vardenafil but a significantly longer half-life of approximately 18 h. This results in enhanced erectile function for up to 36 h. Furthermore, the absorption of tadalafil is not clinically influenced by food. The timing of sexual activity is less critical for tadalafil because of its prolonged duration of effect. Tadalafil is an excellent choice for this patient because he may only have to take this medication once or twice a week. (A) Penile prosthesis is not indicated in mild erectile dysfunction, especially in a young, otherwise healthy man. (B) Sildenafil could be used in this patient but would require more frequent dosing because of the shorter half-life. (D) Vardenafil, like sildenafil, could be used in this patient but would require more frequent dosing because of the shorter half-life. (E) Vacuum erection device would be considered a second-line therapy in this patient after he has failed a trial of at least five attempts of an oral agent such as tadalafil.

38 **The answer is E: QT prolongation.** Long QT syndrome is a congenital disorder in which a genetic mutation leads to a prolonged QT interval on ECG. It may be autosomal dominant or recessive. Erythromycin is reported to also lengthen the QT interval, which may lead to torsades de pointes in this patient. Torsades de pointes is an arrhythmia that is often fatal, so avoidance is key. Neither two drugs that may cause QT prolongation should be used together nor should any such drug be used in a patient with long QT syndrome. (A) Erythromycin is not known to have any interaction with metformin. These two drugs are safe to use together. (B) Erythromycin is not known to have any interaction with ticlopidine. These two drugs are safe to use together. (C) Erythromycin is neither contraindicated in cases of hyperglycemia nor is it known to cause hyperglycemia. (D) Erythromycin is not known to be cardiotoxic, except that it may lead to torsades de pointes as discussed previously. The only heart abnormality that is a contraindication for erythromycin is long QT syndrome.

39 **The answer is E: Seizures.** Imipenem/cilastatin can cause nausea, vomiting, and diarrhea. Eosinophilia and neutropenia are less common than with other lactams. High levels of imipenem may provoke seizures, but meropenem is possibly less likely to do so. Doripenem has not demonstrated any potential to cause seizures in animal studies. (A) Imipenem/cilastatin is not cardiotoxic. (B) Imipenem/cilastatin is not implicated in causing gastrointestinal ischemia. (C) Pulmonary fibrosis is not a side effect of this antibiotic. It is common with an antineoplastic medication, bleomycin. (D) Renal failure is certainly possible with antibiotics; however, the physician must be concerned about new-onset seizures from imipenem/cilastatin.

40 **The answer is C: Inactivation of surfactant.** Daptomycin is indicated for the treatment of complicated skin and skin structure infections and bacteremia caused by *Staphylococcus aureus*, including those with right-sided infective endocarditis. Efficacy of treatment with daptomycin in left-sided endocarditis has not been demonstrated. Additionally, daptomycin is inactivated by pulmonary surfactants; thus, it should never be used in the treatment of pneumonia. (A) Daptomycin does not cause atrial fibrillation. (B) Daptomycin does not cause cardiac arrest. (D) Daptomycin does not cause thromboembolic diseases such as pulmonary embolism. (E) Pulmonary infarct is unlikely to develop in this patient.

41 **The answer is A: Pregnancy complications.** Telavancin is bactericidal against methicillin-resistant *Staphylococcus aureus* (MRSA). The most common adverse reactions reported with telavancin have included taste disturbances, nausea, vomiting, insomnia, and foamy urine. Telavancin is not recommended during pregnancy because of adverse developmental outcomes observed with animal data. In the United States, there is a boxed warning for women of childbearing age to have a pregnancy test prior to use. (B) Telavancin is not associated with thromboembolic complications. (C) QT interval prolongation is possible with this agent if supratherapeutic drug concentrations develop. However, this is unlikely in an otherwise abnormal individual. (D) T wave inversion is unlikely in this patient. (E) Uremic pericarditis does not usually develop following administration of telavancin.

42 **The answer is E: Venous irritation.** Venous irritation: This commonly occurs when quinupristin/dalfopristin is administered through a peripheral rather than a central line. Arthralgia and myalgia: These have been reported when higher levels of the drugs are employed. Hyperbilirubinemia: Total bilirubin is elevated in about 25% of patients, resulting from a competition with the antibiotic for excretion. Interactions: Because of the ability of quinupristin/dalfopristin to inhibit the cytochrome P450 (CYP3A4) isozyme, concomitant administration (A) Arthralgia is more likely to occur following administration of dalfopristan. Arthritis would be an unlikely adverse event. (B) Hyperbilirubinemia is more likely to occur following administration rather than true hepatic failure. (C) Myalgia can occur when higher levels of drug concentration are obtained. (D) Renal failure is not a typical side effect of quinupristin administration.

43 **The answer is B: Ophthalmology.** An ophthalmology consultation should be considered in this patient. Early oxazolidinones had been shown to inhibit monoamine oxidase activity and can precipitate serotonin syndrome in patients concomitantly taking SSRIs. The condition was reversible when the drug was suspended. Irreversible peripheral neuropathies and optic neuritis (causing blindness) is associated with greater than 28 days of use. Thus, the eyes must be examined in this patient. (A) Ophthalmologic concerns are highest in this patient who has been on linezolid for greater than 1 month. (C) This patient is unlikely to have foot-related problems because of medication use. (D) This patient is unlikely to have pulmonary issues related to medication use. (E) There are unlikely to be urologic issues in this patient related to medication use.

44 **The answer is A: DNA gyrase.** Mutations in the bacterial DNA gyrase have been associated with a decreased affinity for fluoroquinolones. Topoisomerase IV also undergoes mutations. Resistance is frequently associated with mutations in both DNA gyrase and topoisomerase IV. (B) Mutations typically occur in both DNA gyrase and topoisomerase IV. (C) Mutations typically occur in DNA topoisomerase IV. (D) Mutations typically occur in DNA topoisomerase IV. (E) Mutations typically occur in DNA topoisomerase IV.

45 **The answer is D: Methyldopa.** A pregnant woman who develops hypertension is at risk for preeclampsia. Preeclampsia is defined as hypertension, proteinuria, and edema. If left untreated, it can progress to eclampsia, which is preeclampsia plus seizures. The only sure cure is delivery of the fetus, but measures can be taken to prolong the pregnancy to allow the fetus to develop as much as possible. Methyldopa is a pregnancy category B drug and has a long history of safety in pregnancy. (A) Atenolol is used in patients with hypertension and a history of heart disease. It is a pregnancy category D drug. (B) Lisinopril is an angiotensin-converting enzyme (ACE) inhibitor. It is a pregnancy category D drug. (C) Losartan is an angiotensin receptor blocker (ARB). It is a pregnancy category D drug. (E) Nifedipine is a calcium channel blocker that affects channels in smooth muscle much more than those in cardiac muscle. It is a pregnancy category C drug.

46 **The answer is A: A 30-year-old man with a history of diabetes mellitus.** Warning to fluoroquinolones about increased risk of tendinitis or tendon rupture that may occur with systemic fluoroquinolone use, not with ophthalmic or otic use. The Achilles tendon is the most frequent tendon associated with the occurrence of tendinitis and tendon rupture. The adverse event can occur during fluoroquinolone treatment or up to several months after completion of therapy. The risk of developing tendinitis or tendon rupture associated with fluoroquinolone use is increased in patients older than 60 years of age; those receiving concomitant corticosteroid therapy; and in patients with kidney, heart, or lung transplants. (B) Patients on corticosteroid therapy are at increased risk of tendinitis/tendon rupture. (C) Patients who are immunosuppressed are at increased risk of tendonitis/tendon rupture. (D) Patients who are renal transplant recipients are at increased risk of tendonitis/tendon rupture. (E) Patients older than the age of 65 years are at increased risk of tendinitis/tendon rupture.

47 **The answer is A: Enhanced production of PABA.** Acquired bacterial resistance to the sulfa drugs can arise from plasmid transfers or random mutations. Organisms resistant to one member of this drug family are resistant to all. Resistance is generally irreversible and may be caused by (1) an altered dihydropteroate synthetase, (2) decreased cellular permeability to sulfa drugs, or (3) enhanced production of the natural substrate, PABA. (B) Resistance to sulfa drugs is caused by decreased cellular permeability to sulfa drugs. (C) Resistance to sulfa drugs is caused by altered dihydropteroate synthetase. (D) Resistance to sulfa drugs is caused by altered dihydropteroate synthetase.

48 **The answer is E: Urinary retention.** Acetylcholine stimulating its various receptors causes bradycardia, increased gastric motility, detrusor muscle contraction, mydriasis, lacrimation, increased bronchial secretions, diaphoresis, salivation, and skeletal muscle contraction. Anticholinergic effects are just the opposite. The only anticholinergic effect listed here is urinary retention. (A) Bradycardia can be caused by cholinergic stimulation of muscarinic receptors on the sinoatrial node of the heart. An anticholinergic's effect on the heart would be tachycardia. (B) Cholinergic stimulation of the gut causes increased motility and secretions, possibly leading to diarrhea. An anticholinergic's effect on the gut would be constipation. (C) Lacrimation is caused by cholinergic stimulation. An anticholinergic would decrease lacrimation. (D) Miosis can be caused by cholinergic stimulation of the pupillary constrictor muscle. An anticholinergic agent would lead to mydriasis caused by the unopposed effect of adrenergic stimulation.

49 **The answer is A: Continue infusion; premedicate with antipyretic for next doses.** Fever and chills occur most commonly 1 to 3 h after starting the IV amphotericin administration, but they usually subside with repeated administration of the drug. Premedication with a corticosteroid or an antipyretic helps to prevent this problem. (B) This is usually a self-limiting problem and will subside with repeated doses of amphotericin. (C) Amphotericin can be continued in this patient. (D) It is unwise to administer an antibiotic to a patient who has a fungal infection. (E) There is no indication to suggest that this patient is anemic. Thus, transfusion of packed red blood cells is not necessary.

50 **The answer is A: Bone marrow depression.** Flucytosine causes reversible neutropenia, thrombocytopenia, and dose-related bone marrow depression. Caution must be exercised in patients undergoing radiation or chemotherapy with drugs that depress bone marrow. Reversible hepatic dysfunction with elevation of serum transaminases and alkaline phosphatase may occur. Gastrointestinal disturbances—such as nausea, vomiting, and diarrhea—are common, and severe enterocolitis may also occur. (B) Severe enterocolitis can occur with this medication. Necrotizing enterocolitis occurs in newborns. (C) Neutropenia, not neutrophilia, can occur with flucytosine. (D) Reversible hepatic dysfunction with elevation of serum transaminases can occur with flucytosine. (E) Thrombocytopenia, not thrombocytosis, can occur with flucytosine.

51 **The answer is D: Coca-Cola.** When ketoconazole is administered orally, it requires gastric acid for dissolution and is absorbed through the intestinal mucosa. Drugs that raise gastric pH (such as antacids) or that interfere with gastric acid secretion (such as H_2-histamine receptor blockers and proton pump inhibitors) impair absorption. Administering acidifying agents, such as cola drinks, before taking the drug can improve absorption in patients with achlorhydria. (A) Calcium carbonate will increase gastric pH and impair absorption of ketoconazole. (B) Calcium citrate will increase gastric pH and lower systemic levels of ketoconazole. (C) Cimetidine will increase gastric pH and lower systemic levels of ketoconazole. (E) Sodium bicarbonate will also increase gastric pH and impair systemic levels of ketoconazole.

52 **The answer is A: Histamine release from mast cells.** Caspofungin is the first approved member of the echinocandin class of antifungal drugs. Caspofungin has activity against *Aspergillus* and most *Candida* species, including those species resistant to azoles. Adverse effects include fever, rash, nausea, and phlebitis. Flushing occurs, which is probably caused by the release of histamine from mast cells. (B) Abdominal imaging is not presented in this question; thus, it is not possible to know whether this patient has any abdominal pathology. (C) Parathyroid adenoma could cause hypercalcemia, which is not related to mast cell release of histamine. (D) Parathyroid hyperplasia could also cause hypercalcemia, which would not be related to mast cell release of histamine. (E) Abdominal imaging is not presented in this question; thus, it is not possible to know whether this patient has any abdominal pathology.

53 **The answer is A: Accumulation in tissues.** Terbinafine is available for oral and topical administration, although its bioavailability is only 40% because of first-pass metabolism. Absorption is not significantly enhanced by food. Terbinafine is greater than 99% bound to

plasma proteins. It is deposited in the skin, nails, and fat. Terbinafine accumulates in breast milk and should not be given to nursing mothers. A prolonged terminal half-life of 200 to 400 h may reflect the slow release from these tissues. (B) Terbinafine is hepatotoxic, not nephrotoxic. (C) Terbinafine is unlikely to result in neuromuscular blockade. (D) Streptomycin is a classic agent that is associated with ototoxicity. (E) Uremia is unlikely to result from administration of terbinafine.

54 **The answer is B: Encephalopathy.** CNS toxicities are the most serious side effects of melarsoprol treatment. Encephalopathy may appear soon after the first course of treatment but usually subsides. In rare cases, however, it may be fatal. Hypersensitivity reactions may also occur, and fever may follow injection. Gastrointestinal disturbances, such as severe vomiting and abdominal pain, can be minimized if the patient is in the fasting state during drug administration and for several hours thereafter. (A) CNS toxicities are the most serious side effect of melarsoprol treatment. (C) Hypercoagulable states are uncommon with melarsoprol treatment. Hemolytic anemia is a possible effect. (D) CNS toxicities, not neuromuscular toxicities, are most concerning for this patient. (E) Renal failure is a less likely sequelae of melarsoprol treatment.

55 **The answer is E: Toxicity of pancreatic cells.** There are some important side effects of pentamidine to know about. Serious renal dysfunction may occur, which reverses on discontinuation of the drug. Other adverse reactions are hypotension, dizziness, rash, and toxicity to cells of the pancreas. (A) Hypotension is a potential adverse effect of pentamidine. (B) Pancreatitis is unlikely to develop in this patient. It is more likely that he will develop a lack of responsiveness of the β-cells of the pancreas to release insulin. (C) There is no evidence to suggest that this patient has pancreatic carcinoma. This disease is common in older men. (D) Pheochromocytoma is unlikely given that this patient does not have sweats, diarrhea, or hypertension.

56 **The answer is A: Cough becomes more productive.** This patient's presentation is consistent with an upper respiratory tract (URT) viral infection. Cough syrups are often preparations containing multiple drugs that each targets a different symptom commonly associated with URT infections such as cough, headache, fever, and nasal congestion. Guaifenesin is an expectorant; its effect is to thin secreted mucus to make it more easily removed by ciliary action and coughing. In this way, guaifenesin will initially make a cough become more productive. (B) Cough syrups often contain an opioid derivative such as dextromethorphan. It appears to work somewhat differently than other opioids but works just as well for cough suppression. (C) Acetaminophen is a common ingredient in cough syrup preparations. Acetaminophen relieves fever apparently by inhibiting cyclooxygenase enzymes in the CNS to prevent production of profebrile prostaglandins. (D) Acetaminophen is a common ingredient in cough syrup preparations. Acetaminophen relieves pain by inhibiting cyclooxygenase enzymes in the CNS to prevent production of pain-stimulating prostaglandins. (E) Guaifenesin is an expectorant. Headache is a rare side effect; and although guaifenesin does not directly lessen the pain of a headache, it will probably not make the pain worse.

57 **The answer is C: Dornase alfa.** The chronic infections that accompany cystic fibrosis lead to an influx of neutrophils that leave behind long strands of DNA when they die. This DNA makes the mucus even thicker than it would otherwise be. Dornase alfa is a recombinant DNase that cleaves DNA strands embedded in the mucus. Cleaving this DNA helps thin the mucus so it can be expectorated. (A) Acetylcysteine is able to cleave disulfide bonds in mucoproteins to thin mucus. Acetylcysteine does not cleave DNA. (B) Bromhexine also thins mucus. It induces secretion of serous (watery) mucus. Bromhexine does not cleave DNA. (D) Guaifenesin thins mucus. It turns a dry cough into a more productive cough. It does not, however, cleave extracellular DNA. (E) Ipratropium is an anticholinergic. It is used to decrease bronchial secretions and relax bronchial smooth muscle in diseases such as asthma and COPD. It does not cleave DNA.

58 **The answer is A: Acetylcysteine.** A common drug used in the treatment of cystic fibrosis is acetylcysteine. The molecule has a free sulfhydryl group that evidently leads to breaks in the disulfide bonds in mucoproteins. This leads to a thinner, more easily managed mucus. Because of its sulfhydryl groups, however, acetylcysteine possesses a sulfuric smell and taste that causes nausea in many patients, especially when administered orally. (B) Bromhexine has been reported to cause mild nausea, but not to the same extent as acetylcysteine. Acetylcysteine, not bromhexine, is known for its unpleasant odor. (C) Calfactant is a derivative of calf pulmonary surfactant. It is used in respiratory distress syndrome and is not known to cause nausea. (D) Dornase alfa cleaves DNA strands that are left behind from neutrophil death in patients with cystic fibrosis. It is not known to cause nausea. (E) Guaifenesin thins mucus and makes it easier to expel. It rarely causes nausea, especially at therapeutic doses.

59 **The answer is C: Renal stone.** Renal stones can form in a patient taking indinavir. The medication is well tolerated, with the usual GI symptoms and headache predominating. Indinavir characteristically causes nephrolithiasis and hyperbilirubinemia. Adequate

hydration is important to reduce the incidence of kidney stone formation, and patients should drink at least 1.5 L of water per day. Fat redistribution is particularly troublesome with this drug. (A) Renal stone formation is more likely than hepatitis. (B) Gallstone pancreatitis is unlikely in this patient. However, hyperbilirubinemia is more common. (D) Small bowel obstruction is unlikely in this patient taking indinavir. (E) Transverse colon colitis is not a plausible diagnosis.

60 **The answer is B: Crystallization in the renal tubules.** Although uncommon during conventional therapy, renal damage is a complication of high-dose methotrexate and its 7-OH metabolite, which can precipitate in the tubules. Alkalinization of the urine and hydration help to prevent this problem. (A) The collecting ducts would be expected to be normal in this patient. (C) The distal tubular cells would be expected to be unchanged in this patient. (D) The glomerulus will be functional in this patient. (E) Proximal tubular cells would appear normal in this patient.

61 **The answer is D: Increased dephosphorylation.** Resistance is associated with (1) an inability to biotransform 6-MP to the corresponding nucleotide because of decreased levels of HGPRT (e.g., in Lesch-Nyhan syndrome, in which patients lack this enzyme), (2) increased dephosphorylation, or (3) increased metabolism of the drug to thiouric acid or other metabolites. (A) Resistance to 6-MP develops because of inability to transform 6-MP to the corresponding nucleotide. (B) Resistance is caused by increased metabolism to other metabolites. (C) Resistance is caused by increased metabolism to thiouric acid. (E) There will be decreased levels of HGPRT.

62 **The answer is B: Paralysis.** Cytarabine has several toxicities. Nausea, vomiting, diarrhea, and severe myelosuppression (primarily granulocytopenia) are the major toxicities associated with ara-C. Hepatic dysfunction is also occasionally encountered. At high doses or with intrathecal injection, ara-C may cause leukoencephalopathy or paralysis. (A) High-dose cytarabine can cause leukoencephalopathy, not cardiac disease. (C) High-dose cytarabine does not typically cause venous stasis or embolism. (D) High-dose cytarabine can cause paralysis, not renal cast formation. (E) Cytarabine at lower doses can cause gastrointestinal and hematologic toxicities. Uremic pericarditis is an unlikely effect.

63 **The answer is D: Prevents release of cholinergic vesicles.** Botox treatment uses botulinum toxin's mechanism to prevent release of cholinergic vesicles in autonomic transmission. The toxin blocks the binding of the vesicle-associated membrane proteins (VAMPs) with the synaptosomal nerve-associated proteins (SNAPs) following the rise in intracellular calcium. The vesicles cannot fuse with the surface membrane, and ACh and cotransmitters cannot be released into the synaptic cleft. (A) Phentolamine binds α-receptors, preventing activation. Phentolamine is a reversible antagonist of α-receptors. (B) Atropine binds muscarinic receptors, preventing activation. When atropine binds to the muscarinic receptor, it prevents actions such as the release of inositol triphosphate (IP3) and the inhibition of adenylyl cyclase caused by muscarinic agonists. (C) Hemicholinium blocks uptake of choline into nerve terminals. Choline is transported from the extracellular fluid into the neuron by the Na^+-dependent membrane choline transporter (CHT) and is required for the formation of ACh. (E) Vesamicol prevents storage of cholinergic vesicles.

64 **The answer is A: Epinephrine.** Lidocaine is a local anesthetic commonly used to numb the skin in cases such as this for nevus removal. It is often administered with epinephrine, which causes local vasoconstriction. This prolongs the action of lidocaine by preventing its diffusion into the bloodstream. The local vasoconstriction caused by epinephrine also leads to blanching of the skin. (B) Levothyroxine is a synthetic form of thyroxine (T4) used to treat hypothyroidism. It does not cause vasodilation (or the accompanying blanching) and is not administered with lidocaine for this purpose. (C) Nifedipine is a vasodilator used to treat hypertension. It does not cause vasodilation (or the accompanying blanching) and is not administered with lidocaine for this purpose. (D) Preparations of lidocaine for routine injection are clear solutions. Phenobarbital is thick and white but is not used for local anesthesia. (E) Sodium bicarbonate is often mixed with lidocaine for injection because it, as felt by some, decreases the initial sting that can accompany an injection of lidocaine. Sodium bicarbonate does not cause vasodilation (or the accompanying blanching) and is not administered with lidocaine for this purpose.

65 **The answer is A: Enhance mucosal resistance.** Misoprostol is sometimes used to inhibit the secretion of gastric acid and to enhance mucosal resistance to injury in patients with gastric ulcer, who are chronically taking nonsteroidal anti-inflammatory agents. Proton pump inhibitors, such as omeprazole, and H_2 antihistamines also reduce the risk of gastric ulcer and are better tolerated than misoprostol, which induces intestinal disorders. (B) Misoprostol does not inhibit gastrin release. It does inhibit gastric acid secretion. (C) Proton pump inhibitors inhibit proton pump secretion. (D) Misoprostol does not inhibit somatostatin release. (E) Misoprostol does not inhibit uric acid secretion.

66 **The answer is E: Serotonin.** Zolmitriptan is used in the treatment of migraine headaches. These agents rapidly and effectively abort or markedly reduce the severity of migraine headaches in about 70% of patients. The triptans are serotonin agonists, acting at a subgroup of serotonin receptors found on small peripheral nerves that innervate the intracranial vasculature. (A) The triptin class of medications acts on the serotonin receptors. (B) Choline receptors are a target for medications to combat Alzheimer disease. (C) Dopamine receptors are a target for medications to combat Parkinson disease. (D) The triptin class of medications acts on the serotonin receptors.

67 **The answer is C: Decrease the dose.** This boy's presentation is consistent with a diagnosis of ADHD. There is nothing wrong with the physician's choice of treatment of amphetamine salts. The reaction exhibited by this patient is called supranormalization and reflects a higher-than-necessary dose. Decreasing the amphetamine salts dose should correct this effect. (A) The physician's diagnosis is most likely correct, and his treatment choice is appropriate. ADHD can be efficaciously treated with amphetamine salts. (B) Because the boy's behavior improved with administration of amphetamine salts, switching to another drug is not necessary. The issue can likely be corrected simply by reducing his dose. (D) This side effect is not inevitable. Simply decreasing the dose will probably solve the problem while still treating the ADHD. (E) This patient is exhibiting supranormalization, which occurs when the amphetamine salts dose is too high. The way to address this problem is to decrease the dose, not increase it.

68 **The answer is B: Do nothing.** This patient's condition fits the qualifications for major depression. The physician has prescribed a selective serotonin reuptake inhibitor (SSRI). As their name suggests, these drugs block the reuptake of serotonin into synaptic vesicles, although the exact way they improve symptoms of depression is not completely understood. It is known, however, that therapy must continue for many weeks before patients notice a change in symptoms. The best response by the physician in this case is to encourage her to continue but make no changes to the fluoxetine dose. (A) Sertraline is another SSRI. Administering a second SSRI will not hasten the onset of the therapeutic effects of fluoxetine. (C) There is an apparently inevitable delay in the onset of action of SSRIs. Increasing the dose of fluoxetine will not hasten the onset of its therapeutic effects. (D) There is an apparently inevitable delay in the onset of action of SSRIs. This fact should be explained to any patients taking an SSRI so they realize a delay is no reason to discontinue the drug. (E) There is an apparently inevitable delay in the onset of action of SSRIs. A delay in the onset of action is no reason to discontinue fluoxetine.

69 **The answer is C: Mirtazapine.** Many drugs carry the side effect of appetite suppression, which is usually seen as an adverse effect. Elderly patients with depression may have a problem with the appetite suppression associated with this medication because of their already poor nutritional status. In addition, many of these patients report problems sleeping at night. Of course, a single drug that addresses all these issues is preferable to multiple drugs. Mirtazapine is a tetracyclic antidepressant that can cause both appetite stimulation and drowsiness; it would probably be the best choice for this patient. (A) Amitriptyline is an antidepressant that can cause drowsiness but is not known to cause appetite stimulation as mirtazapine. Mirtazapine would probably be a better choice to treat this patient. (B) Buspirone is an antidepressant that can cause drowsiness but is not known to cause appetite stimulation as mirtazapine. Mirtazapine would probably be a better choice to treat this patient. (D) Olanzapine causes the desired side effects of drowsiness and appetite stimulation but is not an antidepressant. Olanzapine is an atypical antipsychotic but should not be used to treat psychosis related to dementia in the elderly. (E) Venlafaxine is an antidepressant that can cause drowsiness but is not known to cause appetite stimulation as mirtazapine. Mirtazapine would probably be a better choice to treat this patient.

70 **The answer is E: Promethazine.** There are many receptor types that can be manipulated to decrease nausea. Promethazine is a phenothiazine-like chlorpromazine but has a much lower affinity for dopamine receptors and as such is not used as a neuroleptic. Its primary action is to antagonize H_1 receptors, although its antiemetic properties appear to be related to its central anticholinergic effects. (A) Droperidol is a neuroleptic similar to haloperidol. It can also relieve nausea and vomiting. Droperidol blocks many receptors, primarily dopamine. It does not block histamine receptors. (B) Famotidine is an H_2 antagonist. It is used to treat GERD by inhibiting gastric acid secretion. Famotidine is not an antiemetic. (C) Loratadine is a second-generation H_1 antagonist. Loratadine is an antihistamine used to treat allergic rhinitis and urticaria. It is not an antiemetic. (D) Ondansetron is an antiemetic that works by antagonizing 5-HT_3 receptors both centrally and peripherally. It does not antagonize histamine receptors.

71 **The answer is E: Slows peristalsis.** This patient's presentation suggests ulcerative colitis, a type of inflammatory bowel disease. Pharmacotherapy for ulcerative colitis involves multiple drugs to treat various aspects of the disease. In cases of mild ulcerative colitis, the

frequent diarrhea may be the chief concern. Diphenoxylate may be used in such cases to slow gut motility. (A) Sulfapyridine is an antimicrobial often administered as a compound with mesalamine called sulfasalazine. Diphenoxylate does not possess antimicrobial properties. (B) Many biologics used in the treatment of ulcerative colitis, such as infliximab, bind up TNF-α to prevent its signaling. Diphenoxylate does not block TNF-α signaling. (C) Methotrexate is an inhibitor of dihydrofolate reductase used as an immunosuppressant to treat moderate cases of ulcerative colitis. Diphenoxylate does not inhibit dihydrofolate reductase. (D) Glucocorticoids work in part by increasing lipocortins, which block phospholipase A_2, impairing the inflammatory cells' ability to make prostaglandins. Diphenoxylate does not inhibit phospholipase A_2.

72 **The answer is A: Calcium.** Postprandial (after a meal) chest pain is most likely caused by gastroesophageal reflux disease (GERD), as in this case. The pain is caused by gastric acid irritating the lining of the esophagus. Pantoprazole helps the symptoms of GERD by decreasing the amount of gastric acid through inhibition of proton pumps. Raising the gastric pH in this manner may impair absorption of divalent cations such as magnesium and calcium. Some research suggests that prolonged use of proton pump inhibitors may increase the risk for bone fractures, although this relationship is uncertain. (B) Acarbose, a drug used to treat diabetes mellitus, blocks absorption of carbohydrates. Pantoprazole does not interfere with carbohydrate absorption. (C) Orlistat is a drug that impairs fatty acid absorption by inhibiting gastric and pancreatic lipases. Pantoprazole does not interfere with fatty acid absorption. (D) Vitamin A is a fat-soluble vitamin. Its absorption is decreased in cases of fat malabsorption. Pantoprazole does not interfere with vitamin A absorption. (E) Vitamin D is a fat-soluble vitamin. Its absorption is decreased in cases of fat malabsorption. Pantoprazole does not interfere with vitamin D absorption.

73 **The answer is B: Diarrhea.** Docusate is simply a stool softener. It is used to treat constipation and is generally well tolerated and has few interactions or side effects. One of its few side effects is that too high a dose can cause diarrhea. Docusate does not interact with metoprolol or mirtazapine, so this case of diarrhea cannot be attributed to an interaction between her medications. (A) Too much metoprolol can cause AV block, but neither docusate alone nor docusate with metoprolol is known to cause arrhythmias. Of the adverse reactions listed, diarrhea is the most likely to be caused by docusate. (C) A drop in this patient's metoprolol level may result in hypertension, but this is unlikely because docusate does not interact with metoprolol. Of the adverse reactions listed, diarrhea is the most likely to be caused by docusate. (D) There are many drugs that can cause a skin rash, but docusate is not one of them. Of the adverse reactions listed, diarrhea is the most likely to be caused by docusate. (E) If docusate decreased mirtazapine levels, depression may result, but this is not known to happen. Of the adverse reactions listed, diarrhea is the most likely to be caused by docusate.

74 **The answer is C: Increases water absorption by the stool.** Constipation can have many causes, ranging from decreased gut motility to altered stool consistency. It can often be relieved by modifying one of these factors. Docusate is a surfactant and allows water and lipids to penetrate, bulk up, and soften stool without directly stimulating peristalsis. Docusate is therefore classified as a stool softener, not a laxative. (A) Agents such as polycarbophil and psyllium draw water into the gut lumen to increase the bulk and water content of the stool. Docusate works simply by allowing water to easily enter the stool itself. (B) This response describes the effect of lubiprostone (and cholera toxin). Docusate works simply by allowing water to easily enter the stool itself. (D) A soapsuds enema works in part by irritating the bowel mucosa to stimulate peristalsis. Docusate works simply by allowing water to easily enter the stool itself. (E) Docusate does not directly stimulate the myenteric plexus. By allowing water to easily enter the stool, however, docusate does cause an increase in stool bulk that leads to increased motility.

75 **The answer is E: Xerostomia.** Urge incontinence is caused by inappropriate contractions of the detrusor muscle in the bladder. The detrusor muscle is stimulated by acetylcholine binding to muscarinic receptors. Solifenacin succinate is a competitive antagonist of these receptors. Stimulation of these receptors by acetylcholine also causes peristalsis of the bowel and salivation. Adverse effects of solifenacin, therefore, include constipation and xerostomia. (A) Diarrhea would result from overstimulation of muscarinic receptors. Solifenacin antagonizes these receptors resulting in constipation, not diarrhea. (B) Solifenacin is neither known to cause hypertension nor does it interact with losartan. It may cause torsades de pointes but not hypertension. (C) Photosensitivity is often associated with amiodarone and certain tetracyclines. Solifenacin is not known to cause photosensitivity. (D) Solifenacin is not known to cause restless leg syndrome. Of the side effects listed, xerostomia would be most common.

76 **The answer is D: Gastric acid secretion.** M_1 receptors are found on gastric parietal cells, M_2 receptors on cardiac cells and smooth muscle, and M_3 receptors on

the bladder, exocrine glands, and smooth muscle. Thus, a medication that affects the M_1 receptors will produce a change in gastric acid secretion. Drugs with muscarinic actions preferentially stimulate muscarinic receptors on these tissues; but at high concentration, they may show some activity at nicotinic receptors. (A) Cardiac muscle contractility is mediated by the M_2 receptors. (B) Constipation is mediated by the M_3 receptors. (C) Diarrhea is mediated by the M_3 receptors. (E) Stroke volume is mediated by the M_2 receptors.

77 **The answer is B: Diarrhea.** Bethanechol causes the effects of generalized cholinergic stimulation. These include sweating, salivation, flushing, decreased blood pressure, nausea, abdominal pain, diarrhea, and bronchospasm. Atropine sulfate may be administered to overcome severe cardiovascular or bronchoconstrictor responses to this agent. (A) Bronchoconstriction or bronchospasm can result from cholinergic nervous system stimulation. (C) Dry mouth is a side effect from anticholinergic medications. Salivation is a side effect from cholinomimetic agents. (D) Dry skin can occur with anticholinergic agents. (E) Sigmoid colon stasis can occur with anticholinergic agents. This can lead to constipation.

78 **The answer is E: Pilocarpine.** Pilocarpine is one of the most potent stimulators of secretions (secretagogue) such as sweat, tears, and saliva, but its use for producing these effects has been limited because of its lack of selectivity. The drug is beneficial in promoting salivation in patients with xerostomia resulting from irradiation of the head and neck. Sjögren syndrome, which is characterized by dry mouth and lack of tears, is treated with oral pilocarpine tablets and cevimeline, a cholinergic drug that also has the drawback of being nonspecific. (A) Bethanechol is useful for patients with postoperative urinary retention and neurogenic bowel. (B) Carbachol is useful for patients with ophthalmologic issues such as glaucoma. (C) Although oral liquid intake would be helpful, additional pharmacologic treatment would be more beneficial for this patient. (D) Resection of the parotid gland would unlikely change the symptoms exhibited by this patient.

79 **The answer is A: Cataracts.** An ophthalmic solution of the drug is applied topically to the eye for the chronic treatment of open-angle glaucoma. Echothiophate is not a first-line agent in the treatment of glaucoma. In addition to its other side effects, the potential risk for causing cataracts limits its use. (B) Echothiophate is a treatment of chronic open-angle glaucoma. (C) Echothiophate is a treatment of chronic open-angle glaucoma. (D) Venous nicking of the retina is found in diabetes and hypertension. (E) Uremia is not an expected finding in patients taking a topical ophthalmic medication.

80 **The answer is A: Cycloplegia.** Atropine blocks all cholinergic activity on the eye, resulting in persistent mydriasis (dilation of the pupil), unresponsiveness to light, and cycloplegia (inability to focus for near vision). In patients with narrow-angle glaucoma, intraocular pressure may rise dangerously. (B) Intraocular pressure will increase as a result of administration of atropine. (C) Mydriasis (pupillary dilation) will occur as a result of administration of atropine. (D) Atropine causes unresponsiveness to light.

81 **The answer is B: Cyclopentolate.** Tropicamide and cyclopentolate can be used to create mydriasis. These agents are used similarly to atropine as ophthalmic solutions for mydriasis and cycloplegia. Their duration of action is shorter than that of atropine. Tropicamitolate has a duration of action of 6 h and cyclopentolate has a duration of action of 24 h. (A) Atropine has a short duration of action and would not be useful for this patient. (C) Nicotine is not useful in the treatment of this patient. (D) Tropicamide has a duration of action of 6 h.

82 **The answer is C: Potassium release from intracellular stores.** Succinylcholine increases potassium release from intracellular stores. This may be particularly dangerous in patients with burn and patients with massive tissue damage in which potassium has been rapidly lost from within cells. (A) Iatrogenic fluid overdose will cause hypokalemia, not hyperkalemia. (B) Medication reactions between H_2 blocker and burn eschar will not cause hyperkalemia. (D) This patient has no evidence of succinylcholine overdose.

83 **The answer is A: Ipratropium aerosol.** Ipratropium aerosol is the drug of choice, especially in a patient who cannot tolerate an adrenergic agonist, that would dilate the bronchioles. It would work well in this patient with a history of known COPD and smoking. (B) Mecamylamine is a ganglionic blocker and completely inappropriate in this situation. (C) Nicotine would further aggravate his addiction because this patient is already a known smoker. (D) Oxygen would improve aeration but will not relieve bronchospasm. (E) Scopolamine's main effect is atropinic, and it is the most effective antimotion sickness drug.

84 **The answer is B: Meclizine.** This patient's presentation is consistent with positional vertigo. Vertigo is characterized by a sensation of spinning and, as in this case, may be accompanied by nausea and vomiting. Meclizine is an anti-H_1 antihistamine and anticholinergic drug used to treat vertigo. Although the

mechanism is not completely understood, meclizine appears to dampen signals from the labyrinth and vestibule of the ear. (A) Amlodipine is a dihydropyridine calcium channel blocker. It can be used to treat hypertension, not vertigo, and may in fact cause orthostatic hypotension and postural dizziness. (C) Midodrine can be used to treat dizziness associated with orthostatic hypotension. It is metabolized into the active desglymidodrine, which is an α_1-agonist. This leads to an increase in vascular tone to decrease the risk of orthostatic hypotension. (D) Mirtazapine is a tetracyclic antidepressant that works by antagonizing α_2-receptors to increase norepinephrine release. It has not been shown to be effective in treating vertigo. (E) Ondansetron blocks 5-HT_3 receptors in the chemoreceptor trigger zone to decrease nausea. Although nausea is one of this patient's complaints, treating her nausea with ondansetron will not help the underlying issue of vertigo.

85 **The answer is B: Glucagon release.** β_2-receptors will cause glucagon release. Bronchodilation will occur. Uterine smooth muscle relaxes; and vasodilation, with decrease in peripheral resistance, will occur. Increase muscle and liver glycogenolysis also occurs. (A) Bronchodilation, not bronchoconstriction, occurs with β_2-stimulation. (C) Renin release occurs with stimulation of β_1-receptors. (D) Uterine smooth muscle relaxation occurs with β_2-receptor stimulation. (E) Vasodilation, not vasoconstriction, occurs with β_2-stimulation.

86 **The answer is C: Slow anesthetic metabolism from tissue.** Local anesthetic solutions usually contain 1:100,000 parts epinephrine. The effect of this drug is to greatly increase the duration of the local anesthesia. It does this by producing vasoconstriction at the site of injection, thereby allowing the local anesthetic to persist at the injection site before being absorbed into the circulation and metabolized. Very weak solutions of epinephrine (1:100,000) can also be used topically to vasoconstrict mucous membranes to control oozing of capillary blood. (A) Anesthetics will desensitize pain sensation to allow the procedure to be undertaken pain free. (B) Vasoconstriction will slow bleeding. (D) Vasoconstriction at the site of injection will allow the local anesthetic to persist in tissue for a longer time.

87 **The answer is E: Improved sympathetic outflow to the periphery.** Yohimbine is a selective competitive α_2-blocker. It is found as a component of the bark of the yohimbe tree and is sometimes used as a sexual stimulant. Efficacy of yohimbine for the treatment of impotence has never been clearly demonstrated. Yohimbine works at the level of the CNS to increase sympathetic outflow to the periphery. It directly blocks α_2-receptors and has been used to relieve vasoconstriction associated with Raynaud disease. Yohimbine is contraindicated in CNS and cardiovascular conditions because it is a CNS and cardiovascular stimulant. (A) Yohimbine is a centrally acting α_2-blocker that does not have any effect on the cavernosal artery. (B) Yohimbine has no effect on cavernosal nerve function. (C) Yohimbine's action on the sympathetic outflow should not significantly alter blood pressure. (D) Yohimbine is unlikely to cause priapism.

88 **The answer is A: Aluminum hydroxide.** Multiple factors contribute to acid secretion by parietal cells in gastric mucosa. Gastrin from G cells, histamine from enterochromaffin-like (ECL) cells (acting on H_2 receptors), and acetylcholine from parasympathetic neurons all act directly on parietal cells to induce acid secretion. Prostaglandins from surface mucous cells and somatostatin from D cells directly inhibit acid secretion. Ranitidine is an H_2-receptor antagonist, meaning it blocks the pro-acid effect of endogenous histamine. Aluminum hydroxide is a chemical base that raises the pH by the following reaction to produce water: $H^+ + OH^- \rightarrow H_2O$. (B) Fexofenadine is a second-generation H_1 antagonist. It would not be expected to significantly bind H_2 receptors. (C) Misoprostol is a prostaglandin agonist, not antagonist. It decreases acid by mimicking the inhibitory effect of endogenous prostaglandins. (D) Omeprazole does not bind a receptor. It decreases acid secretion by blocking the proton pump on the lumenal surface of parietal cells. (E) Ranitidine is an H_2 receptor blocker. H_2 receptors are found on gastric parietal cells, and stimulation causes an increase in acid secretion.

89 **The answer is A: Atropine.** Deadly nightshade contains a compound that is metabolized to atropine. Atropine is a cholinergic antagonist, which means that acetylcholine signaling is impaired. Acetylcholine is the neurotransmitter of the peripheral nervous system. Exposure to atropine results in a clinical picture in which the parasympathetic nervous system's (PNS) influence is diminished. The PNS normally leads lacrimation, meiosis, salivation, and bradycardia. The symptoms in these patients are consistent with atropine toxicity. (B) Bethanechol is a direct cholinergic agonist. Exposure would lead to symptoms exactly opposite to those experienced by these patients. (C) Physostigmine is an indirect cholinergic agonist; it blocks degradation of acetylcholine. Exposure would lead to symptoms exactly opposite to those experienced by these patients. (D) Strychnine is a toxin that blocks glycine signaling in the spinal cord. Glycine is an important inhibitory neurotransmitter, so strychnine poisoning results in hyperreflexia and convulsions. (E) Tyramine is a compound

that leads to release of norepinephrine from synaptic vesicles. It is found in foods such as cheeses and beers. If a patient taking a monoamine oxidase inhibitor ingests tyramine, high blood pressure and headaches can result.

90 **The answer is B: Decrease in cerebrovascular resistance.** As a group, inhalational anesthetic agents decrease cerebrovascular resistance, resulting in increased perfusion of the brain. They also cause bronchodilation and decrease both spontaneous minute ventilation (volume of air per unit time moved into or out of the lungs) and hypoxic pulmonary vasoconstriction (increased pulmonary vascular resistance in poorly aerated regions of the lungs, which allows redirection of pulmonary blood flow to regions that are richer in oxygen content). (A) Bronchodilation will result. (C) Increase in brain perfusion will result. (D) Increase in pulmonary vascular resistance will result. (E) Pulmonary vasoconstriction will result.

91 **The answer is A: 5-HT$_3$ antagonist.** The mechanism of action of ondansetron is the antagonism of the 5-HT$_3$ receptor. This blocks serotonin activation of the vomiting center in the medulla, thus producing its antiemetic effect. (B) The mechanism of action of metoclopramide is the antagonism of the D$_2$ receptor. (C) The mechanism of action of cimetidine is the inhibition of the H$_2$ receptor. (D) Sibutramine is a serotonin-norepinephrine reuptake inhibitor used for weight loss. (E) The mechanism of action of aprepitant is the antagonism of substance P. It is used for the treatment of chemotherapy-induced nausea and vomiting.

92 **The answer is D: Misoprostol.** Misoprostol is a synthetic prostaglandin E$_1$ used for the treatment of nonsteroidal anti-inflammatory drug–induced peptic ulcers. Misoprostol inhibits gastric acid secretion from parietal cells at higher doses. At low doses, it increases the production and secretion of gastric mucus. (A) Bismuth is commonly used in triple or quadruple therapy for *Helicobacter pylori*. It is not commonly used to prevent peptic ulcers. (B) Famotidine is an H$_2$-receptor blocker used to decrease gastric acid production. However, misoprostol is the better treatment for nonsteroidal anti-inflammatory drug induced–peptic ulcers. (C) Lansoprazole is a proton pump inhibitor that decreases gastric acid production. However, misoprostol is the better treatment for nonsteroidal anti-inflammatory drug–induced peptic ulcers. (E) Pirenzepine blocks muscarinic (M$_1$ and M$_3$) receptors to decrease gastric acid production. It is rarely used to prevent peptic ulcers.

93 **The answer is D: Omeprazole.** The mechanism of action of omeprazole is irreversible inhibition of H$^+$/K$^+$-ATPase in parietal cells. The secretion of H$^+$ is the last step in acid secretion, and therefore, the irreversible inhibition of this step is the most potent therapy for gastric acid reduction. (A) Bismuth does not prevent the formation of gastric ulcers. Its mechanism of action is to bind to the base of the ulcer and allowing bicarbonate secretion to neutralize stomach pH. (B) Famotidine is a reversible inhibitor of H$_2$ receptors, which decreases the production of gastric acid. It is not as potent as omeprazole. (C) Misoprostol is a prostaglandin E$_1$ analog that, at high doses, decreases the production of gastric acid. It is not as potent as omeprazole. (E) Pirenzepine blocks muscarinic (M$_1$ and M$_3$) receptors to decrease gastric acid production. It is not as potent as omeprazole.

94 **The answer is E: Olsalazine.** Aminosalicylates such as mesalamine are commonly used to treat ulcerative colitis. To be effective, mesalamine must reach the colon. One way to ensure that mesalamine reaches the colon without being absorbed is to conjugate it to another molecule with an azo bond that will only be cleaved by colonic bacterial enzymes. Sulfasalazine and olsalazine are two such formulations. Olsalazine is made of two molecules of mesalamine conjugated together by an azo bond. This bond is cleaved by colonic bacteria, releasing mesalamine on site. (A) Azathioprine is an immunosuppressant. It helps with the symptoms of ulcerative colitis by decreasing the immune response. (B) Cyclosporine is an immunosuppressant. It helps with the symptoms of ulcerative colitis by decreasing the immune response. (C) Sulfasalazine is made up of a molecule of mesalamine connected to a molecule of sulfapyridine, an old sulfa antibiotic. The role of antibiotics in ulcerative colitis is unclear, however, and sulfapyridine causes enough side effects that sulfasalazine is less favorable than other drugs such as olsalazine. (D) Mesalamine is an anti-inflammatory drug used in ulcerative colitis. A large part of an oral dose of mesalamine is absorbed, preventing it from reaching its intended target—the colon. There are many ways to get around this problem, including suppository form, encapsulated extended release form, and conjugation with an azo bond.

95 **The answer is C: Heparin.** Heparin does not cross the placenta, which makes it safe for pregnancy. Heparin is used for anticoagulation in the treatment of a deep vein thrombosis. (A) Abciximab is a monoclonal antibody that is a platelet inhibitor. It is not used in the treatment of a deep vein thrombosis. (B) Aspirin inhibits platelet aggregation and is not used in the treatment of a deep vein thrombosis. It is contraindicated in pregnancy, especially in the third trimester, because of the risk of placental abruption. (D) Streptokinase is a thrombolytic that is not used in the treatment of a deep vein thrombosis. (E) Warfarin is used

to treat a deep vein thrombosis; however, it is contraindicated in pregnancy because of being able to cross the placenta.

96 **The answer is C: Category C.** Pregnancy category A contains drugs that have shown no risk to the fetus in the first trimester of pregnancy in well-controlled human studies. Category B is for drugs that either have had no well-controlled human studies but show no risk in animal studies or drugs that show risk in animal studies but not in well-controlled human studies. Category C is for drugs that show risk in animal models and have had no well-controlled human studies. Category D is for drugs that are known to pose a risk to the fetus but the benefits may outweigh the risks. Category X is for drugs absolutely contraindicated in pregnancy. Category X drugs pose such a great risk to the fetus that no benefit is seen to outweigh the risk. (A) Category A drugs have undergone well-controlled human studies and are shown to be safe in pregnancy. (B) Category B drugs have either shown no risk to fetus in animal models or risk in animal models but not in adequate human studies. (D) Category D drugs are known to pose a risk to the human fetus. In some cases, the benefits may be seen to outweigh the known risks. (E) Category X drugs are known to pose a risk to the human fetus. These drugs are so detrimental to the fetus that no benefit is considered sufficient to outweigh the risk.

97 **The answer is B: Fever.** Halothane anesthesia is associated with significant adverse reactions. This reaction begins as a fever, followed by anorexia, nausea, and vomiting; and patients may exhibit signs of hepatitis. Although the incidence of this reaction is low (approximately 1 in 10,000 individuals), 50% of affected patients may die of hepatic necrosis. (A) Anorexia is the second symptom of halothane sensitivity to occur after fever. (C) Hepatitis is a later symptom of halothane sensitivity. (D) Nausea occurs after fever in halothane sensitivity reactions. (E) Vomiting occurs following anorexia and nausea in patients with halothane sensitivity reactions.

98 **The answer is D: Produces dose-dependent hypotension.** Isoflurane is a very stable molecule that undergoes little metabolism and is not, therefore, toxic to the liver or kidney. Isoflurane does not induce cardiac arrhythmias and does not sensitize the heart to the action of catecholamines. However, like the other halogenated gases, it produces dose-dependent hypotension because of peripheral vasodilation. It has a pungent odor and stimulates respiratory reflexes (e.g., breath-holding, salivation, coughing, and laryngospasm) and is, therefore, not used for inhalation induction. (A) Isoflurane does not cause cardiac arrhythmias. (B) Isoflurane causes peripheral vasodilation and hypotension. (C) Isoflurane has a pungent odor and stimulates laryngospasm. (E) Isoflurane is a very stable molecule and is not significantly metabolized.

99 **The answer is B: Delayed ejaculation.** Loss of libido, delayed ejaculation, and anorgasmia are underreported side effects often noted by clinicians, but these are not prominently featured in the list of standard side effects. One option for managing SSRI-induced sexual dysfunction is to replace the offending antidepressant with an antidepressant having fewer sexual side effects such as bupropion or mirtazapine. (A) Penile sensation is likely to remain unchanged in this patient. (C) Loss of libido is likely in this patient. (D) Orgasm can be impaired in this patient. (E) Ejaculate color will be unaffected in patients taking an SSRI.

100 **The answer is C: 5-HT$_{1B/1D}$ agonist.** Sumatriptan is a 5-HT$_{1B/1D}$ agonist. This causes vasoconstriction of cerebral arteries that are thought to be inflamed during a migraine. It also decreases the activity of the trigeminal nerve, which is proposed to be the cause of some of the pain during migraines. (A) Sumatriptan does not act on 5-HT$_{1A}$ receptors. It is a 5-HT$_{1B/1D}$ agonist. (B) Sumatriptan does not act on 5-HT$_{1A}$ receptors. It is a 5-HT$_{1B/1D}$ agonist. (D) Sumatriptan does act on 5-HT$_{1B}$ receptors, but it is an agonist, not an antagonist. (E) Sumatriptan does not act on 5-HT$_3$ receptors. It is a 5-HT$_{1B/1D}$ agonist.

101 **The answer is A: Albuterol.** The shortness of breath that accompanies an asthma attack is partly caused by narrowing airways because of bronchiolar smooth muscle contraction. These smooth muscles receive both sympathetic and parasympathetic innervation. Parasympathetic stimulation of muscarinic cholinergic receptors leads to bronchoconstriction, whereas sympathetic stimulation of β_2-adrenergic receptors leads to bronchodilation. Albuterol stimulates β_2-receptors to open the airways and relieve an asthma attack. (B) Methacholine is a muscarinic cholinergic receptor agonist. Stimulation of these receptors would lead to further bronchoconstriction and an increase in secretions. (C) Neostigmine is an acetylcholinesterase inhibitor. It would cause an increase in acetylcholine leading to bronchoconstriction and an increase in secretions. (D) Nicotine binds to nicotinic receptors, not the muscarinic receptors found on bronchiolar smooth muscle. It would not cause constriction or dilation of bronchioles. (E) Pilocarpine is a muscarinic cholinergic receptor agonist. Stimulation of these receptors would lead to further bronchoconstriction and an increase in secretions.

102 **The answer is D: Trazodone.** Trazodone is an atypical antidepressant that inhibits serotonin reuptake. It can be used for insomnia as well. A side effect of trazo-

done is priapism. Other side effects include GI upset and sedation. (A) Bupropion is an atypical antidepressant. Common side effects include headaches and a lower seizure threshold but not priapism. (B) Fluoxetine is a selective serotonin reuptake inhibitor. Common side effects include GI distress and decreased libido but not priapism. (C) Maprotiline is an atypical antidepressant. Common side effects include sedation and orthostatic hypotension. (E) Venlafaxine is a serotonin-norepinephrine reuptake inhibitor. Common side effects include GI upset and increased blood pressure.

103 **The answer is B: Furosemide.** Calcium oxalate stones are caused by an increase of calcium, oxalate, or both in the urine. Stone formation can be avoided by preventing high amounts of calcium from being excreted in the urine. Loop diuretics such as furosemide increase renal excretion of calcium, thereby raising the urinary calcium level and predisposing to stone formation. (A) Amiloride inhibits the sodium–potassium exchanger in the distal tubule. It does not raise urinary calcium nearly as much as furosemide and is not associated with an increase in stone formation. (C) Hydrochlorothiazide, by an unknown mechanism, causes calcium retention. It would be a useful drug for this patient because it decreases urinary excretion of calcium. (D) Mannitol is an osmotic diuretic because it is filtered at the glomerulus but minimally reabsorbed. It does not alter calcium handling by the kidney. (E) Spironolactone is an antagonist of aldosterone. Normally, aldosterone causes resorption of sodium from the distal tubules. It does not alter calcium handling by the kidney.

104 **The answer is C: Poikilothermia.** Side effects of antipsychotic agents are important to know about. Blockade of adrenergic receptors causes orthostatic hypotension and light-headedness. The antipsychotics also alter temperature-regulating mechanisms and can produce poikilothermia (condition in which body temperature varies with the environment). In the pituitary, antipsychotics block D_2 receptors, leading to an increase in prolactin release. (A) Orthostatic hypotension is a possible side effect of long-term use of antipsychotic agents. (B) Myocardial infarction is uncommon in patients taking antipsychotic agents. (D) Pulmonary edema is unexpected in this patient. (E) Pulmonary embolism is not a typical side effect of antipsychotic agents.

105 **The answer is C: Neurotoxicity.** Meperidine provides analgesia but is not recommended for long-term use because of its active metabolite, normeperidine, which has significant neurotoxic properties. Unlike morphine, meperidine is not clinically useful in the treatment of diarrhea or cough. Meperidine produces less of an increase in urinary retention than does morphine. (A) Meperidine does not treat cough in clinical applications. (B) Meperidine does not treat diarrhea in clinical applications. (D) Both meperidine and morphine can provide good pain relief. (E) Meperidine does not increase risk of urinary retention.

106 **The answer is B: Familiar short QT syndrome.** Rufinamide in vitro acts at the sodium channels. It is approved for the adjunctive treatment of seizures associated with Lennox–Gastaut syndrome in children older than the age of 4 years and in adults. Rufinamide is a weak inhibitor of CYP2E1 and a weak inducer of CYP3A4 enzymes. Food increases absorption and peak serum concentrations. Serum concentrations of rufinamide are affected by other antiseizure medications. It is induced by carbamazepine and phenytoin and inhibited when given with valproate. Women taking birth control tablets should be counseled that they may not be effective when used concurrently with rufinamide. Adverse effects include the potential for shortened QT intervals. Patients with familial short QT syndrome should not be treated with rufinamide. (A) Rufinamide can be given to patients with egg allergy. (C) Rufinamide can be given to patients with milk allergy. (D) Rufinamide is contraindicated in women taking birth control pills. (E) Rufinamide can be given to women who have had tubal ligation.

107 **The answer is D: Valproic acid.** In utero exposure to valproate, when compared with other commonly used antiepileptic drugs, is associated with an increased risk of impaired cognitive function at 3 years of age. Valproate should not be used in women of childbearing potential. (A) Carbamezapine will produce a child with an approximate IQ of 97. (B) Lamotrigine will produce a child with an approximate IQ of 100. (C) Phenytoin will produce a child with an approximate IQ of 98.

108 **The answer is E: Thalamus.** Deep brain stimulation (DBS) therapy uses a pacemaker-like device to deliver targeted electrical stimulation to the anterior nucleus of the thalamus. The therapy is FDA-approved with conditions for adjunctive treatment for partial-onset seizures in adults with medically refractory epilepsy. DBS is also FDA-approved for treatment of advanced Parkinson disease and essential tremor. (A) DBS provides electrical stimulation to the thalamus. (B) The cerebellum is not stimulated with DBS. (C) DBS provides electrical stimulation to the thalamus. (D) The muscles of the lower extremities are not directly stimulated by DBS. Targeted electrostimulation is centered on the thalamus.

109 **The answer is D: She should be taking high doses of folic acid.** Women with epilepsy are often very concerned about pregnancy and what effect the medications might have on fetal development. Planning is the most important component. All women considering pregnancy should be on high doses of folic acid prior to conception. Divalproex and barbiturates should be avoided. Those women already on divalproex and barbiturates should be switched to other drugs before pregnancy when possible. When seizures are controlled, maintenance medication may be reduced, if possible, to the lowest dose that provides control. If seizures are not controlled, medications and dosages will need to be adjusted prior to pregnancy, if possible. The frequency and severity of seizures may change during pregnancy. (A) Barbiturates should be avoided in pregnancy. (B) Divalproex should be avoided in pregnancy. (C) Maintenance doses should be decreased or stabilized in this patient because her seizure activity is well controlled. (E) She will likely have some changes in seizure activity during pregnancy.

110 **The answer is D: Increase in bradykinins.** The increase in bradykinins has been proposed as the cause of the persistent cough from ACE inhibitors. Bradykinins accumulate because angiotensin-converting enzyme is not able to break down the bradykinins. The ACE inhibitor is switched to an angiotensin receptor blocker to avoid the side effect of a persistent cough. (A) ACE inhibitors do cause a decrease in aldosterone; however, this leads to hyperkalemia, not a persistent cough. (B) ACE inhibitors do cause a decrease in angiotensin; however, through decreased aldosterone, this leads to hyperkalemia, not a persistent cough. (C) ACE inhibitors do cause an increase in angiotensin I; however, this does not lead to a persistent cough. (E) ACE inhibitors do cause an increase in renin; however, this does not lead to a persistent cough.

111 **The answer is C: Nothing was done differently—this outcome is caused by a genetic defect.** This scenario describes a case of malignant hyperthermia. Malignant hyperthermia can be caused by any one of several genetic defects, most of which are autosomal dominant. Most cases involve a mutated ryanodine receptor and are triggered by anesthetic or succinylcholine use during surgery. The signs and symptoms appear to arise from a sudden increase in cellular metabolism. (A) Succinylcholine is a drug that can trigger malignant hyperthermia. It is a commonly used and current neuromuscular blocker. Malignant hyperthermia is not caused by use of outdated drugs. (B) This scenario describes malignant hyperthermia, not an allergic reaction. Allergic reactions can vary but commonly involve hives and, in severe reactions, anaphylaxis. Malignant hyperthermia is not an allergic reaction. (D) A ruptured appendix may produce a high fever, but the rapid rise in temperature with high CO_2 production is more consistent with malignant hyperthermia. A ruptured appendix would not itself cause these symptoms. (E) Malignant hyperthermia is not caused by a drug interaction. It occurs when succinylcholine or certain inhaled anesthetics are used in susceptible people (i.e., those with one of the genetic defects).

112 **The answer is B: Hepatitis.** Tranylcypromine is a monoamine oxidase inhibitor used to treat refractory depression. This agent can cause either hypotension or hypertension. Other effects can include hepatitis. (A) Depression would be more likely to occur than anxiety. (C) Blood glucose levels can be altered with use of this agent. (D) Dry mouth, not salivation, would be expected. (E) Tachycardia, not tachypnea, would be expected.

113 **The answer is B: Flumazenil.** Flumazenil is a benzodiazepine antagonist that acts by blocking the binding site on GABA receptors. In a patient who uses benzodiazepines chronically, flumazenil should be avoided because acute withdrawal can occur, leading to possible seizures or death. This patient never used benzodiazepines in the past. (A) Ammonium chloride is used to acidify the urine as an antidote for amphetamine overdose. (C) *N*-acetylcysteine is used as the antidote for acetaminophen overdose. (D) Naloxone is used for the treatment of opioid overdose. (E) Sodium bicarbonate is used to alkalinize the urine for the treatment of amphetamine and tricyclic antidepressant overdose.

114 **The answer is E: Tacrolimus.** Tacrolimus is an immunosuppressant used for organ transplant recipients. Tacrolimus works by binding to the FK-binding protein, which leads to decreased secretion of IL-2. A side effect of tacrolimus is hyperglycemia, which could lead to this patient's elevated blood glucose. (A) A side effect of azathioprine is bone marrow suppression, not hyperglycemia. (B) A side effect of cyclosporine is nephrotoxicity, not hyperglycemia. (C) A side effect of muromonab is cytokine release syndrome, not hyperglycemia. (D) A side effect of sirolimus is hyperlipidemia, not hyperglycemia.

115 **The answer is E: Toxicity to fetus.** These include postural hypotension, renal insufficiency, hyperkalemia, angioedema, and a persistent dry cough. The potential for symptomatic hypotension with ACE inhibitor therapy requires careful monitoring. ACE inhibitors should not be used in pregnant women because these agents are toxic to the fetus. (A) Although angioedema is an adverse effect of ACE inhibitor therapy, the fact that she has been taking it long term and not had a problem is certainly a positive finding. (B) Hyperkalemia can be easily treated with dietary modifications. (C) Persistent cough may be treated with cough suppressant medications. (D) Renal insufficiency can be monitored by periodic blood chemistries.

116 **The answer is C: A 65-year-old man with heart failure and atrial fibrillation.** Digoxin therapy is indicated in patients with severe left ventricular systolic dysfunction after initiation of ACE inhibitor and diuretic therapy. Digoxin is not indicated in patients with diastolic or right-sided heart failure (HF). Digoxin's major indication is HF with atrial fibrillation. (A) Digoxin is not indicated in patients with right-sided heart failure. (B) Digoxin is not indicated in patients with diastolic heart failure. (D) Digoxin is not indicated for pulmonary-related conditions only. (E) Digoxin is unlikely to be of benefit in this patient with minimal cardiac complaints.

117 **The answer is D: Quinidine.** The clustered symptoms of headache, dizziness, and tinnitus are characteristics of cinchonism, which is caused by quinidine. The other drugs have characteristic adverse effects, but not this particular group of effects. (A) Amiodarone does not typically cause headache and dizziness. (B) Procainamide can cause lupus-like syndrome. (C) Propranolol does not typically cause headache and dizziness. (E) Verapamil does not typically cause headache and dizziness.

118 **The answer is E: Tegaserod.** Tegaserod is a 5-HT_4 serotonin receptor agonist used in the treatment of constipation-predominant irritable bowel syndrome. The 5-HT_4 receptor is thought to help control GI motility; therefore, being an agonist will increase GI motility and prevent constipation. (A) Infliximab is a monoclonal antibody used in the treatment of Crohn disease, not irritable bowel syndrome. (B) Metoclopramide is a dopamine receptor agonist used to treat gastroparesis, not irritable bowel syndrome. (C) Ondansetron is a 5-HT_3 receptor antagonist that is used to treat vomiting, not irritable bowel syndrome. (D) Sulfasalazine is anti-inflammatory used to treat inflammatory bowel diseases, not irritable bowel syndrome.

119 **The answer is D: Magnesium hydroxide.** Of the antacids listed, magnesium hydroxide is the most likely to cause diarrhea. Magnesium is poorly absorbed by the intestinal tract, so it draws water into the feces. When water is added to magnesium hydroxide, it is known as milk of magnesia, which is used as a laxative. (A) Aluminum hydroxide is more likely to cause constipation than diarrhea. (B) Bismuth can lead to darker colored stools but is not likely to cause diarrhea. (C) Calcium carbonate is more likely to cause constipation than diarrhea. (E) Sodium bicarbonate is more likely to cause side effects involving the kidneys and cardiovascular system and has little effect on stool quality.

120 **The answer is D: PDE4 inhibitor.** Chronic obstructive pulmonary disease (COPD) exacerbations account for about 1.5 million emergency department visits every year. Treatment of COPD exacerbation often involves oxygen therapy plus glucocorticoids, bronchodilators, respiratory stimulants, and possibly antibiotics if evidence of an underlying infection exists. To prevent such costly incidents, drugs such as roflumilast have been developed in hopes of decreasing exacerbations. Roflumilast inhibits phosphodiesterase 4 (PDE4) to increase intracellular cAMP. This has the effect of decreasing the activity of inflammatory leukocytes and decreases the average amount of hospital visits for COPD exacerbation in patients with COPD. (A) Glucocorticoids work by blocking arachidonic acid production. This has a strong anti-inflammatory effect because arachidonic acid is the precursor to proinflammatory and bronchoconstrictive molecules (many prostaglandins and leukotrienes). (B) β-Agonists such as albuterol (short acting) and salmeterol (long acting) stimulate bronchiolar β-receptors to cause smooth muscle relaxation, leading to bronchodilation. Roflumilast does not cause bronchodilation. (C) Colchicine is an old drug that inhibits leukocyte chemotaxis by interfering with microtubules. It can be used to treat gout. Roflumilast does not interfere with microtubules. (E) Acetylcysteine is a drug that cleaves disulfide bonds in mucus in order to thin and loosen it. It is used in patients with cystic fibrosis. Roflumilast does not affect the composition of mucus.

121 **The answer is E: Toxic epidermal necrolysis.** This patient's physical findings along with history of sulfamethoxazole use are suggestive of Stevens–Johnson syndrome (SJS). These symptoms in a patient taking a drug with the sulfonamide moiety (also known as sulfa drugs) is worrisome because it may signal the beginning stages of toxic epidermal necrolysis. Toxic epidermal necrolysis (TEN) is characterized by ulcerations of the mucous membranes with blistering and sloughing of the skin. The mortality incidence for TEN is around 30%. (A) Anaphylaxis is the extreme form of a type I hypersensitivity reaction. It presents as shortness of breath from bronchoconstriction, possibly accompanied by shock from vasodilation. The clinical picture in this patient does not suggest this type of hypersensitivity reaction. (B) Her symptoms and history are suggestive of SJS, so the immediate concern is TEN. Sulfamethoxazole is not known to cause lactic acidosis. (C) Her symptoms and history are suggestive of SJS, so the immediate concern is TEN. Sulfamethoxazole is not known to cause rhabdomyolysis. (D) The appearance of a new rash in a patient taking a drug with the sulfonamide moiety is worrisome because it may signal the beginning stages of toxic epidermal necrolysis. Her new symptoms are not likely related to an infection.

122 **The answer is D: Inhibitor of myenteric plexus activity.** Diphenoxylate is an opioid-receptor agonist. It binds

to μ-receptors on the myenteric plexus and, like other opioids, decreases myenteric plexus activity. By inhibiting the myenteric plexus, GI smooth muscle activity is decreased. Stool transit time is increased, and it is thought that this allows more time for water absorption from the feces to decrease diarrhea. (A) Atropine is an example of an anticholinergic that can be used to treat diarrhea. Diphenoxylate does not influence signaling with acetylcholine, although it is commonly administered with atropine that does. (B) Many antidiarrheals (including diphenoxylate) have no antibiotic activity. They simply increase transit time in the bowels to allow for more water reabsorption—any underlying infection will be left to run its course. Inhibiting diarrhea in a patient with an infection may actually lengthen the patient's recovery time. (C) Many antidiarrheals (including diphenoxylate) have no antibiotic activity. They simply increase transit time in the bowels to allow for more water reabsorption—any underlying infection will be left to run its course. Inhibiting diarrhea in a patient with an infection may actually lengthen the patient's recovery time. (E) Clonidine is an example of a sympathetic nervous system stimulant that can be used for diarrhea. Data are limited regarding its efficacy in treating diarrhea, and it is usually only used in refractory cases. Diphenoxylate does not treat diarrhea by modulating sympathetic nervous system activity.

123 **The answer is B: Dextromethorphan.** Dextromethorpan is an opioid used for cough suppression. Dextromethorphan is an agonist of μ-, δ-, and κ-receptors for analgesia, but it has a very low potency. It exhibits its cough suppressant properties by acting centrally on the cough center in the medulla. (A) Butorphanol is an opioid used most commonly for pain control, not cough suppression. (C) Diphenoxylate is an opioid used for diarrhea, not cough suppression. (D) Guaifenesin is an expectorant used for productive coughs, but it is not an opioid. (E) Loperamide is an opioid used for diarrhea, not cough suppression.

124 **The answer is C: Latanoprost.** Latanoprost is a prostaglandin $F_{2\alpha}$ analog that increases the outflow of aqueous humor from the eye. A side effect of latanoprost is causing darkening of the iris, which the patient exhibits with her blue eyes turning brown. (A) Acetazolamide can cause blurry vision, but not darkening of the iris. (B) Epinephrine can cause mydriasis or burn when placed in the eye, but not darkening of the iris. (D) Pilocarpine can cause miosis, but not darkening of the iris. (E) Physostigmine can cause miosis, but not darkening of the iris.

125 **The answer is E: Tramadol.** The patient has a history of seizures, and therefore should avoid tramadol. Tramadol decreases the seizure threshold. In patients without a seizure history, it is very rare for tramadol to cause a seizure. (A) Acetaminophen does not lower the seizure threshold. (B) Butorphanol should not be used in with other opioids because it can lead to withdrawal symptoms, but it does not lower the seizure threshold. (C) Fentanyl can lead to respiratory depression at high doses but does not lower the seizure threshold. (D) Morphine can lead to respiratory depression at high doses but does not lower the seizure threshold.

126 **The answer is B: Cimetidine.** There are many drugs that decrease the amount of acid in the stomach to reduce symptoms of heartburn. One of the stimuli for acid secretion is histamine released from ECL cells binding to H_2 receptors on parietal cells. This binding activates the "proton pumps," which are ATPases on the lumenal surface that force hydrogen ions into the lumen. Cimetidine slows acid production by blocking H_2 receptors. (A) Atropine decreases gastric acid secretion by blocking acetylcholine signaling from the vagus nerve to parietal cells. It is not commonly used to treat GERD because of its systemic anticholinergic side effects. (C) Misoprostol is a prostaglandin analog. Prostaglandins inhibit acid secretion by binding G_i receptors, which lead to a decrease in intracellular cAMP and in turn to decreased H^+/K^+ ATPase activity. It does not interfere with histamine signaling. (D) Octreotide is a somatostatin analog. Although it would decrease gastric acid production, it is not used to treat GERD because of its systemic side effects. (E) Omeprazole decreases the amount of acid secreted by binding to and inhibiting the ATPase on the lumenal surface of parietal cells responsible for pumping hydrogen ions into the lumen. It does not interfere with histamine signaling.

127 **The answer is B: Imipramine.** Imipramine is a tricyclic antidepressant with antimuscarinic properties. This leads to urinary retention and is why it is used in the treatment of enuresis. Usually, bedwetting alarms and desmopressin are tried before imipramine. (A) Citalopram is a selective serotonin reuptake inhibitor that is not used for enuresis. (C) Mirtazapine is an atypical antidepressant that can be used in anorexics for weight gain, but not enuresis. (D) Trazodone is an atypical antidepressant that can be used for insomnia, but not for enuresis. (E) Venlafaxine is a serotonin-norepinephrine reuptake inhibitor that is not used for enuresis.

128 **The answer is D: Methylphenidate.** This boy has ADHD and the first-line treatment is methylphenidate. Methylphenidate increases the presynaptic release of norepinephrine, which increases the activity in the central nervous system. (A) Clomipramine is a tricyclic antidepressant that can also be used for

obsessive-compulsive disorder, not ADHD. (B) Fluoxetine is a selective serotonin reuptake inhibitor used for major depression, not ADHD. (C) Lithium is a mood stabilizer used in the treatment of bipolar disorder, not ADHD. (E) Venlafaxine is a serotonin-norepinephrine reuptake inhibitor that is also used for anxiety, not ADHD.

129 The answer is E: Thick ascending loop of Henle. Ethacrynic acid acts on the $Na^+/K^+/2Cl^-$ cotransport, like furosemide, in the thick ascending loop of Henle. Ethacrynic acid is used in fluid overloaded states such as congestive heart failure, nephrotic syndrome, and pulmonary edema. (A) K^+ sparing diuretics, such as spironolactone, act on the collecting tubule. (B) Mannitol, an osmotic diuretic, acts on the descending loop of Henle and the proximal convoluted tubule. (C) Hydrochlorothiazide acts on the distal convoluted tubule. (D) Acetazolamide, a carbonic anhydrase inhibitor, acts on the proximal convoluted tubule.

130 The answer is A: Gastrointestinal upset. The most common side effect of ibuprofen is gastrointestinal upset. Bleeding and rash are also common. Patients must be aware of these adverse effects. (B) Rash is more common than hives in patients taking ibuprofen. (C) Seizure disorder is uncommon in patients taking ibuprofen. (D) Teratogenicity is unlikely in patients taking ibuprofen. (E) Throat tightness is unexpected in patients taking ibuprofen.

131 The answer is A: Cold extremities. Ergot alkaloids are associated with vasoconstrictive complications. Patients may experience ischemia, cold extremities, and vasospasm. In addition, retroperitoneal fibrosis and cardiac valve fibrosis can also develop. (B) Nausea and vomiting are side effects of ergot alkaloids. (C) Muscle weakness would be expected with an ergot alkaloid. (D) Skin coldness would be expected with an ergot alkaloid. (E) Bradycardia is a side effect of ergot alkaloids.

132 The answer is B: Kidney stones. Topamax can cause dehydration. In a person with a history of kidney stones, this may increase the incidence of stone formation. Further, this medication should not be given to patients with acute myopia and glaucoma. (A) Topamax should not be given to patients with suicidal ideation. (C) Topamax should not be given to patients with acute myopia and glaucoma. (D) Topamax should not be given to patients with hepatic or renal involvement. (E) Topamax can be given to patients with tinnitus.

133 The answer is A: Bradycardia. Adverse effects associated with lidocaine jelly include dizziness, visual disturbances, tremor, bradycardia, and hypotension. (B) Erythema is a side effect of topical lidocaine. (C) Hypotension and bradycardia would be expected with this agent. (D) Temperature change would not be expected with lidocaine jelly. (E) Tinnitus would not be expected with lidocaine jelly.

134 The answer is D: Topiramate. This patient's presentation is consistent with nephrolithiasis or kidney stones. This can be attributed to her seizure medication because she has no prior history of stones. Of the seizure medications listed, only topiramate is known to cause nephrolithiasis. Topiramate is used in the treatment of partial seizures and generalized tonic-clonic seizures as well as for migraine prophylaxis. Its exact mechanism is unknown but appears to block seizure spread rather than raise seizure threshold. (A) Ethosuximide is an anticonvulsant used to treat absence seizures. It is not known to cause nephrolithiasis. (B) Phenobarbital is a CNS depressant used to treat many seizure types. Its major side effects are caused by its CNS depression. It is not known to cause nephrolithiasis. (C) Phenytoin is an anticonvulsant used to treat many types of seizures. One of its more unique side effects is gingival hyperplasia. It is not known to cause nephrolithiasis. (E) Valproic acid is an anticonvulsant used to treat multiple seizure types as well as for migraine prophylaxis. It is not known to cause nephrolithiasis.

135 The answer is E: Spironolactone. Spironolactone is very effective in the treatment of hepatic edema. These patients are frequently resistant to the diuretic action of loop diuretics, although a combination with spironolactone may be beneficial. (A) Acetazolamide would be helpful in treating hypertension but not the ascites and fluid overload. (B) Chlorthalidone would treat hypertension but not markedly improve the edema. (C) Furosemide may improve peripheral fluid edema but have limited success with central ascites fluid removal. (D) Hydrochlorothiazide would be helpful in management of outpatient hypertension without significant peripheral edema.

136 The answer is B: Hydrochlorothiazide. Hydrochlorothi azide is effective in increasing calcium reabsorption, thus decreasing the amount of calcium excreted and decreasing the formation of kidney stones that contain calcium phosphate or calcium oxalate. However, hydrochlorothiazide can also inhibit the excretion of uric acid and cause its accumulation, leading to an attack of gout in some individuals. (A) Furosemide increases the excretion of calcium and can cause an increase in kidney stone formation. (C) Spironolactone neither cause an increase in excretion of urine calcium nor cause gout. (D) Triamterene is a potassium-sparing diuretic that does not cause hypercalciuria. (E) This is a medication side effect that is important for physicians to be aware of.

137 **The answer is A: Constipation.** Ferrous sulfate is one of the iron salts used to provide dietary iron to patients. It is often prescribed for patients who are anemic but may also be used simply for iron supplementation to prevent anemia and other complications of low iron, as in this case. Most iron in the body is found in the hemoglobin of red cells, but many enzymes (e.g., those found in mitochondria) also require iron to function. One of the most common side effects of iron therapy is constipation, and iron supplements may need to be given with a stool softener to counteract this effect. (B) Constipation is a much more common side effect than diarrhea with iron supplementation. Diarrhea may result when the iron supplementation causes significant GI irritation. (C) The estrogen found in many oral contraceptives increases the risk of deep vein thrombosis (DVTs). This is not a side effect of ferrous sulfate. (D) Ferrous sulfate does not generally cause vascular instability of any kind. Hypotension may be caused by many antihypertensive drugs. (E) Ferrous sulfate is not known to cause seizures. Of the side effects listed, constipation is by far the most common.

138 **The answer is A: Location 1.** Location 1 is the proximal convoluted tubule. In this area, acetazolamide acts. This agent is a carbonic anhydrase inhibitor that inhibits bicarbonate reabsorption and acts as a weak diuretic. (B) Location 2 is the descending loop of Henle. (C) Location 3 is the ascending loop of Henle. Loop diuretics such as furosemide act here. (D) Location 4 is the distal convoluted tubule. Thiazide diuretics act here. (E) Location 5 is the collecting duct, and potassium-sparing diuretics act here.

139 **The answer is C: Stage III.** Anesthesia is divided into stages and planes to more accurately measure the depth of a patient's anesthesia. Stage I is characterized by analgesia and amnesia. Stage II is characterized by a loss of consciousness. Stage III is characterized by muscle relaxation, a regular breathing pattern, and loss of the eyelash and corneal reflexes. Stage III is also known as surgical anesthesia and is further subdivided into four planes. Stage IV is characterized by medullary depression and is the overdose stage. There is no stage higher than IV. (A) Stage I is characterized by analgesia and amnesia. The eyelash reflex (blinking of the eyelid when the eyelash is touched) is still present in this stage. (B) Stage II is characterized by loss of consciousness. The eyelash reflex (blinking of the eyelid when the eyelash is touched) is still present in this stage. (D) Stage IV is characterized by medullary depression and is the overdose stage. There is no eyelid reflex but breathing is severely impaired and irregular. (E) There is no stage of anesthesia higher than IV. Stage III is characterized by muscle relaxation, a regular breathing pattern, and loss of the eyelash and corneal reflexes.

140 **The answer is C: Praziquantel.** This patient ingested raw fish and contracted *Clonorchis sinensis*. *C. sinensis* affects the biliary system and can cause cholangitis, which this patient displays. The treatment of choice is praziquantel, which is thought to paralyze the helminth by increasing the cell membranes permeability to calcium. (A) Diethylcarbamazine is used to treat parasitic infections, such as *Toxocara*, but not *Clonorchis*. (B) Ivermectin is used to treat parasitic infections, such as *Onchocerca*, but not *Clonorchis*. (D) Pyrantel pamoate is used to treat parasitic infections, such as *Enterobius* and *Ascaris*, but not *Clonorchis*. (E) Sodium stibogluconate is used to treat parasitic infections, such as *Taenia* and *Diphyllobothrium*, but not *Clonorchis*.

141 **The answer is C: Nifurtimox.** The patient is suffering from an acute infection with *Trypanosoma cruzi*, which causes Chagas disease, and the treatment of choice is nifurtimox. It can be used in the acute stage of the infection but not in the chronic stage when the characteristic dilated cardiomyopathy and megacolon occur. (A) Chloroquine is the treatment of choice for malaria, but resistance has been increasing. (B) Melarsoprol is the treatment of choice for central nervous system invasion by *Trypanosoma gambiense*, but not *T. cruzi*. (D) Sodium stibogluconate is the treatment of choice for *Clonorchis sinensis*. (E) Suramin is the treatment of choice for blood-borne *T. gambiense*, but not *T. cruzi*.

142 **The answer is D: Primaquine.** Primaquine is added to the regimen for treatment of *Plasmodium vivax* and *Plasmodium ovale* to eradicate the dormant stages in the liver. Without primaquine, once the blood stream infection is cleared, it is likely that recurrence will still occur. However, primaquine only will not cure malaria, so both primaquine and quinine is usually prescribed. (A) Chloroquine is used in the treatment of *Plasmodium vivax* to clear the blood stream infection, but it will not affect the hypnozoites in the liver. (B) Clindamycin is used in the treatment of *Babesia*, but not *Plasmodium*. (C) Metronidazole is used to treat *Trichomonas* and *Giardia*, but not *Plasmodium*. (E) Sodium stibogluconate is the treatment of choice for *Clonorchis sinensis*.

143 **The answer is D: Nitrous oxide.** One of the first anesthetic agents was inhaled diethyl ether, often called simple ether. One major drawback to ether was its flammability, which would be especially dangerous in modern operating rooms equipped with electrosurgical devices. Similar molecules were subsequently found and developed in which carbons are halogenated, which decreases flammability (such as halothane and enflurane). Another early inhaled anesthetic that may still be used is nitrous oxide. Nitrous oxide is not a halogenated hydrocarbon and is not flammable (although it is an oxidizer). It is often used in

combination with other anesthetics to increase their efficacy. (A) Enflurane is an inhaled anesthetic containing halogenated carbons. It produces rapid anesthesia and allows quick recovery. (B) Diethyl ether was one of the first anesthetic agents. It was inhaled, but a major drawback was its flammability. (C) Halothane is an inhaled anesthetic containing halogenated carbons. In rare instances, it may result in hepatotoxicity. (E) Propofol is a drug given IV and produces hypnosis, but not analgesia. Its onset is rapid and may cause pain at the injection site.

144 The answer is D: Inhibition of norepinephrine reuptake. Cocaine's peripheral effects are mediated by norepinephrine. Once released, norepinephrine binds to postsynaptic receptors. To halt signaling, norepinephrine is taken up into the presynaptic cell or diffuses away from the synapse to be degraded by COMT and MAO. Cocaine inhibits the reuptake of norepinephrine into the nerve terminals and causes some degree of norepinephrine release. (A) Cocaine does not increase synthesis of norepinephrine. (B) Cocaine does not inhibit COMT. (C) Cocaine does not inhibit MAO. (E) Nicotine stimulates the nicotinic acetylcholine receptors found in autonomic ganglia. Cocaine is not known to interact with acetylcholine receptors.

145 The answer is E: Gas E MAC 105%. The potency of inhaled anesthetics is defined quantitatively as the minimum alveolar concentration (MAC). This is the end-tidal concentration of anesthetic gas needed to eliminate movement among 50% of patients challenged by a standardized skin incision. (Note: MAC is the median effective dose [ED50] of the anesthetic.) MAC is usually expressed as the percentage of gas in a mixture required to achieve the effect. Gas E is nitrous oxide. (A) Gas A is halothane. (B) Gas B is isoflurane. (C) Gas C is sevoflurane. (D) Gas D is desflurane.

146 The answer is B: Alveolar wash-in. This term refers to the replacement of the normal lung gases with the inspired anesthetic mixture. The time required for this process is directly proportional to the functional residual capacity of the lung (the volume of gas remaining in the lungs at the end of a normal expiration) and inversely proportional to the ventilatory rate. It is independent of the physical properties of the gas. As the partial pressure builds within the lung, anesthetic transfer from the lung begins. (A) Anesthetic uptake is the product of gas solubility in the blood, cardiac output, and the anesthetic gradient between alveolar and blood partial pressure gradients. (C) The potency of inhaled anesthetics is defined quantitatively as the minimum alveolar concentration (MAC). (D) Solubility is determined by a physical property of the anesthetic molecule called the blood/gas partition coefficient.

147 The answer is E: Stop paroxetine and begin bupropion. Loss of libido, delayed ejaculation, and anorgasmia are underreported side effects often noted by clinicians, but these are not prominently featured in the list of standard side effects. One option for managing SSRI-induced sexual dysfunction is to replace the offending antidepressant with an antidepressant having fewer sexual side effects such as bupropion or mirtazapine. This would be the best management for this patient. (A) This patient will continue to have sexual dysfunction if the medication is continued. (B) Changing dosing to every other day will reduce therapeutic effect of this medication. (C) It would be easier to change the medication than to begin a course of psychotherapy. (D) It would be easier to change the medication than to begin a course of sexual therapy.

148 The answer is E: Trazodone. Although many antidepressants have been reported to cause priapism, trazodone is perhaps the antidepressant best known for it. Trazodone works primarily by inhibiting serotonin reuptake. Postural hypotension and decreased libido are other possible side effects of trazodone therapy. Trazodone has also been used to decrease alcohol cravings. (A) Bupropion is an antidepressant also used for smoking cessation. It is not known to cause priapism. (B) Duloxetine inhibits serotonin and norepinephrine reuptake. It is not known to cause priapism. (C) Imipramine is a tricyclic antidepressant. It can also be used in some cases of enuresis. It is not known to cause priapism. (D) Sertraline is a selective serotonin reuptake inhibitor. It is not commonly associated with priapism.

149 The answer is B: Bosentan. Bosentan inhibits endothelin-1 receptors and is used in the treatment of pulmonary hypertension. The inhibition of endothelin-1 receptors leads to pulmonary vasodilation, which decreases vascular resistance. (A) Albuterol would be more appropriate to treat asthma, not pulmonary hypertension. (C) Guaifenesin is an expectorant used to treat a productive cough, not pulmonary hypertension. (D) *N*-acetylcysteine is a mucolytic used to treat a productive cough, not pulmonary hypertension. (E) Theophylline is used to treat asthma, not pulmonary hypertension.

Chapter 6

Chemotherapeutic Drugs

QUESTIONS

Select the single best answer.

1 A 5-year-old male patient's parents complain of recurring fever in their son over the course of a month. Past medical history is significant for easy bruisability. A CBC reveals a white blood cell count of 30,000 cells per microliter. A bone marrow biopsy confirms the diagnosis of acute lymphoblastic leukemia. This child is started on a chemotherapeutic regimen. Which of the following chemotherapy drugs acts by causing cross-links to form in DNA?

(A) 5-Fluorouracil
(B) Cyclophosphamide
(C) Cytarabine
(D) Methotrexate
(E) Vincristine

2 A 54-year-old woman with a history of left-sided breast cancer has been in remission for 5 years following paclitaxel therapy coupled with surgical resection. She has now noticed a new lump in her left breast close to where the original tumor was excised. A biopsy reveals recurring cancer. After talking with her physician, she decided to undergo more chemotherapy. Her physician prescribes a drug, which inhibits DNA topoisomerase. Which chemotherapy agent inhibits topoisomerase?

(A) Cisplatin
(B) Docetaxel
(C) Erlotinib
(D) Irinotecan
(E) Vincristine

3 A 26-year-old female with a 2-week history of urinary urgency and frequency presents to her primary care physician for evaluation. Urinalysis reveals nitrates, leukocytes, and red blood cells. The physician selects a quinolone antibiotic for treatment of a presumed urinary tract infection. Which of the following organisms would be most sensitive at the lowest drug concentration?

(A) *Escherichia coli*
(B) *Haemophilus influenzae*
(C) *Neisseria gonorrhoeae*
(D) *Pseudomonas aeruginosa*
(E) *Staphylococcus aureus*

4 A 24-year-old woman who is morbidly obese undergoes a surgical procedure under anesthesia. During the procedure, she is given nitrous oxide. It turns out that after the procedure is completed, the patient learns that she was 10 weeks pregnant while she has that procedure. Which of the following potential risks is possible in the fetus?

(A) Aplastic anemia
(B) Hypotonia
(C) Oral clefts
(D) Thermoregulation abnormalities
(E) Uremia of pregnancy

5 A 20-year-old male college student returns from a trip to India complaining of fever and malaise. A peripheral blood smear confirms the suspicion of malaria. The physician prescribes chloroquine and sends the patient home. What is the problem with this physician's choice of treatment of this patient?

(A) Chloroquine is unnecessary because malaria infection is short lived and benign
(B) He should have also prescribed a drug to treat yellow fever because these diseases are often transmitted together
(C) He should have prescribed primaquine in addition to chloroquine
(D) Primaquine is not the drug of choice—he should have prescribed albendazole
(E) There is nothing wrong with this prescription

6 A 34-year-old male patient with HIV disease presents to the walk-in clinic of the emergency department with pain and blurry vision in his right eye. A dilated ophthalmoscopic exam of the right eye reveals a diffuse retinitis. What is the most appropriate treatment for this patient?

(A) Administer rimantadine
(B) Administer ganciclovir
(C) Administer ribavirin
(D) Temporal artery biopsy
(E) Check HbA_{1c} levels

7 The anesthesiologist is preparing to anesthetize a 30-year-old patient for elective surgery and plans to use inhalational anesthetic agents. Which of the following factors will make the patient more sensitive to these agents?
(A) Age
(B) Hyperpyrexia
(C) Pregnancy
(D) Use of nifedipine for hypertension
(E) Weight

8 A 5-year-old boy is going to undergo tonsillectomy. The procedure will be performed under inhalational anesthesia initially. The boy is very afraid of going to sleep. Which of the following agents would most likely agitate him the most in terms of getting him to sleep for the procedure less quickly and create the most amount of agitation during anesthetic induction?
(A) Desflurane
(B) Halothane
(C) Isoflurane
(D) Nitrous oxide
(E) Sevoflurane

9 A 39-year-old female is scheduled to undergo a laparoscopic cholecystectomy. Induction of anesthesia will be undertaken with fospropofol instead of propofol. Advantages of fospropofol over propofol include which of the following?
(A) Better cerebral perfusion than propofol
(B) Longer half-life than propofol
(C) Lower risk of infection
(D) Lower risk of pain at injection site
(E) Use allowed in hepatic failure

10 Five patients undergo surgery for various reasons. Each patient has a particular prior medical history. Which of the following patients would be most problematic to the anesthesiologist if thiopental is used during the surgery?
(A) A 5-year-old boy with recurrent otitis media
(B) A 7-year-old boy with recurrent sinusitis
(C) A 9-year-old boy with asthma
(D) A 12-year-old boy with anemia of chronic disease
(E) A 15-year-old boy who has never received anesthesia

11 A 57-year-old woman presents to the emergency department with crushing chest pain. She reports having a similar episode 2 weeks ago while shoveling snow, but the pain was much less and it went away as soon as she stopped shoveling. An ECG reveals ST segment elevation, and the doctor administers a fibrinolytic drug. Her symptoms resolve, but later she begins to vomit up blood. Which would be an appropriate medication to give now?
(A) Abciximab
(B) Aminocaproic acid
(C) Anistreplase
(D) Clopidogrel
(E) Urokinase

12 A 24-year-old man complains of night sweats, weight loss, and pruritus over several weeks. Physical exam shows nontender lymphadenopathy. A lymph node biopsy reveals Reed–Sternberg cells. He is started on a chemotherapy regimen including one drug that works primarily by trapping cells in the mitotic (M) phase of the cell cycle. Which drug is this?
(A) Bleomycin
(B) Cisplatin
(C) Etoposide
(D) Methotrexate
(E) Vincristine

13 A 25-year-old man with multiple sexual partners begins to have flulike symptoms. He visits his primary care physician who recommends an HIV screening test based on his history. He is found to have an HIV infection and begins a drug regimen. Which of the following works by blocking the cleavage of the HIV polyproteins?
(A) Darunavir
(B) Delavirdine
(C) Enfuvirtide
(D) Maraviroc
(E) Stavudine

14 A 32-year-old woman found out 1 month ago that she has HIV disease. She began a HAART regimen after learning her HIV status. Now she presents with nausea, vomiting, and abdominal pain. Serum amylase is elevated. If her condition is related to her medications, which drug is most likely the cause of her symptoms?
(A) Efavirenz
(B) Emtricitabine
(C) Nevirapine
(D) Raltegravir
(E) Ritonavir

15 A 22-year-old sexually active man presents to the ambulatory care clinic with dysuria, penile discharge, and a swollen right knee. A joint aspirate of his right knee reveals many neutrophils as well as some gram-negative diplococci. Which is the best choice to treat his condition?

(A) Ceftriaxone
(B) Cephalexin
(C) Dexamethasone
(D) Meropenem
(E) Penicillin G

16 A 58-year-old woman with end-stage cervical cancer has undergone surgery, chemotherapy, and radiation therapy. She has chronic pelvic pain and is being treated with a fentanyl patch. Because of continued intractable pain, she places three patches on at the same time. She is found dead 6 h later by her caretaker. What is the most likely explanation for her death?

(A) Cardiac arrest
(B) Cardiomyopathy
(C) Hypoventilation
(D) Pulmonary edema
(E) Pulmonary embolism

17 A 22-year-old sexually active male presents to his primary care physician with painful urination and urethral discharge. Gram stain of discharge fluid shows gram-negative diplococci. He is given ceftriaxone for gonococcal infection. What additional medication, if any, should he be given?

(A) Aztreonam
(B) Doxycycline
(C) Imipenem/cilastatin
(D) Nitrofurantoin
(E) No additional medication is needed; ceftriaxone is a suitable treatment for this patient

18 A 22-year-old African American man who is a college student plans to travel to Africa for a semester of study abroad. A university student health physician prescribes chloroquine for malaria prophylaxis starting 2 weeks before the trip. Soon after starting the regimen, the patient develops scleral icterus. What is the most likely underlying cause for the icterus?

(A) Biliary sludging
(B) Chloroquine simply turns tears yellow; this is not true icterus
(C) Drug interaction
(D) Enzyme deficiency
(E) Hepatotoxicity of chloroquine

19 A 27-year-old man presents to the urgent care clinic with multiple painful ulcers on the shaft of his penis. Some strains of the causative virus are resistant because of a mutated thymidine kinase enzyme. Which of the following antivirals may be less effective in treating this man's infection if his strain of virus has a mutated thymidine kinase?

(A) Acyclovir
(B) Cidofovir
(C) Foscarnet
(D) Oseltamivir
(E) Rimantadine

20 A 67-year-old woman presents to her primary care physician with a viral infection. She has a 45 pack-year history of smoking, and past medical history includes COPD. The virus causing her infection has a specific M2 ion channel that can be blocked by certain antivirals. With which virus is she infected?

(A) CMV
(B) HSV-1
(C) HSV-2
(D) Influenza A
(E) Influenza B

21 A 64-year-old man who has a history of transient ischemic attacks is taking clopidogrel. He presents to his primary care physician for follow-up. Which of the following should the primary care physician be concerned about in this patient?

(A) Anemia
(B) Leukemia
(C) Lymphoma
(D) Thrombotic thrombocytopenic purpura
(E) Transient ischemic attacks

22 A 45-year-old man with an elevated bleeding time is scheduled to undergo an elective hernia repair in approximately 12 h. He is given vitamin K orally and the bleeding time is still elevated. What is the most likely explanation for this finding?

(A) Interaction of vitamin K with water soluble factors
(B) Need to synthesize new coagulation factors
(C) Subtherapeutic dose of vitamin K given
(D) Toxic effect of vitamin K

23 A 65-year-old man who has already suffered one myocardial infarction because of extensive atherosclerosis is interested in modifying his risk for a second cardiac event. In terms of lipoproteins, which of the following should be modified to reduce the atherogenicity potential?

(A) Chylomicron
(B) High-density lipoprotein
(C) Low-density lipoprotein
(D) Very low-density lipoprotein

24 A 58-year-old woman presents to the ambulatory care clinic with repetitive, uncontrollable lip smacking and puckering. Past medical history includes Type-2 diabetes for which she takes glipizide and metformin, hypercholesterolemia for which she takes lovastatin, bipolar disorder for which she takes haloperidol, and hypertension for which she takes hydrochlorothiazide. Which of her medications is likely causing her symptoms?

(A) Glipizide
(B) Haloperidol
(C) Hydrochlorothiazide
(D) Metformin
(E) Lovastatin

25 A 3-year-old girl presents to the emergency department with a history of recurrent UTIs with costovertebral angle tenderness, high fever, and dysuria. A urine culture grows gram-negative lactose-fermenting rods. The physician suspects *E. coli* pyelonephritis. Ciprofloxacin is highly effective against *E. coli* in vitro, but the physician chooses not to use it in this case. Why would she choose not to prescribe ciprofloxacin?

(A) Ciprofloxacin is bacteriostatic, not bactericidal
(B) Ciprofloxacin is contraindicated in patients younger than 18 years old
(C) Ciprofloxacin is effective against *E. coli* in vitro, but not efficacious in vivo
(D) Ciprofloxacin is nephrotoxic and should not be used to treat kidney infections
(E) The physician should prescribe ciprofloxacin in this case

26 A 32-year-old G2P1 woman in her third trimester presents to the ambulatory care clinic with dysuria and urgency. Urine is nitrite positive and leukocyte esterase positive. A drug commonly used to treat urinary tract infections is trimethoprim–sulfamethoxazole, but the physician is reluctant to use it. What risk is the physician worried about?

(A) Gray baby syndrome
(B) Kernicterus
(C) Limb defects
(D) Premature labor
(E) The physician is being overly cautious; trimethoprim–sulfamethoxazole is the best drug to use in this case

27 A 25-year-old G1P0 woman presents to the emergency department with shaking chills, chest pain, and productive cough. A chest X-ray reveals an area of opacity in the right lower lobe. The physician's choice of antibiotics is limited because some may harm this patient's fetus. Which of the following antibiotics may cause hearing loss in her fetus?

(A) Amoxicillin
(B) Ciprofloxacin
(C) Erythromycin
(D) Doxycycline
(E) Streptomycin

28 A 21-year-old man presents to the ambulatory care clinic with an erythematous, swollen, painful left elbow. History is significant for untreated impetigo on his left forearm. A joint aspirate reveals gram-positive cocci in clusters. The physician begins empiric treatment with vancomycin while the organism is cultured. It is found to be methicillin susceptible. Methicillin is not widely used, but which of the following is an equivalent drug that could be used to treat this man's infection?

(A) Amoxicillin
(B) Ampicillin
(C) Oxacillin
(D) Penicillin G
(E) Penicillin V

29 A 23-year-old woman who underwent a laparoscopic appendectomy is later found to have a wound infection. A culture grows methicillin-resistant *Staphylococcus aureus* (MRSA). What is the principle mechanism this strain uses to avoid the bactericidal properties of methicillin and methicillin-related drugs?

(A) Changes a D-alanine peptidoglycan residue to a D-glycine so methicillin cannot bind
(B) Has altered PBPs that methicillin cannot bind
(C) Prevents methicillin from entering the cell
(D) Pumps methicillin out of the cell
(E) Uses a β-lactamase break down methicillin

30 A 26-year-old sexually active man presents to his primary care physician with a nonpruritic maculopapular rash on his palms. He reports that about 6 weeks ago, he developed a nonpainful ulcer on his penis that healed spontaneously. Benzathine penicillin G is administered. Twelve hours later, he begins to have myalgia, fever, and chills. What is the most likely cause of this new onset of symptoms?

(A) Development of pseudomembranous colitis
(B) Nosocomial infection
(C) Penicillin allergy
(D) Poor drug choice allowed the infection to worsen
(E) Rapid increase of endotoxins in his blood

31 A 25-year-old man presents to the emergency department with severe abdominal pain, rigors, and a temperature of 39°C. For the past 2 days, he has suffered from right lower quadrant pain and only came to the hospital when it suddenly worsened. The physician suspects ruptured appendicitis and administers imipenem with cilastatin. Cilastatin blocks which of the following enzymes to increase imipenem's efficacy?

(A) Bacterial efflux pump
(B) CYP3A4
(C) Dehydropeptidase
(D) Organic anion transporter
(E) Penicillinase

32 A 43-year-old woman who is obese undergoes laparoscopic cholecystectomy following repeated episodes of right upper quadrant pain caused by cholelithiasis. Over the next 48 h, she is found to have an MRSA wound infection. Her physician administers daptomycin. Which of the following laboratory values should she follow most closely as a result of daptomycin administration?

(A) Amylase
(B) Blood urea nitrogen
(C) Creatine kinase
(D) Lipase
(E) Troponin I

33 A 23-year-old woman presents to her primary care physician with dysuria and urgency. Urine is positive for leukocyte esterase and nitrites. Her physician prescribes co-trimoxazole for her UTI. How does co-trimoxazole inhibit bacterial growth?

(A) Inhibition of cell wall synthesis
(B) Inhibition of DNA gyrase
(C) Inhibition of nucleotide synthesis
(D) Inhibition of ribosomes
(E) Inhibition of RNA synthesis

34 A 21-year-old woman college student complains of a skin lesion near her knee on the inside of her thigh. She recently returned from a trip to Africa where she played a handmade goatskin drum. The lesion is painless with a black center. The physician suspects cutaneous anthrax and prescribes oral ciprofloxacin. Which of the following should this patient avoid taking with ciprofloxacin?

(A) Alcohol
(B) Grapefruit juice
(C) Milk
(D) St. John's wort
(E) Ciprofloxacin does not interact with any of these substances

35 A 34-year-old immigrant with HIV disease complains of a productive cough with hemoptysis and night sweats. A sputum smear is positive for acid-fast bacilli. He is placed in isolation and started on isoniazid, rifampin, pyrazinamide, and ethambutol. A few months later, he complains of a loss of his ability to discriminate certain colors. What is causing his vision impairment?

(A) Ethambutol
(B) Isoniazid
(C) Miliary TB
(D) Pyrazinamide
(E) Rifampin

36 A 73-year-old man with overwhelming sepsis requiring intravenous fluid support, pressors, and antibiotics is now beginning to improve clinically. The rationale against the use of a bacteriostatic antibiotic in this patient includes which of the following?

(A) Arrest growth of bacteria
(B) Cause cell death of pathogens
(C) Removal of viable organisms
(D) Requirement for lower doses of medication

37 A 55-year-old woman is hospitalized for treatment of osteomyelitis. The infectious organism is found to be susceptible to gentamicin so she is started on a once-daily dose of intravenous gentamicin. Which of the following symptoms may be a signal to the physician to stop gentamicin therapy?

(A) Eosinophilia
(B) Headache
(C) Nausea
(D) Salivation
(E) Tinnitus

38 A 48-year-old man who is obese and a chronic alcoholic is hospitalized for spontaneous peritonitis. He begins a course of gentamicin as part of an empiric antibiotic regimen. Which of the following medications should the physician avoid prescribing while this patient is taking gentamicin?

(A) Diazepam
(B) Disulfiram
(C) Fomepizole
(D) Furosemide
(E) Omeprazole

39 An 8-month-old female infant is brought to the emergency department by her parents. She is febrile, tachycardic, and hypotensive. Sepsis is suspected and the physician wants to give chloramphenicol but is worried about gray baby syndrome. Why does chloramphenicol sometimes cause gray baby syndrome in infants?

(A) Chloramphenicol's narrow spectrum means empiric therapy is often ineffective
(B) Clindamycin, not chloramphenicol, causes gray baby syndrome
(C) Decreased absorption from the intestines
(D) Decreased conjugation in infant liver
(E) Decreased excretion by infant kidneys

40 A 16-year-old boy presents to the ambulatory care clinic with a persistent dry cough. He had cleaned out a barn attic that was full of bats about 2 weeks ago and has had the cough for 5 days. The physician suspects histoplasmosis. Which would be the best treatment for this patient?
(A) Albendazole
(B) Griseofulvin
(C) Ketoconazole
(D) Nystatin
(E) Penicillin G

41 A 27-year-old man hospitalized following a kidney transplant develops a high fever, tachycardia, and hypotension. Blood cultures grow *Candida albicans*. He is started on amphotericin B and flucytosine. Which of the following describes part of flucytosine's mechanism of action?
(A) Disruption of microtubules
(B) Inhibition of ergosterol synthesis
(C) Inhibition of protein synthesis
(D) Inhibition of thymidylate kinase
(E) Pore formation in the fungal cell membrane

42 A 35-year-old female patient has just received a bone marrow transplant and is taking immunosuppressants. Two days after starting her immunosuppression regimen, she develops dyspnea, chest pain, and hemoptysis. A galactomannan test confirms a diagnosis of aspergillosis. She is given multiple drugs to combat this new infection, one of which is caspofungin. How does caspofungin work?
(A) Inhibition of cell membrane synthesis
(B) Inhibition of cell wall synthesis
(C) Inhibition of ergosterol synthesis
(D) Inhibition of mitotic spindle formation
(E) Inhibition of protein synthesis

43 The rationale behind the lack of use of the antibiotic tetracycline in modern day medicine relates to which of the following?
(A) Altered targets
(B) Efflux
(C) Enzymatic activation
(D) Permeability

44 A 33-year-old woman with nausea, vomiting, and diarrhea after eating a chicken meal at a country picnic presents to the emergency department. Her serum electrolytes are within normal limits. She is placed on amoxicillin and given an antidiarrheal agent. She returns for follow-up in 1 week with worsening of diarrhea and abdominal pain. What is the most likely explanation for these findings?
(A) Basic environment of the stomach
(B) Inability of antibiotic to reach intestinal crypts
(C) Incomplete secretion of antibiotic
(D) Likely fungal infection
(E) Likely viral infection

45 A 71-year-old man with osteomyelitis is treated with aminoglycosides. Blood cultures are drawn and reveal resistance to this antibiotic class. What is the most likely reason for this to occur?
(A) Increased hepatic transaminase activity
(B) Increased phosphodiesterase activity
(C) Presence of plasmid-associated synthesis of acetyltransferase
(D) Uptake of drug into oxygen-dependent transport system

46 A 42-year-old man with a history of recurrent mycoplasma pulmonary infections presents with similar complaints. Sputum culture reveals that the organism present demonstrates resistance to erythromycin and the macrolide antibiotic class. What is the most likely explanation for this finding?
(A) Ability of the organism to take up the antibiotic
(B) Improved affinity of the 50S ribosome for the antibiotic
(C) Plasmid-associated erythromycin esterase
(D) Presence of an influx pump
(E) Sulfonation of guanine

47 A 37-year-old woman with urinary frequency, urgency, and pelvic pain presents to her primary care physician. She has an allergy to quinolones and penicillin. Urinalysis reveals nitrates, leukocytes, and blood. What is the most appropriate treatment for this patient?
(A) Azithromycin
(B) Cefazolin
(C) Clarithromycin
(D) Erythromycin
(E) Levofloxacin

48 A 52-year-old man with recurrent *Pseudomonas* infections now has another infection. Culture and sensitivity now indicate that this pathogen is not sensitive to chloramphenicol. What is the most likely reason for development of resistance?

(A) Facilitated drug penetration to cell membrane
(B) MDR gene
(C) R factor
(D) Thickened cell membrane
(E) Undesirable pH

49 A 44-year-old woman with Crohn's disease in the ileum and right colon is currently maintained on medical therapy including sulfasalazine. Symptoms are currently at baseline with minimal abdominal pain and diarrhea. The most likely reason for improved pain may relate to which of the following compounds/substances?
(A) Phenazopyridine
(B) Sulfamethoxazole
(C) Sulfapyridine
(D) Tetracycline
(E) 5-Aminosalicylate

50 A 54-year-old man with a history of recurrent pulmonary tuberculosis is placed on a multidrug regimen, including isoniazid. Despite long-term therapy with this agent, the treating physician has concerns about resistance. The most likely mechanism for this to occur is which of the following?
(A) Mutation of Acyl A
(B) Mutation of Kat G
(C) Prodrug deactivation
(D) Underexpression of InhA

51 A 34-year-old man with a history of recurrent tuberculosis on a multidrug regimen, including isoniazid. He presents to his primary care physician complaining of paresthesias of his hands and feet. What is the most likely explanation for this finding?
(A) Diabetes mellitus
(B) Lumbar disc disease
(C) Peripheral neuritis
(D) Spinal cord compression
(E) Urinary tract infection

52 A 39-year-old man with HIV disease and active tuberculosis is hospitalized for therapy. He currently takes a protease inhibitor. He complains of cough, dyspnea, and chest pressure. Which of the following is the best treatment adjunct for this patient?
(A) Prednisone
(B) Rifabutin
(C) Rifampin
(D) Ribavirin
(E) Testosterone

53 A 54-year-old man with tuberculosis is maintained on a multidrug regimen including cycloserine. He complains of intermittent chest pressure and dyspnea but this does not limit his daily activities. On a cellular level, which of the following amino acids is blocked by this agent?
(A) D-alanine
(B) D-aspartate
(C) D-glutamate
(D) Para-aminobenzoate
(E) Uracil

54 A 33-year-old sexually active female with a history of recurrent vulvar *Candida* infections presents to her primary care physician for guidance. She has tried treatment with topical miconazole and also with nystatin powder. What is the likely clinical outcome given that she has been treated with both agents?
(A) Miconazole will provide a quicker treatment response
(B) Miconazole will improve concomitant urinary symptoms
(C) No significant difference in clinical outcome will be noted
(D) Nystatin powder will be better tolerated by the patient
(E) Nystatin powder will induce the hepatic cytochrome P450 system

55 A 35-year-old woman with a history of world travel is found to have a hookworm infection. She has begun on therapy with mebendazole therapy orally and now returns home for follow-up. Which of the following statements regarding the pharmacodynamics of this agent is correct?
(A) Best results are obtained with intravenous doses
(B) Hepatic first-pass metabolism is achieved
(C) Low-fat meals enhance absorption
(D) Side effect profile is unfavorable
(E) Use in pregnancy is preferred

56 A 34-year-old man is hospitalized with seizures, headache, and vomiting. CT scan of the brain reveals cysticercosis. What is the most appropriate treatment for this patient?
(A) Albendazole
(B) Niclosamide
(C) Prednisone
(D) Tetracycline
(E) Watchful waiting

57 A 4-year-old boy is hospitalized on the pediatric service with cough, runny nose, and chest pressure. Concern for respiratory syncytial virus is brought up by the treating physician. Treatment with zanamivir is undertaken. Which of the following underlying conditions can worsen bronchospasm in this patient?

(A) Adenoiditis
(B) Asthma
(C) Floppy tongue syndrome
(D) Pharyngitis
(E) Tracheitis

58 Five patients with influenza A are being considered for treatment with either rimantadine or amantadine. Which of the following patients would be better suited to receive treatment with rimantadine?

(A) A 34-year-old woman with epilepsy
(B) A 36-year-old pregnant female
(C) A 36-year-old woman who is postpartum and nursing
(D) A 39-year-old man with chronic diarrhea
(E) A 39-year-old woman with intermittent dizziness and tinnitus

59 A 45-year-old woman complains of facial wrinkles and lines. She heard of a drug for wrinkles from a friend that is a bacterial toxin and works by paralyzing skeletal muscles. What is the mechanism of action of this drug?

(A) ADP-ribosylation of $G_i\alpha$ subunits
(B) ADP-ribosylation of $G_s\alpha$ subunits
(C) Cleaves proteins necessary for vesicle fusion in lower motor neurons
(D) Inactivation of rho GTPases
(E) Inhibition of protein synthesis

60 A 52-year-old female presents with facial wrinkling that has not been satisfactorily treated with creams. She requests information on botulinum toxin A at an acquaintance's recommendation. Botulinum toxin's mechanism of action is most similar to which other bacterial toxin?

(A) Cytolethal distending toxin
(B) Heat-labile enterotoxin
(C) Heat-stable enterotoxin
(D) Shiga toxin
(E) Tetanospasmin

61 A 32-year-old man with hepatitis B refractory to several treatments has begun on a course of lamivudine. The mechanism of action of this medication likely involves which of the following?

(A) HBV DNA polymerase
(B) HBV RNA polymerase
(C) HBV RNA synthetase
(D) HBV RNA transferase

62 A 29-year-old man with recurrent herpes viral infections of the scrotum and penile shaft presents to his primary care physician because the medication is not working for him. He takes oral acyclovir for these outbreaks. Physical examination reveals active genitourinary herpes disease. What is the most likely explanation for the resistance to this medication?

(A) Deficient DNA synthase
(B) Deficient RNA polymerase
(C) Deficient RNA transferase
(D) Deficient thymidine kinase
(E) Deficient uracil synthase

63 A 45-year-old man with HIV disease and herpesvirus has begun on therapy with foscarnet. The medication is administered intravenously. If serum electrolytes are drawn on this patient after 1 week of therapy, which of the following laboratory values would be expected to be abnormal?

(A) Calcium
(B) Chloride
(C) Creatinine
(D) Glucose
(E) Sodium

64 A 25-year-old man with HIV disease presents to his primary care physician for management. His CD4 counts are dramatically lower than normal. He is being considered for therapy with protease inhibitors. Regarding the role of ritonavir in this patient, which of the following statements is true?

(A) Inhibition of CYP4A occurs
(B) This is an excellent single agent for use in therapy
(C) This agent can potentiate therapy when used with other protease inhibitors
(D) This agent is associated with resistance when used in combination with another protease inhibitor

65 Five patients with cancer and/or inflammatory disease are being considered for treatment with single agent methotrexate therapy intravenously. Which of the following patients would be expected to have the greatest objective clinical response to therapy?

(A) A 24-year-old man with Crohn's disease
(B) A 34-year-old man with choriocarcinoma of the testicle
(C) A 39-year-old woman with breast cancer and lymphatic metastasis
(D) A 45-year-old woman with breast cancer and no evidence of lymphatic spread
(E) A 55-year-old man with acute lymphocytic leukemia

66 A 43-year-old man with leukemia is hospitalized for treatment after his prior chemotherapeutic regimen failed to produce remission. Bone marrow biopsy is repeated and indicates the presence of hairy cell leukemia. Treatment with fludarabine has begun. This agent likely works in which of the following ways?

(A) Active as a prodrug
(B) Initiates action via phosphorylation
(C) Methylation
(D) Suppression of bone marrow function
(E) Trabeculation of bone islands

67 A 49-year-old man with advanced squamous cell carcinoma of the skin is treated with topical 5-fluorouracil. He presents to his oncologist for follow-up. In addition to monitoring renal and hepatic function for toxicity, one could theoretically measure levels of which of the following excreted products?

(A) Alanine
(B) Creatinine
(C) Fluoroalanine
(D) Glucose
(E) Hepatic transferase

68 A 42-year-old woman with bilateral metastatic breast cancer undergoes surgery followed by radiation and a cycle of chemotherapy. PET scan still reveals the presence of metastatic disease. She undergoes therapy with a novel chemotherapy agent capecitabine. This medication works through inhibition of which of the following?

(A) DNA synthase
(B) RNA polymerase
(C) RNA transferase
(D) Thymidylate synthase
(E) Uracil transferase

69 A 63-year-old woman presents with a productive cough, shortness of breath, and fever and chills. Past medical history is significant for chronic renal disease. After a standard dose of which of the following drugs would you expect to see the greatest increase in serum drug concentration?

(A) Cefepime
(B) Cyclosporine
(C) Doxycycline
(D) Erythromycin
(E) Nafcillin

70 A 24-year-old male soldier has just returned from a duty tour in Iraq. He complains of a 3-cm diameter nonhealing ulcer on his left forearm. He reports having an insect bite there while in Iraq. Which of the following drugs would be best for this patient?

(A) Primaquine
(B) Praziquantel
(C) Prednisone
(D) Nifurtimox
(E) Sodium stibogluconate

71 A 27-year-old man presented to the clinic for routine abroad trip preparation. He is traveling to the Caribbean in 1 month. Antidiarrheals and antimalarials are prescribed. It is noted that the patient has a history of epilepsy, latent TB, and has contracted malaria once on a prior trip. His vaccines are up to date, and he has no allergies. What medication is contraindicated for this patient?

(A) Chloroquine
(B) Diphenoxylate
(C) Doxycycline
(D) Loperamide
(E) Mefloquine

72 An 18-year-old female plans to take a mission trip to Ghana for 2 weeks during the summer following her senior year of high school. Her doctor recommends starting a regimen of mefloquine before her trip for malaria prophylaxis rather than the traditional chloroquine because of widespread resistance to chloroquine. What is the mechanism of chloroquine resistance?

(A) Antigenic variation
(B) Chloroquine is not an antimalarial in the first place
(C) Increased activity of efflux pumps
(D) Increased protozoal metabolism
(E) Modified target proteins

73 A 4-year-old boy is brought by his mother to the clinic complaining of perianal itching. He spends the weekdays at a daycare center. The mother also brings a strip of adhesive tape from the night before which she had stuck to the child's perianal area as the doctor had ordered on the phone. Microscopic examination of the tape revealed small, white, round worms. Which is the best treatment for this child?

(A) Fluconazole
(B) Mebendazole
(C) Metronidazole
(D) Nifurtimox
(E) Praziquantel

74 A 3-month-old male infant is brought to the emergency department by his parents following a 30-min seizure at home. In the emergency department, the child is not seizing and is afebrile. Prenatal history is insignificant except for a few apparently mild illnesses experienced by his mother. They own three cats. A CT scan of the infant's head reveals intracerebral calcifications and mild ventricular hypertrophy. The infant is given pyrimethamine for toxoplasmosis. Which of the following describes pyrimethamine's mechanism of action?

(A) Inhibition of dihydrofolate reductase
(B) Inhibition of dihydropteroate synthetase
(C) Inhibition of nucleic acid synthesis
(D) Membrane depolarization
(E) Ribosome inhibition

75 A 24-year-old primigravid woman's water breaks at 39 weeks gestation. Twenty-four hours later, she is having regular contractions 3 min apart. Her labor lasts 8 h. At the hospital, she gives birth to a baby boy, who initially appeared healthy. Within the next 12 h, the baby boy begins to have temperature fluctuations, difficulty breathing, and reduced movements. You suspect neonatal sepsis, so IV ampicillin is started. Which additional antibiotic could be given simultaneously to have a synergistic effect in controlling this infection?

(A) Amoxicillin
(B) Cephalexin
(C) Gentamicin
(D) Penicillin G
(E) Penicillin V

76 A 31-year-old woman with HIV disease complains of vulvar itching, burning, and vaginal discharge with rancid odor for 2 months. She presents to the ambulatory care clinic for evaluation. She has had unprotected sexual intercourse with multiple male partners during the past several weeks. The vaginal discharge is yellow-green in color, frothy, and has a pH of 7.0. Vulvovaginal examination reveals vulvar edema and erythema and petechia on the cervix. Wet smear reveals large numbers of mature epithelial cells, white blood cells, and a fusiform protozoan organism. What is the most appropriate treatment for this patient?

(A) Amoxicillin
(B) Ciprofloxacin
(C) Metronidazole
(D) Ofloxacin
(E) Tetracycline

77 A 22-year-old woman with HIV disease notes progressive visual disturbance noted by a decrease in visual acuity. She presents to the ambulatory care clinic for further evaluation and treatment. Funduscopic examination reveals large white areas proximal to the macula with perivascular exudates and hemorrhages. Treatment of this condition involves which of the following agents?

(A) Oral erythromycin
(B) Oral ganciclovir
(C) Oral penicillin
(D) Oral prednisone
(E) Intravenous prednisone

78 A 19-year-old college student man presents to the student health service with a 2-week history of headache, malaise, sore throat, and dry cough, which has become productive over the last 4 days. He states that several of his dorm mates have complained of similar problems in the last few weeks. Pulmonary auscultation reveals scattered coarse rhonchi bilaterally. What is the best treatment for this patient?

(A) Cephazolin
(B) Ciprofloxacin
(C) Oral erythromycin
(D) Intravenous erythromycin
(E) Observation alone

79 A 34-year-old woman complains of fever, fatigue, weight loss, arthralgia, and transient patchy alopecia during the last 3 months. Her review of systems is notable for occasional rhinorrhea and cough that responds well to oral decongestant therapy. Her prior surgical history is notable for cesarean section and tubal ligation at age 31 years. A similar constellation of symptoms occurred 6 months ago during treatment for a cardiovascular disease. Antinuclear antibody testing was positive at her last visit 6 months ago and is still positive at the present time. Presently, her hematocrit is 36% and creatinine is 1.2 mg/dL. The most likely etiology of this constellation of symptoms and findings is related to

(A) Ethosuximide
(B) Oral contraceptives
(C) Hydralazine
(D) Phenytoin
(E) Procainamide

80 A 35-year-old African American male in the military is hospitalized with an MRSA skin infection. The patient starts treatment with an antibiotic and becomes anemic and jaundiced. On peripheral blood smear, Heinz bodies are seen within red blood cells. What is the mechanism of action of the antibiotic given to this patient?

(A) Acts at the 50s ribosomal subunit to inhibit peptide bond formation
(B) Binds to 30s ribosomal subunit and prevents tRNA attachment
(C) Inhibits cell wall formation
(D) Inhibits DNA-dependent RNA polymerase
(E) Inhibits folic acid metabolism

81 A 12-year-old male complains of red plaques covered by silver scales on his elbows and knees. He has one older sister with similar lesions. In each case, the lesions are worse in the winter months. His pediatrician prescribes acitretin. Which of the following may this boy experience as a result of this treatment?
(A) Adrenal insufficiency
(B) Alopecia
(C) Cushing syndrome
(D) Immunosuppression
(E) Striae

82 A 41-year-old man with a history of gastroesophageal reflux disorder and diabetes mellitus is managed with cimetidine and diet/exercise for these disorders. The fact that he takes cimetidine means that the treating physician must be attune to increased effects of which of the following drugs?
(A) Dronabinol
(B) Erythromycin
(C) Ketoconazole
(D) Phenytoin
(E) Rifampin

83 A 35-year-old male with ulcerative colitis has recently been diagnosed with colon cancer. He needs to have a partial colectomy to remove the distal portion of the colon. The patient has no other medical problems. What antibiotic is most appropriate prior to his upcoming colectomy?
(A) Ceftriaxone
(B) Clindamycin
(C) Metronidazole
(D) Neomycin
(E) Trimethoprim–sulfamethoxazole

84 An 18-year-old male college student presents to the emergency room with a fever of 103°F and stiff neck for the past 3 h. After a lumbar puncture and Gram stain, the diagnosis of meningococcal meningitis is established. Unfortunately, his college did not require students to have the meningococcal vaccine. What prophylaxis should be given to his close contacts in the dorm?
(A) Benzathine penicillin G
(B) Ceftriaxone
(C) Penicillin
(D) Rifampin
(E) Trimethoprim–sulfamethoxazole

85 A 41-year-old woman with acute myelogenous leukemia is undergoing a weekly intravenous infusion of chemotherapeutic agents. Upon completion of each cycle, she develops severe nausea and vomiting. A pharmacologic agent is administered intravenously, which seems to decrease nausea in this patient. This agent might have a mechanism of action at which of the following receptors?
(A) 5-HT_1
(B) 5-HT_2
(C) 5-HT_3
(D) Dopamine

86 A 26-year-old sexually active HIV-negative man presents to his primary care physician with a nonpruritic maculopapular rash on his palms. He reports that about 6 weeks ago, he developed a nonpainful ulcer on his penis that healed spontaneously. He is injected with a single dose of benzathine penicillin G intramuscularly and sent home. What, if anything, should have been done differently for this patient's care?
(A) A different antibiotic class should have been used
(B) A different preparation of penicillin G (not benzathine) should have been used
(C) Nothing—the course of action taken is entirely appropriate
(D) Penicillin V should have been given instead of penicillin G
(E) The first shot should have been followed with a second dose 1 week later

87 A 35-year-old man with HIV disease presents to the emergency department with a severe headache and fever for the past 6 h. His fever was measured to be 103°F. He also has chills, stiff neck, and nausea. He is diagnosed with *Cryptococcus neoformans* meningitis and started on amphotericin B. What is the mechanism of action of amphotericin B?
(A) Binds ergosterol
(B) Inhibits cell wall synthesis
(C) Inhibits DNA synthesis
(D) Inhibits ergosterol synthesis
(E) Inhibits squalene epoxidase

88 A 47-year-old male presented with a fungal infection 2 weeks ago and was treated appropriately with an antifungal. However, the man returns today because of noticeable enlargement of his breasts. He read on the Internet that the medication he was given can cause gynecomastia. What antifungal was he most likely given?
(A) Amphotericin B
(B) Caspofungin
(C) Flucytosine
(D) Griseofulvin
(E) Ketoconazole

89 A 31-year-old G3P2002 woman is 30 weeks pregnant and presents for her routine checkup. She has known HIV disease, which she did not have during her two other pregnancies. Her viral load is 1,000 and CD4 count is 455. In order to decrease the likelihood of transmission of HIV disease to her baby, she has been advised to have a cesarean section, not breastfeed, and take an antiviral for HIV disease. What HIV disease medication has been proven to decrease the likelihood of the transmission of HIV disease from the mother to the fetus?

(A) Efavirenz
(B) Enfuvirtide
(C) Indinavir
(D) Lamivudine
(E) Zidovudine

90 A 21-year-old female presented to clinic for lesions on her vulva. The painful and itchy lesions have a red base and are vesicular. She recently has had a new sexual partner. The diagnosis of herpes is established and the patient is started on acyclovir. She becomes resistant to acyclovir and it therefore becomes ineffective. What is the mechanism of resistance for acyclovir?

(A) Lack of thymidine kinase
(B) Lack of viral kinase
(C) Mutated CMV DNA polymerase
(D) Mutation in DNA polymerase
(E) Mutated M_2 protein

91 A 68-year-old man with recurrence of prostate cancer after prostatectomy has been receiving chemotherapy treatments. His last prostate-specific antigen (PSA) was 1.4. The chemotherapy has caused a decrease in production from his bone marrow. His hemoglobin is 9.6 g/dL, hematocrit is 28.1%, and platelet count is 44,000/μL. What medication can be given to stimulate bone marrow production of platelets?

(A) Aldesleukin
(B) Erythropoietin
(C) Filgrastim
(D) Oprelvekin
(E) Sargramostim

92 A 33-year-old man undergoes sinus surgery under general anesthesia. Which of the following anesthetic agents exits the body most quickly after administration?

(A) Enflurane
(B) Halothane
(C) Isoflurane
(D) Nitrous oxide

93 A 5-year-old male patient's parents complain of recurring fever in their son over the course of a month. Past medical history is significant for easy bruisability. A CBC reveals a white blood cell count of 30,000 cells per microliter. A bone marrow biopsy confirms the diagnosis of acute lymphoblastic leukemia. This child is started on a chemotherapeutic regimen. Which of the following chemotherapy drugs interferes with DNA synthesis after its metabolite is incorporated into the growing DNA strand?

(A) 5-Fluorouracil
(B) Cyclophosphamide
(C) Cytarabine
(D) Methotrexate
(E) Vincristine

94 A 54-year-old woman with a history of left-sided breast cancer has been in remission for 5 years following paclitaxel therapy coupled with surgical resection. She has now noticed a new lump in her left breast close to where the original tumor was excised. A biopsy reveals recurring cancer. After talking with her physician, she decided to undergo more chemotherapy. Her physician prescribes a drug, which interferes with microtubules. Which is a chemotherapy drug that disrupts the microtubule assembly?

(A) Cisplatin
(B) Docetaxel
(C) Erlotinib
(D) Irinotecan
(E) Vincristine

95 A 42-year-old woman presents to the emergency department with vaginal bleeding for the past 2 days. Her last menstrual period was 1 week ago and has had regular cycles. She has a history of a hydatidiform mole 8 years ago. A β-hCG is 20,000. The diagnosis of choriocarcinoma is made and she is started on methotrexate. What is the mechanism of action of methotrexate?

(A) Alkylates DNA
(B) Inhibits dihydrofolate reductase
(C) Inhibition of DNA polymerase
(D) Inhibits thymidylate synthase
(E) Inhibits topoisomerase II

96 A 66-year-old man with a history of gout was recently diagnosed with non-Hodgkin's lymphoma. Because of frequent gout attacks, he has been placed on allopurinol. He is started on medication for his lymphoma, and shortly after, he develops GI upset and elevated liver enzymes. Because of taking allopurinol, what medication should have been avoided in this patient?

(A) 5-Fluorouracil
(B) 6-Mercaptopurine
(C) 6-Thioguanine
(D) Bleomycin
(E) Methotrexate

97 A 24-year-old man with Hodgkin's lymphoma presents to the emergency department with chest pain for the past 2 days. An electrocardiogram shows nonspecific changes. An echocardiogram is performed that shows dilation of the left ventricle, and the diagnosis of dilated cardiomyopathy is made. He has been receiving chemotherapy for Hodgkin's lymphoma over the last month. What medication is most likely responsible for his cardiomyopathy?
(A) Bleomycin
(B) Cisplatin
(C) Dactinomycin
(D) Doxorubicin
(E) Vincristine

98 A 70-year-old man presents to clinic because of low-grade fever for the past 2 weeks. He otherwise feels well. On exam, the physician is able to palpate an enlarged spleen. A complete blood count shows a WBC count of 43,000/μL. A peripheral blood smear confirms the diagnosis of chronic myelogenous leukemia. Chromosomal studies are positive for the Philadelphia chromosome. What is the mechanism of action of the medication given to halt the progression of the disease?
(A) Binds to CD20 antigen
(B) Binds to HER-2
(C) Cross-link DNA
(D) Inhibits DNA polymerase
(E) Tyrosine kinase inhibitor

99 A 47-year-old woman with a rheumatoid arthritis comes to clinic for her annual visit. Her arthritis has not worsened over the past 6 months since starting on infliximab. Her arthritis is worst in the joints of her hands. After her morning stiffness ceases, she can usually go through the rest of the day with minimal pain. What is the mechanism of action of infliximab?
(A) Anti-TNF antibody
(B) Directly binds to TNF receptor
(C) Inhibits cyclooxygenase
(D) Inhibits dihydrofolate reductase
(E) TNF receptor that binds TNF

100 A 61-year-old man with osteoarthritis comes to the clinic for follow-up. His arthritis has been worsening over the past year. He has pain constantly throughout the day. He reports the only medication that was effective for him was celecoxib, which was pulled from the market. He is willing to try anything that will improve his pain at this point. What side effect is the reason for the removal of celecoxib from the market?
(A) Increased risk of cardiomyopathy
(B) Increased risk of GI bleeding
(C) Increased risk of pulmonary fibrosis
(D) Increased risk of thrombosis
(E) Increased risk of tuberculosis

101 A 12-year-old boy cuts his hand on a soda can. He has a 5-cm laceration on the palmar aspect of his hand that will require suturing. The emergency department physician injects 1% lidocaine into the wound after careful cleansing with Betadine. The mechanism of action of lidocaine blocks which of the following modalities?
(A) Cerebellar function
(B) Peripheral nervous activity
(C) Pontine function
(D) Spinal reflexes
(E) Temperature sensation

102 A 37-year-old man with a schizophrenia presents to the emergency room with worsening symptoms. He has been hearing voices in his head that tell him to hurt other people. He is scared by these thoughts and wants help. He is currently taking risperidone. The physician changes him to clozapine. What should the physician monitor while the patient is taking clozapine?
(A) BUN/Creatinine
(B) Complete blood counts
(C) Liver function tests
(D) Pulmonary function tests
(E) Thyroid function tests

103 A 25-year-old man with multiple sexual partners begins to have flulike symptoms. He visits his doctor who recommends an HIV screening test based on his history. He is found to have an HIV infection and begins a drug regimen. Which of the following works by inhibiting fusion of the virion with T cells?
(A) Darunavir
(B) Delavirdine
(C) Efavirenz
(D) Maraviroc
(E) Stavudine

104 A 32-year-old woman found out 1 month ago that she has HIV disease. She began a HAART regimen after learning her HIV status. Now she presents with nausea, vomiting, and abdominal pain. Serum amylase is elevated. If her condition is related to her medications, which drug is most likely the cause of her symptoms?
(A) Didanosine
(B) Efavirenz
(C) Emtricitabine
(D) Nevirapine
(E) Raltegravir

105 A 46-year-old woman with chronic pelvic pain caused by endometriosis consults a pain management specialist regarding options for treatment. Which of the following statements is true regarding chronic pain management in this patient?

(A) Hydrocodone is metabolized in the kidney
(B) Hydrocodone is used as an antiemetic
(C) Morphine is the methyl ether of codeine
(D) Morphine and hydrocodone have equal analgesic potency
(E) Morphine will provide cough suppression

106 A 26-year-old man with schizophrenia takes daily codeine for no apparent reason. He does not have issues with upper respiratory disease. Which of the following effects would be least likely to be exhibited by this patient?

(A) Analgesia
(B) Dry cough
(C) Euphoria
(D) Sedation
(E) Tinnitus

107 A 23-year-old G1P0 woman at 34 weeks gestation presents to the labor and delivery floor with contractions. The contractions are intense and occurring regularly every 3 min. The physician wants to slow down the contractions and try to delay labor until betamethasone can be given. What medication would be most appropriate?

(A) Clomiphene
(B) Dinoprostone
(C) Ethinyl estradiol
(D) Mifepristone
(E) Ritodrine

108 When comparing the effects of overdose of meperidine and morphine in the emergency department evaluation of patients, which of the following features would be characteristic of meperidine overdose?

(A) Cerebral blood vessel dilation
(B) Increase in cerebral blood flow
(C) Euphoria
(D) Pain relief
(E) Pupillary dilation

109 A 28-year-old man who suffered a crush injury to his lumbar spine (L4 and L5) with disc herniation is managed with meperidine for pain control. He has been taking this medication for 6 months. In addition to pain relief, which of the following other effects is possible?

(A) Cough
(B) Diarrhea
(C) Neurotoxicity
(D) Tinnitus
(E) Urinary retention

110 The pain of a 57-year-old man with metastatic colorectal cancer to liver, bone, and brain is an inpatient on the oncology service. He is managed with a morphine pump. However, he has become tolerant to morphine. Which of the following might be indicated to ameliorate his pain?

(A) Buprenorphine
(B) Codeine
(C) Fentanyl
(D) Methadone
(E) Meperidine

111 A 28-year-old man presents to the emergency department with diarrhea for the past 2 days. He went on a camping trip 10 days ago. His loose stools are foul smelling and have been associated with abdominal pain and nausea. Stool analysis shows cysts. What is the most appropriate treatment?

(A) Clindamycin
(B) Ivermectin
(C) Metronidazole
(D) Praziquantel
(E) Sulfadiazine

112 A 42-year-old woman who recently immigrated to the United States from Africa presents with diffuse abdominal pain and an unusual rash. The erythematous linear rash spreads from her right upper quadrant to the umbilicus. Laboratory testing confirms the diagnosis of *Toxocara canis* infection. What is the most appropriate treatment?

(A) Diethylcarbamazine
(B) Ivermectin
(C) Mebendazole
(D) Praziquantel
(E) Pyrantel pamoate

113 A 67-year-old woman presents to the emergency department after seizure-like activity. This is her first seizure and a CT scan of her head is performed. The CT scan shows numerous calcified and uncalcified cysts throughout her brain. Her husband does report that they went to a cookout that had a pig roast. What is the most appropriate treatment?

(A) Diethylcarbamazine
(B) Ivermectin
(C) Mebendazole
(D) Praziquantel
(E) Pyrantel pamoate

114 An 8-year-old boy presents to the clinic with an extremely itchy rash for the past 2 days. He is the fourth student from his class to present with the same symptoms. The rash is across his hands, wrists, and elbows bilaterally. Small erythematous papules with obvious burrows, which look like insect bites, are aligned in 8-cm segments. What is the most appropriate treatment?

(A) Diphenhydramine
(B) Doxycycline
(C) Lindane
(D) Permethrin
(E) Topical corticosteroid

115 A 47-year-old man with a history of spina bifida presents to the emergency department with a fever. His temperature was 102°F orally. He has a neurogenic bladder secondary to his spina bifida. A urinalysis showed an infection, and culture grew out vancomycin-resistant *Enterococcus*. He is started on Linezolid. What is the mechanism of resistance of bacteria to vancomycin?

(A) Acetylation of vancomycin
(B) β-Lactamase cleavage of β-lactam ring
(C) D-ala replaced by D-lac in the cell wall
(D) Decreased uptake by bacterial cell
(E) Methylation of rRNA

116 A 32-year-old G2P1001 woman at 36 weeks gestation presents to the emergency room with a high fever. The fever started 2 days ago and has progressively worsened. It has been associated with chills, nausea, vomiting, and full body aches. The resident suggests starting trimethoprim–sulfamethoxazole as part of the empiric coverage of her infection until blood cultures return. What side effect would be a contraindication to starting trimethoprim–sulfamethoxazole in a pregnant woman?

(A) Cartilage damage in fetus
(B) Discoloration of teeth
(C) Gray baby syndrome
(D) Kernicterus
(E) Ototoxicity

117 A 21-year-old woman college student presents to an urgent care clinic with vaginal discharge for the past 3 days. The whitish discharge has a foul odor. A wet prep of the discharge shows squamous cells surrounded by rod-shaped bacteria. The addition of KOH produces a positive whiff test. What is the most appropriate for this patient?

(A) Ceftriaxone
(B) Doxycycline
(C) Metronidazole
(D) Penicillin
(E) Trimethoprim–sulfamethoxazole

118 A 24-year-old sexually active woman presents with vaginal itching and a greenish, frothy vaginal discharge. Her boyfriend is asymptomatic. She is prescribed with metronidazole for *Trichomonas* infection. Which of the following is involved in metronidazole's action?

(A) Blocking folic acid synthesis
(B) Disruption of DNA
(C) Inhibition of PBPs
(D) Inhibition of ribosomes
(E) Inhibition of topoisomerase

119 A 24-year-old woman comes to the emergency department presenting with flank pain and high fever. The pain and fever have been associated with dysuria and increased frequency of urination. She is diagnosed with pyelonephritis and placed on IV antibiotics. After a couple of days, she develops ringing in her ears and feels unbalanced on her feet. What antibiotic was she most likely given?

(A) Ceftriaxone
(B) Ciprofloxacin
(C) Gentamicin
(D) Trimethoprim–sulfamethoxazole
(E) Tetracycline

120 A 17-year-old high school football player presents to clinic with painful burning of his feet. Football practice started 3 weeks ago, and for the past week, he has had blisters and cracking of the skin of his feet. The skin between his toes is erythematous and scaly. He is diagnosed with tinea pedis and started on clotrimazole. What is the mechanism of action of clotrimazole?

(A) Binds ergosterol
(B) Inhibits cell wall synthesis
(C) Inhibits DNA synthesis
(D) Inhibits ergosterol synthesis
(E) Inhibits squalene epoxidase

121 A 27-year-old man has been hospitalized with fatigue and feeling sick for the past 4 months. After many tests and labs, an HIV test is performed and comes back positive. His HIV viral load is 36,000 and CD4 count is 369. He is started on multidrug therapy for his HIV disease. One of the drugs is raltegravir. What is the mechanism of action of raltegravir?

(A) Binds to viral gp41
(B) Inhibits fusion of viral cells to CD4 cells
(C) Inhibits integrase
(D) Inhibits protease
(E) Inhibits reverse transcriptase

122 A 46-year-old man with HIV disease presents to clinic because of a change in the appearance of his face over the past couple of months since he started antiviral therapy. His face looks sunken, particularly in the cheeks. His arms also appear to be wasting, whereas his breast tissue seems larger. He is unsure why this occurred. What medication is most likely responsible for this patients' appearance?

(A) Efavirenz
(B) Enfuvirtide
(C) Nevirapine
(D) Raltegravir
(E) Ritonavir

123 A 43-year-old man with HIV disease presents to the emergency room with blurry vision and eye pain for the past 3 days. His symptoms began in the left eye and now the right eye is involved. His CD4 count is found to be 43. Funduscopic exam confirms the most likely cause for the patients' symptoms is CMV retinitis. What is the most appropriate treatment for CMV retinitis?

(A) Acyclovir
(B) Ganciclovir
(C) Nevirapine
(D) Ribavirin
(E) Ritonavir

124 A 22-year-old man with panic disorder presents to his primary care physician for follow-up. His current medications include Klonopin. Physical examination of the heart, lungs, and abdomen are normal. Which of the following drug interactions is important for the treating physician to be aware of?

(A) Creates anxiety when given with alcohol
(B) Exercise caution when given with -azole antifungals
(C) Hyposalivation is a common side effect
(D) Paradoxical reactions are unusual

125 A 55-year-old man with long-standing bipolar disorder has been treated with numerous agents, which have failed to improve his symptoms. He is started on aripiprazole by his primary care physician. Important treatment warnings for this medication include which of the following?

(A) Hypertension
(B) Leukocytosis
(C) Pneumothorax
(D) Pneumonia, aspiration type
(E) Spermatogenesis abnormality

126 A 13-year-old female presents to her primary care physician with 3 months of hip and leg pain. Imaging tests and immunohistochemistry point to Ewing's sarcoma. She begins a chemotherapy regimen. One of her chemotherapeutic drugs is ifosfamide. Which of the following is a serious potential side effect of ifosfamide therapy?

(A) Anxiety
(B) Diarrhea
(C) Hemorrhagic cystitis
(D) Hepatic failure
(E) Hyperkalemia

127 A 22-year-old African American man who is a college student plans to travel to Africa for a semester of study abroad. A university student health physician prescribes a drug for malaria prophylaxis starting 2 weeks before the trip. Soon after starting the regimen, the patient develops scleral icterus. Which drug was he most likely given?

(A) Amoxicillin
(B) Atovaquone
(C) Chloroquine
(D) Doxycycline
(E) Mefloquine

128 Newer indications for the use of antithrombolytic agents such as heparin may include which of the following?

(A) A 32-year-old man with a clogged dialysis catheter
(B) A 45-year-old man with large pulmonary embolism
(C) A 55-year-old woman with multiple small pulmonary emboli
(D) A 62-year-old man with deep venous thrombosis after pelvic surgery
(E) A 71-year-old man with deep venous thrombosis after colon surgery

129 Five patients are considered for heparin therapy following a thrombotic event. Which of the following patients can safely receive heparin?

(A) A 23-year-old man with head trauma
(B) A 35-year-old woman with intracranial bleeding
(C) A 50-year-old man with brain tumor and metastatic colon cancer
(D) A 65-year-old man with an evolving cerebrovascular accident
(E) A 71-year-old woman with Parkinson's disease and a urinary tract infection

130 A 29-year-old pregnant woman complains of pain and swelling of her left calf. Physical examination reveals a palpable cord in the left calf with swelling. Ultrasound reveals a thrombosis of the popliteal vein. The patient, who was in her second trimester of pregnancy, was treated for 7 days with intravenous unfractionated heparin. The pain resolved during the course of therapy, and the patient was discharged on day 8. Which one of the following drugs would be most appropriate outpatient follow-up therapy for this patient who lives approximately 3 h from the nearest health care facility?

(A) Aspirin
(B) Alteplase
(C) Low-molecular-weight heparin (LMWH)
(D) Unfractionated heparin
(E) Warfarin

131 A 20-year-old woman presents to her primary care physician with heavy menstrual bleeding. An endometrial biopsy revealed no cellular atypia. Her physician prescribes tranexamic acid. What is tranexamic acid's mechanism of action?

(A) Activates plasminogen
(B) Activates platelets
(C) Blocks cyclooxygenase
(D) Inhibits plasmin
(E) Suppresses LH surge

132 A 66-year-old woman with breast cancer presents to the emergency department after seeing blood in her urine for the second straight day. The entire toilet bowl was pink after she urinated. She has had dysuria for about 4 days as well. She has been receiving chemotherapy and radiation of her breast cancer. What chemotherapeutic drug is the most likely cause of her gross hematuria?

(A) Busulfan
(B) Cisplatin
(C) Cytarabine
(D) Doxorubicin
(E) Ifosfamide

133 A 21-year-old man with Hodgkin's lymphoma presents to his primary care physician for follow-up. He has been treated with the MOPP chemotherapy regimen, which includes vincristine. He has responded well, and it is anticipated that he will be cancer free in the near future. What is the mechanism of action of vincristine?

(A) Alkylates DNA
(B) Blocks polymerization of microtubules
(C) Cross-links DNA
(D) Inhibits topoisomerase II
(E) Stabilizes polymerized microtubules

134 A 3-year-old boy with a history of a Wilms tumor presents to the pediatric oncology clinic for follow-up. His right kidney was removed 1 month ago and he recently began chemotherapy. His mother reports he has been doing well. On the neurologic exam, he is found to have absent reflexes. What chemotherapeutic agent is most likely responsible for his areflexia?

(A) Carboplatin
(B) Dactinomycin
(C) Doxorubicin
(D) Vinblastine
(E) Vincristine

135 A 21-year-old woman complains of heavy menstrual bleeding and cramping. She is taking a large class load at a local university and says her periods are interfering with her academic performance. Her physician prescribes a drug that interferes with E2 synthesis in the ovary. Which drug is this?

(A) Danazol
(B) Estradiol valerate
(C) Misoprostol
(D) Naproxen
(E) Pitocin

136 A 46-year-old woman with chronic pelvic pain presents to her primary care physician for evaluation and follow-up. Her urinalysis is normal. Pelvic examination is unremarkable. She has begun on therapy with gabapentin. Important adverse effects of this medication include

(A) Aplastic anemia
(B) Dizziness
(C) Hepatitis
(D) Pancreatitis
(E) Tetany of skeletal muscle

137 A 54-year-old man with chronic low back pain has some exacerbations of pain with lifting. He is placed on tramadol to control his pain. He is also dependent on opioids for pain control. Which of the following is an important issue for the treating physician to be aware of?

(A) Can cause dry skin
(B) Contraindicated in patients with opioid dependence
(C) Contraindicated in patients with nicotine dependence
(D) Recommended in pregnancy

138 A 27-year-old man presents with multiple painful ulcers on the shaft of his penis. The physician wants to prescribe a drug that he can take orally as an outpatient to treat his herpes infection. Which of the following would be the best choice for this patient?

(A) Acyclovir
(B) Cidofovir
(C) Foscarnet
(D) Ganciclovir
(E) Valacyclovir

139 A 67-year-old woman presents to the ambulatory care clinic with a viral infection. She has a 45 pack-year history of smoking, and past medical history includes COPD. The virus causing her infection has a specific M2 ion channel that can be blocked by certain antivirals. Which antiviral blocks the M2 ion channel?

(A) Fomivirsen
(B) Oseltamivir
(C) Rimantadine
(D) Valganciclovir
(E) Zidovudine

140 A 45-year-old man presents to the emergency department after cutting his finger with a handsaw. There is a deep 2-cm long laceration on his right index finger. Bupivacaine is used as local anesthesia for suturing. What nerve function is lost first when bupivacaine is used?

(A) Muscular tone
(B) Pain
(C) Proprioception
(D) Temperature
(E) Touch

141 A 32-year-old woman presents to her primary care physician with 4 months of dry, itchy scalp. She says she has removed large flakes of dead skin many times and has tried scrubbing her hair with more vigor than normal, but the flakes recur and her condition has not improved. A KOH preparation of some of the skin flakes reveals long hyphae accompanied by clusters of small spheres under light microscope. Which of the following would help her condition?

(A) Avoid foods containing gluten
(B) Griseofulvin
(C) Mebendazole
(D) Selenium sulfide
(E) Vancomycin

142 A 54-year-old man complains of painful, swollen joints in his toes and fingers. He has a long history of gout. The metatarsal phalangeal joint of his right great toe is exquisitely tender. He has tried colchicine and allopurinol in the past, but without much relief. His physician now prescribes pegloticase. What is the mechanism of action of pegloticase?

(A) Breaks down urate
(B) Enhances xanthine oxidase
(C) Impair neutrophil chemotaxis
(D) Increases urate excretion
(E) Inhibits xanthine oxidase

143 A graph of the minimal alveolar concentrations (MAC) for various anesthetic agents is shown in the following figure. Which of the following agents would be least potent for use as an anesthetic agent?

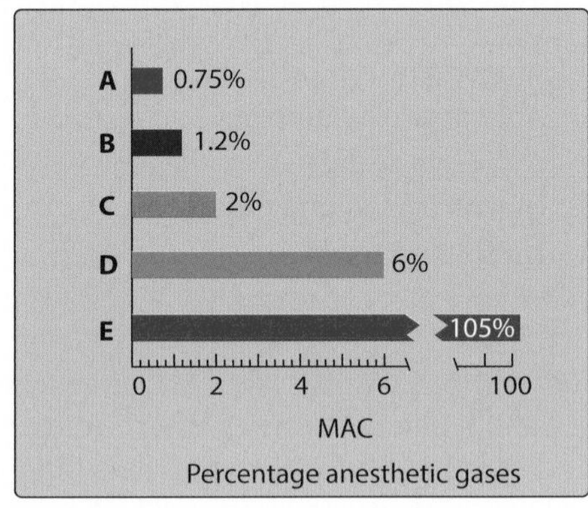

(A) Letter A
(B) Letter B
(C) Letter C
(D) Letter D
(E) Letter E

144 A graph of the blood/gas partition coefficients for various anesthetic agents is shown in the following figure. Which of the following agents would be most soluble in blood?

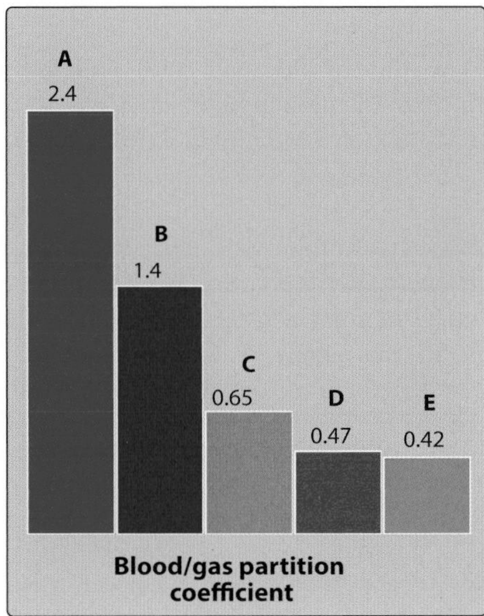

(A) Letter A
(B) Letter B
(C) Letter C
(D) Letter D
(E) Letter E

145 A graph of the alveolar concentration for various anesthetic agents at induction is shown in the following figure. Which of the following agents would have the highest alveolar concentration 10 min after induction?

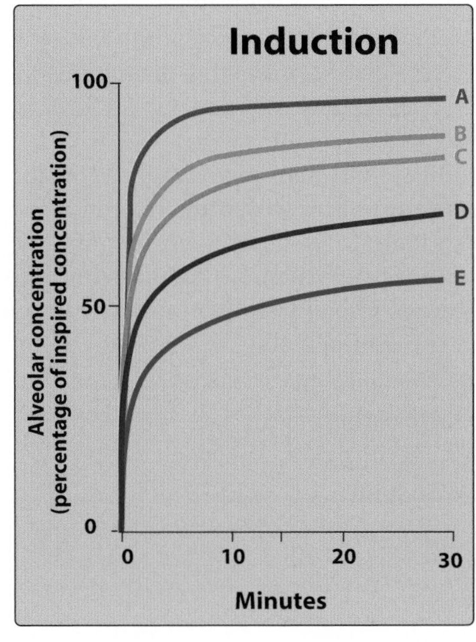

(A) Letter A
(B) Letter B
(C) Letter C
(D) Letter D
(E) Letter E

146 A 49-year-old man with a history of prostate cancer undergoes radical prostatectomy. He is given thiopental as an induction agent for the procedure. At 2 h after induction, where is most of the thiopental redistributed to?

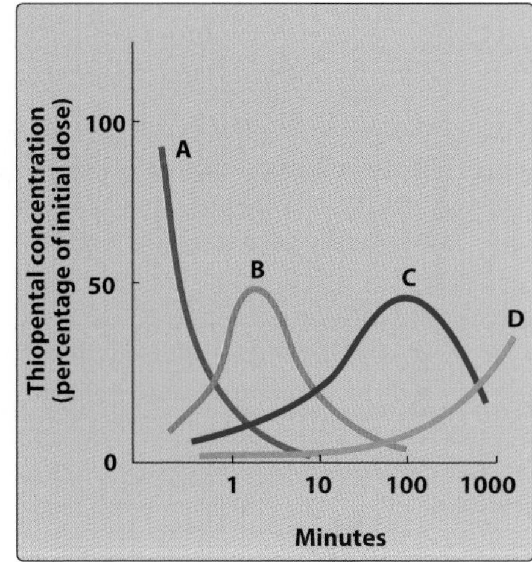

(A) Letter A
(B) Letter B
(C) Letter C
(D) Letter D

147 A 36-year-old man is undergoing opioid withdrawal by his psychiatrist. Which of the following agents depicted in the diagram would represent methadone?

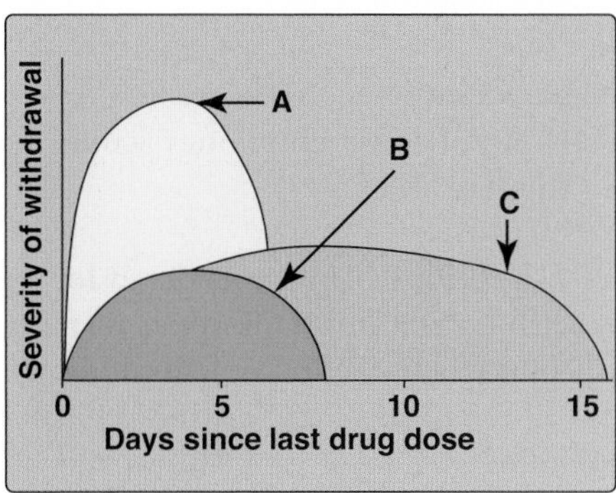

(A) Letter A
(B) Letter B
(C) Letter C
(D) Cannot be determined

148 A 12-year-old boy with meningitis is hospitalized on the pediatrics floor to receive intravenous antibiotics. He is currently on his 10th day of treatment. Which of the following curves represents the concentration of penicillin in the cerebrospinal fluid at this time?

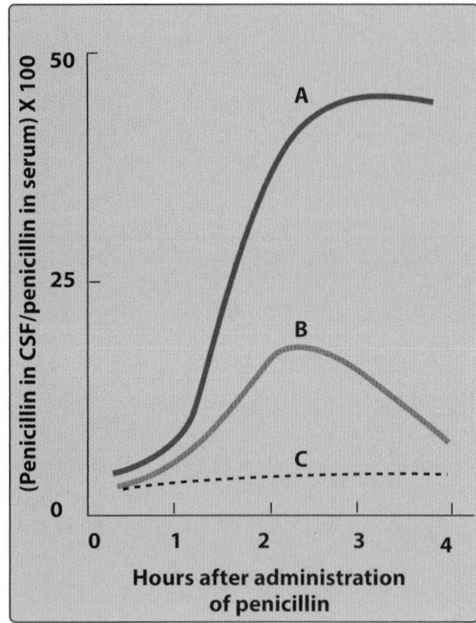

(A) Letter A
(B) Letter B
(C) Letter C
(D) Cannot be determined

149 A 23-year-old woman who underwent an open appendectomy is later found to have a wound infection. A culture grows methicillin-resistant *Staphylococcus aureus* (MRSA). Which of the following antibiotics would be useful in treating this infection?

(A) Ceftriaxone
(B) Dicloxacillin
(C) Nafcillin
(D) Oxacillin
(E) None of these antibiotics would be effective in this case

150 Five patients are being considered for antibiotic therapy with penicillin for an upper respiratory infection with pharyngitis. Which of the following patients is most likely to develop seizures as a result of taking penicillin?

(A) A 19-year-old man with anxiety and history of hernia repair
(B) A 29-year-old woman who takes birth control pills and has seasonal allergies
(C) A 37-year-old man with schizophrenia and manic episodes
(D) A 48-year-old man with epilepsy and chronic renal insufficiency
(E) A 56-year-old woman with diabetes mellitus and hypertension

151 A 39-year-old man who is hospitalized for alcoholic cirrhosis and pancreatitis is placed on aqueous penicillin G to treat a systemic infection that is susceptible to this agent. It is important for the treating physician to monitor which of the following blood levels?

(A) Bicarbonate
(B) Cholesterol
(C) Creatinine
(D) Potassium
(E) Sodium

152 A 13-year-old boy with a known seizure disorder presents to the emergency department with 2 days of nausea and vomiting while on vacation. He has been taking oral phenytoin for 1 year for seizure prophylaxis but has lately been vomiting every time he takes a dose. The ED physician gives him intramuscular (IM) fosphenytoin. Why did she choose to give fosphenytoin in this manner instead of phenytoin?

(A) Fosphenytoin has a much broader therapeutic index
(B) Phenytoin cannot be given IM
(C) Phenytoin is contraindicated in children
(D) Phenytoin was making him nauseous
(E) She made a mistake—phenytoin IM should have been given

153 A 58-year-old man is hospitalized in the medical intensive care unit with a methicillin-resistant bacterial infection. He has begun on a course of intravenous daptomycin. Which of the following laboratory studies needs to be carefully monitored in this patient?

(A) Creatinine
(B) Hemoglobin
(C) Hematocrit
(D) Hepatic transaminases
(E) Sodium

154 A 71-year-old woman is hospitalized with a methicillin-resistant bacterial infection. She has previously demonstrated resistance to multiple antibiotics and has not begun on a course of intravenous telavancin. Which of the following adverse events can occur in this patient?

(A) Diarrhea
(B) Foamy urine
(C) Headache
(D) QT interval shortening
(E) Sleepiness

155 A 78-year-old alcoholic male with mild Alzheimer's disease and poor dental hygiene is to have his remaining teeth extracted. Because of his Alzheimer's disease, he is not a candidate for dentures. He also has a history of mitral valve stenosis with mild cardiac insufficiency. His current medications include captopril, digoxin, and furosemide. Which of the following medications would be the most appropriate for prophylaxis prior to his dental procedure?

(A) Amoxicillin
(B) Co-trimoxazole
(C) Imipenem
(D) Tetracycline
(E) Vancomycin

ANSWERS

1 **The answer is B: Cyclophosphamide.** Cyclophosphamide is one of the drugs used to treat acute lymphoblastic leukemia. This drug is converted to an active metabolite that works by transferring alkyl groups to DNA strands, which then link to each other. Linked DNA strands cannot be replicated. When rapidly dividing cells (such as cancer cells) are unable to replicate this DNA, they undergo apoptosis. (A) 5-Fluorouracil (5-FU) is an antimetabolite that irreversibly inhibits the enzyme thymidylate synthase. Rapidly dividing cells exposed to 5-FU cannot synthesize thymidine and die. (C) Cytarabine is converted to an active metabolite that is incorporated into growing strands of DNA. Other nucleotides cannot be added to strand, and the cell is unable to remove the cytarabine metabolite so DNA synthesis is halted. (D) Methotrexate is a folate antimetabolite. Folate is necessary for precursors to DNA synthesis, so inhibiting folate use by cells slows DNA synthesis and proliferation. (E) Vincristine interferes with microtubules, leading to cell cycle arrest in metaphase.

2 **The answer is D: Irinotecan.** For patients with recurrent cancer, using a different chemotherapeutic agent than was used initially is often favored. This is because of the fact that cancer cells can become resistant to chemotherapy drugs to which they are exposed. In this patient's case, paclitaxel (a microtubule inhibitor) was used during her initial treatment. The physician chose to use irinotecan, an agent that inhibits topoisomerase, this time in hopes to avoid any resistance the cancer cells may have to microtubule inhibitors. (A) Cisplatin is a DNA-binding agent that forms cross-links in DNA strands. It does not interfere with topoisomerase. (B) Docetaxel and paclitaxel are taxanes that inhibit microtubule depolymerization. They do not interfere with topoisomerase. (C) Erlotinib inhibits cell proliferation by blocking the epidermal growth factor receptor. It does not interfere with topoisomerase. (E) Vincristine destabilizes microtubules, inhibiting normal cell cycle progression. It does not interfere with topoisomerase.

3 **The answer is C: *Neisseria gonorrhoeae.*** Quinolone antibiotics are sensitive to all of the pathogens in this question. However, *Neisseria gonorrhoeae* exhibits the highest zone of inhibition in microbiologic susceptibility tests. Thus, the lowest concentration of antibiotic would eradicate this organism. (A) *Escherichia coli* exhibits sensitivity to quinolones in an intermediate manner. (B) *Haemophilus influenzae* exhibits sensitivity to quinolones in a strong manner. (D) *Pseudomonas aeruginosa* exhibits the lowest sensitivity to quinolones of all the pathogens in this question. (E) *Staphylococcus aureus* exhibits sensitivity to quinolones in an intermediate manner.

4 **The answer is A: Aplastic anemia.** Special precautions should be kept in mind when anesthetics and adjunct drugs are administered to a pregnant woman. In early pregnancy, potential effects on organogenesis in the fetus are a major concern. Transient use of nitrous oxide has been reported to cause aplastic anemia in the unborn child. (B) Benzodiazepines should not be used routinely during labor because of risk of hypotonia. (C) Oral clefts have occurred in the fetuses of women who have received benzodiazepines during early pregnancy. (D) Benzodiazepines can result in altered thermoregulation in the newborn. (E) Uremia of pregnancy is not likely to be seen with nitrous oxide use.

5 **The answer is C: He should have prescribed primaquine in addition to chloroquine.** Malaria can be caused by a number of parasites in the *Plasmodium* genus. Most malarial infections are caused by *P. falciparum*, *P. vivax*, or *P. ovale*. *P. vivax* and *P. ovale* are species found primarily in Asia, whereas *P. falciparum* is found primarily in Africa. *P. vivax* and *P. ovale* infect hepatocytes in addition to erythrocytes, whereas *P. falciparum* infects only erythrocytes. This is important because chloroquine will only kill organisms infecting erythrocytes. Because of his travel history, this patient should be suspected of infection with *P. vivax* or *P. ovale* and therefore assumed to have infected hepatocytes as well as erythrocytes. Primaquine is the drug of choice for killing the organisms in hepatocytes and should be given with chloroquine when infection by *P. vivax* or *P. ovale* is suspected. (A) Malaria is a serious infection with high morbidity and mortality. Treatment is often lifesaving. (B) There is no curative drug for yellow fever. Treatment is based on symptom relief. The vector for yellow fever is the *Aedes* mosquito, whereas that for malarial parasites is the *Anopheles* mosquito. Furthermore, yellow fever is endemic to the Americans and Africans, not Asians. (D) Albendazole is used to treat helminthic infections. Either mefloquine or chloroquine plus primaquine should be used in this patient. (E) Either mefloquine (which kills *Plasmodium* organisms in both hepatocytes and erythrocytes) or the combination of chloroquine plus primaquine should be prescribed to a patient with suspected *P. vivax* or *P. ovale* infection.

6 **The answer is B: Administer ganciclovir.** A patient with HIV disease and with blurry vision, eye pain, and retinitis on exam should be suspected to have CMV retinitis. CMV in a healthy person typically causes an asymptomatic infection. In an immunocompromised person, however, the infection can be much more severe. In patients with HIV disease, CMV can infect the retina and cause blindness if untreated. In patients with a bone marrow transplant, CMV can cause a serious lung infection. The treatment for CMV is ganciclovir.

(A) Rimantadine is used to treat influenza A infections. It acts on influenza A's M_2 protein, which is not present in CMV. (C) Ribavirin can be used in RSV and hepatitis C infections. It is not used to treat CMV infections. (D) A temporal artery biopsy would be used to confirm a suspicion of temporal cell arteritis, but this is more common in older patients and would also usually present with jaw claudication and headache. A patient with HIV disease and with blurry vision, eye pain, and retinitis on exam should be suspected to have CMV retinitis and treated with ganciclovir. (E) HbA_{1c} can be used to follow a patient's blood glucose control. The clinical picture here is more closely aligned with CMV retinitis than with diabetic retinopathy. A patient with HIV disease and with blurry vision, eye pain, and retinitis on exam should be suspected to have CMV retinitis and treated with ganciclovir.

7 **The correct answer is C: Pregnancy.** Factors that can decrease minimum alveolar concentration (MAC) (and make the patient more sensitive) include increased age, hypothermia, pregnancy, sepsis, acute ethanol intoxication, concurrent administration of IV anesthetics, and α_2-adrenergic receptor agonists (such as clonidine and dexmedetomidine). (A) This patient is young. Older patients would experience a decrease in MAC. (B) Hypothermia can decrease MAC. (D) Use of α-adrenergic agonists can decrease MAC. (E) Weight will not change MAC.

8 **The answer is B: Halothane.** An anesthetic gas with high blood solubility, such as halothane, dissolves more completely in the blood, and greater amounts of the anesthetic and longer periods of time are required to raise blood partial pressure. This results in increased times of induction and recovery and slower changes in the depth of anesthesia in response to alterations in the concentration of the inhaled drug. The solubility in blood is ranked in the following order: halothane > isoflurane > sevoflurane > nitrous oxide > desflurane. (A) Desflurane is the best agent for this patient because of its rapid induction time. (C) Isoflurane is a poor agent for this patient because of its slow induction time. (D) Nitrous oxide is good agent for this patient because it has a rapid induction time. (E) Sevoflurane is intermediate and would not necessarily be preferred or not preferred as an induction agent in this patient.

9 **The answer is D: Lower risk of pain at injection site.** Because fospropofol is water soluble, the problems associated with lipid-formulated propofol (such as pain at the IV injection site and increased chance for bacterial contamination) are expected to be less frequent. (A) The cerebral perfusion of propofol and fospropofol are the same. (B) The half-life of propofol and fospropofol are the same. (C) The risk of infection is the same for propofol and fospropofol. (E) Both propofol and fospropofol are able to be administered to patients with hepatic failure.

10 **The answer is C: A 9-year-old boy with asthma.** Thiopental has minor effects on the cardiovascular system, but it may contribute to severe hypotension in patients with hypovolemia or shock. All barbiturates can cause apnea, coughing, chest wall spasm, laryngospasm, and bronchospasm. Due to redistribution of thiopental from brain to muscle and adipose tissue, this is a concern for patients with asthma. (A) This child can receive thiopental with minimal fear of complication. (B) This child can receive thiopental with minimal fear of complication. (D) Children with porphyria should not receive thiopental. (E) This child can receive thiopental with minimal fear of complication.

11 **The answer is B: Aminocaproic acid.** This patient is in a state of hyperfibrinolysis, likely because of the fibrinolytic drug she was given. The appropriate drug to administer in this case is aminocaproic acid. Fibrinolytic drugs activate plasminogen into plasmin, which then degrades fibrin and fibrinogen. Aminocaproic acid binds to the active site of plasmin to inhibit its activity. (A) Abciximab is a monoclonal antibody that binds to glycoprotein (Gp) IIb/IIIa on platelets. Gp IIb/IIIa on activated platelets binds fibrinogen and plays a part in platelet aggregation. Administration of abciximab would worsen this patient's bleeding. (C) Anistreplase is a fibrinolytic drug. It eventually leads to the conversion of plasminogen to plasmin, causing further fibrinolysis. Administration of anistreplase would worsen this patient's bleeding. (D) Clopidogrel blocks platelet activation by binding the adenosine diphosphate (ADP) receptor on the platelet membrane. Administration of clopidogrel would worsen this patient's bleeding. (E) Urokinase converts plasminogen to plasmin, causing further fibrinolysis. Administration of urokinase would worsen this patient's bleeding.

12 **The answer is E: Vincristine.** Vincristine is the only drug in this list that inhibits proliferation by blocking mitosis. Vincristine disrupts the formation of microtubules in cells. Microtubules make up the mitotic spindle and are necessary for division after the cell has passed through the G_1, S, and G_2 phases. Vincristine blocks all rapidly dividing cells including cancer cells, bone marrow cells, and intestinal cells. (A) Bleomycin binds DNA and causes strand breaks. It functions primarily in the G_2 phase of the cell cycle. (B) Cisplatin binds DNA to form cross-links in and between the DNA strands. It causes cell cycle arrest in the G_2 phase. (C) Etoposide binds to the DNA-topoisomerase II complex and stabilizes it to

inactivate topoisomerase II. It primarily affects cells in the G_2 phase of the cell cycle. (D) Methotrexate is a folate antimetabolite that interferes with DNA synthesis. It primarily affects cells in the S (DNA synthesis) phase of the cell cycle.

13 **The answer is A: Darunavir.** HIV life cycle involves multiple steps that are targets for drug therapy. Initially, gp120 on the HIV virion must bind the CD4 receptor plus either the CCR5 or CXCR4 coreceptor on a T cell or a macrophage. Next, gp41 on the virion undergoes a conformational change to mediate fusion of the virion and cell membranes. Then, viral reverse transcriptase makes ssDNA copies of the viral RNA. The ssDNA copies are replicated and incorporated into the host genome. mRNA copies made from this viral DNA are translated into polyproteins that must be cleaved by viral protease for the progeny virus to become infective. Darunavir is a protease inhibitor, blocking the cleavage of HIV polyproteins. (B) Delavirdine is a nonnucleoside reverse transcriptase inhibitor. It noncompetitively inhibits viral reverse transcriptase's ability to make a DNA copy of viral RNA. (C) Enfuvirtide is a fusion inhibitor. It binds viral gp41 to prevent the conformational change necessary to fuse the viral and host cell membranes. (D) Maraviroc is a CCR5 antagonist, blocking the ability of virions to bind tightly enough to fuse and enter the host cell. It is useful only in CCR5-trophic (not CXCR4-trophic) viruses. (E) Stavudine is a nucleoside reverse transcriptase inhibitor. It competitively inhibits viral reverse transcriptase's ability to make a DNA copy of viral RNA.

14 **The answer is E: Ritonavir.** A patient on HAART therapy with nausea, vomiting, and abdominal pain with elevated serum amylase likely has pancreatitis. Pancreatitis is a known side effect of many antiretrovirals including ritonavir. Ritonavir should be discontinued in a patient who develops pancreatitis. (A) Efavirenz can cause CNS side effects such as dizziness and insomnia as well as skin rash. It is not known to cause pancreatitis. (B) Emtricitabine can cause GI side effects such as nausea, diarrhea, and abdominal pain. It is not known to cause pancreatitis. (C) Nevirapine can cause a skin rash that may be accompanied by liver damage. A patient taking nevirapine who develops a skin rash should have his or her liver enzymes checked. It is not known to cause pancreatitis. (D) Raltegravir can cause elevated serum lipase, abdominal pain, nausea, and diarrhea. It is not known to cause pancreatitis.

15 **The answer is A: Ceftriaxone.** This patient's presentation is suggestive of infection with *Neisseria gonorrhoeae.* Ceftriaxone is usually the drug of choice for gonorrhea because most strains are now resistant to antibiotics that worked in the past (such as penicillin and fluoroquinolones). A large percentage of patients with gonorrhea also have chlamydia, so this patient should be prescribed an antibiotic to treat chlamydia such as doxycycline. (B) Cephalexin is second-generation cephalosporin and has not been shown to be effective against *Neisseria gonorrhoeae.* Cephalexin can be used in some cases of pneumonia, otitis media, and streptococcal pharyngitis. (C) Dexamethasone would reduce the swelling in this patient's knee but works by suppressing the immune system. His overall condition would deteriorate with dexamethasone administration. (D) Meropenem would certainly kill *Neisseria gonorrhoeae*, but to prevent the development of resistance, this drug is used in infections when other antibiotics have failed or in patients so sick that they are at risk of death without empiric treatment. (E) Although used successfully in the past, most strains of *Neisseria gonorrhoeae* are now resistant to penicillin.

16 **The answer is C: Hypoventilation.** The transmucosal preparation of fentanyl is used in the treatment of patients with cancer and with breakthrough pain who are tolerant to opioids. The transdermal patch must be used with caution because death resulting from hypoventilation has been known to occur. The transdermal patch creates a reservoir of the drug in the skin. Hence, the onset is delayed 12 h, and the offset is prolonged. (A) This patient likely died from pulmonary hypoventilation, which led to respiratory arrest. (B) This patient has no underlying reason to have cardiomyopathy. (D) This patient has no clinical features of pulmonary edema. (E) Although cancer predisposes to thrombosis development, this patient does not have any findings to suggest that she has suffered a pulmonary embolism.

17 **The answer is B: Doxycycline.** This patient presents with a *Neisseria gonorrhoeae* infection, which is treatable with ceftriaxone. It is also important to remember that a very high percentage of patients with a gonococcal infection also have a chlamydial infection, and chlamydia is not treatable with ceftriaxone. Doxycycline is the drug of choice for chlamydial infections and should be coadministered with ceftriaxone whenever either of the two infections is diagnosed. (A) Aztreonam is not effective in treating chlamydia. Aztreonam is often used in lieu of aminoglycosides in patients with renal insufficiency. (C) Imipenem is a broad-spectrum antibiotic usually reserved for microbes resistant to conventional treatment and empirically in life-threatening infections. Minimizing its use helps prevent development of resistance against it. Cilastatin is added to prevent renal breakdown of imipenem. (D) Nitrofurantoin is not known to be effective against chlamydia. It is used in certain cases of urethritis and cystitis. (E) As mentioned previously,

a high percentage of patients infected with *Neisseria gonorrhoeae* are coinfected with *Chlamydia trachomatis*. A patient diagnosed with either infection should be treated for both with ceftriaxone and doxycycline or equivalent.

18 **The answer is D: Enzyme deficiency.** A patient of African, Middle Eastern, or South Asian descent taking chloroquine who develops jaundice should be suspected of glucose-6 phosphate dehydrogenase (G6PD) deficiency. This enzyme is involved in the pentose phosphate pathway, which is particularly important in erythrocytes to maintain stores of glutathione. When erythrocytes are unable to produce enough glutathione, oxidative stressors (such as chloroquine) will cause a hemolytic anemia leading to jaundice and scleral icterus. (A) Ceftriaxone is a drug that can cause biliary sludging, more appropriately pseudocholelithiasis. This is usually asymptomatic and produces no jaundice. (B) Chloroquine does not change the color of secretions. An example of a drug that does is rifampin, which can turn urine, tears, saliva, and sweat to red-orange. (C) Drug interactions should always be considered. However, a patient of African, Middle Eastern, or South Asian descent taking chloroquine who develops jaundice should first be suspected of G6PD deficiency. (E) Chloroquine is not known to be hepatotoxic. It causes jaundice not by impairing hepatic handling of bilirubin but by leading to an overproduction of bilirubin from the hemolytic anemia.

19 **The answer is A: Acyclovir.** Genital herpes is usually caused by herpes simplex virus type 2 (HSV-2), although it can also be caused by HSV-1. In either case, the virus uses a thymidine kinase as a preliminary step in DNA synthesis. Viral thymidine kinase is structurally different from human thymidine kinase and has a much higher affinity for acyclovir. Viral thymidine kinase phosphorylates acyclovir, which (after a few more steps) is incorporated into growing DNA strands but has no 3′-OH group to which more nucleotides can be added. This results in impaired DNA synthesis in cells infected with HSV-1 or HSV-2. A mutation in HSV thymidine kinase can greatly decrease its affinity to acyclovir, providing resistance to the drug. (B) Cidofovir is usually used to treat CMV infections but can be used in acyclovir-resistant HSV infections. Cidofovir is similar to acyclovir in that it competes with nucleotides in DNA synthesis, but cidofovir does not need to be activated by thymidine kinase. (C) Foscarnet is also used for CMV or HSV infections. It interacts with viral DNA polymerase to inhibit DNA synthesis. It does not need to be activated by thymidine kinase. (D) Oseltamivir is used to treat infections with influenza viruses. It inhibits influenza A and B neuraminidase and does not need to be activated by thymidine kinase. (E) Rimantadine was used to treat influenza A infections, but most viral strains are now resistant. It is not activated by a thymidine kinase.

20 **The answer is D: Influenza A.** M2 ion channels are found only in strains of influenza A. This ion channel is important in the uncoating of the viral genome. By blocking the M2 channel, uncoating is inhibited and the virus is unable to replicate. The adamantanes such as amantadine and rimantadine block the M2 ion channel. Most strains of influenza A have mutated ion channels, however, and are now resistant to the adamantanes. (A) CMV does not possess the M2 ion channel. CMV infections are commonly treated with ganciclovir. (B) HSV-1 does not possess the M2 ion channel. HSV infections are commonly treated with acyclovir. (C) HSV-2 does not possess the M2 ion channel. HSV infections are commonly treated with acyclovir. (E) Influenza B does not possess the M2 ion channel. Influenza B infections and adamantane-resistant influenza A infections are commonly treated with oseltamivir or zanamivir.

21 **The answer is D: Thrombotic thrombocytopenic purpura.** Clopidogrel is a thienopyridine that blocks platelet aggregation. Life-threatening hematologic adverse reactions are possible. Thrombotic thrombocytopenic purpura is one such reaction that the physician must be aware of. (A) Thrombocytopenia is more likely to result than anemia in this patient. (B) Aplastic anemia rather than leukemia could result in this patient. (C) Aplastic anemia rather than lymphoma could result in this patient. (E) This agent may prevent transient ischemic attacks.

22 **The answer is B: Need to synthesize new coagulation factors.** Vitamin K has a slow response because it takes about 24 h to synthesize new coagulation factors. Thus, it is not surprising that this individual still has an elevated bleeding time at 12 h. This is not a toxic or subtherapeutic effect of this agent. (A) Vitamin K acts on vitamin K–dependent clotting factors. (C) This is not a subtherapeutic effect of vitamin K. (D) This is not a toxic effect of vitamin K.

23 **The answer is C: Low-density lipoprotein.** Plasma lipids and proteins can be atherogenic. Low-density lipoprotein (LDL) has the highest atherogenicity and should be lowered to normal levels when elevated. LDL is strongly correlated to increased risk of heart disease. (A) Chylomicrons are at low risk of atherogenicity. (B) High-density lipoproteins are at the lowest risk of atherogenicity. (D) Very low-density lipoproteins are at high risk of atherogenicity but not as high as LDL.

24 **The answer is B: Haloperidol.** This patient's presentation suggests tardive dyskinesia (TD). TD may be irreversible and is associated with use of the typical neuroleptics such as haloperidol. The mechanism for TD is unclear, but the incidence is much lower with atypical neuroleptics. Long-term use and high doses seem to contribute to the development of TD, but it can occur even in the short term and at low doses. (A) Glipizide is a sulfonylurea drug used to increase insulin secretion following meals. Any side effects are generally mild. Glipizide is not associated with TD. (C) Hydrochlorothiazide is a diuretic that decreases ion and water uptake early in the distal tubule. It also increases calcium reabsorption and potassium excretion, so the concentration of these ions may need to be monitored. It is not associated with TD. (D) Metformin decreases blood glucose in part by inhibiting gluconeogenesis. A worrisome but rare side effect is severe lactic acidosis. It is not associated with TD. (E) Lovastatin blocks cholesterol synthesis by inhibiting the rate-limiting enzyme HMG-CoA reductase. A serious but rare side effect is rhabdomyolysis. It is not associated with TD.

25 **The answer is B: Ciprofloxacin is contraindicated in patients younger than 18 years old.** Pyelonephritis is a serious infection that can result in kidney failure or scarring if not treated properly. Most cases are caused by *E. coli*. Ciprofloxacin is bactericidal and efficacious against *E. coli* in vivo. It is contraindicated in children and adolescents because of risk of joint and cartilage damage. There are other safer drugs for use in children that are just as efficacious as ciprofloxacin would be. (A) Ciprofloxacin is bactericidal. It works by inhibiting bacterial DNA gyrase, which ultimately leads to cell death. (C) Ciprofloxacin is efficacious in vivo in treating *E. coli* pyelonephritis and can be used in adults. Even in adults, there is risk of rare tendon rupture. (D) Ciprofloxacin is not particularly nephrotoxic. Even drugs that are nephrotoxic such as aminoglycosides can be used to treat kidney infections under proper supervision. (E) The physician could use ciprofloxacin to treat pyelonephritis but would likely get the same result using another drug or drug combination without the risk of cartilage and joint problems.

26 **The answer is B: Kernicterus.** Trimethoprim–sulfamethoxazole is effective against all of the most common bacteria causing urinary tract infections (UTIs) and is widely used in their treatment. It is contraindicated in pregnancy (especially late pregnancy) because it easily crosses the placenta and displaces bilirubin from plasma proteins. This increases the risk of kernicterus in the newborn. Trimethoprim–sulfamethoxazole can also cause kernicterus in newborns and is secreted in breast milk, so it should not be given to breastfeeding women. (A) Gray baby syndrome is caused by chloramphenicol administration to newborns and infants. Whether it causes harm to the unborn fetus is not known. Trimethoprim–sulfamethoxazole does not cause gray baby syndrome. (C) Thalidomide is a drug that can cause limb defects if exposure happens at the right time. By the third trimester, the limbs have already formed so any potential harm to the fetus would not involve limb defects. (D) Cocaine use causes vasospasm, which can lead to premature labor. Trimethoprim–sulfamethoxazole is not known to cause premature labor. (E) The physician is right to be cautious about using trimethoprim–sulfamethoxazole in this case. The risks may outweigh the benefits, so other drugs must also be considered.

27 **The answer is E: Streptomycin.** Although treatment would depend ultimately on sputum culture findings, empiric treatment is advised while avoiding drugs that may harm the fetus. Ototoxic drugs include the aminoglycosides such as streptomycin. Streptomycin is known to cross the placenta. It belongs in pregnancy category D. As such, it should be used only in cases where the potential benefits outweigh the obvious risks. It would not be the first drug of choice in this patient's case. (A) Amoxicillin is in pregnancy category B. All the penicillins are generally considered safe in pregnancy. Amoxicillin is not known to be ototoxic. (B) Ciprofloxacin is a fluoroquinolone in pregnancy category C. Ciprofloxacin is thought to potentially cause problems in cartilage development but not known to be ototoxic. (C) Erythromycin is in pregnancy category B. It is not associated with birth defects or ototoxicity. (D) Doxycycline is a tetracycline antibiotic and belongs to pregnancy category D. It is associated with causing tooth discoloration in exposed persons younger than 8 years of age. It is not known to be ototoxic.

28 **The answer is C: Oxacillin.** This patient's infection is most likely caused by *Staphylococcus aureus*. Most strains in the United States have penicillinases rendering them resistant to the β-lactam penicillins and aminopenicillins. Methicillin is a β-lactam antibiotic with a bulky side chain that make it a poor substrate for penicillinases. Oxacillin and nafcillin are two more examples of methicillin-like β-lactam antibiotics. (A) Amoxicillin is an aminopenicillin. Aminopenicillins have more activity against gram-negative organisms than penicillin. (B) Ampicillin is susceptible to degradation by penicillinases, which are likely found in the strain of *S. aureus* infecting this patient. (D) Penicillin G is for parenteral use only because it is inactivated by stomach acid. (E) Penicillin V has a slight modification making it acid stable so it can be taken orally.

29 **The answer is B: Has altered PBPs that methicillin cannot bind.** Methicillin, oxacillin, and nafcillin are β-lactam antibiotics related to penicillin. They have a bulky side chain that makes them poor targets for β-lactamase enzymes that break down and deactivate penicillins. Like penicillins, they work by inhibiting the so-called penicillin-binding proteins (PBPs, also known as transpeptidases), which are enzymes bacteria used to make their peptidoglycan cell wall. MRSA strains have altered PBPs with lower affinity for penicillins and methicillin. (A) This response illustrates the mechanism of vancomycin resistance. Vancomycin requires two terminal D-alanine residues in tandem on the peptide segment of the peptidoglycan cell wall in order to bind and inhibit the cross-linking enzyme. Methicillin does not require this sequence for action. (C) This response describes one method bacteria use to avoid damage by aminoglycosides. β-Lactam antibiotics do not need to enter the cell—they work within the layer of the cell wall to inhibit transpeptidases found there. (D) Efflux pumps that remove toxic compounds from bacterial cells work against most antibiotics, but this is not the principal mechanism behind methicillin resistance. (E) β-Lactamases that could deactivate penicillin are the reason methicillin and its equivalents were developed. Methicillin cannot be broken down by β-lactamases.

30 **The answer is E: Rapid increase of endotoxins in his blood.** This patient's presentation is consistent with secondary syphilis. Penicillin is the drug of choice for treatment of syphilis. One issue in the treatment of syphilis with penicillin is that the rapid lysis of spirochetes releases large amounts of endotoxin into the bloodstream. These endotoxins stimulate cytokine release from immune system cells, leading to the symptoms of fever, chills, and myalgia. This is termed the Jarisch-Herxheimer reaction. It will usually resolve within 24 h. (A) Penicillin can cause pseudomembranous colitis, but very rarely. Clindamycin and amoxicillin are more common causes. Pseudomembranous colitis normally presents with diarrhea. (B) The patient's condition makes this option unlikely. A new onset of fever, chills, and myalgia following penicillin treatment of syphilis is very common and simply represents the Jarisch-Herxheimer reaction. (C) A penicillin allergy would have a different presentation, possibly including urticaria and wheezing. Allergies do not typically present as fever and chills. (D) Penicillin G is the drug of choice for secondary syphilis. The Jarisch-Herxheimer reaction is actually a sign that the infection is being rapidly cleared, not worsening.

31 **The answer is C: Dehydropeptidase.** Imipenem is a broad-spectrum antibiotic often used empirically when prompt treatment is essential and susceptibilities of the bacteria to more narrow spectrum antibiotics are not known. Imipenem is primarily metabolized in the kidneys by the enzyme dehydropeptidase. Cilastatin is not an antibiotic but serves to inhibit dehydropeptidase activity to slow renal imipenem metabolism. (A) Imipenem inhibits bacterial cell wall synthesis by blocking transpeptidase enzymes as do penicillins. It does not need to enter the cytoplasm to exert its effects, so blocking efflux pumps would not increase its efficacy. (B) Cytochrome P450 3A4 (CYP3A4) is not important in the metabolism of imipenem. Cilastatin does not inhibit CYP3A4. (D) The organic anion transporters aid in the excretion of negatively charged organic molecules into the urine. Probenecid is a drug that interferes with these transporters and can be used to slow the elimination of penicillin in the urine. (E) Imipenem is a β-lactam but is inherently resistant to degradation by penicillinases. Clavulanic acid is an example of a penicillinase inhibitor commonly given with a penicillin to prevent its breakdown.

32 **The answer is C: Creatine kinase.** Daptomycin is a lipopeptide antibiotic that causes depolarization of bacterial cells leading to cell death. It does not need to enter the cytoplasm to be effective. A principal side effect is myopathies including myalgia and rhabdomyolysis. Serum creatine kinase (CK) can be used to monitor myopathies. Greatly elevated CK levels accompanied by myopathy are an indication to stop daptomycin therapy. (A) Amylase is an enzyme found in the pancreas and is used as indicators to pancreatic health. Daptomycin is not known to cause pancreatitis. (B) Blood urea nitrogen (BUN) is used as a measure of kidney function. Daptomycin is not known to cause renal failure, except indirectly via rhabdomyolysis. (D) Lipase is an enzyme found in the pancreas and is used as indicators pancreatic health. (E) Troponin I is a protein specific to cardiac muscle and is used as a marker in cases such as myocardial infarction. Cardiac may be a daptomycin-related side effect, but this is rare and the relationship is unclear.

33 **The answer is C: Inhibition of nucleotide synthesis.** Co-trimoxazole is actually a combination of two drugs, trimethoprim and sulfamethoxazole (SMX-TMP). Each inhibits a separate stage of the tetrahydrofolate synthesis pathway that bacteria require to synthesize nucleotides. Alone, neither trimethoprim nor sulfamethoxazole is very effective at stopping bacterial growth. Only when used together are they significantly efficacious for therapeutic use. Care must be taken because sulfamethoxazole contains the sulfonamide group known to cause hypersensitivity reactions in susceptible patients. (A) β-Lactams such as penicillins and cephalosporins inhibit cell wall synthesis. These drugs inactivate bacterial transpeptidase enzymes. SMX-TMP does not interfere with cell wall synthesis.

(B) Fluoroquinolones work by inhibiting bacterial DNA gyrase. The human equivalent enzyme, topoisomerase, is not significantly affected by fluoroquinolones. SMX-TMP does not inhibit DNA gyrase. (D) Bacterial ribosomes are impaired by many antibiotics. This group includes the tetracyclines, macrolides, and aminoglycosides. SMX-TMP does not interfere with ribosomes. (E) Rifampin binds bacterial (but not human) RNA polymerase to inhibit RNA synthesis. SMX-TMP does not interfere with RNA synthesis.

34 **The answer is C: Milk.** Ciprofloxacin is a fluoroquinolone drug that can be used to treat anthrax infections. Most fluoroquinolones including ciprofloxacin have a structure that allows them to chelate divalent and trivalent cations. Once they chelate an ion, they cannot be absorbed from the gut and are excreted. Patients should not take supplements and foods that contain large amounts of divalent and trivalent cations at the same time as their ciprofloxacin dose. Dairy products contain high amounts of calcium, and so she should not drink milk with ciprofloxacin. (A) Some drugs such as metronidazole produce a disulfiram-like effect. Disulfiram inhibits aldehyde dehydrogenase, allowing acetaldehyde from alcohol metabolism to build up. High levels of acetaldehyde cause nausea and headaches. (B) Grapefruit juice is an inhibitor of cytochrome P450 3A4 and so should be avoided with drugs that are metabolized by this enzyme. Ciprofloxacin is not, so there is no interaction between ciprofloxacin and grapefruit juice. (D) St. John's wort is an activator of cytochrome P450 3A4 and so should be avoided with drugs that are metabolized by this enzyme. Ciprofloxacin is not, so there is no interaction between ciprofloxacin and St. John's wort. (E) This statement is untrue. Ciprofloxacin chelates divalent and trivalent cations. This inhibits its absorption. Ciprofloxacin should not be taken with anything (such as milk) that contains large amounts of divalent or trivalent cations.

35 **The answer is A: Ethambutol.** This patient's presentation is consistent with an active tuberculosis infection. Ethambutol is not normally given as first-line therapy, but because of his HIV status, he is started on quadruple therapy. Ethambutol is notable for its ability to cause optic neuritis, which may manifest as impaired ability to discriminate colors as in this patient's case. Vision usually returns to normal after a few weeks of discontinuation of ethambutol. (B) Isoniazid can cause optic neuritis but much less commonly than ethambutol. Isoniazid's major adverse reaction is hepatitis. (C) Miliary tuberculosis is extremely unlikely in this case because the patient is taking four antituberculosis drugs. This patient's presentation and history point to ethambutol toxicity. (D) Pyrazinamide is not known to cause optic neuritis. Its major adverse effect is, like isoniazid, hepatitis. (E) Rifampin is not known to cause optic neuritis. Rifampin is known for its ability to induce cytochrome P450 3A4 thereby increasing the rate that substrates of CYP3A4 are metabolized.

36 **The answer is A: Arrest growth of bacteria.** Bacteriostatic agents arrest bacterial growth and replication of bacteria. This will limit the spread of infection; but in this seriously ill patient, a more aggressive bactericidal action would be more appropriate. (B) A bactericidal agent will cause cell death of pathogens, which is certainly needed in this critically ill patient. (C) A bactericidal agent will cause cell death and allow for removal of viable organisms from circulation. (D) Because of the bactericidal nature of the medication, it is possible that a lower dose given for a shorter time period may be possible.

37 **The answer is E: Tinnitus.** Aminoglycosides such as gentamicin are known to be ototoxic and nephrotoxic. A once-daily dose is intended to cause a sufficiently low trough of drug concentration to allow damaged renal and ear cells to recover. Patients must still be carefully monitored for signs and symptoms of ototoxicity and nephrotoxicity. Tinnitus may be an early symptom of ototoxicity, and nephrotoxicity will likely follow if the patient continues receiving the same dose. (A) This is a potential nonserious adverse reaction to gentamicin. (B) This reaction does not represent the onset of any serious, irreversible condition. (C) This reaction is not a serious one such as permanent hearing loss that may follow tinnitus. (D) This side effect is transient and reversible and not a reason to stop gentamicin administration.

38 **The answer is D: Furosemide.** Gentamicin is known to be ototoxic and nephrotoxic. Combining gentamicin with another ototoxic or nephrotoxic drug greatly increases the risk that such an adverse reaction may occur. Furosemide can also be ototoxic. This patient may have ascites that furosemide could correct, but furosemide should not be given concomitantly with gentamicin. (A) A benzodiazepine such as diazepam may be useful to prevent an alcoholic from developing delirium tremens. Diazepam can be used with gentamicin. (B) Disulfiram may be useful if this patient desires to quit drinking once he leaves the hospital. It would likely not be useful to this patient while he is hospitalized, but it could be used with gentamicin without any problems. (C) Fomepizole inhibits alcohol dehydrogenase and may be useful if this patient had consumed methanol or ethylene glycol to prevent formation of toxic metabolites. It can be given with gentamicin. (E) Omeprazole is a proton pump inhibitor that may be useful if this patient complains of heartburn. It can be safely given with gentamicin.

39 **The answer is D: Decreased conjugation in infant liver.** Chloramphenicol is a broad-spectrum antibiotic often used as empiric treatment in cases of sepsis. It is metabolized and inactivated via conjugation in the liver by glucuronyl transferase. The glucuronyl conjugate is easily excreted by the kidneys. Neonates and infants have decreased glucuronyl transferase activity, allowing chloramphenicol to build up to toxic levels. This is the supposed mechanism behind gray baby syndrome. (A) Chloramphenicol is a broad-spectrum antibiotic. Gray baby syndrome does not result from failure of chloramphenicol to halt the infection. (B) Chloramphenicol is the drug associated with gray baby syndrome. Clindamycin is one drug known for its ability to cause pseudomembranous colitis. (C) Intestinal absorption is not a factor in gray baby syndrome. Chloramphenicol can be given orally and is absorbed from the intestines. It appears to be the high level of unconjugated chloramphenicol in infants that leads to gray baby syndrome. (E) Infant kidneys are able to excrete conjugated chloramphenicol just as well as adult kidneys. The issue in gray baby syndrome appears to be impaired conjugation in the liver.

40 **The answer is C: Ketoconazole.** Histoplasmosis is a fungal infection caused by the dimorphic fungus *Histoplasma capsulatum*. Although it is found in the soil of the entire Ohio River basin, spores appear to be more concentrated in bird and bat droppings. This patient likely stirred up a large number of spores while cleaning an area frequented by bats, enough spores to cause an infection. A common treatment for histoplasmosis is ketoconazole for less serious infections or amphotericin B for more serious systemic infections. (A) Albendazole is an antihelminthic. It works by interfering with helminth microtubules, ultimately leading to paralysis of the worm. It would not be useful in treating a fungal infection. (B) Griseofulvin is an antifungal used for topical infections. Although it is administered orally, it deposits in keratin-containing tissues. It would not be as useful as ketoconazole in treating a pulmonary fungal infection such as histoplasmosis. (D) Nystatin is too toxic for systemic use. It is used for superficial candidiasis and would not be used to treat a pulmonary infection. (E) Penicillin G is a β-lactam antibiotic used to treat some gram-positive bacterial infections. It would not be useful against *Histoplasma capsulatum*.

41 **The answer is D: Inhibition of thymidylate kinase.** Flucytosine is metabolized to 5-fluorouracil (5-FU) by the enzyme cytosine deaminase in fungal cells. This conversion does not occur in human cells. 5-FU inhibits the enzyme thymidylate kinase, which is necessary for DNA synthesis. Resistance to flucytosine develops rapidly if used alone. It is generally used in combination therapy for serious *Candida* and *Cryptococcus* infections. (A) Griseofulvin is an antifungal that interferes with microtubules impairing the mitotic spindle. It concentrates in keratin-containing tissues and is used for superficial rather than for systemic fungal infections. (B) The -azole drugs such as fluconazole and ketoconazole inhibit ergosterol synthesis. Ergosterol is a vital component to fungal cell membranes, much like cholesterol in mammalian cell membranes. (C) Antibiotics such as tetracyclines, macrolides, and aminoglycosides work by inhibiting prokaryotic protein synthesis. These antibiotics are not useful against fungi because fungi are eukaryotes. (E) Amphotericin B and nystatin bind ergosterol in fungal cell membranes and lead to pore formation. Fungal cell homeostasis is interrupted as the membrane becomes permeable to important ions and molecules. Flucytosine does not form membrane pores.

42 **The answer is B: Inhibition of cell wall synthesis.** Caspofungin is an echinocandin that inhibits fungal cell wall synthesis by blocking formation of β-D-glucan. Only fungi use β-D-glucan in their cell walls, so echinocandins are fungi specific. Common side effects of caspofungin include fever and elevated liver enzymes. Echinocandins are commonly used against aspergillosis and candidiasis. (A) Caspofungin inhibits cell wall synthesis, not cell membrane synthesis. As mammalian and fungal cell membranes are similar in makeup, this would not be a good drug target because any drug that affects fungal cell membranes would likely affect human cell membranes. (C) Ketoconazole, itraconazole, and fluconazole are examples of drugs that inhibit ergosterol synthesis. Ergosterol is an important component of fungal cell membranes, as cholesterol is to mammalian cell membranes. (D) Griseofulvin disrupts microtubules, the main components of the mitotic spindle. Caspofungin does not affect the mitotic spindle. (E) Antibiotics such as tetracyclines, macrolides, and aminoglycosides work by inhibiting prokaryotic protein synthesis. These antibiotics are not useful against fungi because fungi are eukaryotes.

43 **The answer is B: Efflux.** Tetracycline was effective against gynecologic infection because of *Bacteroides*, but now these organisms are resistant because of the presence of plasmid-mediated protein that promotes efflux of the drug. (A) Alteration in the target enzyme, DNA gyrase, has resulted in resistance to fluoroquinolones. (C) Enzymatic activation such as which occurs with β-lactamases can destroy antibiotic activity. (D) Enterobacter is largely resistant to cephalosporins by producing β-lactamases. However, resistant organisms may also have altered porin channels through which cephalosporins do not pass.

44 **The answer is B: Inability of antibiotic to reach intestinal crypts.** Most of the penicillins are incompletely absorbed after oral administration, and they reach the intestine in sufficient amounts to affect the composition of the intestinal flora. However, amoxicillin is almost completely absorbed. Consequently, it is not an appropriate therapy for the treatment of *Shigella*- or *Salmonella*-derived enteritis because therapeutically effective levels do not reach the organisms in the intestinal crypts. Absorption of all the penicillinase-resistant penicillins is decreased by food in the stomach, because gastric emptying time is lengthened, and the drugs are destroyed in the acidic environment. (A) The stomach environment is acidic and can destroy certain drugs. (C) Most penicillins are incompletely absorbed following oral administration. (D) This patient likely has a bacterial infection with *Salmonella* or *Shigella*. (E) This patient likely has a bacterial infection with *Salmonella* or *Shigella*.

45 **The answer is C: Presence of plasmid-associated synthesis of acetyltransferase.** Resistance to aminoglycosides can be caused by (1) decreased uptake of drug when the oxygen-dependent transport system for aminoglycosides is absent and (2) plasmid-associated synthesis of enzymes (e.g., acetyltransferases, nucleotidyltransferases, and phosphotransferases) that modify and inactivate aminoglycoside antibiotics. Each of these enzymes has its own aminoglycoside specificity; therefore, cross-resistance is not an invariable rule. (A) Hepatic transaminase activity is the normal liver enzyme activity. (B) This mechanism of resistance of aminoglycosides does not include phosphodiesterase activity. (D) Decreased uptake of drug into oxygen-dependent transport system contributes to antibiotic resistance.

46 **The answer is C: Plasmid-associated erythromycin esterase.** Resistance to erythromycin is becoming a serious clinical problem. For example, most strains of staphylococci in hospital isolates are resistant to this drug. Several mechanisms have been identified: (1) the inability of the organism to take up the antibiotic or the presence of an efflux pump, both of which limit the amount of intracellular drug; (2) a decreased affinity of the 50S ribosomal subunit for the antibiotic, resulting from the methylation of an adenine in the 23S bacterial ribosomal RNA; and (3) the presence of a plasmid-associated erythromycin esterase. (A) Resistance is caused by inability of the organism to take up the antibiotic. (B) Decreased affinity of the 50S ribosomal subunit for the antibiotic can contribute to resistance. (D) The presence of an efflux pump contributes to aminoglycoside resistance. (E) Methylation of an adenine in the 23S bacterial ribosomal subunit can contribute to antibiotic resistance.

47 **The answer is C: Clarithromycin.** Erythromycin and azithromycin are primarily concentrated and excreted in an active form in the bile. Partial reabsorption occurs through the enterohepatic circulation. Inactive metabolites are excreted into the urine. In contrast, clarithromycin and its metabolites are eliminated by the kidney as well as the liver, and it is recommended that the dosage of this drug be adjusted in patients with compromised renal function. (A) Azithromycin is concentrated and excreted by the liver. (B) This patient is likely going to have an allergy to cefazolin as she has an allergy to penicillin. (D) Erythromycin is concentrated and excreted by the liver. (E) This patient would be expected to have an allergy to levofloxacin.

48 **The answer is C: R factor.** Resistance to chloramphenicol is conferred by the presence of an R factor that codes for an acetyl coenzyme A transferase. This enzyme inactivates chloramphenicol. Another mechanism for resistance is associated with an inability of the antibiotic to penetrate the organism. This change in permeability may be the basis of multidrug resistance. (A) It is likely that the drug is less able to penetrate the pathogen cell membrane. (B) MDR gene is the multidrug resistance gene and is usually present in cancer cells. (D) This pathogen creates resistance through R-factor mediation. (E) The mechanism of drug resistance is not related to pH change.

49 **The answer is E: 5-Aminosalicylate.** Sulfasalazine is not absorbed when administered orally or as a suppository and, therefore, is reserved for treatment of chronic inflammatory bowel disease (e.g., Crohn's disease or ulcerative colitis). Local intestinal flora split sulfasalazine into sulfapyridine and 5-aminosalicylate, with the latter exerting the anti-inflammatory effect. (A) Phenazopyridine is a urinary analgesic agent that is not concentrated in the GI tract. (B) Sulfamethoxazole is an antibiotic agent that is not concentrated in the GI tract. (C) Although sulfapyridine is a breakdown product of sulfasalazine, it does not have active anti-inflammatory activity. (D) Tetracycline is an antibiotic agent that is not concentrated in the GI tract.

50 **The answer is B: Mutation of Kat G.** Isoniazid resistance is associated with several different chromosomal mutations, each of which results in one of the following: mutation or deletion of Kat G (producing mutants incapable of prodrug activation), varying mutations of the acyl carrier proteins, or overexpression of InhA. Cross-resistance does not occur between isoniazid and other antitubercular drugs. (A) Isoniazid resistance does not involve chromosomal mutations of Acyl A. (C) Mutations capable of prodrug activation are associated with development of resistance to isoniazid. (D) Overexpression of InhA is a possible mechanism of isoniazid resistance.

51 **The answer is C: Peripheral neuritis.** Isoniazid is associated with development of peripheral neuritis (manifesting as paresthesias of the hands and feet), which is the most common adverse effect and appears to be caused by a relative pyridoxine deficiency. Most of the toxic reactions are corrected by supplementation of 25 to 50 mg/d of pyridoxine (vitamin B_6). Isoniazid can achieve levels in breast milk that are high enough to cause a pyridoxine deficiency in the infant unless the mother is supplemented with the vitamin. (A) Although diabetes mellitus can cause peripheral neuropathy, it is unlikely in this patient because there is no indication that blood sugar levels are abnormal. (B) History in this question gives no indication of lumbar disc abnormality. No evidence of imaging study to suggest this finding is provided. (D) No history of trauma is provided in this question to suggest spinal cord compression. (E) This patient does not have any urinary symptoms; thus, urinary tract infection is unlikely.

52 **The answer is B: Rifabutin.** Rifabutin, a derivative of rifampin, is the preferred drug for use in patients with tuberculosis and human immunodeficiency virus (HIV) disease who are concomitantly treated with protease inhibitors or nonnucleoside reverse transcriptase inhibitors because it is a less potent inducer of cytochrome P450 enzymes. Rifabutin has adverse effects similar to those of rifampin but can also cause uveitis, skin hyperpigmentation, and neutropenia. (A) This patient would benefit from an antituberculosis agent that will have limited hepatic side effects. (C) Rifampin is not the preferred treatment for this patient with HIV disease. (D) Ribavirin would not likely be of benefit to this patient with tuberculosis. (E) Testosterone is not helpful because this patient has HIV disease and tuberculosis.

53 **The answer is A: D-alanine.** Cycloserine is an orally effective, tuberculostatic agent that appears to antagonize the steps in bacterial cell wall synthesis involving D-alanine. It distributes well throughout body fluids including the CSF. Cycloserine is metabolized, and both parent and metabolite are excreted in urine. (B) D-aspartate is not inhibited by cycloserine. (C) D-glutamate is not inhibited by cycloserine. (D) Para-aminobenzoate is not inhibited by cycloserine. (E) Uracil is not inhibited by cycloserine.

54 **The answer is C: No significant difference in clinical outcome will be noted.** Topical use is associated with contact dermatitis, vulvar irritation, and edema. Miconazole is a potent inhibitor of warfarin metabolism and has produced bleeding in warfarin-treated patients even when applied locally to the vaginal area. No significant difference in clinical outcomes is associated with any -azole or nystatin in the treatment of vulvar candidiasis. Induction of hepatic cytochrome P450 activity by griseofulvin. (A) Both agents will provide quick and equivalent treatment responses. (B) Neither agent will improve urinary symptoms. (D) Both agents will be equally well tolerated by the patient. (E) Griseofulvin induces the hepatic cytochrome P450 system.

55 **The answer is B: Hepatic first-pass metabolism is achieved.** Mebendazole is nearly insoluble in aqueous solution. Little of an oral dose (that is chewed) is absorbed, unless it is taken with a high-fat meal. It undergoes first-pass metabolism to inactive compounds. Mebendazole is relatively free of toxic effects, although patients may complain of abdominal pain and diarrhea. It is, however, contraindicated in pregnant women because it has been shown to be embryotoxic and teratogenic in experimental animals. (A) The best results with mebendazole are obtained after oral administration. (C) High-fat meals enhance absorption of mebendazole. (D) The side effect profile of mebendazole is favorable and usually involves gastrointestinal complaints such as abdominal pain and diarrhea. (E) Use of this agent in pregnancy is contraindicated because of potential teratogenic effects.

56 **The answer is A: Albendazole.** Cysticercosis is caused by *Taenia solium* larvae. Infection produces cysticerci in the brain (causing seizures, headache, and vomiting) and in the eyes. The disease follows ingestion of eggs from human feces. Cysticercosis is diagnosed by CT scan or biopsy. Therapy: praziquantel, albendazole, and/or surgery. (B) Niclosamide is the treatment of choice for Taeniasis. (C) Corticosteroids are beneficial in reducing inflammation and swelling as an adjunct to albendazole therapy. (D) Antibiotic therapy with tetracycline is not indicated for this patient with cysticercosis. (E) Observation is not recommended for this acutely ill patient.

57 **The answer is B: Asthma.** Zanamivir is not associated with GI disturbance because it is administered directly to the airways. Irritation of the respiratory tract does occur, however. Zanamivir should be avoided in individuals with severe reactive asthma or chronic obstructive respiratory disease because bronchospasm may occur with the risk of fatality. Neither drug has been reported to have clinically significant drug interactions. (A) Reactive airway disease, not upper airway conditions, such as adenoiditis, predisposes this patient to increased bronchospasm. (C) Floppy tongue syndrome is not associated with increased risk of bronchospasm. (D) Pharyngitis is an upper airway condition not associated with increased risk of bronchospasm. (E) Isolated tracheitis is not associated with bronchospasm.

58 The answer is E: A 39-year-old woman with intermittent dizziness and tinnitus. The drug should be employed cautiously in patients with psychiatric problems, cerebral atherosclerosis, renal impairment, or epilepsy. Rimantadine causes fewer CNS reactions because it does not efficiently cross the blood–brain barrier. For this patient with some mild CNS complaints of tinnitus and dizziness, rimantadine would be the preferred agent. Both drugs cause GI intolerance. Amantadine and rimantadine should be used with caution in pregnant and nursing mothers because they have been found to be embryotoxic and teratogenic in rats. (A) Both drugs should be used with caution in patient with epilepsy. (B) Both agents are potentially embryotoxic and teratogenic. (C) Both agents should not be used in patients who are nursing. (D) Both agents can cause diarrhea.

59 The answer is C: Cleaves proteins necessary for vesicle fusion in lower motor neurons. The toxin described in the stem is botulinum toxin. Botulinum toxin works by cleaving the proteins necessary for vesicle fusion in lower motor neurons. Under the influence of this toxin, vesicles containing acetylcholine cannot fuse with the membrane and therefore cannot release neurotransmitter onto the motor end plate. This leads to a flaccid paralysis of the muscles involved and can diminish wrinkles. (A) This response describes the function of pertussis toxin. The $G_i\alpha$ subunit normally inhibits production of cAMP. ADP-ribosylation inactivates the $G_i\alpha$ subunit, resulting in increased cAMP production. This does not cause skeletal muscle paralysis. (B) This response describes cholera toxin. ADP-ribosylation activates the $G_s\alpha$ subunit, which also results in increased cAMP production. This does not cause skeletal muscle paralysis. (D) This response describes *Clostridium difficile* toxins A and B. Rho GTPases are involved in many aspects of cellular function, including vesicular trafficking, cell polarity, and regulation of apoptosis. These toxins do not cause skeletal muscle paralysis. (E) This response describes diphtheria toxin. Diphtheria toxin ADP-ribosylates the elongation factor 2, which is necessary for protein synthesis. This does not cause skeletal muscle paralysis.

60 The answer is E: Tetanospasmin. Botulinum toxin works by cleaving the proteins necessary for vesicle fusion in lower motor neurons. Under the influence of this toxin, vesicles containing acetylcholine cannot fuse with the membrane and therefore cannot release neurotransmitter onto the motor end plate. Tetanospasmin is almost identical. It also inhibits neurotransmitter vesicle fusion, but it inhibits membrane fusion of GABA- and glycine-containing vesicles in inhibitory interneurons. (A) Cytolethal distending toxin is produced by *Campylobacter* species. It inactivates cyclin-dependent kinase 1, stopping the cell cycle in G2. (B) Heat-labile enterotoxin is one of the toxins produced by enterotoxigenic *Escherichia coli*. It ADP-ribosylates the $G_s\alpha$ subunit, leading to an increased cAMP concentration. (C) Heat-stable enterotoxin is another toxin produced by enterotoxigenic *E. coli*. It activates guanylate cyclase, causing an increased cGMP concentration. (D) Shiga toxin is produced by *Shigella dysenteriae* and enterohemorrhagic *E. coli* O157:H7. It inhibits protein synthesis by irreversibly inactivating ribosomes through cleavage of part of the 60S subunit.

61 The answer is A: HBV DNA polymerase. Lamivudine must be phosphorylated by host cellular enzymes to the triphosphate (active) form. This compound competitively inhibits HBV DNA polymerase at concentrations that have negligible effects on host DNA polymerase. As with many nucleotide analogs, the intracellular half-life of the triphosphate is many hours longer than its plasma half-life. (B) Lamivudine is a competitive inhibitor of HBV DNA polymerase. (C) Lamivudine is a competitive inhibitor of HBV DNA polymerase. (D) Hepatitis B is a DNA virus.

62 The answer is D: Deficient thymidine kinase. Resistance can be found with several viral strains to acyclovir. Altered or deficient thymidine kinase and DNA polymerases have been found in some resistant viral strains and are most commonly isolated from immunocompromised patients. Cross-resistance to the other agents in this family occurs. Cytomegalovirus (CMV) is resistant because it lacks a specific viral thymidine kinase. (A) Altered or deficient DNA polymerase is a reason for resistance to acyclovir. (B) Altered or deficient thymidine kinase is found in some resistant viral strains. (C) RNA transferase is not deficient in patients with herpes viral resistant strains. (E) Deficient uracil synthase is not a mechanism of resistance for herpes viral strains.

63 The answer is A: Calcium. Foscarnet is poorly absorbed orally and must be injected IV. It must also be given frequently to avoid relapse when plasma levels fall. It is dispersed throughout the body, and greater than 10% enters the bone matrix from which it slowly leaves. The parent drug is eliminated by glomerular filtration and tubular secretion into the urine. Adverse effects include nephrotoxicity, anemia, nausea, and fever. Because of chelation with divalent cations, hypocalcemia and hypomagnesemia are also seen. In addition, hypokalemia, hypophosphatemia and hyperphosphatemia, seizures, and arrhythmias have been reported. (B) Chloride is not a divalent cation and would be expected to be normal in this patient. (C) Serum creatinine levels would be expected to be normal in this patient. (D) Serum glucose levels would be expected to be normal in this patient. Glucose is not a divalent cation. (E) Sodium is not a divalent cation and would be expected to be normal in this patient.

64 **The answer is C: This agent can potentiate therapy when used with other protease inhibitors.** Ritonavir is no longer used as a single protease inhibitor but instead is used as a pharmacokinetic enhancer or "booster" of other protease inhibitors. Ritonavir is a potent inhibitor of CYP3A, and concomitant ritonavir administration (at low doses) increases the bioavailability of the second protease inhibitor, often allowing for longer dosing intervals. The resulting higher C_{min} levels of the "boosted" protease inhibitors also help to prevent the development of resistance. (A) Ritonavir inhibits CYP3A. (B) Ritonavir is no longer used as a single protease inhibitor. (D) Ritonavir is associated with a lower rate of resistance when used in combination with another protease inhibitor.

65 **The answer is A: A 24-year-old man with Crohn's disease.** Methotrexate, usually in combination with other drugs, is effective against acute lymphocytic leukemia, choriocarcinoma, Burkitt lymphoma in children, breast cancer, and head and neck carcinomas. In addition, low-dose methotrexate is effective as a single agent against certain inflammatory diseases, such as severe psoriasis and rheumatoid arthritis as well as Crohn disease. All patients receiving methotrexate require close monitoring for possible toxic effects. (B) Choriocarcinoma is usually treated with multidrug chemotherapy. (C) Metastatic breast cancer or locally advanced breast cancer is best treated with multiagent chemotherapy. (D) This patient with localized breast cancer would best respond to combination chemotherapy. (E) Acute leukemia responds better to multiagent chemotherapy than single agents.

66 **The answer is B: Initiates action via phosphorylation.** Fludarabine is the 5′-phosphate of 2-fluoroadenine arabinoside, a purine nucleotide analog. It is useful in the treatment of chronic lymphocytic leukemia and may replace chlorambucil, the current drug of choice. Fludarabine is also effective against hairy cell leukemia and indolent non-Hodgkin lymphoma. Fludarabine is a prodrug, the phosphate being removed in the plasma to form 2-F-ara-A, which is taken up into cells and again phosphorylated (initially by deoxycytidine kinase). (A) Fludarabine is inactive as a prodrug and becomes activated by phosphorylation. (C) This agent becomes activated by phosphorylation. (D) This agent can cause bone marrow suppression but this is not a mechanism of action of fludarabine. (E) Fludarabine does not cause trabeculation of bone islands.

67 **The answer is C: Fluoroalanine.** Because of its severe toxicity to the GI tract, 5-FU is given IV or, in the case of skin cancer, topically. The drug penetrates well into all tissues, including the CNS. 5-FU is rapidly metabolized in the liver, lung, and kidney. It is eventually converted to fluoroalanine, which is removed in the urine, and to CO_2, which is exhaled. (A) Fluoroalanine can be measured because it is excreted in urine and into CO_2. (B) Creatinine is a good marker of renal function but is not a direct measure of 5-FU excretion. (D) Urine glucose levels would be elevated in patients with diabetes mellitus whose serum glucose levels are above 180 mg/dL. (E) Hepatic transferase levels would be elevated in patients with liver failure. This is not a direct indicator of hepatic toxicity from 5-FU.

68 **The answer is D: Thymidylate synthase.** After being absorbed, capecitabine, which is itself nontoxic, undergoes a series of enzymatic reactions, the last of which is hydrolysis to 5-FU. This step is catalyzed by thymidine phosphorylase, an enzyme that is concentrated primarily in tumors. Thus, the cytotoxic activity of capecitabine is the same as that of 5-FU and is tumor specific. The most important enzyme inhibited by 5-FU (and, thus, capecitabine) is thymidylate synthase. (A) Capecitabine is hydrolyzed to 5-FU. Thus, 5-FU is what created the cytotoxic effects of this agent. (B) This agent inhibits thymidylate synthase. (C) This agent does not inhibit RNA transferase. (D) Capecitabine does not inhibit uracil transferase.

69 **The answer is A: Cefepime.** Many drugs are renally excreted and may reach much higher than expected serum concentrations in patients with renal disease. Most β-lactam antibiotics are largely excreted unchanged in the urine. Cefepime, a cephalosporin, is an example—about 85% of a dose is excreted unchanged in the urine. Of the drugs listed, cefepime would be expected to reach the highest above normal drug concentration in this patient. (B) Cyclosporine and its metabolites are excreted mostly in the bile. Its concentration would not be expected to rise as high above normal as cefepime's would in this patient. (C) Doxycycline is excreted mostly in the bile. Its concentration would not be expected to rise as high above normal as cefepime's would in this patient. (D) Erythromycin is excreted mostly in the bile. Its concentration would not be expected to rise as high above normal as cefepime's would in this patient. (E) Nafcillin is excreted mostly in the bile. Its concentration would not be expected to rise as high above normal as cefepime's would in this patient.

70 **The answer is E: Sodium stibogluconate.** A nonhealing ulcer following an insect bite in the Middle East is consistent with cutaneous leishmaniasis.

Leishmaniasis is caused by protozoans transmitted by the bite of sand flies. If left untreated, cutaneous leishmaniasis can progress to the much more deadly visceral leishmaniasis. Sodium stibogluconate is used to treat cutaneous leishmaniasis, although its mechanism of action is still unclear. (A) Primaquine is used to kill the hypnozoites of *Plasmodium vivax* and *Plasmodium ovale* that persist in hepatocytes. It is not used to treat leishmaniasis. (B) Praziquantel is used to treat flatworm infections by increasing the permeability of their cell membranes to calcium ions leading to spastic paralysis of the worms. It is not used to treat leishmaniasis. (C) Prednisone is a corticosteroid. It should generally not be used in infections because it impairs the immune response. (D) Nifurtimox is used to treat trypanosomiasis. It inhibits DNA synthesis in the trypanosomes. It is not used to treat leishmaniasis.

71 **The answer is E: Mefloquine.** Mefloquine is contraindicated for patients with a history of epilepsy, psychiatric disorders, arrhythmia, cardiac conduction defects, or sensitivity to related drugs. Weekly dosing may cause nausea, vomiting, dizziness, sleep and behavioral disturbances, epigastric pain, diarrhea, headache, and rash. Reports of more severe reactions include depression, confusion, acute psychosis, and seizures. It is an effective antimalarial for many strains of chloroquine-resistant *P. falciparum* and is used mostly in malaria-endemic regions where resistance to chloroquine is prevalent. (A) Chloroquine is the standard treatment in sensitive *P. falciparum* and other species of human malaria parasites. Although chloroquine is usually well tolerated, it is recommended to be used with caution in patients who have a history of neurologic disorders. (B) Diphenoxylate is an antidiarrheal. It is an opioid that has no analgesic properties in standard doses. High doses can have CNS effects and prolonged use can lead to opioid dependence. (C) Doxycycline is an antibiotic with modest antimalarial properties. The mechanism of action is unknown, but it cannot be used as a single agent in the treatment of malaria. Side effects include infrequent GI symptoms, candidal vaginitis, and photosensitivity. (D) Loperamide is a nonprescription antidiarrheal agent. It does not cross the blood–brain barrier. It has no analgesic properties or potential for addiction.

72 **The answer is C: Increased activity of efflux pumps.** Chloroquine works by inhibiting conversion of heme to hemozoin causing a buildup of heme, which poisons the malarial parasites. In order to be effective, chloroquine must remain in the parasite's food vacuole. Resistance occurs when efflux pumps remove chloroquine from the food vacuoles so that chloroquine is unable to reach therapeutic concentrations. (A) Antigenic variation is a mechanism by which infectious organisms evade the immune system. Chloroquine resistance is accomplished by the increased activity of efflux pumps. (B) Chloroquine is an antimalarial and was a mainstay of malaria treatment before widespread resistance arose. It is now reliable only in and around Central America. (D) Chloroquine is not inactivated by protozoal metabolism. Chloroquine resistance is accomplished by the increased activity of efflux pumps. (E) Chloroquine is not inactivated by modification of target proteins. It binds heme polymerase, and resistance is accomplished by the increased activity of the flux pumps.

73 **The answer is B: Mebendazole.** This child has an *Enterobius vermicularis*, or "pinworm," infection. A simple way to ascertain infection is by the adhesive tape test described in the question stem. This test should be done at night to maximize the chance of collecting worms for identification. A single dose of mebendazole is sufficient to treat this type of infection. (A) Fluconazole is an antifungal. It would not be useful for treating an *Enterobius* infection. (C) Metronidazole is used to treat certain bacterial and parasitic infections but is not effective in treating an *Enterobius* infection. Mebendazole is the best choice in this case. (D) Nifurtimox is a drug used to treat trypanosomiasis, the infection caused by the *Trypanosoma cruzi* parasite. It would not be useful for treating an *Enterobius* infection. (E) Praziquantel is used to treat schistosomal infections. It would not be the best choice for treating an *Enterobius* infection.

74 **The answer is A: Inhibition of dihydrofolate reductase.** Toxoplasmosis is caused by infection by the organism *Toxoplasma gondii*. This parasite can be transmitted to humans through contact with cat feces and can cross the placenta in pregnant women, leading to congenital toxoplasmosis. As with this infant, congenital infection can cause seizures and hydrocephalus. Treatment involves pyrimethamine and sulfadiazine, which both interfere with folic acid metabolism in the parasite. Pyrimethamine blocks dihydrofolate reductase to prevent folate recycling, whereas sulfadiazine blocks dihydropteroate synthetase (an enzyme involved in folic acid synthesis). (B) Sulfadiazine inhibits the enzyme dihydropteroate synthetase. Pyrimethamine inhibits dihydrofolate reductase. (C) Nifurtimox is an antiparasitic that inhibits nucleic acid synthesis and is used to treat *Trypanosoma cruzi* infection. Pyrimethamine inhibits dihydrofolate reductase. (D) Praziquantel, used to treat schistosomal infections, causes membrane depolarization and parasite paralysis. Pyrimethamine inhibits dihydrofolate reductase. (E) Antibacterials such as the aminoglycosides and macrolides inhibit ribosomal function. Pyrimethamine inhibits dihydrofolate reductase.

75 The answer is C: Gentamicin. Synergy is a term used to describe a situation when the combined effect of two or more drugs simultaneously is greater than can be explained by arithmetically adding the individual effects. A fine example is the synergistic effect when a penicillin such as ampicillin is combined with an aminoglycoside such as gentamicin. Synergy occurs in this case because ampicillin and gentamicin employ different, unrelated mechanisms of action. (A) Amoxicillin is a β-lactam antibiotic as is ampicillin. They both work by inhibiting the same enzymes involved in cell wall synthesis and would compete with each other rather than work together. (B) Cephalexin is a β-lactam antibiotic as is ampicillin. They both work by inhibiting the same enzymes involved in cell wall synthesis and would compete with each other rather than work together. (D) Penicillin G is a β-lactam antibiotic as is ampicillin. They both work by inhibiting the same enzymes involved in cell wall synthesis and would compete with each other rather than work together. (E) Penicillin V is a β-lactam antibiotic as is ampicillin. They both work by inhibiting the same enzymes involved in cell wall synthesis and would compete with each other rather than work together.

76 The answer is C: Metronidazole. *Trichomonas vaginalis* is a protozoan organism that lives in the urethra and vagina. This organism can freely be transmitted during sexual intercourse. Symptoms of infection include vulvar itching, burning, copious discharge with rancid odor, dysuria, and dyspareunia. Examination may reveal edema and erythema of the vulva and petechiae of the upper vagina and cervix. The secretions are often yellow-green with a pH of greater than 6.5. Wet smear will reveal the *Trichomonas* organism. Treatment is by oral metronidazole, and 1-day therapy regimens will result in a 90% cure rate. (A) Amoxicillin is not an appropriate treatment choice for *Trichomonas vaginalis*. (B) Ciprofloxacin is a quinolone antibiotic that will not effectively treat *Trichomonas vaginalis*. (D) Ofloxacin is an infrequently used quinolone antibiotic that will not effectively treat *Trichomonas vaginalis*. (E) Tetracycline is not an effective treatment of vaginal candidiasis.

77 The answer is B: Oral ganciclovir. Treatment of CMV retinitis involves ganciclovir, foscarnet, and cidofovir. The drugs are given as an initial induction phase and then a later lifelong phase. Ganciclovir can also be given in an intraocular implantable form. (A) Oral erythromycin is not indicated in the treatment of CMV retinitis. (C) Oral penicillin is not useful in the management of CMV retinitis. (D) Oral corticosteroids are unproven in the treatment of CMV retinitis. (E) Intravenous prednisone is not of value in the treatment of CMV retinitis.

78 The correct answer is C: Oral erythromycin. The patient described has *Mycoplasma pneumoniae* infection. This is a common cause of respiratory tract infections in college-aged students, especially among those who reside in close surroundings such as college dormitories. Symptoms include headache, fever, malaise, sore throat, and cough, which often becomes productive. Treatment of choice is oral erythromycin. (A) Cephazolin is expensive and provides no better coverage against this organism than erythromycin. (B) Ciprofloxacin is also expensive and not an appropriate medication of choice for this infection. (D) Intravenous erythromycin should be reserved for severely ill patients. (E) Although this disease will resolve spontaneously without therapy in 4 weeks, antibiotics will shorten the disease course.

79 The answer is E: Procainamide. Several drugs can cause a syndrome resembling systemic lupus erythematosus (SLE). The syndrome is most common with procainamide, which induces the presence of antinuclear antibodies in up to 75% of individuals within a few months. There is a genetic predisposition to drug-induced lupus determined by drug acetylation rates. Typical symptoms include systemic complaints and arthralgias. The initial therapeutic approach is withdrawal of the offending drug. (A) Although ethosuximide has been reported to cause drug-induced SLE, case reports have been mainly anecdotal. (B) Drug-induced lupus is exceedingly rare with the use of oral contraceptives. (C) Hydralazine is the second most common cause of drug-induced SLE and induces antinuclear antigen positivity in up to 30% of patients taking this medication. (D) Phenytoin has not been shown in clinical studies to cause a lupus-like reaction.

80 The answer is E: Inhibits folic acid metabolism. The patient is suffering from hemolysis secondary to G6PD deficiency. This is an adverse reaction seen in patients who take trimethoprim–sulfamethoxazole. It is more commonly seen in African Americans. Look for the symptoms of hemolysis, such as anemia and jaundice. (A) This is the mechanism of action of clindamycin. A common side effect is *C. difficile* infection. (B) This is the mechanism of action of tetracyclines. Common side effects are discoloration of children's teeth and disruption of bone synthesis. (C) This is the mechanism of action of vancomycin. Common side effects are nephrotoxicity, ototoxicity, and red man syndrome. (D) This is the mechanism of action of rifampin. Common side effects are hepatotoxicity and red-orange body fluids.

81 The answer is B: Alopecia. This describes a case of psoriasis. The plaques are caused by a proliferation of keratinocytes in the skin that produce leukocyte-attracting chemokines. These circumstances lead to the thickened, scaly skin of psoriasis accompanied by characteristic inflammation. Acitretin is a vitamin A analog that, by an incompletely understood mechanism, retards keratinocyte proliferation. Alopecia is a common (>50%) side effect of acitretin therapy, similar to vitamin A toxicity. (A) Adrenal insufficiency can result from sudden cessation of glucocorticoid therapy. This side effect is not associated with acitretin. (C) Cushing syndrome is caused by excess glucocorticoids in the body. The most common cause of Cushing syndrome is iatrogenic—because of glucocorticoids prescribed by physicians. Acitretin does not cause Cushing syndrome. (D) Immunosuppression may be caused by administration of glucocorticoids of other immune system modifiers. Acitretin does not modify the immune system. (E) Striae can be a complication of Cushing syndrome, or having a too high glucocorticoid level in the body. Acitretin does not lead to formation of striae.

82 **The answer is D: Phenytoin.** It is important to know that particular medicines that inhibit the P450 system can increase effects of other medications. For patients taking the H_2 blocker cimetidine, there will be increased effects of quinidine, phenytoin, tricyclic antidepressants, and warfarin. (A) Dronabinol's effects will be increased in the presence of the protease inhibitor ritonavir. (B) Erythromycin's effects are increased in the presence of ritonavir. (C) Ketoconazole's effects are increased in the presence of ritonavir. (E) Rifampin's effects are increased in the presence of ritonavir.

83 **The answer is D: Neomycin.** Neomycin is an aminoglycoside that is commonly used for bowel surgeries. Neomycin is not absorbed from the GI tract and sterilizes the intestines by killing the bacteria, especially gram negative. (A) Ceftriaxone would be more appropriate for gram-negative bacteria causing health care–associated pneumonia, meningitis, and gonorrhea. (B) Clindamycin is commonly used to treat anaerobes above the diaphragm. (C) Metronidazole is commonly used to treat anaerobes below the diaphragm but is not preferred over Neomycin prior to bowel surgery. (E) Trimethoprim–sulfamethoxazole is commonly used to treat gram-positive and -negative bacteria but is not preferred over Neomycin prior to bowel surgery.

84 **The answer is D: Rifampin.** The prophylaxis for a meningococcal infection is rifampin and should be given to all close contacts. It works by inhibiting DNA-dependent RNA polymerase in bacteria and is lipophilic, so it can cross the blood–brain barrier. (A) Benzathine penicillin G is used as prophylaxis and the treatment of syphilis. (B) Ceftriaxone is used as prophylaxis for gonorrhea. (C) Penicillin is used as endocarditis prophylaxis in dental surgeries. (E) Trimethoprim–sulfamethoxazole is used as prophylaxis for *Pneumocystis jiroveci* and recurrent UTIs.

85 **The answer is C: 5-HT$_3$.** Antagonists at the 5-HT$_3$ receptor include agents such as ondansetron, which is highly effective in the treatment of nausea and vomiting associated with chemotherapy. This agent inhibits receptors for 5-HT$_3$ in the area postrema, which will prevent nausea and vomiting and might have an added effect by reducing peripheral sensation of pain. (A) The 5-HT$_1$ receptors cause smooth muscle contraction especially in the carotid artery. (B) The 5-HT$_2$ receptors cause vascular and smooth muscle contraction and cause platelet aggregation. (D) The dopamine receptors play a minor role in the treatment of chemotherapy-associated nausea and vomiting.

86 **The answer is C: Nothing—the course of action taken is entirely appropriate.** This patient's presentation is consistent with secondary syphilis. Penicillin is the drug of choice for treatment of syphilis. In an otherwise healthy person, a single intramuscular shot of benzathine penicillin G is curative. The benzathine preparation allows for a continuous, slow diffusion of penicillin into the blood over a matter of weeks. This provides an efficacious and convenient antibiotic regimen and avoids problems with patient adherence. (A) Penicillin is an excellent drug for the treatment of syphilis. Resistance is minimal and penicillin is effective, inexpensive, and generally well tolerated. (B) Benzathine penicillin G is the best option for the treatment of syphilis because of its ease and efficacy. A single IM dose of another preparation would likely not maintain a sufficiently high drug level to eradicate the infection. (D) Benzathine penicillin G is the drug of choice for secondary syphilis. Penicillin V is an oral preparation of penicillin and would require many more doses than the single IM shot of benzathine penicillin G. (E) In an otherwise healthy person, a single IM shot of benzathine penicillin G is curative. More shots may be necessary in immunocompromised individuals and pregnant women.

87 **The answer is A: Binds ergosterol.** The mechanism of action of amphotericin B is binding to ergosterol, which disrupts the cell membrane forming pores. The pores allow the leakage of electrolytes from the fungal cell. (B) The mechanism of action of caspofungin is the inhibition of cell wall synthesis by inhibiting the synthesis of β-glucan. (C) The mechanism of action of flucytosine is inhibiting fungal DNA synthesis. (D) The mechanism of action of the -azoles (e.g., fluconazole) is inhibiting ergosterol synthesis. (E) The mechanism of action of terbinafine is the inhibition of the enzyme squalene epoxidase.

88 **The answer is E: Ketoconazole.** Ketoconazole causes gynecomastia by the inhibition of the testosterone. Other side effects are liver toxicity, rash, GI upset, and inhibition of cytochrome P450. (A) Common side effects of amphotericin B are fever/chills, nephrotoxicity, arrhythmias, anemia, and hypotension. Gynecomastia is not a common side effect. (B) Common side effects of caspofungin are GI upset and flushing of the skin. Gynecomastia is not a common side effect. (C) Common side effects of flucytosine are GI upset and bone marrow suppression. Gynecomastia is not a common side effect. (D) Common side effects of griseofulvin are GI upset, confusion, headaches, and induction of cytochrome P450. Gynecomastia is not a common side effect.

89 **The answer is E: Zidovudine.** Zidovudine, a nucleoside reverse transcriptase inhibitor, has been proven to decrease the likelihood of transmission of HIV disease from mother to fetus. It is given to the mother during pregnancy and delivery and to the infant for 6 weeks. (A) Efavirenz is a nonnucleoside reverse transcriptase inhibitor. It has not been proven to decrease the likelihood of transmission of HIV disease like zidovudine. (B) Enfuvirtide is a fusion inhibitor. It is used in patients with persistent viral replication despite therapy. (C) Indinavir is a protease inhibitor. It has not been proven to decrease the likelihood of transmission of HIV disease like zidovudine. (D) Lamivudine is a nucleoside reverse transcriptase inhibitor. It is also used for the treatment of hepatitis B.

90 **The answer is A: Lack of thymidine kinase.** The mechanism of action of acyclovir is the inhibition of DNA polymerase by being monophosphorylated by HSV thymidine kinase and then triphosphorylation is achieved using cellular enzymes. Therefore, the mechanism of resistance is by HSV lacking thymidine kinase. (B) The lack of viral kinase is one of the mechanisms of resistance for ganciclovir. (C) The mutation of CMV DNA polymerase is one of the mechanisms of resistance for ganciclovir. (D) The mutation of DNA polymerase is the mechanism of resistance for foscarnet. (E) The mutation of the M_2 protein is the mechanism of resistance for amantadine.

91 **The answer is D: Oprelvekin.** Oprelvekin is a recombinant interleukin-11, which stimulates megakaryocyte progenitor cells to produce platelets. Oprelvekin is an alternative to platelet transfusions in patients with chronically low platelets. (A) Aldesleukin is a recombinant interleukin-2 used for renal cell carcinoma and metastatic melanoma. (B) Erythropoietin stimulates hematopoietic stem cells for the production of red blood cells. (C) Filgrastim is a recombinant granulocyte colony-stimulating factor used to stimulate the proliferation of granulocytes in the bone marrow. (E) Sargramostim is a recombinant granulocyte-macrophage colony-stimulating factor used to stimulate granulocyte and macrophage production in the bone marrow.

92 **The answer is D: Nitrous oxide.** When the administration of an inhalation anesthetic is discontinued, the body becomes the "source" that drives the anesthetic into the alveolar space. The same factors that influence attainment of steady state with an inspired anesthetic determine the time course of clearance of the drug from the body. Thus, nitrous oxide exits the body faster than halothane. (A) Enflurane exits the body slowly. (B) Halothane exits the body slowly. (C) Isoflurane exits the body slowly.

93 **The answer is C: Cytarabine.** Cytarabine is converted to an active metabolite that is incorporated into growing strands of DNA. Other nucleotides cannot be added to strand, and the cell is unable to remove the cytarabine metabolite so DNA synthesis is halted. When rapidly dividing cells (such as cancer cells) are unable to replicate this DNA, they undergo apoptosis. (A) 5-Fluorouracil (5-FU) is an antimetabolite that irreversibly inhibits the enzyme thymidylate synthase. Rapidly dividing cells exposed to 5-FU cannot synthesize thymidine and die. (B) Cyclophosphamide is converted to an active metabolite that works by transferring alkyl groups to DNA strands, which then link to each other. Linked DNA strands cannot be replicated. (D) Methotrexate is a folate antimetabolite. Folate is necessary for precursors to DNA synthesis, so inhibiting folate use by cells slows DNA synthesis and proliferation. (E) Vincristine interferes with microtubules, leading to cell cycle arrest in metaphase.

94 **The answer is E: Vincristine.** For patients with recurrent cancer, using a different chemotherapeutic agent than was used initially is often favored. This is caused by the fact that cancer cells can become resistant to chemotherapy drugs to which they are exposed. In this patient's case, paclitaxel (a microtubule inhibitor) was used during her initial treatment. Although both paclitaxel and vincristine interfere with microtubules, they bind to different sites and have differing mechanisms of action. Paclitaxel stabilizes microtubules, but vincristine disrupts microtubules leading to their dissolution. (A) Cisplatin is a DNA-binding agent that forms crosslinks in DNA strands. It does not interfere with microtubules. (B) Docetaxel and paclitaxel are taxanes, which inhibit microtubule depolymerization. They stabilize, not disrupt, microtubules. (C) Erlotinib inhibits cell proliferation by blocking the epidermal growth factor receptor. It does not interfere with microtubules. (D) Irinotecan is an agent that inhibits topoisomerase. It does not interfere with microtubules.

95 **The answer is B: Inhibits dihydrofolate reductase.** Methotrexate is an analog of folic acid that inhibits dihydrofolate reductase. This leads to decreased DNA and protein synthesis. Methotrexate is used in the treatment of choriocarcinoma. (A) The mechanism of action of busulfan is the alkylation of DNA. (C) The mechanism of action of cytarabine is the inhibition of DNA polymerase through pyrimidine antagonism. (D) 5-Fluorouracil is a pyrimidine analog that inhibits thymidylate synthase to decrease DNA and protein synthesis. (E) The mechanism of action of etoposide is the inhibition of topoisomerase II.

96 **The answer is B: 6-Mercaptopurine.** 6-Mercaptopurine is metabolized by xanthine oxidase, which is inhibited by allopurinol. This increases the toxicity of 6-mercaptopurine. Side effects of 6-mercaptopurine include bone marrow suppression, liver toxicity, and GI upset. (A) 5-Fluorouracil is primarily metabolized by the liver. There is no contraindication to taking allopurinol. (C) 6-Thioguanine is similar to 6-mercaptopurine in mechanism of action, but it is metabolized in the liver. There is no contraindication to taking allopurinol. (D) Bleomycin is metabolized by CYP450. There is no contraindication to taking allopurinol. (E) Methotrexate is metabolized primarily in the liver. There is no contraindication to taking allopurinol.

97 **The answer is D: Doxorubicin.** Doxorubicin is used for the treatment of Hodgkin's lymphoma. A side effect of the medication is dose-dependent cardiomyopathy. (A) The main side effect of bleomycin to monitor for is pulmonary fibrosis. (B) The main side effect of cisplatin to monitor for is nephrotoxicity. (C) The main side effect of dactinomycin to monitor for is myelosuppression. (E) The main side effect of vincristine to monitor for is neurotoxicity.

98 **The answer is E: Tyrosine kinase inhibitor.** The patient will start therapy with imatinib, which is a tyrosine kinase inhibitor. The development of tyrosine kinase inhibitors in the treatment of chronic myelogenous leukemia with a positive Philadelphia chromosome (9:22 translocation) has improved survival drastically. (A) Rituximab is a monoclonal antibody that binds to CD20 on B cells is used in the treatment of B-cell lymphomas. (B) Trastuzumab is a monoclonal antibody that binds to HER-2 and used in the treatment of HER-2–positive metastatic breast cancer. (C) The mechanism of action of cisplatin is cross-linking DNA. It is used in the treatment of testicular and ovarian tumors. (D) Cytarabine inhibits DNA polymerase and is used in the treatment of acute myelogenous leukemia.

99 **The answer is A: Anti-TNF antibody.** Infliximab is a monoclonal antibody that binds directly to tumor necrosis factor (TNF), which does not allow binding to the TNF receptor. The binding of TNF to the TNF receptor activates the inflammatory cascade. (B) The mechanism of adalimumab is the direct binding to the TNF receptor. It does not bind to TNF directly. (C) The mechanism of aspirin is the inhibition of cyclooxygenase. It is also used in the treatment of arthritis as an anti-inflammatory. (D) The mechanism of action of methotrexate is the inhibition of dihydrofolate reductase. It is used in the treatment of rheumatoid arthritis. (E) Etanercept is a recombinant form of the TNF receptor that binds TNF. This decreases the amount of TNF that binds to the TNF receptor attached to the cell membrane of native cells.

100 **The answer is D: Increased risk of thrombosis.** Celecoxib is a selective COX-2 inhibitor. It was developed to protect the gastric mucosa from COX-1 inhibition that is seen from other nonsteroidal anti-inflammatory drugs. However, COX-2 normally increases prostaglandin I_2, which causes anticoagulation. The decrease of prostaglandin I_2 leads to a hypercoagulable state and an increased risk of thrombosis. (A) Doxorubicin leads to an increased risk of dilated cardiomyopathy, but this is dose dependent. Doxorubicin has not been removed from the market. (B) Celecoxib was developed because of an increased risk of GI bleeding from COX-1 inhibition. Celecoxib protects the GI mucosa. (C). Bleomycin and busulfan lead to increased risk of pulmonary fibrosis. They have not been removed from the market. (E) Infliximab increases the risk of reactivation of latent tuberculosis. This is the reason for getting a PPD test prior to starting infliximab.

101 **The answer is E: Temperature sensation.** Delivery techniques include topical administration, infiltration, ring blocks, peripheral nerve blocks, and neuraxial (spinal, epidural, or caudal) blocks. The small, unmyelinated nerve fibers that conduct impulses for pain, temperature, and autonomic activity are most sensitive to the action of local anesthetics. (A) Cerebellar function is unchanged after lidocaine administration. (B) Lidocaine blocks autonomic activity. (C) Lidocaine does not alter pontine function. (D) Lidocaine does not alter spinal reflexes.

102 **The answer is B: Complete blood counts.** Clozapine can lead to agranulocytosis, which requires frequent white blood cell monitoring. Initially, monitoring should be weekly and then less often when signs of agranulocytosis are not present. (A) The concern with clozapine is agranulocytosis, not kidney failure; therefore, BUN/creatinine does not need to be monitored frequently. (C) The concern with clozapine is agranulocytosis, not liver toxicity; therefore, liver function tests do not need to be monitored frequently. (D) The concern with clozapine is agranulocytosis, not pulmonary toxicity; therefore, pulmonary function tests do not need to be monitored frequently. (E) The concern with clozapine is agranulocytosis, not thyroid toxicity; therefore, thyroid function tests do not need to be monitored frequently.

103 **The answer is D: Maraviroc.** HIV life cycle involves multiple steps that are targets for drug therapy. Initially, gp120 on the HIV virion must bind the CD4 receptor plus either the CCR5 or CXCR4 coreceptor on a T cell or a macrophage. Next, gp41 on the virion undergoes a conformational change to mediate fusion of the virion and cell membranes. Then, viral reverse transcriptase makes ssDNA copies of the viral RNA. The ssDNA copies are replicated and incorporated into the host genome. mRNA copies made from this viral DNA are translated into polyproteins that must be cleaved by viral protease for the progeny virus to become infective. Maraviroc inhibits fusion of the virion and T-cell membranes by blocking the CCR5 coreceptor. It is useful only in CCR5-trophic (not CXCR4-trophic) viruses. (A) Darunavir is a protease inhibitor. It blocks the last step in HIV replication—cleavage of the polyproteins into functional proteins. Darunavir does not inhibit membrane fusion. (B) Delavirdine is a nonnucleoside reverse transcriptase inhibitor. It noncompetitively inhibits viral reverse transcriptase's ability to make a DNA copy of viral RNA. Delavirdine does not inhibit membrane fusion. (C) Efavirenz is a nonnucleoside reverse transcriptase inhibitor. It noncompetitively inhibits viral reverse transcriptase's ability to make a DNA copy of viral RNA. Efavirenz does not inhibit membrane fusion. (E) Stavudine is a nucleoside reverse transcriptase inhibitor. It competitively inhibits viral reverse transcriptase's ability to make a DNA copy of viral RNA. Stavudine does not inhibit membrane fusion.

104 **The answer is A: Didanosine.** A patient on HAART therapy with nausea, vomiting, and abdominal pain with elevated serum amylase likely has pancreatitis. Pancreatitis is a known side effect of many antiretrovirals including didanosine. Didanosine should be discontinued in a patient who develops pancreatitis. (B) Efavirenz can cause CNS side effects such as dizziness and insomnia as well as a skin rash. It is not known to cause pancreatitis. (C) Emtricitabine can cause GI side effects such as nausea, diarrhea, and abdominal pain. It is not known to cause pancreatitis. (D) Nevirapine can cause a skin rash that may be accompanied by liver damage. A patient taking nevirapine who develops a skin rash should have his or her liver enzymes checked. It is not known to cause pancreatitis. (E) Raltegravir can cause elevated serum lipase, abdominal pain, nausea, and diarrhea. It is not known to cause pancreatitis.

105 **The answer is D: Morphine and hydrocodone have equal analgesic potency.** Hydromorphone is preferred over morphine in patients with renal dysfunction because of less accumulation of active metabolites compared to morphine. Hydrocodone is the methyl ether of hydromorphone but is a much weaker analgesic than hydromorphone. The analgesic potency of oral hydrocodone is approximately that of morphine. Hydrocodone is often combined with acetaminophen or ibuprofen to treat moderate-to-severe pain. It is also used as an antitussive. Hydrocodone is metabolized in the liver to several metabolites, one of which is hydromorphone. (A) Hydrocodone is metabolized in the liver. (B) Hydrocodone can be used as an antitussive. (C) Hydrocodone is the methyl ether of hydromorphone. (E) Hydrocodone can be used as an antitussive.

106 **The answer is E: Tinnitus.** The analgesic actions of codeine are derived from its conversion to morphine by the CYP450 2D6 enzyme system, whereas the drug's antitussive effects are caused by the codeine itself. Thus, codeine is a much less potent analgesic than morphine. Codeine's analgesic potency is approximately 30% that of morphine. Codeine shows good antitussive activity at doses that do not cause analgesia. At commonly used doses, the drug has a lower potential for abuse than morphine. (A) Codeine can have a significant analgesic effect. (B) Codeine can cause dry coughing spells. (C) Codeine can cause significant euphoria. (D) Codeine can cause significant sedation.

107 **The answer is E: Ritodrine.** Terbutaline is a β_2-agonist that decreases uterine contractions by relaxing uterine smooth muscle. It should only be used to delay labor for no more than 72 h. In that time, steroids can be given to promote lung maturity. (A) Clomiphene is used to induce ovulation, not delay labor. (B) Dinoprostone is a prostaglandin E_2 analog used to induce labor, not delay labor. (C) Ethinyl estradiol is an estrogen analog used for hormone replacement for postmenopausal women. (D) Mifepristone is used to terminate pregnancy, not delay labor.

108 **The answer is E: Pupillary dilation.** Meperidine causes a depression of respiration similar to that of morphine, but it has no significant cardiovascular action when given orally. On IV administration, meperidine produces a decrease in peripheral resistance and an increase in peripheral blood flow, and it may cause an increase in cardiac rate. As with morphine, meperidine dilates cerebral vessels, increases CSF pressure, and contracts smooth muscle (the latter to a lesser extent than does morphine). Meperidine does not cause pinpoint pupils but rather causes the pupils to dilate because of an anticholinergic action. (A) Both meperidine and morphine cause cerebral blood vessel

dilation. (B) Both meperidine and morphine cause increase in cerebral blood flow. (C) Both meperidine and morphine cause euphoria. (D) Both meperidine and morphine provide pain relief.

109 **The answer is C: Neurotoxicity.** Meperidine provides analgesia but is not recommended for long-term use because of its active metabolite, normeperidine, which has significant neurotoxic properties. Unlike morphine, meperidine is not clinically useful in the treatment of diarrhea or cough. Meperidine produces less of an increase in urinary retention than does morphine. (A) Meperidine is not useful in the treatment of clinical cough. (B) Meperidine is not useful in the treatment of diarrhea. (D) Meperidine is unlikely to cause otologic symptoms. (E) Meperidine is unlikely to cause urinary retention.

110 **The answer is C: Fentanyl.** Fentanyl is used in anesthesia. It produces analgesia and is usually injected epidurally. However, its analgesic action is also beneficial in patients with cancer. It is available as a transdermal patch and an oral transmucosal preparation. (A) Buprenorphine, like methadone, is used in opiate detoxification and could precipitate withdrawal. (B) Codeine shows cross-tolerance with morphine and thus would not be effective. (D) Methadone, like buprenorphine, is used in opiate detoxification and could precipitate withdrawal. (E) Meperidine shows cross-tolerance with morphine and thus would not be effective.

111 **The answer is C: Metronidazole.** The patient is most likely suffering from giardiasis that he acquired while camping. After entering parasitic cells, metronidazole forms toxic metabolites that destroy DNA. (A) Clindamycin is used to treat parasitic infections such as *Babesia*, but not *Giardia*. (B) Ivermectin is used to treat parasitic infections such as *Onchocerca*, but not Giardia. (D) Praziquantel is used to treat parasitic infections such as *Taenia* and *Diphyllobothrium*, but not *Giardia*. (E) Sulfadiazine is used to treat parasitic infections such as *Toxoplasma*, but not *Giardia*.

112 **The answer is A: Diethylcarbamazine.** The patient is most likely suffering from visceral larva migrans caused by *Toxocara canis*. The first-line treatment is diethylcarbamazine. The mechanism of action is the inhibition of arachidonic acid metabolism in helminths. (B) Ivermectin is used to treat parasitic infections such as *Onchocerca*, but not *Toxocara*. (C) Mebendazole is used to treat parasitic infections such as *Enterobius* and *Ascaris*, but not *Toxocara*. (D) Praziquantel is used to treat parasitic infections such as *Taenia* and *Diphyllobothrium*, but not *Toxocara*. (E) Pyrantel pamoate is used to treat parasitic infections such as *Enterobius* and *Ascaris*, but not *Toxocara*.

113 **The answer is C: Mebendazole.** The patient has neurocysticercosis from *Taenia solium* most likely caused by undercooked pork. The first-line treatment for neurocysticercosis is mebendazole. (A) Diethylcarbamazine is used to treat parasitic infections such as *Toxocara*, but not neurocysticercosis. (B) Ivermectin is used to treat parasitic infections such as *Onchocerca*, but not neurocysticercosis. (D) If the patient has just cysticercosis from *Taenia solium*, the treatment of choice is praziquantel. (E) Pyrantel pamoate is used to treat parasitic infections such as *Enterobius* and *Ascaris*, but not neurocysticercosis.

114 **The answer is D: Permethrin.** This patient most likely has scabies and the treatment of choice is permethrin. Permethrin is neurotoxic to parasites by prolonging sodium channel activation. (A) Diphenhydramine, an antihistamine, will not kill the *Sarcoptes* mite, but may help with the itch. (B) Doxycycline is an antibiotic used to treat Lyme disease caused by *Borrelia* ticks. It is not a treatment for scabies. (C) Lindane was a treatment for scabies; however, toxicity and resistance have decreased its usefulness. (E) Topical corticosteroids are used for dermatitis but not for scabies.

115 **The answer is C: D-ala replaced by D-lac in the cell wall.** The resistance of bacteria to vancomycin occurs via a replacement of D-ala in the terminal chain of the bacterial cell wall to D-lac. This is effective because the mechanism of action of vancomycin is binding to D-ala-D-ala chain of the cell wall, which inhibits cell wall formation. (A) The mechanism of resistance to chloramphenicol is by acetylation. (B) The mechanism of resistance to penicillin is by β-lactamase cleaving the β-lactam ring of penicillin. (D) The mechanism of resistance to tetracyclines and quinolones is by decreased uptake by bacterial cells. (E) The mechanism of resistance to macrolides is by methylation of rRNA. This inhibits binding to the ribosome.

116 **The answer is D: Kernicterus.** Sulfonamides in pregnancy can cause kernicterus. Sulfamethoxazole cross the blood–placental barrier and competes with bilirubin in the binding to albumin. This increases free bilirubin in fetus and leads to kernicterus. (A) The side effect of cartilage damage in the fetus is more likely seen with fluoroquinolones. (B) Tetracyclines are more likely to cause discoloration of the fetus' teeth. (C) Gray baby syndrome is most commonly associated with chloramphenicol. (E) The most likely side effect of aminoglycosides in pregnancy is fetal ototoxicity.

117 **The answer is C: Metronidazole.** This patient has bacterial vaginosis as evident by a wet prep with clue cells and a positive whiff test. The treatment of choice for bacterial vaginosis is metronidazole. She should be

advised not to drink alcohol while on metronidazole because of the possibility of a disulfiram-like reaction. (A) Ceftriaxone is not the treatment of choice for bacterial vaginosis. It would be first line for *Chlamydia*. (B) Doxycycline is not the treatment of choice for bacterial vaginosis. It would be first line for gonorrhea. (D) Penicillin is not the treatment of choice for bacterial vaginosis. It would be first line for primary syphilis. (E) Trimethoprim–sulfamethoxazole is not the treatment of choice for bacterial vaginosis. It would be first line for a urinary infection.

118 **The answer is B: Disruption of DNA.** Metronidazole is an antibiotic effective against anaerobes and some Protozoa, including *Trichomonas vaginalis*. These organisms carry out the reaction necessary for partial metronidazole reduction. Once reduced, metronidazole disrupts DNA molecules. Resistance to metronidazole is rare. (A) Sulfamethoxazole and trimethoprim both block bacterial folic acid synthesis, which itself is necessary for DNA synthesis. Metronidazole does not block folic acid synthesis. (C) β-Lactam antibiotics such as penicillins and cephalosporins inhibit the penicillin-binding proteins (PBPs). These enzymes are necessary for bacterial cell wall synthesis. (D) Many antibacterials impair ribosome function, including aminoglycosides, tetracyclines, and clindamycin. Metronidazole does not work by interfering with ribosomes. (E) Fluoroquinolones inhibit bacterial topoisomerase. Metronidazole does not work by inhibition of this enzyme.

119 **The answer is C: Gentamicin.** The patient was most likely given gentamicin. A side effect of gentamicin is ototoxicity, which this patient is experiencing as evidenced by her tinnitus and poor balance. Aminoglycosides are toxic to the sensory cells within the ear. (A) A common side effect of ceftriaxone is nephrotoxicity, not ototoxicity. (B) A common side effect of ciprofloxacin is tendonitis, not ototoxicity. (D) A common side effect of trimethoprim–sulfamethoxazole is nephrotoxicity, not ototoxicity. (E) A common side effect of tetracycline is GI upset, not ototoxicity.

120 **The answer is D: Inhibits ergosterol synthesis.** The mechanism of action of clotrimazole is the inhibition of fungal ergosterol synthesis. This increases the permeability of the fungal cell wall, which leads to cell death. Clotrimazole can be used in the treatment of athlete's foot or tinea pedis. (A) The mechanism of action of amphotericin B is binding to ergosterol in the fungal cell membrane. (B) The mechanism of action of caspofungin is the inhibition of cell wall synthesis by inhibiting the synthesis of β-glucan. (C) The mechanism of action of flucytosine is inhibiting fungal DNA synthesis. (E) The mechanism of action of terbinafine is the inhibition of the enzyme squalene epoxidase.

121 **The answer is C: Inhibits integrase.** Raltegravir is a newer antiviral used for HIV therapy. Raltegravir inhibits the HIV enzyme integrase, which is used to integrate the viral DNA into the human DNA. It is usually always used in combination therapy. (A) Enfuvirtide is a fusion inhibitor that binds to viral gp41 to prevent the fusion of viral cells to CD4 cells. (B) Enfuvirtide is a fusion inhibitor that inhibits the fusion of viral cells to CD4 cells by binding to viral gp41. (D) Indinavir inhibits protease, which prevents the maturation of viral cells. (E) Reverse transcriptase inhibitors can be broken down into nucleoside and nonnucleoside; examples are zidovudine and efavirenz, respectively.

122 **The answer is E: Ritonavir.** The patient is suffering from lipodystrophy, which is most commonly associated with protease inhibitors used for HIV therapy. Ritonavir is a protease inhibitor. Protease inhibitors are thought to inhibit lipid metabolism leading to lipodystrophy. Lipodystrophy has been associated with nucleoside reverse transcriptase inhibitors; however, it is more common with protease inhibitors. (A) Efavirenz is a nonnucleoside reverse transcriptase inhibitor that is more likely to cause bone marrow suppression, not lipodystrophy. (B) Enfuvirtide is a fusion inhibitor that is more likely to cause injection site reactions, not lipodystrophy. (C) Nevirapine is a nonnucleoside reverse transcriptase inhibitor that is more likely to cause bone marrow suppression, not lipodystrophy. (D) Raltegravir is an integrase inhibitor that is more likely to cause GI upset, not lipodystrophy.

123 **The answer is B: Ganciclovir.** Ganciclovir is the treatment of choice for CMV and CMV retinitis. CMV infections are more common in the immunocompromised. If ganciclovir fails, foscarnet is the best alternative. Ganciclovir works by inhibiting viral DNA polymerase. (A) Acyclovir is commonly used to treat herpes and zoster infections, but not CMV. (C) Nevirapine is a nonnucleoside reverse transcriptase inhibitor used to treat HIV, but not CMV. (D) Ribavirin is used to treat respiratory syncytial virus and hepatitis C, but not CMV. (E) Ritonavir is protease inhibitor used to treat HIV, but not CMV.

124 **The answer is B: Exercise caution when given with -azole antifungals.** Klonopin is a benzodiazepine used to treat panic disorder. Interactions include potentiation of CNS depression when used with alcohol. Caution must be exercised with drugs that inhibit CYP450 such as -azole antifungals. (A) This agent creates CNS depression when given with alcohol. (C) Hypersalivation is a common side effect of Klonopin. (D) Paradoxical reactions are common adverse reactions of Klonopin.

125 **The answer is D: Pneumonia, aspiration type.** Aripiprazole is indicated for the treatment of manic or mixed bipolar disorder. Important warnings include risk of hypotension, aspiration pneumonia, seizures, diabetes, and leukopenia. (A) Hypotension would be expected with the use of this agent. (B) Leukopenia would be expected with the use of this agent. (C) Aspiration pneumonia is a known warning for use of this agent. (E) Spermatogenesis abnormality, although a possibility, is an unlikely challenge for a 55-year-old man.

126 **The answer is C: Hemorrhagic cystitis.** Hemorrhagic cystitis is a potentially severe side effect of cyclophosphamide and ifosfamide. These drugs can also cause other bladder pathology including hematuria and fibrosis. The damage to the bladder is attributed to a toxic metabolite called acrolein. To lessen the toxicity of these drugs, physicians may also coadminister mesna. Mesna binds to acrolein in the urine, rendering it inactive. It also prevents the formation of more acrolein from other cyclophosphamide and ifosfamide metabolites. (A) Stimulant drugs such as amphetamines can cause anxiety. Anxiety is not a known side effect of ifosfamide. (B) Substances such as cholinomimetics and many antibiotics cause GI upset and diarrhea. However, these are not side effects of ifosfamide. (D) Hepatic failure is a potential serious side effect of acetaminophen toxicity. Ifosfamide is not known to damage the liver. (E) High doses of ifosfamide may lead to hypokalemia, hypomagnesemia, hypophosphatemia, and low bicarbonate. Hyperkalemia has not been associated with ifosfamide use.

127 **The answer is C: Chloroquine.** G6PD deficiency is more common in patients of African, Middle Eastern, or South Asian descent. This enzyme is involved in the pentose phosphate pathway, which is particularly important in erythrocytes to maintain stores of glutathione. G6PD deficiency by itself does not cause any problems, but it makes red blood cells more susceptible to oxidative stress. There are many oxidating drugs that can cause hemolysis and jaundice in patients who have G6PD deficiency including chloroquine. (A) Amoxicillin is a β-lactam antibiotic commonly used to treat bacterial ear infections and upper respiratory tract infections. It is not indicated for malaria prophylaxis nor does it cause significant hemolysis in patients with G6PD deficiency. (B) Atovaquone is an antiprotozoal drug. It may be used in conjunction with proguanil for malaria prophylaxis but is not known to cause significant hemolysis in patients with G6PD deficiency. (D) Doxycycline is used to treat many bacterial infections. Although it is not used to treat malaria, it is used for malaria prophylaxis. It is not known to cause significant hemolysis in patients with G6PD deficiency. (E) Mefloquine is an antimalarial used both to treat the disease and for prophylaxis. It is not known to cause significant hemolysis in patients with G6PD deficiency.

128 **The answer is A: A 32-year-old man with a clogged dialysis catheter.** Originally used for the treatment of deep vein thrombosis and serious pulmonary embolism, thrombolytic drugs are now being used less frequently for these conditions. Their tendency to cause bleeding has also blunted their use in treating acute myocardial infarction or peripheral arterial thrombosis. However, thrombolytic agents are helpful in restoring catheter and shunt function, by lysing clots causing occlusions. Thrombolytic agents are also used to dissolve clots that result in strokes. (B) This is one of the original uses of heparin. (C) This is an example of one of the original uses of heparin. (D) Deep venous thrombosis is an original use of heparin and has shown significant success in this area. (E) This is an example of an original use of heparin.

129 **The answer is E: A 71-year-old woman with Parkinson's disease and a urinary tract infection.** Hemorrhage is a major side effect of heparin. For example, a previously unsuspected lesion, such as a peptic ulcer, may hemorrhage following injection of a thrombolytic agent. These drugs are contraindicated in patients with healing wounds, pregnancy, a history of cerebrovascular accident, brain tumor, head trauma, intracranial bleeding, and metastatic cancer. Continued presence of thrombogenic stimuli may cause rethrombosis after lysis of the initial clot. (A) Heparin is contraindicated in patients with head trauma. (B) Heparin is contraindicated in patients with intracranial bleeding. (C) Heparin is contraindicated in patients with brain tumors and metastatic cancer. (D) Heparin is contraindicated in patients with an evolving cerebrovascular accident.

130 **The answer is C: Low-molecular-weight heparin (LMWH).** Low-molecular-weight heparin (LMWH) has a reliable dose response and can be administered subcutaneously by selected patients who have been taught home injection techniques. LMWH does not cross the placenta and shows no teratogenic effects. (A) Aspirin, which inhibits platelet aggregation, has little effect on venous thrombosis, which is composed of fibrin with only a few platelets. (B) Alteplase is not indicated for deep vein thrombosis. (D) Unfractionated heparin is not indicated for outpatient therapy. (E) Warfarin is teratogenic and is contraindicated in pregnant patients.

131 **The answer is D: Inhibits plasmin.** Heavy menstrual bleeding, or menorrhagia, can have many causes. Often, neoplasm must be ruled out. Hormonal medication can be used to control heavy bleeding by minimizing or eliminating a woman's menstrual periods. Hormonal methods have the added effect of contraception, which may or may not be desired. In cases where a patient wishes to control bleeding and maintain fertility, tranexamic acid may be used. This drug is a plasmin inhibitor, which controls bleeding by impairing clot breakdown. Patients who are hypercoagulable should not take tranexamic acid because of the risk of clot formation. (A) Urokinase and streptokinase are drugs that activate plasminogen into plasmin to help break down clots. Tranexamic acid does just the opposite. (B) Many endogenous substances activate platelets, including ADP, platelet-activating factor, thromboxane A_2, and von Willebrand factor. Tranexamic acid, however, does not act on platelets. (C) As far as the clotting cascade goes, blocking cyclooxygenase would decrease the production of the platelet activator thromboxane A_2. This would result in excess bleeding and is not the desired effect or the mechanism of tranexamic acid's action. (E) Hormonal contraceptives (primarily progestins) block the LH surge and may decrease or even eliminate menstruation by mimicking the pregnant state. Tranexamic acid works instead by inhibition of plasmin and is not hormonal.

132 **The answer is E: Ifosfamide.** Ifosfamide is an alkylating agent used in the treatment of various cancers, including breast cancer. A side effect of ifosfamide is hemorrhagic cystitis, which this patient has with gross hematuria and dysuria. To help prevent hemorrhagic cystitis, hydration and mesna can be used with ifosfamide. (A) A common side effect of busulfan is pulmonary fibrosis, not hemorrhagic cystitis. (B) A common side effect of cisplatin is nephrotoxicity, not hemorrhagic cystitis. (C) A common side effect of cytarabine is leukopenia, not hemorrhagic cystitis. (D) A common side effect of doxorubicin is cardiomyopathy, not hemorrhagic cystitis.

133 **The answer is B: Blocks polymerization of microtubules.** Vincristine blocks the polymerization of microtubules so mitosis cannot occur. It is used as part of the MOPP treatment regimen for Hodgkin's lymphoma. The use of chemotherapeutic agents has led to a very favorable prognosis for young people diagnosed with Hodgkin's lymphoma. (A) The mechanism of action of busulfan is the alkylation of DNA. (C) The mechanism of action of cisplatin is cross-linking DNA. (D) The mechanism of action of etoposide is the inhibition of topoisomerase II. (E) The mechanism of action of paclitaxel is the stabilization of polymerized microtubules not allowing anaphase to occur.

134 **The answer is E: Vincristine.** Vincristine is part of the chemotherapy regimen for a Wilms tumor. One of the side effects that should be monitored for is peripheral neuropathy. This can present as foot drop, paralysis, or in this case, areflexia. When neurologic symptoms are present, the dose of the drug needs to be reduced or even stopped to prevent permanent damage. (A) Carboplatin would be likely to cause acoustic nerve damage, but not areflexia. (B) Dactinomycin can be used in the treatment of a Wilms tumor; however, it is more likely to cause myelosuppression, not areflexia. (C) Doxorubicin would be more likely to lead to cardiomyopathy, not areflexia. (D) Vinblastine has a similar mechanism of action as vincristine and can be used in the treatment of a Wilms tumor. However, it is more likely to cause myelosuppression, not areflexia.

135 **The answer is A: Danazol.** Heavy menstrual bleeding, or menorrhagia, can have many causes. Often, neoplasm must be ruled out. One way to decrease pain and excessive bleeding during menstruation is to decrease the amount of circulating estradiol (E2). Danazol causes a decrease in the ovarian production of E2 precursors to decrease E2 production. (B) Estradiol valerate is a synthetic estrogen used in hormonal contraceptives. When used with a progestin, it decreases menstrual symptoms by halting the menstrual cycle altogether. (C) Misoprostol is a prostaglandin E1 analog. It causes cervical softening and may be used for induction of labor or medical abortions. It does not interfere with E2 synthesis. (D) Naproxen is a nonsteroidal anti-inflammatory drug (NSAID). NSAIDs work by inhibiting cyclooxygenase to inhibit production of proinflammatory cytokines. (E) Pitocin is an analog of the hormone oxytocin. It causes strong uterine contractions and may be used for induction of labor or medical abortions. It does not interfere with E2 synthesis.

136 **The answer is B: Dizziness.** Gabapentin is useful in the treatment of chronic neuropathic pain. Side effects can include dizziness, peripheral edema, GI upset, ataxia, and visual disturbances. (A) Aplastic anemia is not a side effect of gabapentin. (C) Hepatitis is not a side effect of gabapentin. (D) Pancreatitis is not a side effect of gabapentin. (E) Tetany is not a result of treatment with gabapentin.

137 **The answer is B: Contraindicated in patients with opioid dependence.** Tramadol is useful in the management of chronic mild-to-moderate pain. This medication should not be given to patients who are opioid dependent. Further, it should not be given to patients who are drug abusers. (A) Tramadol can cause itchy skin. (C) Tramadol can be given to patients with nicotine dependence. (D) Tramadol is contraindicated in pregnancy. Of note, this patient is a man.

138 **The answer is E: Valacyclovir.** Genital herpes is usually caused by herpes simplex virus type 2 (HSV-2), although it can also be cause by HSV-1. In either case, the virus uses a thymidine kinase as a preliminary step in DNA synthesis. Viral thymidine kinase is structurally different from human thymidine kinase and has a much higher affinity for acyclovir. Viral thymidine kinase phosphorylates acyclovir, which (after a few more steps) is incorporated into growing DNA strands but has no 3′-OH group to which more nucleotides can be added. This results in impaired DNA synthesis in cells infected with HSV-1 or HSV-2. Acyclovir's poor oral bioavailability led to the development of valacyclovir, which works in the same way but has a much higher oral bioavailability. It would be the best choice in this patient. (A) Acyclovir would be active against the virus of this man's infection, but its oral bioavailability is very poor. Valacyclovir is a prodrug that is activated to become acyclovir in vivo and has a much higher oral bioavailability. (B) Cidofovir is usually used to treat CMV infections but can be used in acyclovir-resistant HSV infections. Cidofovir is similar to acyclovir in that it competes with nucleotides in DNA synthesis and has a similarly low oral bioavailability. (C) Foscarnet is also used for CMV or HSV infections. It interacts with viral DNA polymerase to inhibit DNA synthesis. It also has poor oral bioavailability and would not be the best choice to use in this patient. (D) Ganciclovir is active against herpes types 1 and 2, but its oral bioavailability is very poor. Valacyclovir has a much higher oral bioavailability.

139 The answer is C: Rimantadine. M2 ion channels are found only in strains of influenza A. This ion channel is important in the uncoating of the viral genome. By blocking the M2 channel, uncoating is inhibited and the virus is unable to replicate. The adamantanes, such as amantadine and rimantadine, block the M2 ion channel. Unfortunately, most strains of influenza A have mutated ion channels and are now resistant to the adamantanes. (A) Fomivirsen can be used to treat CMV infections. It binds to a specific mRNA sequence that prevents translation of CMV proteins. (B) Oseltamivir is used against the flu virus but does not work by blocking the M2 channel. Instead, it is a neuraminidase inhibitor and prevents newly formed virions from leaving infected cells. (D) Valganciclovir is converted in vivo to ganciclovir, which impairs CMV DNA synthesis. It does not block the M2 channel nor is it used against flu virus. (E) Zidovudine is a nucleoside reverse transcriptase inhibitor used to treat HIV infections. It does not block the M2 channel nor is it used against flu virus.

140 The answer is B: Pain. Pain is the first sensation lost when using local anesthesia. This is because pain is carried by very small diameter unmyelinated and small myelinated nerve fibers. The smaller the diameter of the nerve fibers, the quicker the nerve is blocked. The order of loss is pain > temperature > touch > proprioception > muscular tone. (A) Muscular tone is the last function to be lost because it is carried by the largest diameter myelinated nerve fibers. (C) Proprioception is carried by large diameter myelinated nerve fibers. (D) Temperature is carried by small diameter myelinated nerve fibers; however, they are larger than the small unmyelinated fibers carrying pain signals. (E) Touch is carried by large diameter myelinated nerve fibers.

141 The answer is D: Selenium sulfide. A long history of a flaky scalp that does not improve with normal scrubbing and washing is suspicious for *Malassezia furfur*. This is supported by the finding under microscopy of a "spaghetti and meatballs" appearance after digestion with KOH. The hyphae and spheres are parts of the *Malassezia* fungus. One of the chief complaints of *Malassezia* infection is pruritic dandruff, as in this patient's case. Infection with *Malassezia furfur* is called tinea versicolor. A common treatment for tinea versicolor is selenium sulfide shampoo. (A) Avoiding foods containing gluten would help control symptoms of celiac disease as well as a skin manifestation of celiac disease called dermatitis herpetiformis. This patient's case would not be affected by avoiding gluten. (B) Griseofulvin can be used to treat fungal infections of the nails (onychomycosis). It has not been shown to be effective against *Malassezia* infections. (C) Mebendazole is useful in treating many types of parasitic worm infections. It has not been shown to be effective against *Malassezia* infections. (E) Vancomycin is an antibacterial effective against gram-positive organisms. It has not been shown to be effective against *Malassezia* infections.

142 The answer is A: Breaks down urate. Gouty arthritis occurs when uric acid crystals cause joint irritation and inflammation. The level of uric acid in the blood is not a reliable predictor of who will suffer a gout attack—some patients have relatively high levels of serum urate but may never have an attack, whereas others with relatively low levels can suffer an attack. Regardless of the baseline serum urate level, patients who are symptomatic may find relief from lowering the amount of urate in the blood. Pegloticase is a recombinant uricase enzyme, which is found naturally in many animals but the human version is mutated and defective. It can relieve gout symptoms by breaking down urate into a metabolite that is more easily excreted. (B) Xanthine oxidase is the enzyme responsible for urate production as part of purine metabolism. Enhancing this enzyme would not help this patient. (C) Colchicine is an old drug that has been used to treat gout flairs by blocking neutrophil chemotaxis to decrease overall inflammation. Pegloticase does not impair neutrophil chemotaxis. (D) Probenecid is a drug used to treat gout that increases urate excretion in the kidney tubules. Pegloticase does not increase urate excretion. (E) Allopurinol is a drug used to treat gout that works by inhibiting xanthine oxidase. Pegloticase does not inhibit xanthine oxidase.

143 **The answer is E: Letter E.** Nitrous oxide has the highest minimal alveolar concentration (MAC) of all agents shown in the diagram. Thus, it is the least potent anesthetic agent. (A) Letter A represents halothane and has the lowest MAC and the highest potency. (B) Letter B represents isoflurane. (C) Letter C represents sevoflurane with a MAC of 2%. (D) Letter D represents desflurane with a MAC of 6%.

144 **The answer is A: Letter A.** Halothane has the highest blood/gas partition coefficient and is the most soluble in blood of all agents shown in the diagram. (B) Letter B represents isoflurane. (C) Letter C represents sevoflurane. (D) Letter D represents nitrous oxide. (E)Letter E represents desflurane.

145 **The answer is A: Letter A.** Nitrous oxide has the highest alveolar concentration 10 min after induction. (B) Letter B represents desflurane. (C) Letter C represents sevoflurane. (D) Letter D represents isoflurane. (E) Letter E represents halothane.

146 **The answer is C: Letter C.** Letter C represents adipose tissue. Initially, thiopental is redistributed to blood, then brain, and then to muscle with peak levels. (A) Letter A represents blood. (B) Letter B represents brain. (D) Letter D represents adipose tissue.

147 **The answer is C: Letter C.** Methadone is represented by letter C. This agent has symptoms that last longer but they are less severe than that of heroin withdrawal. Methadone is well-absorbed orally. (A) Letter A represents heroin. (B) Letter B represents buprenorphine, which is used in opioid detoxification because it has a short duration of withdrawal symptoms but they can be severe. (D) This information can be determined from the graphs.

148 **The answer is C: Letter C.** On the 10th day of administration of penicillin for meningitis, the meninges are minimally inflamed. Because inflammation allows for easier drug penetration into the CSF and there is little inflammation present, CSF levels of antibiotic at this time will be low. (A) This curve represents the antibiotic concentration in the CSF on the first day of treatment. (B) This curve represents the antibiotic concentration in the CSF on the fifth day of treatment. (D) This information can be determined from the information provided.

149 **The answer is E: None of these antibiotics would be effective in this case.** Methicillin, oxacillin, dicloxacillin, and nafcillin are β-lactam antibiotics related to penicillin. They have a bulky side chain that makes them poor targets for β-lactamase enzymes that break down and deactivate penicillins. MRSA strains are resistant in a different way, however. They have altered PBPs with lower affinity for β-lactam antibiotics. None of the β-lactam antibiotics are effective against MRSA because of this, and vancomycin is often the drug of choice in such cases. (A) Ceftriaxone is a third-generation cephalosporin. Cephalosporins are β-lactam antibiotics and are ineffective against MRSA because of altered PBPs. (B) Dicloxacillin is one of the antistaphylococcal penicillins. Dicloxacillin is a β-lactam antibiotic and is ineffective against MRSA because of altered PBPs. (C) Nafcillin is one of the antistaphylococcal penicillins. Nafcillin is a β-lactam antibiotic and is ineffective against MRSA because of altered PBPs. (D) Oxacillin is one of the antistaphylococcal penicillins. Oxacillin is a β-lactam antibiotic and is ineffective against MRSA because of altered PBPs.

150 **The answer is D: A 48-year-old man with epilepsy and chronic renal insufficiency.** The penicillins are irritating to neuronal tissue, and they can provoke seizures if injected intrathecally or if very high blood levels are reached. Patients with epilepsy are particularly at risk. When indicated, dosage adjustments for patients with renal dysfunction further minimize the risk for seizure. (A) This patient has no renal dysfunction or history of epilepsy and would not likely develop seizures from penicillin. (B) This patient has no risk factors for seizures and should have no adverse effects if given penicillin. (C) This patient has no contraindication to penicillin. (E) Diabetes mellitus and hypertension do not represent contraindications to penicillin use.

151 **The answer is D: Potassium.** Penicillins are generally administered as the sodium or potassium salt. Toxicities may be caused by the large quantities of sodium or potassium that accompany the penicillin. For example, sodium excess may result in hypokalemia. This can be avoided by using the most potent antibiotic, which permits lower doses of drug and accompanying cations. Treatment with aqueous penicillin G has a high potassium load, which must be taken into account while monitoring electrolytes. (A) Hyperkalemia can result from aqueous penicillin G treatment. (B) Cholesterol levels are likely to be normal in this patient. (C) Creatinine levels should be unaffected following penicillin G administration. (E) Sodium excess can result in hypokalemia.

152 **The answer is B: Phenytoin cannot be given IM.** Phenytoin can be used for seizure prophylaxis or to

abort seizures. It is a sodium channel blocker to inhibit action potentials. Fosphenytoin is a prodrug that is metabolized to phenytoin. Both have a narrow therapeutic index, meaning the toxic dose is not much higher than the therapeutic dose. One major benefit to fosphenytoin is its stability in solution and the fact that is does not form a precipitate when given IM as phenytoin does. This patient received an IM dose in order to avoid a seizure because he was unable to keep the oral preparation down. (A) Both phenytoin and fosphenytoin have a narrow therapeutic index. Because of its formulation, fosphenytoin has fewer local effects but is still metabolized to phenytoin and causes the same side effects as phenytoin. (C) Phenytoin is FDA approved for use in children the same as it is in adults. IM fosphenytoin was given because the patient could not take the oral form, and phenytoin cannot be given IM. (D) Although nausea and vomiting can be side effects of phenytoin therapy, this patient had already been taking oral phenytoin for 1 year before this episode of nausea began. Fosphenytoin also causes nausea and vomiting. (E) Phenytoin forms a precipitate and cannot be given IM. Fosphenytoin is stable as an IM injection and has the same effect as phenytoin on seizure prophylaxis because fosphenytoin is metabolized into phenytoin.

153 **The answer is D: Hepatic transaminases.** The most common adverse effects reported in clinical trials included constipation, nausea, headache, myalgias, and insomnia. Increased hepatic transaminases and also elevations in creatine phosphokinases occurred, suggesting weekly monitoring of these enzymes, while the patient is receiving daptomycin. (A) Daptomycin has a more significant effect on hepatic function than renal function. (B) Daptomycin does not affect hemoglobin levels. (C) Daptomycin does not affect hematocrit levels. (E) Serum sodium levels are usually normal in patients taking daptomycin.

154 **The answer is B: Foamy urine.** The most common adverse reactions reported with telavancin have included taste disturbances, nausea, vomiting, insomnia, and foamy urine. Telavancin is not recommended during pregnancy because of adverse developmental outcomes observed with animal data. In the United States, there is a boxed warning for women of childbearing age to have a pregnancy test prior to use. Because telavancin may prolong the QTc interval, use should be avoided in patients with a history of QTc prolongation, uncompensated heart failure, severe left ventricular hypertrophy, or patients receiving other medications that may prolong the QTc interval. (A) Telavancin is associated with nausea and vomiting. (C) Telavancin may cause insomnia. (D) Telavancin can cause QT interval prolongation. (E) Telavancin can cause insomnia.

155 **The answer is A: Amoxicillin.** Multiple tooth extractions can lead to bacteremia, and the mitral valve stenosis and cardiac insufficiency place him at risk for developing endocarditis. The present American Heart Association guidelines indicate amoxicillin (2 g given 1 h before procedure). For penicillin-allergic patients, cephalexin, cefadroxil, clindamycin, clarithromycin, or azithromycin are alternative medications listed as prophylactic regimens for dental procedures. (B) Clotrimazole is not an appropriate agent for prophylaxis in this patient. (C) Imipenem is also inappropriate because it is broad spectrum and can only be given intravenously. (D) Tetracycline is not considered to be an alternative prophylaxis agent in this patient. (E) Vancomycin is not an alternative medication currently listed as a prophylactic regimen for dental procedures.

Chapter 7

Inflammation, Immune Pharmacology, and Toxicology

QUESTIONS

Select the single best answer.

1 A 6-year-old boy presents to his pediatrician for follow-up of recurrent hay fever and asthma. He usually has two to three attacks per week. For symptom control, he uses an albuterol inhaler, but his parents would like to try something more. They would like him to take something that would lessen the amount of attacks he has. Although corticosteroids would probably work best for prophylaxis, they are contraindicated in children. Which of the following drugs would decrease the amount of asthma attacks by preventing an arachidonic acid derivative from binding to its receptor?

(A) Aspirin
(B) Celecoxib
(C) Ipratropium
(D) Montelukast
(E) Zileuton

2 A 15-year-old female presents to her primary care physician complaining of runny nose and itchy eyes. She said that she first had these symptoms during the spring a few years ago, but each year, they have been bothering her more. You know there are multiple ways to interfere with the signaling that is causing her symptoms. Which of the following drugs would prevent the release of the main chemical mediator in her case?

(A) Cromolyn sodium
(B) Diphenhydramine
(C) Ranitidine
(D) Loratadine
(E) Theophylline

3 A 52-year-old overweight male steamroller operator presents to his primary care physician complaining of itchy, watery eyes and runny nose in the springtime. He says that he has had this problem for as long as he can remember but does not like going to doctors. His wife finally convinced him to come today to see what his physician might be able to do for him. What is the most appropriate treatment for this patient?

(A) Albuterol
(B) Diphenhydramine
(C) Epinephrine
(D) Hydroxyzine
(E) Loratadine

4 Intravenous atropine at low doses is commonly used by oral surgeons during surgical procedures to remove impacted wisdom teeth. The rationale behind the use of this agent in this situation likely involves which of the following beneficial effects?

(A) Antispasmodic for gastrointestinal tract relaxation
(B) Drying effect on the oral mucous membranes
(C) Induction of tachycardia to increase cardiac output
(D) Pupillary dilation to produce unresponsiveness to darkness
(E) Reduction of urinary tract motility to reduce voiding during the procedure

5 A 45-year-old woman has just received a kidney transplant. She is placed on several immunosuppressants to prophylactically prevent her body rejecting the donor organ. Which of the following immunosuppressants interferes with T-cell activation by modifying the activity of calcineurin?

(A) Cyclosporine
(B) Methotrexate
(C) Prednisolone
(D) Sirolimus
(E) Temsirolimus

6 A 39-year-old man with chronic allergic rhinitis and nasal congestion takes an over-the-counter nasal spray containing oxymetazoline. Over the next few days, he has significant improvement in his symptoms. Which of the following is the most likely mechanism of action of this agent?
(A) Increased nasal blood flow
(B) Increased intranasal arterial pressure
(C) Receptor stimulation on nasal vasculature
(D) Transmembrane conductance change
(E) Understimulation of inflamed nasal membranes

7 A 63-year-old man with glaucoma maintained on a regimen of topical medications with an exacerbation of his symptoms. He complains of difficulty with his vision in both eyes and has headaches. Which of the following drugs is the most appropriate treatment for this patient?
(A) Bimatoprost
(B) Latanoprost
(C) Pilocarpine
(D) Tetracycline
(E) Travoprost

8 A 59-year-old man with hypertension, gastroesophageal reflux disorder, AIDS, seizure disorder, and depression is currently maintained on multiple medications, including propranolol. He does not have his medication list at his current office visit with his primary care physician. His blood pressure is 180/100 mm Hg. The patient states that he is taking all of his medications as scheduled. Which of the following drugs is the most likely explanation of this finding?
(A) Cimetidine
(B) Fluoxetine
(C) Paroxetine
(D) Rifampin
(E) Ritonavir

9 A 33-year-old man spends the morning outside gardening in the sun on a warm spring day. He develops a tension headache, and the only medication he has at home is aspirin. After taking two regular-sized aspirin tablets, there was an increase in his respiration rate. What is the reason for the increased respirations?
(A) Salicylates are agonists at the CO_2 receptors in the carotid bodies
(B) Salicylates at this dose directly stimulate the respiratory center of the brain
(C) Salicylates shift the oxygen dissociation curve to the right
(D) Salicylate uncoupling of oxidative phosphorylation

10 A 26-year-old man presents to the emergency department with severe right lower quadrant pain. Physical exam reveals rebound tenderness and decreased bowel sounds. An emergent appendectomy is performed. Postsurgically, he is given an NSAID along with morphine for pain control. Which of the following NSAIDs is commonly used as an adjunct to opioids postsurgically?
(A) Acetaminophen
(B) Celecoxib
(C) Ibuprofen
(D) Ketorolac
(E) Naproxen

11 A 22-year-old woman ingests an entire bottle of acetaminophen in an attempted suicide. She unexpectedly feels well for the next 24 h, at which time her boyfriend discovers what she has done and takes her to the ER. The toxic metabolite of acetaminophen exerts its deleterious effect by what mechanism?
(A) Depletion of endogenous antioxidant
(B) Hapten formation leading to autoantibody production
(C) Inhibition of cytochrome C oxidase
(D) Ischemia from decreased hepatic blood flow
(E) Paralysis of gall bladder causing bile stasis

12 A 60-year-old man with agitation is hospitalized on the medicine service for hyponatremia. He is being treated with intravenous fluids and haloperidol. He develops new onset of tremors and difficulty with ambulation and gait disturbance. What is the most likely explanation for these findings?
(A) Iatrogenic
(B) Infection
(C) Neoplastic process
(D) Viral encephalitis

13 A 62-year-old man with Parkinson's disease on levodopa and carbidopa presents to his primary care physician for follow-up. He is following his prescribed course of medications. He is stable in terms of his motor function but recently has begun to have visual and auditory hallucinations. What is the most likely explanation for these findings?

(A) Drug toxicity
(B) Overactivity of dopamine at basal ganglia receptors
(C) Subtherapeutic dosing with low plasma levels of medication
(D) Underlying undiagnosed subclinical dementia
(E) Underlying undiagnosed upper respiratory tract infection

14 A 48-year-old woman with 2-year history of rheumatoid arthritis has not had sufficient relief with methotrexate alone. Her physician prescribes a biologic TNF-α inhibitor that consists of a recombinant human IgG fused to TNF-α receptor. Which of the following drugs is this?
(A) Adalimumab
(B) Certolizumab
(C) Etanercept
(D) Golimumab
(E) Infliximab

15 A 42-year-old woman with a 1-year history of rheumatoid arthritis comes to see her primary care physician complaining of worsening symptoms. She has been taking leflunomide. IL-1 and TNF-α are two key cytokines involved in the negative sequelae of rheumatoid arthritis. Which of the following drugs is a recombinant form of an endogenous IL-1 antagonist?
(A) Abatacept
(B) Anakinra
(C) Methotrexate
(D) Hydroxychloroquine
(E) Rituximab

16 A 21-year-old male presents to the clinic with 6 weeks of painful, bloody stools. Flexible sigmoidoscopy reveals erythema and friability with pseudopolyps. Which of the following drugs used for ulcerative colitis has both anti-inflammatory and antibacterial properties?
(A) Azathioprine
(B) Cyclosporine
(C) Sulfasalazine
(D) Mesalamine
(E) Olsalazine

17 A 5-year-old boy is brought to his primary care physician by his parents who say that he often has trouble catching his breath when he has been playing hard outside. He is allergic to peanuts. At the moment, he is breathing fine. Which of the following drugs is commonly used to diagnose suspected asthma?
(A) Albuterol
(B) Methacholine
(C) Neostigmine
(D) Nicotine
(E) Pilocarpine

18 A 34-year-old man is a chronic alcoholic and is in and out of a rehabilitation center on a monthly basis. His physician administers a blocker of aldehyde dehydrogenase. Which of the following effects is most likely to be exhibited by this patient following administration?
(A) Bradycardia
(B) Elation
(C) Euphoria
(D) Nausea
(E) Urticaria

19 A 39-year-old man is a chronic alcoholic and is in and out of a rehabilitation center on a monthly basis. His physician administers a blocker of aldehyde dehydrogenase and the patient becomes violently ill with nausea, vomiting, chills, sweats, and hyperventilation. The same reaction occurs 1 week later after medication administration and was felt to be intolerable by the patient. Which of the following is the next best course of action to take?
(A) Continue aldehyde dehydrogenase at full dose
(B) Continue aldehyde dehydrogenase at full dose with 6 oz of beer
(C) Discontinue aldehyde dehydrogenase and administer naltrexone
(D) Discontinue aldehyde dehydrogenase and administer alprazolam
(E) Discontinue aldehyde dehydrogenase and begin intensive psychotherapy

20 A mother brings her 4-year-old son to the emergency department after discovering him eating her iron supplement. Which of the following should be administered to chelate the excess iron in his body?
(A) EDTA
(B) Deferoxamine
(C) Dimercaprol
(D) Penicillamine
(E) Succimer

21 A 27-year-old medical student has recurrent sinusitis and takes an over-the-counter agent. Unfortunately, he fell asleep while taking his final examination of the anatomy course. Which of the following agents is most likely to cause this adverse effect?
(A) Doxycycline
(B) Doxylamine
(C) Doxazosin
(D) Diphenhydramine
(E) Hydroxyzine

22 A 22-year-old female accounting student requires a daily cup of coffee upon arising and another cup as she finishes her first class of the day. She prefers to drink caffeinated products. Which of the following is the most plausible mechanism of action of this product?

(A) Blockade of adenosine receptors
(B) Decrease in cyclic adenosine monophosphate
(C) Decrease in cyclic guanosine monophosphate
(D) Stimulation of phosphodiesterase
(E) Transportation of intracellular calcium

23 A 63-year-old woman with congestive heart failure begins to have lower extremity swelling. She starts taking a diuretic and the swelling improves significantly. Over the next few days, however, she develops ringing in her ears. Which of the following diuretics is she taking?

(A) Acetazolamide
(B) Furosemide
(C) Hydrochlorothiazide
(D) Mannitol
(E) Spironolactone

24 A 32-year-old anesthesiology resident injects himself with ketamine after he is served with divorce papers from his wife. In addition to being suspended from his hospital because of his actions, he would likely exhibit which of the following behaviors?

(A) Hypersensitivity to pain
(B) Loss of consciousness
(C) Normal-appearing gait
(D) Slurred speech
(E) Tranquil affect

25 A 48-year-old woman pricks her finger on a rose bush while pruning. A few days later, she develops small, red lesions near the wound and a red track ascending her hand toward her trunk. Her doctor prescribes itraconazole for the sporotrichosis. What is the mechanism of action of this medication?

(A) Disrupts fungal cell membrane by forming pores (nystatin, amphotericin B)
(B) Disrupts fungal microtubules (griseofulvin)
(C) Inhibits conversion of lanosterol to ergosterol
(D) Inhibits squalene monooxygenase (terbinafine)
(E) Is converted to 5-fluorouracil in fungal cells (flucytosine)

26 A 52-year-old man undergoes three surgical procedures in a 2-week period involving debridement of a deep skin abscess. Each surgical anesthesia procedure involves the use of halothane. Which of the following pathologic processes is possible as a result of the surgical procedures?

(A) Cholelithiasis
(B) Hepatic necrosis
(C) Nephrolithiasis
(D) Steatorrhea
(E) Tinnitus

27 Recent studies into the pathogenesis of halothane-induced malignant hyperthermia indicate which of the following as the likely implicating cause?

(A) Drug toxicity
(B) Excitation–contraction coupling defect
(C) Myoplasmic sodium defect
(D) Oxygen–hemoglobin concentration deficit
(E) Neural overmodulation

28 Thiopental is used as an anesthetic agent during surgery to repair a small-bowel obstruction in a 78-year-old man. Approximately 1 day after his surgery, toxicology studies still reveal some thiopental present in the bloodstream. What is the most likely explanation for this finding?

(A) Hepatitis
(B) Hepatic insufficiency
(C) Physiologic metabolism
(D) Renal failure
(E) Trauma to bowel vasculature

29 A 39-year-old man who suffered a work-related injury has chronic back pain. A morphine pain pump was implanted to control his chronic pain. Formerly, he had chronic diarrhea which is now much improved. What is the most likely explanation for this finding?

(A) Improved gastrointestinal motility
(B) Improved intestinal circular muscle tone
(C) Weakened anal sphincter tone
(D) Weakened rectal balloon dilation pressure
(E) Weakened transverse colonic musculature

30 A 71-year-old man who has chronic back pain after falling from a first-floor apartment 25 years ago is managed with a morphine pump for his chronic pain. He also had a long history of chronic diarrhea that preceded his accident. The pump has been in place for 22 years. Which of the following effects will still likely be maintained by the device at this time?

(A) Analgesia
(B) Constipation
(C) Euphoria
(D) Pupil dilation
(E) Sedation

31 A 23-year-old man is a driver who is involved in a motor vehicle accident. He is brought to the emergency department for evaluation. He is found to have a blood alcohol level of 850 mg/dL. Because of the way the body handles ethanol, the conventional "half-life" to describe its metabolism does not apply. Which of the following drugs at therapeutic concentrations exhibits the same property?

(A) Ibuprofen
(B) Phenytoin
(C) Simvastatin
(D) Tolbutamide
(E) Valproic acid

32 A 17-year-old man is brought to the emergency department with severe right lower quadrant pain that he first felt around his umbilicus. His white blood cell count is 12,000/μL of blood. He is taken to the operating room for emergent laparoscopic appendectomy. About an hour into the surgery, his body temperature spikes and CO_2 production rises uncontrollably. What is the next step in the treatment of this patient?

(A) Acetaminophen
(B) Bromocriptine
(C) Dantrolene
(D) Diazepam
(E) Naproxen

33 An 18-year-old woman presents to her primary care physician after experiencing a one-sided headache for the fourth time in the last 2 years. Her headaches have all been similar in nature. She says the pain is worst right behind her eye and that she feels nauseous and cannot stand bright lights or loud noises while she is having a headache. The physician prescribes sumatriptan. What is the mechanism of action of this medication?

(A) Blocking cyclooxygenase enzymes in the CNS
(B) Blocking serotonin-mediated nociceptive signaling
(C) Blocking synthesis of proinflammatory prostaglandins around nerve endings
(D) Stimulating μ-receptors in the brain
(E) Stimulating κ-receptors in the brain

34 A 63-year-old woman with a history of cardiac arrhythmia maintained on quinidine presents to her primary care physician complaining of frequency, urgency, and dysuria. Urine culture reveals >100,000 CFU/mL of *Escherichia coli*. She is given a prescription for ciprofloxacin 500 mg to be taken twice daily for 7 days. Which of the following sequelae could be problematic for this patient?

(A) Asystole
(B) Myocardial infarction
(C) Pulmonary edema
(D) Pulmonary embolism
(E) QT interval prolongation

35 A 59-year-old man with a long history of cardiac arrhythmia is maintained on procainamide. He presents to his primary care physician complaining of malaise, fevers, and nausea. Physical examination reveals a bilateral malar rash with erythema. What is the most likely diagnosis?

(A) Contact dermatitis
(B) Cutaneous skin reaction to sun exposure
(C) Discoid lupus erythematosus
(D) Lupus-like syndrome
(E) Systemic collagen vascular disease

36 A 24-year-old sexually active woman presents to her primary care physician with vaginal itching and a greenish, frothy vaginal discharge. Her boyfriend is asymptomatic. She is prescribed metronidazole for *Trichomonas vaginalis*. Which of the following should be told to avoid while taking metronidazole?

(A) Alcohol
(B) Aspirin
(C) Caffeine
(D) Grapefruit juice
(E) Operating heavy machinery

37 A 33-year-old female is brought to the emergency department by her mother. The patient had a sudden onset of fever and her temperature is now 40°C (104°F). She has no sick contacts. The mother mentions that she is on a medication for schizophrenia but could not remember the name. A complete blood count shows 250 neutrophils per microliter. Which of the following medications is she likely taking?

(A) Clozapine
(B) Olanzapine
(C) Quetiapine
(D) Risperidone
(E) Haloperidol

38 A 13-year-old female presents with 3 months of easy bruisability and bone pain. Complete blood count shows extreme leukocytosis. She is diagnosed with ALL and begins a chemotherapy regimen. One of her chemotherapeutic drugs is cyclophosphamide. What should also be given to avoid a potentially serious side effect of cyclophosphamide?

(A) Mesna
(B) Methylene blue
(C) *N*-acetylcysteine
(D) Ibuprofen
(E) Succimer

39 A 3-year-old girl was found by her mother chewing on some weeds in their flower garden. The mother rushed her to the hospital along with a portion of the weed. The emergency department physician identifies the weed as deadly nightshade, which contains atropine. Which of the following physiologic changes will be expected because of this patient's atropine exposure?

(A) Bradycardia
(B) Decreased gastric acid secretion
(C) Increased bronchial secretions
(D) Increased salivation
(E) Miosis

40 A 43-year-old Caucasian woman complains that her irises have been darkening. She says that she has been taking a drug for years to treat her glaucoma. Which of the following drugs is most likely causing the increased pigmentation of her irises?

(A) Acetazolamide
(B) Epinephrine
(C) Latanoprost
(D) Pilocarpine
(E) Timolol

41 A 24-year-old G1P0 woman arrives at the hospital in labor at 39 weeks gestation. She denies an epidural, stating her desire to give birth naturally. After 5 h of labor, the baby has begun its descent through the birth canal when the patient requests pain relief. Which of the following opioids would be best to administer?

(A) Butorphanol
(B) Codeine
(C) Dextromethorphan
(D) Methadone
(E) Morphine

42 A 16-year-old female was rescued from a house fire and transported to the emergency department. She has no serious burns but is beginning to show signs of cyanide toxicity. She is given sodium nitrite as an antidote. How will sodium nitrite help in this case?

(A) Changing urine pH
(B) Chelating cyanide
(C) Chemically inactivating cyanide
(D) Oxidation of iron in hemoglobin
(E) Regenerating a damaged enzyme

43 A 37-year-old man is found to have hypercholesterolemia during a routine checkup. The physician prescribes lovastatin and counsels the patient to make healthy dietary and lifestyle changes to keep his cholesterol under control. Two weeks later, he returns complaining of severe muscle pain, possibly caused by his lovastatin therapy. He insists that he is taking the medication exactly as prescribed, but the physician knows that lovastatin is metabolized by the cytochrome P450 3A4. What else may he be using that would explain his condition?

(A) Barbiturate abuse
(B) Grapefruit juice
(C) Griseofulvin
(D) Phenytoin
(E) St. John's wort supplement

44 A 6-year-old boy cuts his hand on the training wheel of his bicycle. The wound is 1.5 cm in size and the bleeding stops with direct pressure. One of the steps of blood clotting involved platelet aggregation through activation of collagen. Platelet release of granules is mediated by the release of mediators. Which of the following mediators, if activated, will likely cause bleeding to continue?

(A) Adenosine diphosphate
(B) Dopamine
(C) Serotonin
(D) Thrombin
(E) Thromboxane A_2

45 A 33-year-old woman who is 20 weeks pregnant with a porcine heart valve is at risk for thromboembolism. Which of the following is the best agent to use in this situation?

(A) Heparin
(B) Streptokinase
(C) TED stockings
(D) Warfarin sodium

46 A 78-year-old woman with ovarian cancer and pancreatitis is hospitalized for acute treatment of a massive pulmonary embolism. She is immediately given an intravenous dose of alteplase once the diagnosis of pulmonary embolism was made. Characteristics of this agent include which of the following?

(A) Acts on free plasminogen
(B) High antigenicity
(C) Low fibrin specificity
(D) Long half-life
(E) Success at clot resolution

47 A 29-year-old woman presents to her primary care physician for a regular yearly checkup. She has a history of a seizure disorder and has been taking an antiseizure medication for 8 years. She is also taking an oral contraceptive. She is in good health but complains that her gums seem to be overgrowing her teeth. Which of the following medications is likely responsible for her chief complaint?

(A) Estrogen analog
(B) Lamotrigine
(C) Phenytoin
(D) Progesterone analog
(E) Valproic acid

48 A 4-year-old boy is brought to the emergency department who was found drinking antifreeze while the father was working on their car. A primary component of antifreeze is ethylene glycol, an alcohol converted to toxic metabolites by the liver enzyme alcohol dehydrogenase. To prevent toxicity, the physician could administer ethanol, which would compete with ethylene glycol for the enzyme. In order to avoid administering ethanol to this patient, the physician could instead give which of the following drugs that would also prevent metabolism of ethylene glycol?

(A) Bicarbonate
(B) Disulfiram
(C) Fomepizole
(D) Furosemide
(E) Methanol

49 A 66-year-old man with a history of recurrent pulmonary infections and hypertension is managed with ethacrynic acid, which controls his hypertension well. He is often hospitalized and placed on gentamicin for his recurrent pulmonary infections. Which of the following adverse effects must the treating physician be keenly aware of?

(A) Dizziness
(B) Hearing loss
(C) Nausea
(D) Vertigo
(E) Vomiting

50 A 38-year-old man who is obese complains of an extremely painful, swollen metatarsophalangeal joint of his left big toe. He presents to his primary care physician for evaluation. He has had two similar attacks in the past 4 years. The physician prescribes probenecid. Which of the following describes probenecid's mechanism of action?

(A) Anti-inflammatory
(B) Inhibition of leukocyte migration
(C) Inhibition of urate reabsorption
(D) Inhibition of xanthine oxidase
(E) Upregulation of urate metabolism

51 A 27-year-old man with recurrent asthma attacks is being considered for preventative therapy with cromolyn sodium. This agent is not effective as an acute treatment of an asthma attack because of the lack of which of the following properties?

(A) Anti-inflammatory
(B) Bronchodilator
(C) Immune modulator
(D) Mast cell stabilizer
(E) Neutrophil inhibitor

52 A 52-year-old man with asthma treated with a β_2-agonist via inhaler has been having difficulty with therapy because of persistent changes in blood pressure, nausea, vomiting, and hypomagnesemia. Which of the following medications would be best for this patient?

(A) β_2-Agonist via inhaler every other day
(B) β_2-Agonist via inhaler every third day
(C) β_2-Agonist via inhaler twice daily
(D) Change to ipratropium
(E) Change to epinephrine

53 A 48-year-old man with a known history of asthma takes daily theophylline. He is found unconscious in his bathroom with an open bottle of theophylline that is now empty nearby. He is found by EMS to be apneic and pulseless. What is the most likely cause of death in this patient?

(A) Apnea
(B) Cardiac arrhythmia
(C) Pulmonary embolism
(D) Seizures
(E) Tetany

54 A 34-year-old man with allergic rhinitis presents to his primary care physician for treatment. He is prescribed diphenhydramine and develops dry eyes and mouth within 2 days. His symptoms of rhinitis are approximately 75% better. He calls his physician asking what he should do. The most appropriate management for this patient is which of the following?

(A) Continue medication at current dose
(B) Discontinue diphenhydramine
(C) Start therapy with chlorpheniramine in addition to diphenhydramine
(D) Surgical consultation for rhinoplasty
(E) Surgical consultation for septoplasty

55 A 26-year-old man with a chronic cough takes codeine for cough suppression. He presents to his primary care physician for follow-up. The patient admits to taking this medication three times daily even when he does not have symptoms. The treating physician must be concerned about which of the following effects?

(A) Addiction
(B) Diarrhea
(C) Euphoria
(D) Excessive anxiety
(E) Sweating

56 A 64-year-old alcoholic man who has not had access to alcohol for days is brought to the hospital by family. He is extremely agitated and reports seeing spiders on the walls that he wants to kill. His temperature is 39°C, pulse is 96 beats/minute, and blood pressure is 152/88 mm Hg. He is given a benzodiazepine, which mimics the effects of alcohol on his brain. Which of the following types of receptor to benzodiazepines is acted upon?
(A) G_i receptor
(B) G_s receptor
(C) G_q receptor
(D) Ion channel
(E) Transcription factor

57 A 19-year-old male college student develops sore throat, chills, and fever. Instead of going to the student health service for care, he takes a few of his roommates' amoxicillin antibiotics. Over the next few hours, he develops a maculopapular rash on his palms and swelling of his lips. What is the most likely explanation for this finding?
(A) DNA gyrase
(B) Penicilloic acid
(C) RNA synthase
(D) Telomerase
(E) Transferase

58 A 52-year-old man with organic impotence is in the preoperative holding area before surgery. He is given intravenous vancomycin over 20 min and begins to develop fever, chills, and redness at the injection site. What is the most appropriate course of action for the physician to take?
(A) Administer anticholinesterase inhibitor
(B) Administer corticosteroids
(C) Immediate intubation for airway protection
(D) Immediately discontinue vancomycin
(E) Slow the infusion rate over 2 h

59 A 33-year-old man with a history of chronic epididymo-orchitis is treated with long-term tetracycline antibiotic therapy. During the 3 months of therapy, he develops discoloration of his teeth. What is the most likely explanation for this finding?
(A) Binding to tissues with calcium content
(B) Drug toxicity effect
(C) Inhibition of folate synthesis
(D) Inhibition of hepatic enzymes
(E) Inhibition of osteoclast activity

60 A 42-year-old female who is obese and with a history of gallstones and cholecystitis complains of superficial skin swelling and itching. Physical examination by the primary care physician reveals skin erythema, tenderness, and swelling consistent with cellulitis. The patient is given a prescription for erythromycin. Which of the following effects must the treating physician be keenly aware of?
(A) Cholestatic jaundice
(B) Mild abdominal discomfort
(C) Nausea
(D) Tinnitus
(E) Vomiting

61 A 37-year-old woman is brought to the emergency department by a friend after consuming an entire month's supply of amitriptyline. She is tachycardic, drowsy, nauseous, and has a headache. Which of the following could the physician administer to help this patient?
(A) Bicarbonate
(B) Dimercaprol
(C) Methylene blue
(D) Naloxone
(E) Vitamin K

62 A 52-year-old woman with a history of recurrent urinary tract infections complains of easy bruising as well as chronic fatigue. She is maintained on daily antibiotic prophylaxis with trimethoprim. Which of the following hematologic effects is likely as a result of long-term therapy with trimethoprim?
(A) Aplastic anemia
(B) Megaloblastic anemia
(C) Microcytic anemia
(D) Normocytic anemia
(E) Pernicious anemia

63 A 24-year-old man is admitted for an emergent appendectomy. While in the operating room, the anesthesiologist finds that he must use a much higher than expected anesthetic dose to anesthetize this patient. After the surgery, the patient admits to barbiturate abuse. What is the correct term for the fact that his history of barbiturate abuse led to a greater anesthetic requirement?
(A) Addiction
(B) Cross-dependence
(C) Cross-tolerance
(D) Dependence
(E) Tolerance

64 A 48-year-old man presents to the emergency department in the morning with urticaria and difficulty breathing following a bee sting received while gardening. He is treated, recovers, and is sent home. Later that evening, his symptoms return and he is treated again in the emergency department. He denies having been stung again. What should have been given to this patient to avoid his return to the emergency department?

(A) Diphenhydramine
(B) Epinephrine
(C) Loratadine
(D) Prednisolone
(E) The patient is likely mistaken; he probably was stung a second time

65 A 13-year-old male has begun having spells of wheezing and difficulty breathing while playing outside. He is diagnosed with asthma and given an inhaler to treat acute attacks. His medication is working well, but he would also like something to prevent attacks from happening. Which of the following drugs would be best to add to his regimen?

(A) Albuterol
(B) Epinephrine
(C) Ipratropium
(D) Isoproterenol
(E) Salmeterol

66 A 33-year-old man with a history of asthma comes into the emergency department after getting stung by a bee. The treating physician wants to give epinephrine subcutaneously. Which of the following contraindications to this medication is noted?

(A) Diabetes mellitus
(B) Narrow-angle glaucoma
(C) Pulmonary failure
(D) Thyroid disease
(E) Age older than 80 years

67 A 27-year-old man with HIV disease and hepatitis B is hospitalized for treatment of his hepatitis B. He has begun on intravenous treatment with interferon. After administration, he develops fever, chills, and myalgias. Physical examination reveals that the lungs are clear to auscultation bilaterally. What is the most likely explanation for this reaction?

(A) Expected adverse event
(B) Drug toxicity
(C) Underlying atypical pneumonia
(D) Underlying bacterial pneumonia
(E) Underlying viral pneumonia

68 A 44-year-old man with acute lymphocytic leukemia is undergoing a multiagent chemotherapy protocol. Agents used include methotrexate. The cycle of medication will last 6 weeks. Which of the following tissues is most likely to experience toxic effects as a result of this therapy?

(A) Buccal mucosa
(B) Long bones, legs
(C) Epidermal layer, skin
(D) Small bones, face
(E) Teeth

69 A 54-year-old man with an attack of gout approximately 4 months ago was placed on allopurinol. He now presents to his primary care physician complaining of a skin rash on his arms. Allopurinol was discontinued 3 months ago. What is the most likely explanation for this finding?

(A) Contact dermatitis
(B) Dermatitis herpetiformis
(C) Hypersensitivity
(D) Squamous cell carcinoma
(E) Telangiectasia

70 A 22-year-old man with seasonal allergic rhinitis takes an antihistamine for relief of symptoms. It is successful for him over 90% of the time. Histamine is a natural amine formed by the decarboxylation of which of the following amino acids?

(A) L-arginine
(B) Heparin
(C) Histidine
(D) Lysine
(E) Tyrosine

71 A 52-year-old man who works as an air traffic controller has seasonal allergies. Currently, he is very symptomatic but cannot miss work because of staffing issues. Which of the following agents would be best suited for this patient?

(A) Chlorpheniramine
(B) Diphenhydramine
(C) Doxylamine
(D) Fexofenadine
(E) Hydroxylamine

72 A 39-year-old man with long-standing allergies has no health insurance and simply takes over-the-counter diphenhydramine for symptom relief. He has no other medical problems but uses this medication up to four times per day. Which of the following effects of this medication is possible to be experienced by this patient?

(A) Appetite enhancement
(B) Dizziness
(C) Hypotension
(D) Reflex bradycardia
(E) Urinary retention

73 A local municipality is alerted that low doses of carbon tetrachloride have been dumped into the drinking water. A public health alert is transmitted to all residents of this town. Which of the following signs and symptoms should these residents be aware of?

(A) Convulsions
(B) Eye irritation
(C) Nausea
(D) Stupor
(E) Vomiting

74 A 22-year-old woman is investigated by authorities after the accidental death of her 4-year-old child. It appears that the child would not go to sleep and the mother used chloroform to make the child sleepy. What is the most likely explanation for this accidental death?

(A) Myocardial infarction
(B) Toxic dose of chloroform via inhalation
(C) Underlying pulmonary hypertension
(D) Underlying pulmonary venous thrombosis
(E) Ventricular septal defect with overriding aorta

75 A 55-year-old man with a 40 pack-year history of smoking develops agranulocytosis and some leukemic features. His physical examination of the heart, lungs, and abdomen are within normal limits. Should this disease relate to a potential toxic exposure, which of the following should be considered most likely?

(A) Benzene
(B) Ethylene alcohol
(C) Carbon tetrachloride
(D) Methanol
(E) Toluene

76 A 44-year-old man is found dead in his home by the police. Reports indicate that the man was heating his one-room apartment with a kerosene space heater. He was found because other people in the apartment complex that he lives at developed headache, lethargy, and confusion. What is the most likely explanation for these findings?

(A) Carbon monoxide poisoning
(B) Clustering of community-acquired pneumonia
(C) Cyanide exposure
(D) Silica dust exposure

77 A 13-year-old female complains of an itchy, runny nose during the fall season. She says she experienced similar symptoms around the same time last year. Her family history is significant for hay fever in her mother. Which of the following would be the best choice to treat this patient?

(A) Aspirin
(B) Epinephrine
(C) Montelukast
(D) Naproxen
(E) Terbutaline

78 A 57-year-old man with a history of intermittent angina normally takes sublingual nitroglycerin when attacks occur. He states that he does not take this medication because it makes him feel "funny. . . itch uncontrollably. . . and have pain radiating to his toes." These symptoms have never been witnessed by his family members who are with him all the time. What is the best course of action for the treating physician to take?

(A) Consultation with psychiatrist
(B) Consultation with behavioral medicine physician
(C) Encourage patient to take medication and explore reasons for noncompliance
(D) Switch to another antianginal agent
(E) Treatment with antipsychotic agent

79 An 18-year-old college student is hanging shelves in his dorm room. He accidentally hits his thumb with the hammer, which subsequently becomes swollen and red. He takes some aspirin for the pain. Many enzymes and other proteins are activated in response to injury leading to inflammation. Production of which of the following mediators is inhibited by aspirin?

(A) HAT
(B) IκB
(C) NO
(D) NF-κB
(E) PGE_2

80 A 19-year-old female is brought to the emergency department by a friend concerned with a change in her behavior during a party. The patient is agitated, anxious, and exhibits paranoid reactions to the physical exam. Her pulse is 120 beats/minute and her blood pressure is 150/100 mm Hg. She also complains of "bugs" crawling all over her skin, although there is nothing there. Which of the following drugs has she most likely taken?

(A) Cocaine
(B) Heroin
(C) LSD
(D) Methanol
(E) Propofol

81 A 31-year-old woman smoker expresses a desire to quit smoking. She has a 10 pack-year history of smoking but no other health issues. She wants to try varenicline, a drug she recently heard about, to help her quit. Which of the following side effects of varenicline is she most likely to encounter?

(A) Abnormal dreams
(B) Gastric ulcers
(C) Pancreatitis
(D) Photosensitivity
(E) Seizures

82 A 45-year-old woman undergoes a complete hysterectomy for leiomyomas and dysfunctional uterine bleeding. The surgeon wants to prescribe a pain relief medication following the procedure, but the patient's serum creatinine is 1.2 mg/dL. Which of the following pain relief medications should the surgeon avoid prescribing?
(A) Acetaminophen
(B) Codeine
(C) Hydrocodone
(D) Ketorolac
(E) Oxycodone

83 A 43-year-old man undergoes a kidney transplantation. His physician prescribes azathioprine for graft rejection prophylaxis. His past medical history is significant for gouty arthritis. Which of the following antigout drugs should he avoid while taking azathioprine?
(A) Allopurinol
(B) Colchicine
(C) Indomethacin
(D) Prednisolone
(E) Probenecid

84 A 31-year-old woman is planning to take a 7-day cruise to the Caribbean islands. She has never been on a ship before and fears developing motion sickness. She purchases scopolamine transdermal patch. When is the best time for her to place the patch to maximize drug efficacy?
(A) After nausea first begins
(B) After nausea occurs for 2 h
(C) After vomiting occurs
(D) After short-term memory fails
(E) Prior to the onset of symptoms

85 A 22-year-old woman is interested in taking oral contraceptives for the prevention of pregnancy. The most likely benefit in terms of disease prevention from oral contraceptives is which of the following?
(A) Decreased risk of colon cancer
(B) Decreased risk of ectopic pregnancy
(C) Decreased risk of infiltrating ductal carcinoma of the breast
(D) Decreased risk of medullary carcinoma of the thyroid
(E) Decreased risk of teratoma of the uterus

86 A 29-year-old woman has a positive pregnancy test. She presents to her primary care physician for confirmation. She has a history of recurrent urinary tract infections, headaches, seizure disorder, and pulmonary embolus. Her current medications include acetaminophen, ciprofloxacin, warfarin, valproic acid, and methotrexate. Which of the following medications could be maintained at its current dose during her pregnancy?
(A) Acetaminophen
(B) Ciprofloxacin
(C) Methotrexate
(D) Valproic acid
(E) Warfarin

87 A 20-year-old female with a history of substance abuse has delivered a child whose weight is less than the 10th percentile. Other findings include small head and flat midface. The patient has an atrial septal defect. Which of the following substances may have caused these symptoms?
(A) Alcohol
(B) Cocaine
(C) Marijuana
(D) Opioids
(E) Tobacco

88 A 26-year-old alcoholic man is trying to quit drinking. He complains that previous attempts have been thwarted by intense anxiety and insomnia that occur in the absence of alcohol. These symptoms disappear when he resumes alcohol use. Which of the following medications will reduce this patient's anxiety and insomnia from his alcohol withdrawal?
(A) Acamprosate
(B) Disulfiram
(C) Methadone
(D) Methanol
(E) Naltrexone

89 A 69-year-old man with exercise-induced angina presents to his primary care physician for follow-up. The angina is worsening and is now present at rest. The patient is not taking any medications. Isosorbide dinitrate sublingual is prescribed for the patient. Which of the following interactions must the physician warn this patient about?
(A) Cold extremities
(B) Hot extremities
(C) Severe hypotension with sildenafil
(D) Tinnitus
(E) Vertigo

90 A 35-year-old African American male in the military is hospitalized with an MRSA skin infection. The patient starts treatment with an antibiotic and becomes anemic and jaundiced. On peripheral blood smear, Heinz bodies are seen within red blood cells. What is the mechanism of action of the antibiotic given to this patient?

(A) Acts at the 50s ribosomal subunit to inhibit peptide bond formation
(B) Binds to 30s ribosomal subunit and prevents tRNA attachment
(C) Inhibits cell wall formation
(D) Inhibits DNA-dependent RNA polymerase
(E) Inhibits folic acid metabolism

91 A 6-year-old boy from Connecticut presents to the emergency department with a bulls-eye–shaped rash on his upper left arm after he went hiking with his family a couple of days ago. He also has had intermittent fevers and muscle aches. The blood test for Lyme disease is positive. He has a history of hearing loss in his left ear from trauma. What side effect would prevent the physician from treating the boy with doxycycline?

(A) Discoloration of teeth
(B) Megaloblastic anemia
(C) Nephrotoxicity
(D) Ototoxicity
(E) Worsening leg cramps and myalgias

92 A 28-year-old female presents with a 4 × 5 cm purulent ulcer on her abdomen following a spider bite. A wound culture grows MRSA, so intravenous vancomycin is started. While receiving her first dose of vancomycin, her face, neck, and chest flushed red. This reaction can best be described as

(A) Non-hypersensitivity mast cell degranulation
(B) Type I hypersensitivity reaction
(C) Type II hypersensitivity reaction
(D) Type III hypersensitivity reaction
(E) Type IV hypersensitivity reaction

93 A 22-year-old man has taken an overdose of sleeping pills after learning that he did not receive the job he has recently been interviewed for. He is found by his roommate conscious but not able to completely follow commands. The roommate calls the local poison control center. Instructions are given to self-administer syrup of ipecac while waiting for the rescue squad to respond. This agent has a mechanism of action that involves which of the following?

(A) Stimulating the gag reflex
(B) Stimulating the trigger zone of chemotaxis
(C) Suppressing gastric outlet pressures
(D) Suppressing the gag reflex
(E) Suppressing the motor cortex

94 A 19-year-old man is brought to the emergency room after being found by the police to be disruptive in a shopping mall. He states that he is hearing voices and seeing Jesus Christ. The police apprehended him because he was acting violently. He arrives in the emergency department and is combative. His blood pressure is 190/90 mm Hg. His core body temperature is 39°C. The most likely explanation for these findings is overdose of which of the following?

(A) Alcohol
(B) Cocaine
(C) Marijuana
(D) Phencyclidine piperidine
(E) Quailudes

95 A 17-year-old man presents to the emergency department with a persistent cough and nasal congestion. He has been taking various prescription cough and cold medicines but did not know their names. A urine drug screen is positive for amphetamines. When confronted with this information, he vehemently denies amphetamine use. What is the best explanation?

(A) He had a false positive because of codeine use
(B) He had a false positive because of ephedrine use
(C) He had a false positive because of marijuana use
(D) He is lying about drug use
(E) His urine sample was mixed up with another patient's

96 A 6-year-old boy is brought to his primary care physician with a history of hay fever and asthma. He usually has two to three attacks per week. For symptom control, he uses an albuterol inhaler, but his parents would like to try something more. They would like him to take something that would lessen the amount of attacks he has. Although corticosteroids would probably work best for prophylaxis, they are contraindicated in children. He is instead given montelukast. How does montelukast works?

(A) Blocks leukotriene receptors
(B) Blocks muscarinic acetylcholine receptors
(C) Inhibits COX-1 and COX-2
(D) Inhibits COX-2 only
(E) Inhibits lipoxygenase

97 A 52-year-old overweight man steamroller operator comes to you complaining of itchy, watery eyes and runny nose in the springtime. He says that he has had this problem for as long as he can remember but does not like going to doctors. His wife finally convinced him to come today see what you might be able to do for him. You prescribe cetirizine. Which of the following describes cetirizine's mechanism of action?

(A) Inhibits β_2-receptors
(B) Inhibits H_1 receptors
(C) Stimulates α_1-receptors
(D) Stimulates β_2-receptors
(E) Stimulates H_1 receptors

98 A 43-year-old woman with multiple sclerosis has not been treated with medication because of only having mild symptoms. Now, she has bilateral lower extremity weakness and urinary complaints. She has begun on mitoxantrone. Which of the following adverse effects must the treating physician be aware of?
(A) Anxiety
(B) Hepatitis
(C) Hypopyrexia
(D) Improved muscle strength
(E) Leukocytosis

99 A 22-year-old man college student does poorly on a course examination and decides to attempt suicide. He finds a bottle of barbiturates in his mother's medicine cabinet. He takes 2 of the 30 pills in the bottle. Which of the following effects is most likely to be exhibited by the patient?
(A) Anesthesia
(B) Coma
(C) Death
(D) Hypnosis
(E) Sedation

100 A 36-year-old man is brought to the emergency department after being involved in a one-car motor vehicle accident where his car struck a telephone pole. He is a known chronic alcoholic. He smells alcohol on his breath, and his blood alcohol level is 300 mg/dL. Which of the following treatments should be given to him if he goes into alcohol withdrawal?
(A) Buspirone
(B) Lorazepam
(C) Pentobarbital
(D) Phenytoin
(E) Watchful waiting with saline intravenous infusion

101 A 45-year-old woman has just received a kidney transplant. She is placed on several immunosuppressants to prophylactically prevent her body from rejecting the donor organ. Which of the following immunosuppressants interferes with T-cell activation by inhibition of mTOR?
(A) Azathioprine
(B) Cyclosporine
(C) Methotrexate
(D) Prednisolone
(E) Sirolimus

102 You have been monitoring a 62-year-old man who is a retired small business owner over the past year and have noted a slowly changing intraocular pressure bilaterally. You have started him on physostigmine to treat his open-angle glaucoma. How does physostigmine affect intraocular pressure?
(A) Lowers pressure by decreasing aqueous humor secretion
(B) Lowers pressure by decreasing aqueous humor synthesis
(C) Lowers pressure by increasing aqueous humor outflow
(D) Raises pressure by decreasing aqueous humor outflow
(E) Raises pressure by increasing aqueous humor secretion

103 A 34-year-old man presents to the emergency department with fevers, chills, muscle aches, and headaches for the past 16 h. His son has been sick for the past week and unable to attend daycare. He did not receive the influenza vaccine this year. A nasal swab is performed and he is diagnosed with influenza. He is started on oseltamivir. What is the mechanism of action of oseltamivir?
(A) Blocks viral uncoating via M_2 protein
(B) Inhibits IMP dehydrogenase
(C) Inhibits neuraminidase
(D) Inhibits reverse transcriptase
(E) Inhibits viral DNA polymerase

104 A 43-year-old woman with a history of hypertension drinks one to two cups of coffee per day. She has been doing this for 3 months. As a result of her continued behavior, which of the following effects of coffee is most likely for her?
(A) Decrease in fatigue
(B) Decrease in mental alertness
(C) Tolerance
(D) Tremors
(E) Withdrawal

105 A 58-year-old woman who is obese comes to the emergency department with diaphoresis and crushing chest pain that radiates to her left arm. The physician orders an ECG and checks her cardiac enzymes to confirm his suspicion of myocardial infarction. Because of the quick response and intervention, she survives and is ultimately discharged with a prescription for low-dose daily aspirin to inhibit platelet aggregation. Which of the following enzymes is the intended target of aspirin in this patient?
(A) Cyclooxygenase
(B) Lipoxygenase
(C) Phospholipase A_2
(D) Prostacyclin synthase
(E) Thromboxane synthase

106 A 65-year-old man with end-stage renal disease because of diabetes recently underwent a renal transplant. He has been responding well to the transplant and his creatinine has stabilized around 2.1 mg/dL. He was placed on immunosuppressive therapy with muromonab. What is the mechanism of action of muromonab?

(A) Binds to CD3 on T cells
(B) Binds to FK-binding protein
(C) Binds to IL-2 receptors on T cells
(D) Binds to mTOR
(E) Inhibits calcineurin

107 A 5-year-old boy presents to the emergency room with abdominal pain, nausea, and three episodes of bloody emesis. His mother is concerned because she saw him playing near the open medicine cabinet and her prenatal vitamins were opened. What is the most appropriate treatment for the child's overdose?

(A) Aminocaproic acid
(B) Deferoxamine
(C) Dimercaprol
(D) Penicillamine
(E) Succimer

108 A 24-year-old woman medical student with a history of depression presents to the emergency department with tachycardia and shallow breathing. After her initial presentation, she begins to become confused and has a seizure. An ECG is performed and shows QT prolongation. An arterial blood gas shows metabolic acidosis. She has been taking antidepressants for a couple of years, but her depression is worsening. She had a test yesterday and told her mother that she felt she did poorly. There is concern that she has overdosed on her medication. What is the most appropriate treatment?

(A) Ammonium chloride
(B) Atropine
(C) Flumazenil
(D) *N*-acetylcysteine
(E) Sodium bicarbonate

109 A 38-year-old man who is a chronic coffee drinker for 20 years drinks approximately seven cups of coffee per day. He suddenly decides to stop drinking coffee. Which of the following effects may he exhibit?

(A) Lethargy
(B) Migraine
(C) Nausea
(D) Tinnitus
(E) Vomiting

110 A 29-year-old man who is a known alcoholic is able to purchase phencyclidine from another user of this substance. He takes a "triple dose" of the substance. Which of the following effects is likely to be observed?

(A) Eyes remain open
(B) Loss of consciousness
(C) Numbness of extremities
(D) Rapid, normal gait
(E) Rapid, normal speech

111 A 48-year-old woman with obsessive-compulsive disorder presents to her primary care physician for evaluation. She states that her symptoms have worsened during the last 6 months and desires treatment. She has begun on sertraline. Which of the following precautions must be exercised by the physician?

(A) Associated with hepatic carcinoma
(B) Observe for volume overload
(C) Potentiate actions of antibiotics
(D) Suicidal tendencies

112 A 29-year-old man with recurrent allergic rhinitis presents to his primary care physician for evaluation. He states that his symptoms are more problematic lately and desires treatment. He has begun on fexofenadine. Which of the following adverse reactions is possible in this patient?

(A) Anxiety
(B) Cough
(C) Headache
(D) Otitis media
(E) Upper respiratory infection

113 A 53-year-old man spends his mornings outside gardening. He frequently develops tension headaches, and the only medication he keeps at home is aspirin. After taking two regular-sized aspirin tablets almost daily for a few weeks, which of the following side effects is he most at risk for?

(A) Angina
(B) Insomnia
(C) Hypercoagulability
(D) Nephrolithiasis
(E) Tinnitus

114 A 19-year-old G1P0 woman at 34 weeks gestation lost her eyeglasses for a day. Constant squinting causes her to develop a headache. She asks her doctor for a pain reliever. Which of the following drugs may disrupt her fetus' circulatory system?

(A) Acetaminophen
(B) Codeine
(C) Hydrocodone
(D) Morphine
(E) Ketorolac

115 A 22-year-old woman ingests an entire bottle of acetaminophen in an attempted suicide. She unexpectedly feels well; and when her boyfriend discovers what she has done, he takes her to the emergency department. Which of the following drugs should be given in the ER?

(A) Acetylsalicylic acid
(B) Acetylcysteine
(C) Bicarbonate
(D) Fomepizole
(E) Penicillamine

116 A 42-year-old woman with a 1-year history of rheumatoid arthritis comes to see you complaining of worsening symptoms. She has been taking leflunomide. You know that IL-1 and TNF-α are two key cytokines involved in the negative sequelae of rheumatoid arthritis. You decide to give her anakinra to interfere with IL-1 signaling. Which of the following is the most common side effect of anakinra administration?

(A) Blurry vision
(B) Diarrhea
(C) Headache
(D) Injection site reaction
(E) Nausea

117 A 48-year-old woman with 2-year history of rheumatoid arthritis has not had sufficient relief with methotrexate alone. Her physician prescribes etanercept to help control her symptoms. How does etanercept work?

(A) Depletes substance P
(B) Inhibition of COX enzymes
(C) Inhibition of leukocyte chemotaxis
(D) Inhibition of TNF-α signaling
(E) Prevents production of arachidonic acid

118 A 25-year-old male comes to the emergency department with crushing, substernal chest pain. The pain radiates up to his jaw and down to his right arm. He has never had chest pain like this before. An ECG shows ST elevations in leads I, II, and AVF. A detailed history reveals that he had used cocaine 2 h prior to the onset of chest pain. Which of the following medications is contraindicated in the treatment of myocardial infarction caused by his cocaine use?

(A) ACE inhibitors
(B) Aspirin
(C) β-Blockers
(D) Calcium channel blockers
(E) Nitroglycerin

119 A 56-year-old alcoholic man consumes a six-pack of beer before going to bed. After being absorbed from his gut, blood carries the alcohol through the portal vein into the liver where it can be metabolized. Ethanol is metabolized in multiple steps by various enzymes, including alcohol dehydrogenase. Which of the following describes a characteristic of this enzyme?

(A) Acts on acetaldehyde
(B) Acts on acetate
(C) Inhibited by disulfiram
(D) Inhibited by fomepizole
(E) Produces acetate

120 An 18-year-old man is brought to the emergency department by a friend after smoking crack cocaine because he was "acting funny." His temperature is 38°C (100.4°F), pulse is 110 beats/minute, and he appears agitated. Which of the following is an effect of cocaine intoxication?

(A) Hypercoagulability
(B) Hypocoagulability
(C) Hypothermia
(D) Vasoconstriction
(E) Vasodilation

121 A 59-year-old man with a history of depression cuts his wrists in a suicide attempt. He is brought to the local emergency department for care. He has bilateral medial 3-cm lacerations through the skin and subcutaneous tissues that will require sutures. A review of his prior medical history indicates an allergy to 2% lidocaine. The most likely explanation for this is which of the following?

(A) Allergic
(B) Mast cell mediated
(C) Neurogenic
(D) Psychogenic
(E) Vascular induced

122 A 44-year-old man who is a chronic smoker and takes bupropion takes 10 pills at once in an attempted suicide. Which of the following effects is possible as a result of this overdose?

(A) Dry mouth
(B) Nervousness
(C) Seizures
(D) Sexual dysfunction
(E) Sweating

123 A 56-year-old man with chronic pain injects himself with morphine, which he obtained from a friend who is an emergency department nurse. He is found dead in his apartment by the police. What is the most likely cause of death?

(A) Congestive heart failure
(B) Hepatitis
(C) Respiratory depression
(D) Pulmonary edema
(E) Pulmonary embolism

124 A 19-year-old man who is a known heroin addict is brought to the emergency department because of an apparent overdose. The reason why addicts enjoy heroin is because of its conversion to which of the following substances?
(A) Dopamine
(B) Epinephrine
(C) Morphine
(D) Norepinephrine
(E) Serotonin

125 A 52-year-old man with chronic low back pain following an automobile accident desires pain relief. He has significant gastroesophageal reflux and abdominal pain. Which of the following agents may improve his pain but worsen his gastrointestinal symptoms?
(A) Choline magnesium trisalicylate
(B) Celecoxib
(C) Ketorolac
(D) Naproxen sodium
(E) Salsalate

126 A 26-year-old woman presents to her primary care physician complaining of seasonal allergies. She has done well without medications for some time but now has worsening of her symptoms. She is given a prescription for fexofenadine. Which of the following adverse effects must be considered in this patient?
(A) Flank pain
(B) Headache
(C) Otitis externa
(D) Pulmonary bacterial infection
(E) Tinnitus

127 A 34-year-old man with seasonal allergic rhinitis that has been refractory to oral antihistamines is now placed on Singulair, a leukotriene receptor blocker, to see if this will improve symptoms. Important interactions with this medication include which of the following?
(A) Ampicillin
(B) Chloramphenicol
(C) Rifampin
(D) Tetracycline

128 A 21-year-old male college student presents to the emergency department with hives over his chest and arms. The history and physical exam reveals that he used a new laundry detergent and he was having an allergic reaction. The physician wants to prescribe an antihistamine that will not sedate the patient because he has to study for a test. What is the most appropriate treatment?
(A) Chlorpheniramine
(B) Dimenhydrinate
(C) Diphenhydramine
(D) Fexofenadine
(E) Ipratropium

129 A 13-year-old boy with moderate asthma presents to the clinic for follow-up. His symptoms appear to be better controlled since adding salmeterol to his regimen. He has had to use his rescue inhaler once over the past 2 weeks during exertion. His breathing at night has improved as well. How does salmeterol exhibit its beneficial effects for asthma?
(A) Long-acting β_1-agonist
(B) Long-acting β_1-antagonist
(C) Long-acting β_1- and β_2-agonist
(D) Long-acting β_2-agonist
(E) Long-acting β_2-antagonist

130 A 28-year-old woman presents to the emergency department in an acute asthma exacerbation. Her asthma developed in her 20s after she had recurrent upper respiratory infections. She was doing well, but she twisted her ankle yesterday and was taking aspirin to reduce the inflammation. She is diagnosed with aspirin-induced asthma. What is the most appropriate long-term treatment for her condition?
(A) Albuterol
(B) Cromolyn
(C) Ipratropium
(D) Theophylline
(E) Zafirlukast

131 A 23-year-old man victim of a motor vehicle accident is brought to the emergency department. He is found to have a blood alcohol level of 850 mg/dL. Because of the way the body handles ethanol, the conventional "half-life" to describe its metabolism does not apply. Which of the following drugs at therapeutic concentrations exhibits the same property?
(A) Aspirin
(B) Ibuprofen
(C) Simvastatin
(D) Tolbutamide
(E) Valproic acid

132 A mother brings her unconscious 14-year-old son to the emergency department. He was found in his bedroom by his mother appearing agitated and sweaty. He complains of a feeling of ants crawling under his skin and a dry mouth. The mother suspects that he has been abusing his brother's prescription ADHD medicine, showing an empty pill bottle. What should he be given now?

(A) Ammonium chloride
(B) Epinephrine
(C) Flumazenil
(D) Pilocarpine
(E) Theophylline

133 A 53-year-old man with chronic neuropathic back pain and depression is managed with amitriptyline. He has recently complained of urinary frequency and was given a prescription for Ditropan. He now complains of acute abdominal pain and is unable to pass flatus or bowel movement. What is the most likely explanation of this finding?

(A) Alcoholic hepatitis
(B) Pancreatitis
(C) Paralytic ileus
(D) Supratherapeutic dose of medication (overdose)
(E) Normal finding

134 A 19-year-old man attempts suicide after failing all of his college courses. He goes home and takes more than 90 digoxin tablets (0.25 mg each), ingesting them about 3 h prior to presentation at the emergency department. He is brought to the hospital by his brother. Vital signs are as follows: pulse is 50 beats/minute, and the electrocardiogram indicates third-degree heart block. Serum electrolytes are normal. Which of the following is the most important therapy to initiate in this patient?

(A) Amiodarone
(B) Digoxin immune Fab
(C) Lidocaine
(D) Potassium salts
(E) Verapamil

135 A 63-year-old man presents to the emergency department with altered mental status after ingesting an entire bottle of acetaminophen. The patient's heart rate is 120 beats/minute, blood pressure is 100/58 mm Hg, and respiration rate is 28/minute. His aspartate aminotransferase and alanine aminotransferase are 4,128 IU and 3,978 IU, respectively. What is the most appropriate treatment for this patient?

(A) Ammonium chloride
(B) Flumazenil
(C) *N*-Acetylcysteine
(D) Naloxone
(E) Sodium bicarbonate

136 A 64-year-old man is brought to the emergency department unconscious. He undergoes a CT of the chest, which reveals a pulmonary embolism. He is considered for immediate therapy with heparin. Because the man is unconscious, a history cannot be obtained from him. Which of the following would represent a contraindication to heparin therapy?

(A) Alcoholism
(B) Drug abuse
(C) Hypertension
(D) Immune deficiency state
(E) Recent surgery to remove genital warts

137 A 74-year-old woman with a history of atrial fibrillation presents to the emergency department after bowel movement with bright red blood. Her blood pressure is 88/56 mm Hg with a pulse of 118 beats/minute. She is on warfarin for anticoagulation and a stat INR is 7.2. The decision is made to start transfusing blood. What is the most appropriate treatment to reverse the warfarin?

(A) Fresh frozen plasma
(B) Platelet transfusion
(C) Protamine sulfate
(D) Vitamin K
(E) Whole blood transfusion

138 A 36-year-old woman grocery store manager with a fair complexion and blue eyes presents to her primary care physician for a routine exam. She mentions a friend of hers who is taking bimatoprost to increase the length and amount of her eyelashes and asks if you would recommend it for her. Her past medical history is significant for migraine headaches. Which of the following is a side effect you should warn her about?

(A) New-onset glaucoma
(B) Permanent darkening of the irises
(C) Stevens–Johnson syndrome
(D) Weight gain
(E) Worsening of migraines

139 A 6-year-old boy presents to the emergency department with an altered mental status. He is hyperventilating, has a rash on his hands, and a high fever. His mother has been giving him an antipyretic for his fever for the past 2 days. The patient's liver enzymes are elevated. His mental status continues to decline. What is the mechanism of action of the most likely medication given to this child by his mother?

(A) Inhibits phospholipase A_2
(B) Irreversibly inhibits cyclooxygenases 1 and 2
(C) Reversibly inhibits cyclooxygenases 1 and 2
(D) Reversibly inhibits cyclooxygenase 2
(E) Reversibly inhibits H_1 histamine receptors

140 A 51-year-old alcoholic man presents to the emergency department with severe pain in his right big toe. The pain is so unbearable that even the sheets touching it at night caused him excruciating pain. The toe is erythematous, edematous, and tender. The diagnosis of gout is made after negatively birefringent crystals are seen from joint aspirate. The patient is given colchicine. What is the mechanism of action of colchicine?

(A) Inhibits microtubule polymerization
(B) Inhibits reabsorption of uric acid
(C) Inhibits xanthine oxidase
(D) Irreversibly inhibits cyclooxygenase
(E) Reversibly inhibits cyclooxygenase

141 A 24-year-old G1P0 woman arrives at the hospital in labor at 39 weeks gestation. She denies an epidural, stating her desire to give birth naturally. After 5 h of labor, the baby has begun its descent through the birth canal when the patient requests pain relief. Which is a serious potential side effect for the fetus if an opioid is given to the mother for analgesia?

(A) Diarrhea
(B) Hallucinations
(C) Hyperthermia
(D) Respiratory depression
(E) Restlessness

142 A 53-year-old woman with chronic low back pain presents to the emergency department with pain in her left hand. The pain is a 10/10 and began acutely after she tried to catch herself after a fall. Her hand is edematous and bruised. An X-ray confirms a scaphoid bone fracture. She is given opioid pain medications to treat her pain. She has a history of chronic narcotic use for her low back pain. Which of the following side effects from the chronic use of opioids will the patient not develop a tolerance?

(A) CNS depression
(B) Constipation
(C) Nausea
(D) Pain response
(E) Respiratory depression

143 A 56-year-old man who is an alcoholic presents to the emergency department with altered mental status. Blood tests reveal normal creatinine but hyperammonemia. He is admitted to the hospital for treatment. He has several comorbidities that are being managed well as an outpatient. His wife brings a list of his home medications, which includes bimatoprost, simvastatin, alprostadil, aspirin, and lisinopril. Which of the following should be held (not given to him) during his hospital stay?

(A) Alprostadil
(B) Ascorbic acid
(C) Bimatoprost
(D) Lisinopril
(E) Simvastatin

144 A 33-year-old man with schizophrenia presents to the ambulatory clinic for follow-up. He has been taking haloperidol for years but has been developing extrapyramidal system symptoms recently. He also tells the physician that he knows that the rabbits in his yard have small cameras in their eyes and are being used by the FBI to spy on him. The physician decides to switch him to chlorpromazine. What is a common side effect of chlorpromazine?

(A) Agranulocytosis
(B) Corneal deposits
(C) Diabetes insipidus
(D) Hypertension
(E) Hypothyroidism

145 A 13-year-old boy complains of nausea and vomiting when he takes long road trips with his family. His family is getting ready to leave on another such trip, so he asks if there is anything he can take to lessen his nausea. The physician prescribes an antinausea drug with anticholinergic activity. Which of the following drugs is this?

(A) Dimenhydrinate
(B) Droperidol
(C) Marijuana
(D) Ondansetron
(E) Palonosetron

146 A 45-year-old man who smokes three packs of cigarettes per day has a desire to quit smoking. He begins therapy with varenicline. Which of the following symptoms is likely to be attributed to use of this medication?

(A) Attention deficit disorder
(B) Diarrhea
(C) Flatulence
(D) Hepatitis
(E) Tachypnea

147 A 24-year-old man presents to the primary care clinic for follow-up of his asthma. He has had asthma since he was 8 years old and requires daily treatment for his symptoms. He often has nighttime awakenings with coughing spells. On physical exam, diffuse wheezing is heard bilaterally. He is willing to try anything to improve his symptoms. The physician decides to add cromolyn to his regimen. What is the mechanism of action of cromolyn?

(A) Blocks leukotriene receptors
(B) Inhibits endothelin-1 receptors
(C) Mast cell stabilizer
(D) Muscarinic antagonist
(E) Phosphodiesterase inhibitor

148 A 34-year-old man with exercised-induced asthma is searching for a bronchodilator that will allow him to run in a marathon. The event will take him approximately 6 h and 30 min to complete. The following diagram shows five bronchodilators. Which of the following agents will provide him with the most efficacious therapy during his run?

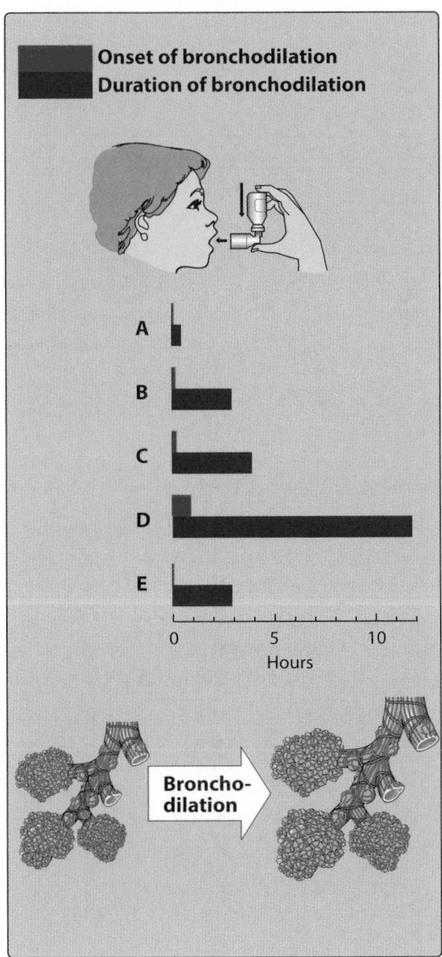

(A) Letter A
(B) Letter B
(C) Letter C
(D) Letter D
(E) Letter E

149 A 39-year-old man with a history of smoking three packs of cigarettes per day for the last 15 years is trying to stop smoking. His primary care physician gives him a choice of various modalities to stop smoking, including a nicotine patch, nicotine gum, continued smoking, or hypnotherapy. The following figure is a graph of blood concentration of nicotine in three of the treatment options mentioned. Which of the following would best represent nicotine gum?

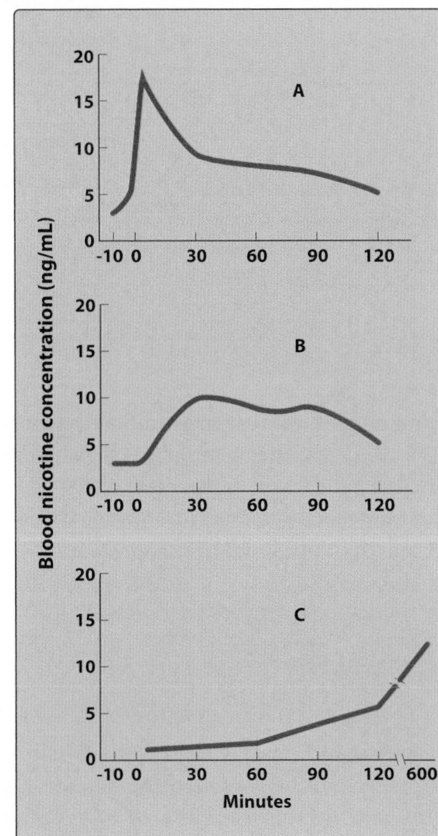

(A) Figure A
(B) Figure B
(C) Figure C
(D) Cannot be determined

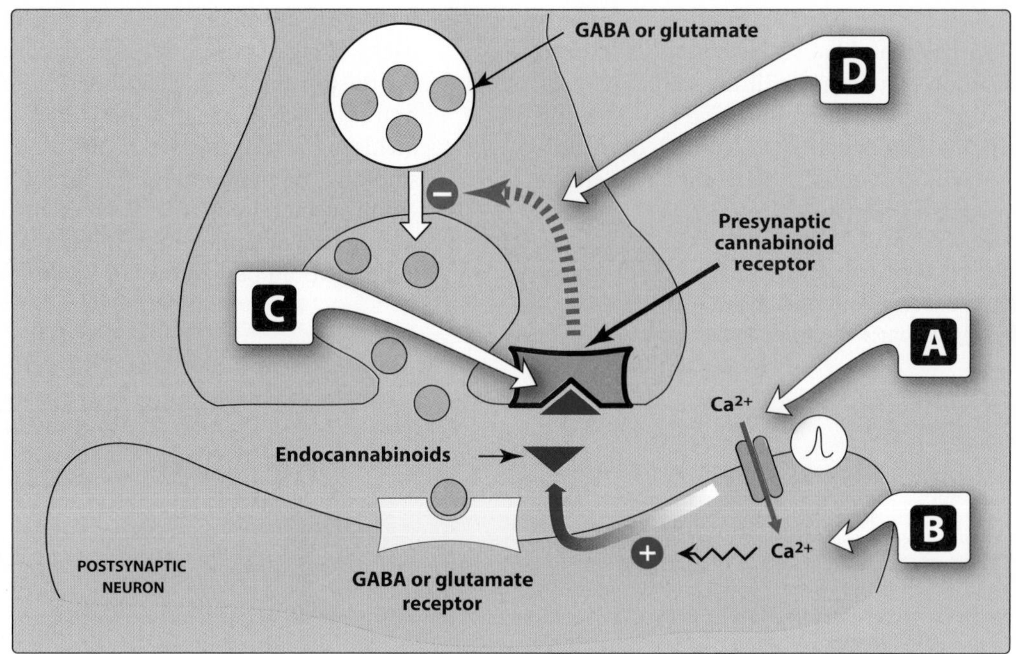

150 A diagram of the cannabinoid receptor is presented above. A researcher is considering the efficacy for intractable pain from bone metastasis. In which of the following steps is excitation of the postsynaptic receptor causing depolarization and calcium influx?

(A) Letter A
(B) Letter B
(C) Letter C
(D) Letter D

151 A 38-year-old man who is obese complains of an extremely painful, swollen metatarsophalangeal joint of his left big toe. He has had two similar attacks in the past 4 years. The physician prescribes febuxostat. Which of the following describes febuxostat's mechanism of action?

(A) Anti-inflammatory
(B) Inhibition of leukocyte migration
(C) Inhibition of urate reabsorption
(D) Inhibition of xanthine oxidase
(E) Upregulation of urate metabolism

152 A 68-year-old man with congestive heart failure presents to the emergency department with dehydration. He has been vomiting and had diarrhea for the past 36 h. He does not feel feverish or have any sick contacts. His blood pressure is 106/78 mm Hg with a pulse of 82 beats/minute. His digoxin level is 4.1 (normal 1.0 to 2.6). What other symptoms may be experienced with digoxin toxicity?

(A) Blurry yellow vision
(B) Impotence
(C) Lupus-like syndrome
(D) Prolongation of the AV refractory period
(E) Pulmonary fibrosis

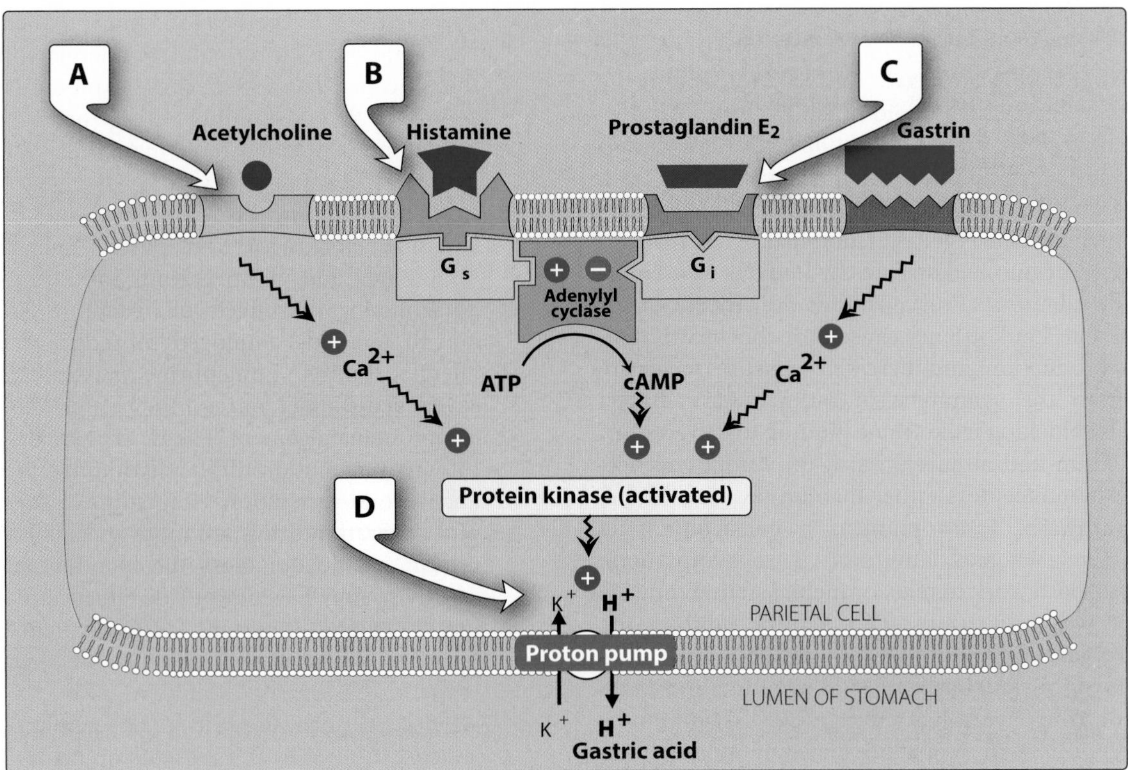

153 A 52-year-old man with a long history of gastroesophageal reflux disease and peptic ulcer disease has been taking multiple medications to control symptoms. His physician places him on misoprostol. This agent works at which of the following sites?

(A) Letter A
(B) Letter B
(C) Letter C
(D) Letter D

154 A 31-year-old woman with a sore throat, cough, and rhinitis presents to the ambulatory care clinic for evaluation. She has no known allergies, although she has never taken antibiotics. She is given a prescription for penicillin and develops a maculopapular rash on her hands and swelling of her tongue. The most likely explanation for these findings is

(A) Arachidonic acid
(B) Macrophages
(C) Penicillin
(D) Penicilloic acid
(E) Xanthine oxidase

155 A 43-year-old man with overwhelming sepsis has been receiving intravenous gentamicin for 3 months. He now complains of hearing loss. What is the most likely explanation for this finding?

(A) Destroyed hair cells in the organ of Corti
(B) Edema of the pinnae
(C) Low peak plasma levels but toxic to the ear
(D) Otitis externa
(E) Vestibular toxicity

ANSWERS

1 **The answer is D: Montelukast.** Arachidonic acid is the precursor for the eicosanoids such as prostaglandins and leukotrienes. First, phospholipase A_2 cleaves cell membrane phospholipids to release arachidonic acid. Arachidonic acid can then be converted into prostaglandins by cyclooxygenase (inhibited by aspirin and celecoxib) or into leukotrienes by lipoxygenase (inhibited by zileuton). Prostaglandins are drivers of inflammation. Leukotrienes cause bronchoconstriction, mucus production, and increased vessel permeability leading to the symptoms of asthma. Montelukast works by blocking leukotriene binding to its receptor. Ipratropium and albuterol work on autonomic nervous system receptors rather than on the arachidonic acid pathways. Ipratropium is a parasympathetic antagonist, whereas albuterol is a sympathetic agonist—both work to relax bronchial smooth muscle and decrease secretions. (A) Aspirin inhibits the cyclooxygenase enzymes COX-1 and COX-2. It does not prevent a signaling molecule from binding to its receptor. (B) Celecoxib is a selective COX-2 inhibitor. It does not prevent a signaling molecule from binding to its receptor. (C) Ipratropium is a parasympathetic antagonist. It blocks acetylcholine from binding to muscarinic receptors but does not block arachidonic acid derivatives from binding to their receptors. (E) Zileuton inhibits lipoxygenase to decrease the amount of leukotriene synthesized. It does not prevent a signaling molecule from binding its receptor.

2 **The answer is A: Cromolyn sodium.** This patient has a classic history of allergic rhinitis, commonly called hay fever. Symptoms are caused by itching and vasodilation from histamine binding to H_1 receptors. The histamine is released from mast cells as they degranulate, which is caused by antigen linking two IgE molecules attached to their cell membrane. Mast cells must be "sensitized" before they can react this way, which occurs when IgE made by plasma cells attaches to receptors on mast cell membranes. Mast cell stabilizers such as cromolyn sodium prevent the release of histamine. (B) Diphenhydramine is a first-generation antihistamine. It does not prevent the release of histamine but is an antagonist for H_1 receptors. (C) Ranitidine is an H_2-receptor blocker. H_2 receptors are found on gastric parietal cells. Stimulation causes an increase in acid secretion. H_2 receptors are not important in allergic reactions. (D) Loratadine is a second-generation antihistamine. It does not prevent the release of histamine but is an antagonist for H_1 receptors. Second-generation antihistamines have higher specificity for H_1 receptors (therefore fewer side effects) than first-generation antihistamines. (E) Theophylline is a functional antagonist: It does not block histamine receptors but elicits physiologic responses that are opposite those caused by histamine.

3 **The answer is E: Loratadine.** Itchy, watery eyes with runny nose in spring is likely allergic rhinitis, commonly called hay fever. These symptoms are caused primarily by histamine acting on H_1 receptors. Histamine is released from mast cells when they encounter the antigen to which they have been sensitized. Interrupting histamine release (i.e., cromolyn sodium), blocking H_1 receptors (diphenhydramine, loratadine, and hydroxyzine), and physiologically antagonizing the effects of histamine (epinephrine) are all methods employed to reduce symptoms of allergic rhinitis. Epinephrine may be useful for a severe acute attack but not the best choice for chronic symptom management. The H_1 antagonists are divided into first-generation (diphenhydramine, hydroxyzine) and second-generation (loratadine) drugs. The second-generation drugs are more specific for the H_1 receptor and do not cross the blood–brain barrier as readily so they have fewer side effects (such as drowsiness). This is important for the patient because he operates heavy equipment. Of the options listed, loratadine is the best choice. (A) Albuterol is a noradrenergic agonist used in the treatment of asthma attacks. It binds to β_2-receptors on smooth muscle in the airways, causing relaxation and dilation. Albuterol would not be effective in treating symptoms of allergic rhinitis. (B) Diphenhydramine would control this patient's symptoms but would likely make him drowsy and unsuited to perform his job. (C) Epinephrine would help counteract his symptoms but not as well as an H_1 antagonist. (D) Hydroxyzine would control the patient's symptoms but would likely make him drowsy and unsuited to perform his job.

4 **The answer is B: Drying effect on the oral mucous membranes.** Atropine blocks the salivary glands, producing a drying effect on the oral mucous membranes. This could be very beneficial to the oral surgeon who is removing impacted wisdom teeth. This agent is commonly infused intravenously at low doses. (A) This agent has an antispasmodic effect on the gastrointestinal tract but this is not the reason that an oral surgeon would use this medication. (C) This agent induces bradycardia at low doses as would be given to this patient. (D) The pupillary response to atropine occurs to light, not darkness. (E) The reduction of urinary tract motility is an effect of atropine but is not the reason that an oral surgeon would use this medication.

5 **The answer is A: Cyclosporine.** Cyclosporine forms a complex with protein called cyclophilin. This complex then binds the calcium-calmodulin-calcineurin complex to inhibit it from dephosphorylating NF-AT. Calcineurin is normally activated by binding calcium-calmodulin, and its role in dephosphorylating NF-AT allows NF-AT to enter the nucleus and transcribe genes necessary for T- and B-cell activation. (B) Methotrexate is a folate antimetabolite. It blocks cell proliferation by inhibiting DNA synthesis, not by modulating calcineurin. (C) Prednisolone is not known to modify calcineurin's activity. It is a glucocorticoid and inhibits many pathways necessary for inflammation and immune system function. (D) Sirolimus forms a complex with FKBP, which then inhibits mTOR. Sirolimus does not affect calcineurin activity. (E) Temsirolimus is metabolized into sirolimus. It does not affect calcineurin activity.

6 **The answer is C: Receptor stimulation on nasal vasculature.** Oxymetazoline is found in many over-the-counter short-term nasal spray decongestant products (applied every 12 h) as well as in ophthalmic drops for the relief of redness of the eyes associated with swimming, colds, and contact lenses. The mechanism of action of oxymetazoline is direct stimulation of receptors on blood vessels supplying the nasal mucosa and the conjunctiva to reduce blood flow and decrease congestion. Oxymetazoline is absorbed in the systemic circulation regardless of the route of administration and may produce nervousness, headaches, and trouble sleeping. (A) Nasal blood flow is reduced by administration of oxymetazoline. (B) Decrease in intranasal arterial pressure may occur. (D) The mechanism of this agent does not involve transmembrane conductance change. (E) The mechanism of this agent does not involve understimulation of inflamed nasal membranes.

7 **The answer is C: Pilocarpine.** These drugs neither affect the ability of the eye to focus for near vision nor change pupil size as do the cholinergic drugs. When administered in the eye, the onset is about 30 min, and the effects last for 12 to 24 h. However, in an acute attack of glaucoma, pilocarpine is still the drug of choice. The blockers are only used to treat this disease chronically. (A) Bimatoprost is a topical or systemic carbonic anhydrase inhibitor used to treat glaucoma. (B) Latanoprost is a topical or systemic carbonic anhydrase inhibitor used to treat glaucoma. (D) Tetracycline is not a treatment of glaucoma. (E) Travoprost is a topical or systemic carbonic anhydrase inhibitor used to treat glaucoma.

8 **The answer is D: Rifampin.** Drugs that interfere with, or inhibit, the metabolism of propranolol, such as cimetidine, fluoxetine, paroxetine, and ritonavir, may potentiate its antihypertensive effects. Conversely, those that stimulate or induce its metabolism, such as barbiturates, phenytoin, and rifampin, can decrease its effects. In this case, the patient is taking rifampin; and it is affecting the metabolism of propranolol and inducing rapid metabolism, which is minimizing its antihypertensive effects. (A) Cimetidine potentiates the antihypertensive effects of propranolol. (B) Fluoxetine potentiates the antihypertensive effects of propranolol. (C) Paroxetine potentiates the antihypertensive effects of propranolol. (E) Ritonavir potentiates the antihypertensive effects of propranolol.

9 **The answer is D: Salicylate uncoupling of oxidative phosphorylation.** At low therapeutic dose (antiplatelet dose), aspirin has no effect on respiratory rate. At high therapeutic dose (anti-inflammatory dose), however, salicylates uncouple oxidative phosphorylation. This uncoupling leads to an increase in CO_2 production, which causes a secondary increase in respiratory rate by stimulating chemoreceptors such as those found in the carotid bodies. Above high therapeutic dose, aspirin directly stimulates the respiratory center. (A) Salicylates are not agonists at CO_2 receptors. (B) Salicylates only stimulate the respiratory center above high therapeutic dose. (C) Salicylates can lead to a metabolic acidosis, which would shift the oxygen dissociation curve to the right, but this itself would not cause an increase in the respiration rate.

10 **The answer is D: Ketorolac.** Ketorolac is an NSAID but has poor anti-inflammatory properties. Its main use is as an analgesic and can be used in place of or in addition to opioids. It carries a high risk of toxicity and should not be used for more than 5 days in any patient. (A) Acetaminophen is used as an analgesic but is not an NSAID. (B) Celecoxib is a selective COX-2 inhibitor that is used when gastric ulceration is a concern. It is not commonly used as an adjunct to opioids. (C) Ibuprofen is an NSAID but is not commonly used postsurgically for pain management because bleeding is a complication. (E) Naproxen is an NSAID but is not commonly used postsurgically for pain management because bleeding is a complication.

11 **The answer is A: Depletion of endogenous antioxidant.** Acetaminophen metabolism follows one of two pathways in the liver. Most (more than 90%) undergoes phase II metabolism directly and is excreted via the kidney. The remainder undergoes phase I metabolism by CYP1A2 or CYP2E1 to produce NAPQI, the toxic metabolite of acetaminophen. NAPQI requires glutathione for its next step of metabolism. Excess acetaminophen in the body produces so much NAPQI that liver glutathione (a natural, endogenous antioxidant) is depleted. Oxidative damage then occurs. (B) Halothane type II hepatotoxicity involves hapten formation leading to autoantibody production. (C) Cyanide inhibits cytochrome C oxidase. This leads to blockage of the electron transport chain in the mitochondria. (D) Neither acetaminophen nor its metabolites produce appreciable ischemia. Ischemic damage in the liver is rare regardless because of its dual blood supply. (E) Neither acetaminophen nor its metabolites cause paralysis of the gall bladder.

12 **The answer is A: Iatrogenic.** Parkinsonian symptoms infrequently follow viral encephalitis or multiple small vascular lesions. Drugs such as the phenothiazines and haloperidol, whose major pharmacologic action is blockade of dopamine receptors in the brain, may also produce parkinsonian symptoms. These drugs should not be used in patients with Parkinson's disease. This patient is being given haloperidol to treat agitation, which likely caused the parkinsonian symptoms. (B) This process is not caused by an underlying infection. Parkinsonian symptoms can follow viral encephalitis. (C) There is no reason to suggest underlying malignancy in this patient. (D) Parkinsonian symptoms can follow viral encephalitis; however, in this patient, there is no reason to suggest this diagnosis.

13 **The answer is B: Overactivity of dopamine at basal ganglia receptors.** Visual and auditory hallucinations and abnormal involuntary movements (dyskinesias) may occur. These CNS effects are the opposite of parkinsonian symptoms and reflect the overactivity of dopamine at receptors in the basal ganglia. Levodopa can also cause mood changes, depression, psychosis, and anxiety. (A) There is no indication to suggest drug toxicity in this patient. (C) There is no suggestion that this patient is not taking his medications appropriately. (D) There is no indication of underlying dementia in this patient. (E) This patient does not have any upper respiratory complaints in the history.

14 **The answer is C: Etanercept.** All of the options listed are biologic TNF-α inhibitors. TNF-α is a signaling molecule that stimulates leukocyte activation, bone reabsorption, and cartilage degradation. Blocking TNF-α significantly improves symptoms of rheumatoid arthritis. Etanercept is a recombinant human IgG molecule fused to a recombinant TNF-α receptor molecule. The TNF-α receptor moiety binds up endogenous TNF-α to prevent it from stimulating its normal downstream effects. (A) Adalimumab is simply recombinant human IgG directed against TNF-α. (B) Certolizumab is the Fab fragment of humanized IgG directed against TNF-α. (D) Golimumab is a monoclonal antibody directed against TNF-α. (E) Infliximab is also a monoclonal antibody directed against TNF-α.

15 **The answer is B: Anakinra.** IL-1ra (interleukin-1 receptor antagonist) is a natural blocker of the IL-1 receptor. As an antagonist, IL-1ra blocks the effects of IL-1. In rheumatoid arthritis, these effects include bone and cartilage destruction in the joints. Anakinra is a recombinant form of IL-1ra. It must be administered daily and mimics the effects of IL-1ra, blocking IL-1 signaling. It is not very effective when used alone. (A) Abatacept is a recombinant CTLA4 fused to IgG. CTLA4 binds to B7 to prevent docking to CD28, which is the costimulatory signal needed for T-cell activation. (C) Methotrexate is a folate antimetabolite. It helps with the symptoms of rheumatoid arthritis by decreasing leukocyte proliferation. (D) Hydroxychloroquine is a weak base that acts on lysosomes by raising the pH. This impairs antigen processing and slows the immune response. (E) Rituximab is a human–mouse chimeric IgG molecule against CD20, which is necessary for B-cell activation.

16 **The answer is C: Sulfasalazine.** Aminosalicylates such as mesalamine are commonly used to treat ulcerative colitis. To be effective, mesalamine must reach the colon. One way to ensure that mesalamine reaches the colon without being absorbed is to conjugate it to another molecule with an azo bond that will only be cleaved by colonic bacterial enzymes. Sulfasalazine and olsalazine are two such formulations. Sulfasalazine is made up of a molecule of mesalamine connected to a molecule of sulfapyridine, an old sulfa antibiotic. The role of antibiotics in ulcerative colitis is unclear; however, sulfapyridine causes enough side effects that sulfasalazine is less favorable than other drugs such as olsalazine. (A) Azathioprine is an immunosuppressant. It helps with the symptoms of ulcerative colitis by decreasing the immune response. (B) Cyclosporine is an immunosuppressant. It helps with the symptoms of ulcerative colitis by decreasing the immune response. (D) Mesalamine is an anti-inflammatory drug used in ulcerative colitis. A large part of an oral dose of mesalamine is absorbed, preventing it from reaching its intended target: the colon. There are many ways to get around this problem, including suppository form, encapsulated extended-release form, and conjugation with an azo bond. (E) Olsalazine is made up of two molecules of mesalamine conjugated together by an azo bond. This bond is cleaved by colonic bacteria, releasing mesalamine on site.

17 **The answer is B: Methacholine.** Patients with airway hyperreactivity will react to lower doses of an inhaled cholinergic agent. Methacholine is commonly used to diagnose asthma in this way. It binds to muscarinic receptors on bronchiolar smooth muscle, causing bronchoconstriction. Methacholine is a synthetic choline ester that is degraded by cholinesterase more slowly than acetylcholine. (A) Albuterol is used in the treatment of asthma. It is an adrenergic β_2-agonist and causes relaxation of bronchial smooth muscle. (C) Neostigmine is an acetylcholinesterase inhibitor. It is used in the treatment of myasthenia gravis and neuromuscular blockade reversal. Neostigmine's half-life is too long to be useful in diagnosing asthma. (D) Nicotine binds to nicotinic receptors, not the muscarinic receptors found on bronchiolar smooth muscle. It would not be useful in causing bronchoconstriction.

(E) Pilocarpine is used in the treatment of glaucoma. Its half-life is too long to be useful in diagnosing asthma.

18 **The answer is D: Nausea.** Disulfiram blocks the oxidation of acetaldehyde to acetic acid by inhibiting aldehyde dehydrogenase. This results in the accumulation of acetaldehyde in the blood, causing flushing, tachycardia, hyperventilation, and nausea. Disulfiram has found some use in the patient seriously desiring to stop alcohol ingestion. A conditioned avoidance response is induced so that the patient abstains from alcohol to prevent the unpleasant effects of disulfiram-induced acetaldehyde accumulation. (A) This patient would likely exhibit tachycardia. (B) This patient would likely feel quite ill with nausea, flushing, and even vomiting. (C) This patient would likely feel quite ill from the accumulation of acetaldehyde in the blood. (E) Urticaria would be unlikely in this patient.

19 **The answer is C: Discontinue aldehyde dehydrogenase and administer naltrexone.** Naltrexone is a long-acting opiate antagonist that should be used in conjunction with supportive psychotherapy. Naltrexone is better tolerated than disulfiram and does not produce the aversive reaction that disulfiram does. It may work well in this patient who had difficulty taking aldehyde dehydrogenase. (A) It would not be prudent to continue aldehyde dehydrogenase in this patient. (B) Administration of aldehyde dehydrogenase with a beer does not treat the alcohol abuse in this patient. (D) Alprazolam is not a good choice because this patient does not exhibit anxiety features. (E) Intensive psychotherapy may be considered in addition to naltrexone in this patient.

20 **The answer is B: Deferoxamine.** Chelating agents are (usually) organic compounds that can form multiple coordinate bonds with metal ions by wrapping around them. Chelating the ions prevents toxicity because a chelated ion is inactive chemically and metabolically. Of the agents listed, deferoxamine is commonly used for iron chelation. (A) Ethylenediaminetetraacetic acid is more commonly used for chelation of mercury and lead ions. (C) Dimercaprol is used for chelation of arsenic, mercury, gold, and lead ions. (D) Penicillamine is used for chelation of copper, arsenic, and gold ions. (E) Succimer is used for chelation of lead ions.

21 **The answer is D: Diphenhydramine.** Some antihistamines with sedating properties, such as diphenhydramine, are effective in treating mild types of insomnia. However, this agent has numerous undesirable side effects (such as anticholinergic effects) that it is less useful than the benzodiazepines. Some sedative antihistamines are marketed in numerous over-the-counter products. Diphenhydramine is a classic example. (A) Doxycycline is a prescription antibiotic. (B) Doxylamine is a prescription antihistamine. (C) Doxazosin is a prescription α-blocker. (E) Hydroxyzine is a prescription antihistamine.

22 **The answer is A: Blockade of adenosine receptors.** Several mechanisms have been proposed for the actions of methylxanthines, including translocation of extracellular calcium, increase in cyclic adenosine monophosphate and cyclic guanosine monophosphate caused by inhibition of phosphodiesterase, and blockade of adenosine receptors. The latter most likely accounts for the actions achieved by the usual consumption of caffeine-containing beverages. (B) There is an increase in cyclic adenosine monophosphate. (C) There is an increase in cyclic guanosine monophosphate. (D) There is an inhibition of phosphodiesterase. (E) There is translocation of intracellular calcium.

23 **The answer is B: Furosemide.** Ototoxicity, which often presents as tinnitus, is a known side effect of loop diuretics such as furosemide. This is especially true when given with other ototoxic drugs (such as aminoglycoside antibiotics), in patients with renal disease, when given in high doses, or with rapid intravenous administration. (A) Acetazolamide is a carbonic anhydrase inhibitor. It is not known to be ototoxic. (C) Hydrochlorothiazide inhibits sodium reabsorption in the distal tubule. It is not known to be ototoxic. (D) Mannitol is an osmotic diuretic. It is filtered in the glomerulus but very little is reabsorbed, so it provides osmotic gradient to retain water in the tubules. It is not known to be ototoxic. (E) Spironolactone is a competitive antagonist of aldosterone, which normally causes sodium reabsorption in the distal tubule.

24 **The answer is D: Slurred speech.** Ketamine causes dissociative anesthesia (insensitivity to pain without loss of consciousness) and analgesia. In this state, it produces numbness of extremities, staggered gait, slurred speech, and muscular rigidity. Sometimes, hostile and bizarre behavior is seen. At increased dosages, anesthesia, stupor, and coma may result but, strangely, the eyes may remain open. (A) This patient would be expected to have insensitivity to pain without loss of consciousness. (B) This patient would not have loss of consciousness. (C) This patient will exhibit staggered gait. (E) This patient may exhibit hostile and bizarre behavior.

25 **The answer is C: Inhibits conversion of lanosterol to ergosterol.** Sporotrichosis is caused by the dimorphic fungi *Sporothrix schenckii*. *Sporothrix* and other

fungi stabilize their cell membranes with ergosterol (which is not found in humans) in the same way that mammalian cell membranes are stabilized with cholesterol. Many antifungals target ergosterol synthesis or ergosterol itself. The -azole antifungals such as itraconazole inhibit a fungal cytochrome P450 enzyme responsible for the last step in ergosterol synthesis: conversion of lanosterol to ergosterol. (A) Nystatin and amphotericin B are examples of antifungals that disrupt the fungal cell membrane by binding ergosterol and causing pore formation. Itraconazole does not lead to membrane pore formation. (B) Griseofulvin is an antifungal that disrupts fungal cell microtubules. It is particularly useful in skin and nail infections because it is concentrated in keratin. Itraconazole does not disrupt microtubules. (D) Terbinafine is an antifungal that works by inhibition of squalene monooxygenase. This enzyme normally produces lanosterol, which is then converted to ergosterol. Itraconazole does not inhibit squalene monooxygenase. (E) Flucytosine is an antifungal that is converted to 5-fluorouracil (an antimetabolite) in fungal cells. This conversion does not occur in human cells. Itraconazole does not undergo this conversion.

26 **The answer is B: Hepatic necrosis.** This patient is at risk for hepatic necrosis. There are toxic reactions that some patients (especially females) develop after halothane anesthesia. This reaction begins as a fever, followed by anorexia, nausea, and vomiting; and patients may exhibit signs of hepatitis. Although the incidence of this reaction is low (approximately 1 in 10,000 individuals) 50% of affected patients may die of hepatic necrosis. To avoid this condition, halothane anesthesia is not repeated at intervals of less than 2 to 3 weeks. (A) This patient is not at increased risk of cholelithiasis. (C) This patient is not at increased risk of nephrolithiasis. (D) This patient is not at risk for steatorrhea. (E) This patient is not at risk for tinnitus.

27 **The answer is B: Excitation–contraction coupling defect.** In susceptible individuals for malignant hyperthermia (MH), these drugs can induce a drastic and uncontrolled increase in skeletal muscle oxidative metabolism, which overwhelms the body's capacity to supply oxygen, remove carbon dioxide, and regulate body temperature eventually leading to circulatory collapse and death if not treated immediately. Recent investigations have identified a dramatic increase in the myoplasmic calcium ion concentration. Strong evidence indicates that MH is caused by an excitation–contraction coupling defect. Ligand-gated membrane channel is modulated by inhaled anesthetics. (A) Malignant hyperthermia is not a drug toxicity event. (C) Myoplasmic calcium ion concentration defect is the culprit. (D) Malignant hyperthermia is not caused by an oxygen–hemoglobin concentration deficit. (E) Malignant hyperthermia is not caused by neural overmodulation.

28 **The answer is C: Physiologic metabolism.** The short duration of anesthetic action is caused by the decrease of barbiturate concentration in the brain to a level below that is necessary to produce anesthesia. These drugs may remain in the body for relatively long periods of time after their administration, because only about 15% of the dose of barbiturates entering the circulation is metabolized by the liver per hour. Thus, metabolism of thiopental is much slower than its tissue redistribution. (A) This patient has no evidence of hepatitis. (B) This patient has no evidence of hepatic failure. (D) This patient has no evidence of renal failure. (E) This patient has no evidence of bowel ischemia.

29 **The answer is B: Improved intestinal circular muscle tone.** Morphine relieves diarrhea and dysentery by decreasing the motility and increasing the tone of the intestinal circular smooth muscle. Morphine also increases the tone of the anal sphincter. Overall, morphine and other narcotics produce constipation, with little tolerance developing. A nonprescription laxative combination of the stool softener docusate with the stimulant laxative senna has been used successfully to treat this opioid-induced constipation. (A) Gastrointestinal motility will decrease. (C) Anal sphincter tone will increase. (D) Rectal balloon dilation pressure will increase. (E) Transverse colonic musculature tone will increase.

30 **The answer is B: Constipation.** Repeated use produces tolerance to the respiratory depressant, analgesic, euphoric, and sedative effects of morphine. However, tolerance usually does not develop to the pupil-constricting and constipating effects of the drug. Physical and psychological dependence readily occur with morphine and with some of the other agonists. (A) Tolerance develops to the analgesic effects of morphine. (C) Tolerance develops to the euphoric effects of morphine. (D) Tolerance develops to the pupil-constricting effects of morphine. (E) Tolerance develops to the sedative effects of morphine.

31 **The answer is B: Phenytoin.** Ethanol undergoes zero-order elimination, meaning the same amount is eliminated per unit time regardless of its concentration in the blood. Most drugs undergo first-order elimination in which proportionately higher amounts of drug are eliminated when their blood concentration is higher. The duration of first-order type drugs is therefore explained by their half-life or the time it takes for half of the drug to be eliminated. A drug undergoing zero-order elimination cannot be

described in terms of half-lives, because its duration of action depends only on the absolute amount of drug in the body (twice as much drug will last twice as long). All drugs would likely undergo zero-order metabolism at high enough concentrations because their eliminating enzymes would be saturated. However, only a few drugs saturate their respective metabolic enzymes at therapeutic concentrations. These include phenytoin, ethanol, and aspirin. (A) Ibuprofen undergoes first-order elimination. Its half-life is between 2 and 4 h. (C) Simvastatin undergoes first-order elimination. Its half-life is approximately 2 h. (D) Tolbutamide undergoes first-order elimination. Its half-life is between 4.5 and 6.5 h. (E) Valproic acid undergoes first-order elimination. Its half-life is between 6 and 16 h.

32 **The answer is C: Dantrolene.** This scenario describes a case of malignant hyperthermia. Malignant hyperthermia can be caused by any one of several genetic defects, most of which are autosomal dominant. Most cases involve a mutated ryanodine receptor and are triggered by anesthetic or succinylcholine use during surgery. The signs and symptoms appear to arise from a sudden increase in cellular metabolism. Dantrolene is the drug used to treat malignant hyperthermia. It is believed to inhibit calcium release from the sarcoplasmic reticulum. By paralyzing the muscle in this way, muscle cell metabolism is drastically decreased. (A) Acetaminophen has antipyretic and analgesic effects. It can be used for mild pain and fevers but is not useful in malignant hyperthermia. (B) Bromocriptine is a dopamine agonist that can be used to treat neuroleptic malignant syndrome. Neuroleptic malignant syndrome in some ways resembles malignant hyperthermia, but their pathophysiologies are very different. Bromocriptine is not useful for treating malignant hyperthermia. (D) Diazepam is a benzodiazepine that can be used to treat serotonin syndrome. Serotonin syndrome in some ways resembles malignant hyperthermia, but their pathophysiologies are very different. Diazepam is not useful for treating malignant hyperthermia. (E) Naproxen is a nonsteroidal anti-inflammatory drug (NSAID). It can be used to decrease pain, inflammation, and fever, but these are not hallmarks of malignant hyperthermia.

33 **The answer is B: Blocking serotonin-mediated nociceptive signaling.** This clinical scenario describes a woman having migraine headaches. Because migraine pathophysiology is not completely understood, the mechanisms of medications used to treat them are also not completely understood. It is known, however, that sumatriptan stimulates serotonin receptors, which leads to inhibition of inflammation and vasodilation; and it inhibits serotonin stimulation of receptors on nociceptive neurons. (A) The cyclooxygenase (COX-1 and COX-2) enzymes are responsible for production of proinflammatory prostaglandins. The nonsteroidal anti-inflammatory drugs (NSAIDs) and acetaminophen block COX activity. (C) Acetaminophen only works on central COX enzymes, so it has analgesic and antipyretic effects but is not an anti-inflammatory drug. (D) The opioids bind to μ- and κ-receptors. Stimulation of either receptor results in analgesia, respiratory depression, and miosis. (E) Stimulation of μ-receptors additionally results in euphoria, whereas stimulation of κ-receptors results in dysphoria.

34 **The answer is E: QT interval prolongation.** Caution should be exerted when combining several drugs with effects on the QT interval (e.g., quinidine with levofloxacin) or when giving these drugs combined with -azole antifungals (fluconazole and itraconazole). The latter are known to inhibit drug metabolism, leading to large increases in plasma drug concentrations. (A) Asystole is unlikely in this patient. (B) The QT prolongation is more common than myocardial infarction in this setting. (C) Pulmonary edema is unlikely in this patient. (D) Pulmonary embolism would not be expected in this patient.

35 **The answer is D: Lupus-like syndrome.** With chronic use, procainamide causes a high incidence of side effects, including a reversible lupus erythematosus–like syndrome that develops in 25% to 30% of patients. Toxic concentrations of procainamide may cause asystole or induction of ventricular arrhythmias. Central nervous system (CNS) side effects include depression, hallucination, and psychosis. (A) This patient has no evidence to suggest contact dermatitis from an exposure. (B) The history of this patient does not describe excessive sun exposure. (C) This patient does not have discoid lupus erythematosus. (E) This patient does not likely have a collagen vascular disease.

36 **The answer is A: Alcohol.** Metronidazole is one of the few drugs with disulfiram-like side effects. Disulfiram inhibits acetaldehyde dehydrogenase, which is the enzyme needed to break down acetaldehyde produced in ethanol metabolism. High levels of acetaldehyde lead to nausea, vomiting, and headache. Patients taking metronidazole should be advised to avoid alcohol because of this side effect. (B) Metronidazole and aspirin are not known to interact. It should be fine for her to take aspirin while on metronidazole. (C) Metronidazole and caffeine are not known to interact. It should be fine for her to consume caffeine while taking metronidazole. (D) Grapefruit juice is known to inhibit some cytochrome P450 enzymes and can alter the metabolism of many drugs. However, grapefruit juice is not known to interfere with the metabolism of metronidazole. (E) Patients taking seda-

tives, such as benzodiazepines, or medications that cause drowsiness, such as diphenhydramine, should avoid operating heavy machinery. Metronidazole is not known to cause drowsiness or sedation.

37 **The answer is A: Clozapine.** This patient's sudden onset of high fever in the absence of sick contacts is attributable to her extremely low neutrophil count. Agranulocytosis is a known side effect of clozapine therapy, and patients taking clozapine should be monitored frequently to make sure their white blood cell count does not drop too low. With a neutrophil count this low, opportunistic infections leading to sepsis will rapidly take a person's life. Clozapine should be stopped as soon as signs or symptoms of agranulocytosis appear. Once the medication is discontinued, the white blood cell count will generally recover in 1 to 4 weeks. (B) Olanzapine has been associated with agranulocytosis but not to the same extent that clozapine has. A well-known side effect of olanzapine therapy is weight gain. (C) Quetiapine has also been shown to cause agranulocytosis, but the likelihood of developing agranulocytosis is much lower with quetiapine than with clozapine. (D) Risperidone has also been associated with agranulocytosis but not to the same extent as clozapine. (E) Haloperidol has also been associated with agranulocytosis but not to the same degree as clozapine. Extrapyramidal symptoms are more common side effects of haloperidol.

38 **The answer is A: Mesna.** Hemorrhagic cystitis is a potentially severe side effect of cyclophosphamide and ifosfamide. These drugs can also cause other bladder pathology including hematuria and fibrosis. The damage to the bladder is attributed to a toxic metabolite called acrolein. Mesna binds to acrolein in the urine, rendering it inactive. It also prevents the formation of more acrolein from other cyclophosphamide and ifosfamide metabolites. (B) Methylene blue is a reducing agent that can be used to treat methemoglobinemia. It is not useful in the treatment of cyclophosphamide-induced hemorrhagic cystitis. (C) The *N*-acetylcysteine is used to regenerate glutathione in the liver following toxic exposure to acetaminophen. It is also used in patients with cystic fibrosis to break up the thick mucus of the airway. It is not useful in the treatment of cyclophosphamide-induced hemorrhagic cystitis. (D) Ibuprofen is a nonsteroidal anti-inflammatory drug (NSAID) used to treat pain and inflammation. It is not useful in treating the underlying cause of cyclophosphamide-induced hemorrhagic cystitis. (E) Succimer is used in children to chelate lead ions in cases of lead exposure. It is not useful in the treatment of cyclophosphamide-induced hemorrhagic cystitis.

39 **The answer is B: Decreased gastric acid secretion.** Atropine is an antimuscarinic anticholinergic agent. Muscarinic receptors are found on the pupillary constrictor muscle, on gastrointestinal cells, on the sinoatrial (SA) node of the heart, and on many exocrine glands. The parasympathetic nervous system stimulates these receptors by releasing acetylcholine. (A) Tachycardia would be expected. (C) Decreased bronchial secretions occur. (D) Decreased salivation occurs. (E) Mydriasis occurs.

40 **The answer is C: Latanoprost.** Glaucoma is caused by an increase in intraocular pressure. There are many drugs used to lower intraocular pressure that work by decreasing aqueous humor synthesis, decreasing aqueous humor secretion, or increasing the outflow of aqueous humor. Prostaglandins such as latanoprost increase the outflow of aqueous humor—the only class of drugs used to treat glaucoma that can cause increased iris pigmentation. Long-term prostaglandin use in the eye can also cause eyelash lengthening. (A) Acetazolamide is a carbonic anhydrase inhibitor. In addition to treating glaucoma, it is also used as a diuretic. It is not known to cause iris darkening. (B) Epinephrine is an α-adrenergic agonist. Epinephrine should not be used in close-angle glaucoma. It decreases aqueous humor synthesis in open-angle glaucoma by causing vasoconstriction. It is not known to cause iris darkening. (D) Pilocarpine is a cholinomimetic. It increases outflow of aqueous humor by contracting the ciliary muscle to open the trabecular meshwork. It is not known to cause iris darkening. (E) Timolol is a β-adrenergic antagonist. It decreases aqueous humor secretion. It is not known to cause iris darkening.

41 **The answer is A: Butorphanol.** A major concern with opioids during birthing is respiratory depression of the newborn. All opioids cause respiratory depression to some degree; but of the options listed, butorphanol causes the least. Butorphanol is only a partial agonist μ-receptor, and it is the activation of the μ-receptors that is responsible for respiratory depression. Butorphanol would be the best opioid to administer in this case because it will relieve her pain without causing too much respiratory depression in the neonate. (B) Codeine is metabolized in the liver to morphine, which is a complete μ-receptor agonist. Both would treat her pain but likely cause dangerous respiratory depression in the neonate. (C) Dextromethorphan is used for its antitussive properties. It has not been shown to be very efficacious in pain management, and it also causes respiratory depression. (D) Methadone can be used in pain management but is also commonly used to treat opioid dependence and withdrawal. Like most opioids, it causes significant respiratory depression. (E) Codeine is metabolized in the liver to morphine, which is a complete μ-receptor agonist that can cause respiratory depression in the neonate.

42 **The answer is D: Oxidation of iron in hemoglobin.** Cyanide has a much higher affinity for Fe^{3+} than Fe^{2+}. Sodium nitrite oxidizes some of the iron in hemoglobin to Fe^{3+} (methemoglobin), which then acts as a sink for the cyanide to prevent the cyanide-disrupting metabolism in other body tissues. Of course, too much nitrite will cause excessive oxidation of hemoglobin and will do more harm than good, but this is true of any medication. After the nitrite is administered, sodium thiosulfate is given to convert the cyanide-methemoglobin complex back into hemoglobin and thiocyanate, which is excreted in the urine. (A) The urine's pH is changed to trap toxic ions in the urine for more rapid excretion. Examples include acidifying urine to hasten amphetamine excretion and alkalinizing urine to hasten salicylate excretion. (B) Chelators are used to bind up metal ions, such as succimer for lead toxicity or dimercaprol for mercury toxicity. Nitrites do not chelate cyanide. (C) Nitrites do not chemically react directly with cyanide. Nitrites oxidize the iron in heme to raise the iron's affinity for cyanide. (E) Pralidoxime use following organophosphate poisoning is an example of enzyme regeneration. Nitrites do not serve to regenerate any enzyme.

43 **The answer is B: Grapefruit juice.** Lovastatin (and other statin drugs) is known to cause myopathies including rhabdomyolysis, especially at high plasma concentrations. Assuming this patient was indeed taking his lovastatin as directed, his muscle pain could be caused by a cytochrome P450 3A4 (CYP3A4) inhibitor, causing a high plasma concentration of lovastatin. Common CYP3A4 inhibitors include protease inhibitors (-navirs), isoniazid, cimetidine, ketoconazole, erythromycin, grapefruit juice, and sulfonamides. (A) Barbiturates are inducers of CYP3A4. These drugs increase the liver's ability to metabolize lovastatin, leading to subtherapeutic levels of lovastatin. This would manifest as persistent hypercholesterolemia, not as a myopathy. (C) Griseofulvin is also an inducer of CYP3A4. (D) Phenytoin is also an inducer of CYP3A4. (E) St. John's wort supplement is an inducer of CYP3A4.

44 **The answer is B: Dopamine.** Dopamine release will unlikely stimulate platelet aggregation and will lead to continuous bleeding. Receptors on the surface of the adhering platelets are activated by the collagen of the underlying connective tissue. This causes morphologic changes in platelets and the release of platelet granules containing chemical mediators, such as adenosine diphosphate (ADP), thromboxane A_2, serotonin, platelet-activation factor, and thrombin. (A) Adenosine diphosphate will stimulate platelet aggregation. (C) Serotonin will stimulate platelet aggregation. (D) Thrombin will stimulate platelet aggregation. (E) Thromboxane A_2 will stimulate platelet aggregation.

45 **The answer is A: Heparin.** Heparin is the anticoagulant of choice for treating pregnant women with prosthetic heart valves or venous thromboembolism because this agent does not cross the placenta. Heparin has a rapid onset of action. (B) Streptokinase would not be a preferred agent and can cross the placenta. (C) TED stockings may be helpful, but heparin is the preferred pharmacologic agent. (D) Warfarin sodium can cross the placenta and should not be given in pregnancy.

46 **The answer is E: Success at clot resolution.** Alteplase is known as tissue plasminogen activator. It is superior to streptokinase at clot dissolution. It can improve clinical outcome when administered early in the suspicion of massive pulmonary embolism. (A) Streptokinase acts on free plasminogen. (B) Alteplase has low antigenicity. (C) Alteplase has high fibrin specificity. (D) Alteplase has a short half-life of about 5 min.

47 **The answer is C: Phenytoin.** This patient's chief complaint is gingival hyperplasia. Although many drugs can cause gingival hyperplasia, it is most often associated with phenytoin. The mechanism behind the gingival overgrowth is unclear. A contributing factor appears to be poor oral hygiene. Gingival hyperplasia is also more likely to occur during long-term use. This is reversible if phenytoin is withdrawn. (A) Estrogens are not known to cause gingival hyperplasia, but the absence of estrogen (e.g., following ovariectomy) appears to contribute to gingival hyperplasia. (B) Lamotrigine is not known to cause gingival hyperplasia. Lamotrigine is known for causing a rash and may rarely lead to Stevens–Johnson syndrome. (D) Progesterones are not known to cause gingival hyperplasia but, as with estrogens, sudden drops (e.g., postpartum) may contribute to gingival hyperplasia. (E) Valproic acid is not known to cause gingival hyperplasia. More common side effects of valproic acid are changes in appetite and gastrointestinal disturbances.

48 **The answer is C: Fomepizole.** Ethylene glycol is metabolized to oxalic acid (among other molecules) by the enzyme alcohol dehydrogenase, the same enzyme responsible for converting ethanol into acetaldehyde and methanol into formaldehyde. Acetaldehyde, formaldehyde, and oxalic acid are all toxic. Because ethanol is less toxic than methanol or acetaldehyde, it can be used to inhibit their metabolism by competing with them for the active site on alcohol dehydrogenase. However, an even better option is, usually, fomepizole, which inhibits the enzyme altogether to prevent the formation of toxic metabolites. (A) Bicarbonate would have no significant effect on the metabolism of ethylene glycol. It is used to

alkalinize the urine to ion trap weak acids (such as salicylates) for secretion. (B) Disulfiram inhibits the second enzyme in alcohol metabolism—aldehyde dehydrogenase. It can be used to dissuade alcoholics from drinking because with it, ethanol will be metabolized to acetaldehyde and no further. A buildup of acetaldehyde produces severe nausea and headaches. (D) Furosemide is a loop diuretic. It would have no significant effect on ethylene glycol metabolism and would not be helpful in this patient. (E) Methanol, like ethanol, would compete with ethylene glycol for metabolism to decrease the toxic metabolites of ethylene glycol. However, the metabolites of methanol are even more toxic than those of ethylene glycol. There is no medical use for methanol.

49 **The answer is B: Hearing loss.** Hearing can be affected adversely by the loop diuretics, particularly when used in conjunction with the aminoglycoside antibiotics. Permanent damage may result with continued treatment. Ethacrynic acid is most likely to cause deafness. Vestibular function is less likely to be disturbed, but it, too, may be affected by combined treatment with the antibiotic. (A) Vestibular function is preserved in this patient. Thus, dizziness is unlikely. (C) Nausea often goes along with vestibular dysfunction which is unlikely in this patient. (D) Vertigo is unlikely in this patient as vestibular function is likely to be intact. (E) Vomiting is unlikely in this patient.

50 **The answer is C: Inhibition of urate reabsorption.** Probenecid works on the renal tubules by interfering with organic acid secretion and reabsorption. Its exact mechanism is not known, but probenecid inhibits urate reabsorption to lower blood urate levels. It also inhibits renal excretion of many penicillins and cephalosporins, so probenecid can be used to prolong their half-life. (A) NSAIDs are common anti-inflammatory drugs used for acute gout attacks. They can help with the pain and inflammation associated with an attack but will not increase urate excretion. (B) Colchicine is a drug used in gout to inhibit leukocyte migration. Specifically, colchicine interferes with microtubules. It has no effect on urate excretion. (D) Allopurinol is an example of a drug that inhibits xanthine oxidase. Xanthine oxidase converts xanthine into urate, so inhibition decreases urate production. (E) Humans lack a uricase enzyme, which can be found in other animals allowing them to break down urate. There is to pathway for urate metabolism in humans.

51 **The answer is B: Bronchodilator.** Cromolyn is an effective prophylactic anti-inflammatory agent. However, it is not useful in managing an acute asthma attack because it is not a direct bronchodilator. This agent can block the initiation of immediate and delayed asthmatic reactions. For use in asthma, cromolyn is available as a nebulized solution. (A) Cromolyn is an anti-inflammatory agent. (C) Cromolyn possesses the ability to modulate the immune system. (D) Cromolyn possesses the ability to stabilize mast cells. (E) Cromolyn can inhibit neutrophil function as part of its anti-inflammatory properties.

52 **The answer is D: Change to ipratropium.** Anticholinergic agents are generally less effective than β_2-adrenergic agonists. The anticholinergic agents block the vagally mediated contraction of airway smooth muscle and mucus secretion. Inhaled ipratropium, a quaternary derivative of atropine, is useful in patients who are unable to tolerate adrenergic agonists. Ipratropium is slow in onset and nearly free of side effects. (A) The β_2-agonist is causing side effects so it should be discontinued. (B) Changing the frequency of administration of the β_2 agonist may not only decrease the side effect but also decrease the efficacy of this therapy. (C) This patient has difficulty with once daily therapy, thus doubling the dose will increase the likelihood of side effects. (E) Ipratropium is a better selection than epinephrine for this patient.

53 **The answer is B: Cardiac arrhythmia.** Previously the mainstay of asthma therapy, theophylline has been largely replaced with β_2-agonists and corticosteroids because of a narrow therapeutic window, its high side effect profile, and potential for drug interactions. The FDA no longer recommends this drug for acute bronchospasm or status asthmaticus. Overdose may cause seizures or potentially fatal arrhythmias. (A) The most likely cause of death from theophylline overdose is fatal cardiac arrhythmia, not apnea. (C) This agent is not associated with an increase in thromboembolism formation. (D) Although seizures can occur with theophylline therapy, the most common cause of death from overdose is fatal cardiac arrhythmia. (E) Tetany would not be expected with overdose of theophylline.

54 **The answer is A: Continue medication at current dose.** In general, anticholinergic side effects of the first-generation antihistamines, such as diphenhydramine (dry eyes/mouth, difficulty urinating and/or defecating) are transient and may resolve in 7 to 10 days. Constipation associated with chronic use of the first-generation antihistamines is not transient and may require treatment with a stool softener, especially in more susceptible patients. (B) This side effect will likely improve in 7 to 10 days. (C) It is not wise to begin therapy with a second anticholinergic agent in a patient who is already having difficulty with one agent. (D) This patient does not need a surgical procedure at this time. His medical therapy is working well except for this side effect that will likely abate with time. (E) There is no indication to perform a septoplasty in this patient.

55 **The answer is A: Addiction.** Codeine is the gold standard treatment for cough suppression because of its long history of availability and use. Codeine decreases the sensitivity of cough centers in the central nervous system to peripheral stimuli and decreases mucosal secretion. These therapeutic effects occur at doses lower than those required for analgesia but still incur common side effects, such as constipation, dysphoria, and fatigue as well as having addictive potential. (B) Constipation is a typical side effect of codeine therapy. (C) Dysphoria is a typical side effect of codeine therapy. (D) Fatigue is a common side effect of increasing doses of codeine therapy. (E) Sweating is not a side effect of codeine therapy.

56 **The answer is D: Ion channel.** Benzodiazepines (and alcohol) stimulate GABA receptors, which have an inhibitory effect on neurons. GABA receptors are chloride ion channels. When stimulated, they allow an influx of chloride ions that hyperpolarizes the cell. These channels are downregulated in chronic alcoholics such that normal brain function requires alcohol to sufficiently stimulate the remaining GABA receptors to maintain proper inhibition of excess activity. Absence of GABA inhibition leads to the symptoms of delirium tremens exhibited in this patient. (A) G_i receptors are a type of G protein–coupled receptor (GPCR). Stimulation of G_i receptors causes a decrease of cAMP inside the cell, which leads to many downstream effects. α_2-Adrenergic receptors are an example of G_i receptors. (B) G_s receptors are a type of GPCR. Stimulation of G_s receptors causes an increase of cAMP inside the cell which leads to many downstream effects. The β_1- and β_2-adrenergic receptors are examples of G_s receptors. (C) G_q receptors are a type of GPCR. Stimulation of G_q receptors causes an increase of calcium and diacylglycerol inside the cell, which lead to many downstream effects. α_1-Adrenergic receptors are an example of G_q receptors. (E) Transcription factors are molecules that, once activated, bind DNA sequences to influence transcription of genes. Many transcription factors are hormone receptors, such as the glucocorticoid receptor and the thyroid hormone receptor. Benzodiazepines do not act on any transcription factors.

57 **The answer is B: Penicilloic acid.** The major antigenic determinant of penicillin hypersensitivity is its metabolite penicilloic acid, which reacts with proteins and serves as a hapten to cause an immune reaction. Approximately 5% of patients have some kind of reaction, ranging from maculopapular rash (the most common rash seen with ampicillin hypersensitivity) to angioedema (marked swelling of the lips, tongue, and periorbital area) and anaphylaxis. Among patients with mononucleosis who are treated with ampicillin, the incidence of maculopapular rash approaches 100%. (A) DNA gyrase is inhibited by the quinolone class of antibiotics. (C) RNA synthase is not the hapten that causes an immune reaction in this case of hypersensitivity. (D) Telomerase is an enzyme that breaks down the ends of chromosomes. (E) Transferase can be either DNA related or RNA related and is not a mechanism of action of penicillin hypersensitivity.

58 **The answer is E: Slow the infusion rate over 2 h.** Side effects are a serious problem with vancomycin and include fever, chills, and/or phlebitis at the infusion site. Flushing ("red man syndrome") and shock result from histamine release associated with a rapid infusion. If an infusion-related reaction occurs, slow the infusion rate to administer vancomycin over 2 h, increase the dilution volume, and/or pretreat with an antihistamine 1 h prior to administration. In addition, reactions can be treated with antihistamines and steroids. (A) An anticholinesterase inhibitor should not be given. This patient needs to have increased fluids given and slowing of the infusion rate of vancomycin. (B) Corticosteroids are of benefit in allergic reactions; this is more of a rapid infusion reaction than an allergic reaction. (C) Intubation is not necessary in this case. (D) Vancomycin does not need to be discontinued. The infusion rate needs to be slowed down.

59 **The answer is A: Binding to tissues with calcium content.** The tetracyclines concentrate in the liver, kidney, spleen, and skin; and they bind to tissues undergoing calcification (e.g., teeth and bones) or to tumors that have a high calcium content (e.g., gastric carcinoma). Deposition in the bone and primary dentition occurs during calcification in growing children. This causes discoloration and hypoplasia of the teeth and a temporary stunting of growth. (B) The binding of antibiotic to calcified tissue is not a drug toxicity effect. (C) Tetracyclines do not inhibit folate synthesis. (D) Tetracyclines do not impair hepatic transaminases. (E) Tetracyclines do not inhibit osteoclast activity.

60 **The answer is A: Cholestatic jaundice.** Cholestatic jaundice is a possible side effect. This side effect occurs especially with the estolate form of erythromycin, presumably as the result of a hypersensitivity reaction to the estolate form (the lauryl salt of the propionyl ester of erythromycin). It has also been reported for other forms of the drug. (B) Mild abdominal discomfort is possible with erythromycin but is usually self-limiting. (C) Nausea is another mild side effect of erythromycin and is also self-limiting. (D) Tinnitus and ototoxicity is possible with supratherapeutic doses of erythromycin. (E) Vomiting is usually self-limiting with erythromycin.

61 **The answer is A: Bicarbonate.** Amitriptyline is a tricyclic antidepressant (TCA). A major consequence of TCA overdose is metabolic acidosis. Bicarbonate can

be given to counteract this acidosis as well as protect against TCA-induced arrhythmias. Gastric lavage and administration of activated charcoal may also be useful in TCA toxicity. (B) Dimercaprol is a chelating agent used to remove toxic metal ions from the body. It is used in cases of gold, mercury, and arsenic toxicity. (C) Methylene blue is an antioxidant. It is used to reverse the oxidation of iron in cases of methemoglobinemia. (D) Naloxone is an opioid-receptor antagonist. It can be used to reverse opioid overdose by competing with and blocking receptors. (E) Vitamin K is important in the γ-carboxylation of clotting factors II, VII, IX, and X as well as proteins C and S. Warfarin blocks vitamin K recycling, thereby slowing production of these factors. Vitamin K may be given to reverse warfarin toxicity.

62 **The answer is B: Megaloblastic anemia.** Trimethoprim can have hematologic side effects. Megaloblastic anemia, leukopenia, and thrombocytopenia may occur. All these effects may be reversed by the concurrent administration of folinic acid, which protects the patient and does not enter the microorganism. Hemolytic anemia may occur in patients with glucose 6-phosphate dehydrogenase deficiency caused by the sulfamethoxazole. (A) Aplastic anemia is not a common side effect of trimethoprim therapy. (C) Microcytic anemia is associated with chronic blood loss and iron deficiency states. (D) This patient is likely to have megaloblastic anemia caused by folate deficiency. (E) Pernicious anemia is often associated with deficiency of vitamin B_{12}.

63 **The answer is C: Cross-tolerance.** This patient has developed a tolerance to barbiturates that has also led to anesthetic tolerance. This phenomenon is called cross-tolerance. Cross-tolerance occurs when a patient who has developed tolerance to one drug or drug class (such as the barbiturates in this case) exhibits tolerance to another drug or drug class (such as the anesthetics in this case) that both have similar properties. (A) Addiction refers to a psychological craving for a substance. Physiologic dependence may or may not be present. Addiction to one substance does not necessarily lead to tolerance in another. (B) Cross-dependence refers to a situation in which withdrawal symptoms caused by dependence on one substance are prevented by administration of another related substance. An example is the use of methadone to prevent withdrawal symptoms following cessation of heroin. (D) This scenario does not describe simple dependence. Dependence is defined as physiologic requirement of the drug for normal function, usually accompanied by tolerance. (E) This scenario does not describe simple tolerance. When tolerance developed to one substance leads to tolerance in a related substance, the correct term is "cross-tolerance."

64 **The answer is D: Prednisolone.** An allergic reaction can present in two phases: early and late. The early phase appears within minutes and is caused by the release of preformed molecules such as histamine and heparin during mast cell degranulation. The late phase appears many hours after the initial exposure. The delay occurs because of late-phase molecules such as prostaglandins and leukotrienes that are not stored inside mast cells; they are synthesized later by enzymes that are upregulated beginning when mast cells degranulate. Corticosteroids such as prednisolone block the synthesis of the enzymes, which are responsible for the production of late-phase mediators. (A) Diphenhydramine is a first-generation antihistamine. It blocks H_1 receptors to prevent the downstream effects of histamine. Diphenhydramine would not affect the late phase, which is mediated by prostaglandins and leukotrienes. (B) Epinephrine is a physiologic antagonist of mast cell degranulation and is useful for treating the effects of all mediators made by mast cells. However, it would not prevent the late-phase reaction as prednisolone would. (C) Loratadine is a second-generation antihistamine. It blocks H_1 receptors to prevent the downstream effects of histamine. Loratadine would not affect the late phase, which is mediated by prostaglandins and leukotrienes. (E) There is insufficient evidence to make this claim. A corticosteroid such as prednisolone would likely have prevented the late-phase reaction in this patient.

65 **The answer is E: Salmeterol.** Treatment of acute asthma attacks commonly involves short-acting β_2-adrenergic agonists such as albuterol, epinephrine, or isoproterenol or an anticholinergic such as ipratropium. These agents are useful in acute attacks because of their rapid onset, but they are not as useful for the chronic treatment of asthma. Salmeterol is a long-acting β_2-adrenergic agonist that can be used to achieve symptom control until an effective, chronic corticosteroid dose can be established. (A) Albuterol is a short-acting β_2-adrenergic agonist. It is useful for the treatment of acute asthma attacks but not as useful as salmeterol for asthma prophylaxis. (B) Epinephrine is a short-acting β_2-adrenergic agonist. It is useful for the treatment of acute asthma attacks but not as useful as salmeterol for asthma prophylaxis. (C) Ipratropium is an anticholinergic used in conjunction with a β_2-adrenergic agonist to reduce bronchial secretions and bronchial smooth muscle tone in asthma attacks. It has not been shown to be effective for asthma prophylaxis. (D) Isoproterenol is a short-acting β_2-adrenergic agonist. It is useful for the treatment of acute asthma attacks but not as useful as salmeterol for asthma prophylaxis.

66 **The answer is B: Narrow-angle glaucoma.** Contraindications to epinephrine include narrow-angle glaucoma, cardiac failure, shock, and brain damage.

Pregnancy and active labor are also contraindications. (A) Diabetes mellitus is a precaution, not a contraindication. (C) Cardiac failure, not pulmonary failure, is a contraindication. (D) Hyperthyroidism is a precaution to this medication, not a contraindication. (E) Age is not a limiting factor for epinephrine.

67 **The answer is A: Expected adverse event.** Adverse effects include flulike symptoms on injection, such as fever, chills, myalgias, arthralgias, and GI disturbances. Fatigue and mental depression are common. These symptoms subside with subsequent administrations. The principal dose-limiting toxicities are bone marrow suppression including granulocytopenia, neurotoxicity characterized by somnolence, and behavioral disturbances. (B) This reaction is an expected adverse event of administration of interferon. (C) This patient does not have evidence of an underlying atypical pneumonia on history and physical examination. (D) This patient has no evidence to suggest an underlying bacterial pneumonia. (E) There is no evidence to suggest an underlying viral pneumonia.

68 **The answer is A: Buccal mucosa.** In addition to nausea, vomiting, and diarrhea, the most frequent toxicities occur in tissues that are constantly renewing. Thus, methotrexate causes stomatitis, myelosuppression, erythema, rash, urticaria, and alopecia. Some of these adverse effects can be prevented or reversed by administering leucovorin, which is taken up more readily by normal cells than by tumor cells. (B) The long bone tissue does not constantly renew, thus they are somewhat resistant to toxicities. (C) The epidermal layer of the skin is somewhat resistant to the effects of chemotherapy. (D) The small bones of the face do not constantly renew, thus they are resistant to the toxicities of these chemotherapeutic agents. (E) Teeth are not rapidly dividing tissues and are resistant to methotrexate chemotherapy.

69 **The answer is C: Hypersensitivity.** Allopurinol is well tolerated by most patients. Hypersensitivity reactions, especially skin rashes, are the most common adverse reactions, occurring in approximately 3% of patients. The reactions may occur even after months or years of chronic administration, and allopurinol therapy should be discontinued. (A) There is no evidence to suggest a contact hypersensitivity in this patient. This is a hypersensitivity reaction to allopurinol. (B) There is no evidence to suggest dermatitis herpetiformis in this patient. (D) This patient does not describe a history of sun exposure to suggest squamous cell carcinoma. (E) Telangiectasia would produce a more localized reaction.

70 **The answer is C: Histidine.** Histamine is an amine formed by the decarboxylation of the amino acid histidine by histidine decarboxylase, an enzyme that is expressed in cells throughout the body, including central nervous system (CNS) neurons, gastric mucosa parietal cells, mast cells, and basophils. In mast cells, histamine is stored in granules as an inactive complex composed of histamine and the polysulfated anion, heparin, along with an anionic protein. If histamine is not stored, it is rapidly inactivated by amine oxidase enzymes. (A) L-arginine is an amino acid precursor to the production of nitric oxide. (B) Heparin is not an amino acid. (D) Lysine is not a precursor of histamine. (E) Tyrosine is a precursor to dopamine and norepinephrine.

71 **The answer is D: Fexofenadine.** This patient would benefit from the use of an antihistamine agent. However, his job requires that he be alert. Thus, selection of an agent that does not cause sedation would be most important. Fexofenadine will provide symptom relief for this patient and not cause sedation. (A) Chlorpheniramine is a sedating antihistamine agent that is ill suited for this patient because it will cause sedation. (B) Diphenhydramine would cause significant sedation and should not be given to this patient because of sedative properties. (C) Doxylamine is a sedating antihistamine and should not be prescribed to this patient because of its sedative effects. (E) Hydroxylamine is a sedating antihistamine and would be ill suited for this patient because of sedation.

72 **The answer is E: Urinary retention.** Diphenhydramine is an over-the-counter antihistamine agent. It provides good symptom relief of allergic symptoms but can be associated with urinary retention, dry mouth, and sinus tachycardia. These effects may be dose related. (A) Appetite suppressant effects are noted with H receptors that have an effect on the serotonin pathway. (B) Dizziness can be seen with the use of the antihistamine promethazine. (C) Hypotension can be seen with the use of the antihistamine promethazine. (D) Reflex tachycardia can be seen with the use of the antihistamine promethazine.

73 **The answer is B: Eye irritation.** Individuals can be exposed to carbon tetrachloride through consumption of contaminated drinking water. Although transient, low-level inhalation of carbon tetrachloride can produce irritation of the eyes and respiratory system. Higher levels, whether inhaled or ingested, can produce nausea, vomiting, stupor, convulsions, coma, and death from CNS depression. (A) Convulsions can occur at higher levels of carbon tetrachloride ingestion or inhalation. (C) Nausea can occur at higher levels of carbon tetrachloride ingestion or inhalation. (D) Stupor only occurs at high levels of carbon tetrachloride ingestion/inhalation. (E) Eye irritation and respiratory symptoms occur at low levels of carbon tetrachloride ingestion/inhalation.

74 The answer is B: Toxic dose of chloroform via inhalation. The adverse effects associated with chloroform exposure are similar to those with carbon tetrachloride. Exposures can occur through ingestion or inhalation, and toxic dose will result in nausea, vomiting, dizziness, headaches, and stupor. Chloroform can also sensitize the heart to catecholamine-induced arrhythmias. (A) Myocardial infarction is unlikely in a young child with no evidence of prior cardiac disease. (C) There is no evidence to suggest that this child had any underlying pulmonary disease process. (D) Deep venous thrombosis, venous stasis disease, and hypercoagulable states were not discussed in this case. (E) There is no evidence to suggest ventricular septal defect with overriding aorta in this patient.

75 The answer is A: Benzene. Approximately half of the national exposure to benzene occurs through tobacco smoke. Chronic benzene exposure in humans produces hematopoietic toxicities, of which the most serious are agranulocytosis and leukemia, particularly acute myelogenous leukemia. Nonoccupational exposures to benzene can occur as a result of combustion of fossil fuels, including automobile gasoline, and by consumption of contaminated water. (B) Ethylene alcohol in toxic dose can cause CNS reactions such as sedation. (C) Carbon tetrachloride exposure in low doses produces respiratory symptoms and eye irritation. (D) Methanol in toxic doses can cause CNS reactions such as sedation. (E) Toluene exposure can produce seizures, tremors, and CNS depression.

76 The answer is A: Carbon monoxide poisoning. This patient has carbon monoxide poisoning. It is a natural by-product of the combustion of carbonaceous materials, and common sources of this gas include automobiles, poorly vented furnaces, fireplaces, wood-burning stoves, kerosene space heaters, and charcoal grills. The symptoms of carbon monoxide intoxication are consistent with hypoxia, with the brain and heart showing the greatest sensitivity. Symptoms include headache, dyspnea, lethargy, confusion, and drowsiness, whereas higher exposure levels can lead to seizures, coma, and death. The management of a carbon monoxide–poisoned patient includes prompt removal from the source of carbon monoxide and institution of 100% oxygen by nonrebreathing face mask or endotracheal tube. In patients with severe intoxication, oxygenation in a hyperbaric chamber is recommended/followed. (B) There is no reason to suggest an epidemic of pneumonia. The reason is that there is a clearly identified source of the problem. In this case, the kerosene stove is the culprit. (C) Cyanide exposure quickly binds to many metalloenzymes, thereby rendering them inactive. Its principal toxicity occurs as a result of the inactivation of the enzyme cytochrome oxidase. (D) Silicosis is a progressive lung disease that results in fibrosis and, often, emphysema. Silicosis is currently incurable, and the prognosis is often poor.

77 The answer is C: Montelukast. This patient's presentation and history suggest that seasonal allergies are causing her symptoms. Allergy symptoms are the result of mediators released because of a type 1 hypersensitivity reaction in which an allergen simultaneously binds two IgE molecules on a mast cell's surface. This simultaneous binding initially causes mast cell degranulation, releasing histamine, and leads to the later conversion of arachidonic acid to leukotrienes. Montelukast is a leukotriene receptor inhibitor and would be the most useful of the drugs listed to treat this patient. (A) Aspirin is a nonsteroidal anti-inflammatory drug (NSAID) and blocks the conversion of arachidonic acid to prostaglandins by cyclooxygenase enzymes. Aspirin would not help this patient's symptoms and may actually worsen them by forcing excess arachidonic acid down the leukotriene path. (B) Epinephrine would be more useful to treat a severe hypersensitivity reaction than for routine treatment of allergy symptoms. Epinephrine does not block the immediate actions of histamine or leukotrienes. (D) Naproxen is an NSAID and blocks the conversion of arachidonic acid to prostaglandins by cyclooxygenase enzymes. Naproxen would not help this patient's symptoms and may actually worsen them by forcing excess arachidonic acid down the leukotriene path. (E) Terbutaline is a β_2-adrenergic agonist and causes dilation of bronchiolar smooth muscle. It would not relieve this patient's itchy, runny nose.

78 The answer is C: Encourage patient to take medication and explore reasons for noncompliance. This patient is having some difficulty in taking his medications. The reasons for this are not well understood. It may be caused by a behavioral problem with the patient or a medication side effect (less likely). The physician must explore the reasons for noncompliance before consideration of any other treatment choice. (A) The physician should first explore reasons for patient noncompliance. (B) Consultation with a behavioral medicine physician could be considered if an underlying behavioral problem is uncovered. (D) This patient is responding well to nitroglycerin. There is no reason to switch medications. (E) There is no indication to begin an antipsychotic agent in this patient. There is no obvious underlying psychiatric disturbance.

79 The answer is E: PGE_2. Inflammation is a cellular response with many triggers. Some examples are infection, chemical stress, and (as in this case) physical stress. The first step is phosphorylation of IκB, an inhibitory protein whose role is to bind NF-κB and keep it inactive in the cytoplasm. Phosphorylation of IκB causes dissociation from NF-κB. The NF-κB then enters the nucleus where it activates histone acetyltransferase (HAT) and acts as a transcription factor for COX-2 and iNOS. COX-2 is an enzyme responsible for the sustained production of inflammatory prostaglandins such as PGE_2 following injury. Aspirin has anti-inflammatory action because it is an irreversible inhibitor of COX-2. COX-2 is an enzyme induced by NF-κB and is responsible for the sustained production of inflammatory prostaglandins following injury. (A) HAT can be activated by NF-κB. By acetylating histones, it promotes a more open configuration of DNA, thereby facilitating transcription of genes. Its action is not interrupted by aspirin. (B) When IκB is bound to NF-κB, IκB hides the nuclear localization signal domain on NF-κB to keep it inactive in the cytoplasm. Aspirin does not act on IκB. (C) iNOS is an enzyme inducible by NF-κB. iNOS produces nitric oxide (NO), which is a potent vasodilator. Aspirin does not inhibit NO production. (D) When IκB is bound to NF-κB, IκB hides the nuclear localization signal domain on NF-κB to keep it inactive in the cytoplasm. Aspirin does not act on NF-κB.

80 **The answer is A: Cocaine.** This patient's behaviors and physical findings are consistent with a CNS stimulant toxicity. Of the drugs listed, cocaine is the most likely candidate. In the CNS, cocaine causes dopamine release as well as inhibits dopamine reuptake. Patients with cocaine toxicity may present with anxiety, confusion, paranoia, hallucinations, tachycardia, and hypertension. Treatment is largely supportive in nature, but benzodiazepines can be used to control seizures. (B) Heroin toxicity causes respiratory depression and miosis. This patient's presentation does not appear to be caused by heroin. (C) A patient on LSD may appear physically similar to one on cocaine (sleepless, hypertensive, and tachycardic) but would not likely be as anxious and would report more dreamlike feelings and more vivid sensations. (D) Methanol, like ethanol, is a CNS depressant. Toxicity is caused by this CNS depression as well as methanol's metabolism into formic acid. Formic acid causes hypoxia from mitochondrial inhibition and metabolic acidosis. This patient's presentation does not appear to be caused by methanol. (E) Propofol is a CNS depressant with a similar mechanism of action to benzodiazepines and barbiturates. Propofol toxicity would cause respiratory depression, hypotension, and bradycardia.

81 **The answer is A: Abnormal dreams.** Varenicline is thought to decrease nicotine cravings by stimulating neuronal nicotinic acetylcholine receptors (nAChRs). This provides a moderate level of stimulation in the place of nicotine, making quitting easier. It also blocks the full effects of nicotine by competing with the binding sites in cases where a patient on varenicline does smoke. Although all of the options listed are side effects that have been reported with varenicline, abnormal dreams is the most common. These occur in about 10% of patients. (B) Gastric ulcers have been reported with varenicline but much less commonly than abnormal dreams. Of the side effects listed, abnormal dreams appears to be by far the most common. (C) Pancreatitis has been reported with varenicline but much less commonly than abnormal dreams. Pancreatitis is more commonly caused by some nucleoside reverse transcriptase inhibitors such as didanosine. Of the side effects listed, abnormal dreams appears to be by far the most common. (D) Photosensitivity has been reported with varenicline but much less commonly than abnormal dreams. Of the side effects listed, abnormal dreams appears to be by far the most common. (E) Seizures have been reported with varenicline but much less commonly than abnormal dreams. Of the side effects listed, abnormal dreams appears to be by far the most common.

82 **The answer is D: Ketorolac.** Any patient with a serum creatinine level this high should avoid all nephrotoxic drugs. Nonsteroidal anti-inflammatory drugs (NSAIDs) such as ketorolac can decrease renal blood flow, exacerbating mild renal failure. This occurs because NSAIDs block prostaglandin synthesis, and prostaglandins are responsible for dilation of the afferent arteriole. Opioids and acetaminophen do not block peripheral prostaglandin synthesis and so do not affect renal blood flow. (A) Acetaminophen blocks prostaglandin synthesis centrally but not peripherally. It is hepatotoxic in high doses but is not nephrotoxic. (B) Codeine is an opioid analgesic and cough suppressant. Although it can reach toxic levels in patients with severe renal failure, it is not nephrotoxic and would not be contraindicated in this case. (C) Hydrocodone is an opioid analgesic. Although it can reach toxic levels in patients with severe renal failure, it is not nephrotoxic and would not be contraindicated in this case. (E) Oxycodone is an opioid analgesic. Although it can reach toxic levels in patients with severe renal failure, it is not nephrotoxic and would not be contraindicated in this case.

83 **The answer is A: Allopurinol.** Azathioprine is metabolized in part by the enzyme xanthine oxidase. This is the same enzyme responsible for converting xanthine into uric acid, which can lead to attacks of gout. Allopurinol, an antigout drug, works by inhibiting xanthine oxidase. This would lead to azathioprine toxicity in this patient, so he should avoid taking allopurinol while on azathioprine. (B) Colchicine prevents white blood cells from mounting an

inflammatory response by impairing microtubule formation. Colchicine does not interact with azathioprine. (C) Indomethacin is an NSAID and works by inhibiting cyclooxygenase enzymes. Indomethacin does not interact with azathioprine. (D) Prednisolone is a glucocorticoid and blocks synthesis of inflammatory mediators. Prednisolone does not interact significantly with azathioprine. (E) Probenecid acts by increasing the renal excretion of uric acid. It does not interact with azathioprine.

84 **The answer is E: Prior to the onset of symptoms.** Although similar to atropine, therapeutic use of scopolamine is limited to prevention of motion sickness (for which it is particularly effective) and to blocking short-term memory. As with all such drugs used for motion sickness, it is much more effective prophylactically than for treating motion sickness once it occurs. The amnesic action of scopolamine makes it an important adjunct drug in anesthetic procedures. (A) Scopolamine is efficacious in the prevention of motion sickness. (B) Scopolamine should be given prior to the onset of symptoms. (C) Administration of scopolamine after vomiting limits its efficacy. (D) Short-term memory loss can occur with scopolamine.

85 **The answer is B: Decreased risk of ectopic pregnancy.** Cardiovascular complications, increased gallbladder disease, and benign hepatic tumor are all disadvantages to the pill in addition to the requirement of having to take a medication every day. There is a decreased risk of ectopic pregnancy in patients who are taking oral contraceptives. (A) The risk of colon carcinoma is not decreased with the use of oral contraceptives. (C) The risk of infiltrating breast cancer is not decreased with birth control pills. (D) The risk of medullary carcinoma of the thyroid is not decreased by birth control pills. (E) The risk of uterine teratoma is not decreased by birth control pills.

86 **The answer is A: Acetaminophen.** Analgesics such as acetaminophen, ibuprofen, and codeine are considered safe during pregnancy. Antibiotics such as penicillins, erythromycin, and cephalosporins are also considered safe in pregnancy. These medications usually do not require dose adjustments. (B) Ciprofloxacin is contraindicated during pregnancy. (C) Methotrexate is contraindicated during pregnancy. (D) Valproic acid is contraindicated during pregnancy. (E) Warfarin is contraindicated during pregnancy.

87 **The answer is A: Alcohol.** Of the substances listed, only alcohol has been consistently associated with a "syndrome" involving intrauterine growth retardation; abnormal facies; and cardiac abnormalities, most commonly atrial septal defects. (B) Cocaine has been associated with growth restriction, placental abruption, and CNS effects. (C) Marijuana has not been proven to be teratogenic. (D) Opioids are not proven to be teratogenic. (E) Although associated with IUGR and other problems of pregnancy, it does not fit with the presented case.

88 **The answer is A: Acamprosate.** Ethyl alcohol, commonly referred to simply as alcohol, has an overall depressive effect on the CNS. Ethanol stimulates GABA receptors, leading to a decrease in cellular excitability. Chronic CNS depression in this manner leads to an increase in excitatory neurotransmitters to compensate for the alcohol's depressive effect. In the sudden absence of alcohol, the excess excitatory neurotransmitters cause this patient's anxiety and insomnia. Acamprosate appears to block the excitatory neurotransmissions so alcoholics taking it become less dependent on alcohol for normal function. (B) Disulfiram causes nausea and headache in people who drink while taking disulfiram. It can also be used for alcoholism but would not decrease the symptoms of this patient. (C) Methadone is used to treat opioid withdrawal, not alcoholism. Methadone would not decrease this patient's anxiety and insomnia as well as acamprosate would. (D) Methanol is a highly toxic alcohol and has no medical use. It would not decrease this patient's anxiety and insomnia. (E) Endogenous opioids apparently play an important role in alcoholism. By blocking opioid receptors, naltrexone decreases the positive feelings associated with drinking. Naltrexone would not, however, decrease this patient's anxiety and insomnia.

89 **The answer is C: Severe hypotension with sildenafil.** Patients who take nitrates for angina are at risk for severe hypotension when they combine this with sildenafil (Viagra). All physicians must warn patients about this important interaction because it can be life threatening. (A) Cold extremities are unlikely to be seen with the use of nitrates. Headaches are more common. (B) Hot extremities are uncommon with the use of nitrates. Weakness is more common. (D) Tinnitus is uncommon with the use of nitrates. Rash is more common. (E) Vertigo is uncommon with the use of nitrates. Dizziness is more common.

90 **The answer is E: Inhibits folic acid metabolism.** The patient is suffering from hemolysis secondary to G6PD deficiency. This is an adverse reaction seen in patients who take trimethoprim–sulfamethoxazole. It is more commonly seen in African Americans. Look for the symptoms of hemolysis, like anemia and jaundice. (A) This is the mechanism of action of clindamycin. A common side effect is *Clostridium difficile* infection. (B) This is the mechanism of action of tetracyclines. Common side effects are discoloration of children's teeth and disruption of bone synthesis. (C) This is the mechanism of action of vancomycin.

Common side effects are nephrotoxicity, ototoxicity, and red man syndrome. (D) This is the mechanism of action of rifampin. Common side effects are hepatotoxicity and red-orange body fluids.

91 **The answer is A: Discoloration of teeth.** Doxycycline should not be prescribed to children younger than age 8 years because of the risk of discoloration of teeth. Other side effects are GI upset, inhibition of bone growth, and photosensitivity. (B) Trimethoprim, not doxycycline, can cause megaloblastic anemia because of its mechanism of inhibiting folate metabolism. (C) Vancomycin, aminoglycosides, and sulfamethoxazole are known to be nephrotoxic, not doxycycline. (D) Vancomycin and aminoglycosides are known to be ototoxic, not doxycycline. (E) Fluoroquinolones are known to cause leg cramps and myalgias in kids, not doxycycline.

92 **The answer is A: Non-hypersensitivity mast cell degranulation.** The scenario described the case of the so-called red man syndrome known to sometimes occur with vancomycin administration. This is a flushing of the skin caused by mast cell degranulation but is not a hypersensitivity reaction and does not involve IgE. An anti-H_1 antihistamine may be used to decrease the erythema associated with vancomycin administration even though this is not a hypersensitivity reaction. This rash may also be avoided by administering vancomycin slowly over a longer period of time. (B) A type I hypersensitivity reaction is characterized by an antigen cross-linking two IgE molecules on the surface of the mast cell leading to mast cell degranulation. Red man syndrome is not an example of a type I hypersensitivity reaction. (C) A type II hypersensitivity reaction is characterized by autoantibodies, which bind to the patient's own cells. Red man syndrome is not an example of a type II hypersensitivity reaction. (D) A type III hypersensitivity reaction is characterized by the deposition of large amounts of immune complexes in tissues. Red man syndrome is not an example of a type III hypersensitivity reaction. (E) A type IV hypersensitivity reaction is mediated by cytotoxic T cells and takes at least 48 h to develop. Red man syndrome is not an example of a type IV hypersensitivity reaction.

93 **The answer is B: Stimulating the trigger zone of chemotaxis.** Ipecac is a mixture of alkaloids that induce vomiting by stimulating the chemotactic trigger zone, which causes gastrointestinal irritation and afferent input to the vomiting center. This agent produces vomiting in most patients within 20 min and is useful for removing toxins that have slow gastric transit times. (A) Ipecac does not stimulate the gag reflex. (C) Ipecac does not suppress gastric outlet pressures. (D) Ipecac does not suppress the gag reflex. (E) Ipecac does not suppress the motor cortex.

94 **The answer is D: Phencyclidine piperidine.** Phencyclidine piperidine (PCP) is associated with auditory and visual hallucinations as well as alterations of body images and distortion of time and space. Findings on physical examination may include hypertension, tachycardia, hyperthermia, and nystagmus. (A) Alcohol abuse does not produce findings exhibited by this patient. (B) Cocaine abuse produces intense euphoria and is often followed by acute depression. (C) Marijuana produces euphoria, relaxation, and sleepiness as well as orthostatic hypotension and tachycardia. (E) Quailudes do not typically produce findings exhibited by this patient.

95 **The answer is B: He had a false positive because of ephedrine use.** Ephedrine is a vasoconstrictor used to treat nasal congestion and can cause a false-positive amphetamine drug test. Codeine, present in many cough medicines, would cause a positive drug test for opioids. This patient's recent use of prescription cough and cold medicines could be expected to produce false positives in a urine drug screen in this manner. (A) This patient likely has ingested codeine, which is an opioid. Codeine would cause a positive urine opioid screen but not a positive amphetamine screen. (C) Abuse of one substance is often accompanied by abuse of another, but marijuana use would not cause a false positive for amphetamines. Ephedrine use is the best explanation for this patient's positive amphetamine test. (D) This patient may indeed be lying about drug use, but his history of cold medicine use would raise the suspicion for ephedrine ingestion. Ephedrine use is the best explanation for this patient's positive amphetamine test. (E) Although this is a theoretical possibility, other more likely causes should be investigated first. Ephedrine use is the best explanation for this patient's positive amphetamine test.

96 **The answer is A: Blocks leukotriene receptors.** Arachidonic acid is the precursor for the eicosanoids such as prostaglandins and leukotrienes. First, phospholipase A_2 cleaves cell membrane phospholipids to release arachidonic acid. Arachidonic acid can then be converted into prostaglandins by cyclooxygenase (inhibited by aspirin and celecoxib) or into leukotrienes by lipoxygenase (inhibited by zileuton). Prostaglandins are drivers of inflammation. Leukotrienes cause bronchoconstriction, mucus production, and increased vessel permeability leading to the symptoms of asthma. Montelukast works by preventing leukotrienes from binding to their receptors. Ipratropium works on autonomic nervous system receptors rather than on the arachidonic acid pathways. Ipratropium is a parasympathetic antagonist and works to relax bronchial smooth muscle and decrease secretions. (B) Ipratropium is a parasympathetic antagonist that blocks acetylcholine from binding to muscarinic

receptors. Montelukast does not block acetylcholine receptors. (C) Aspirin inhibits the cyclooxygenase enzymes COX-1 and COX-2. Montelukast does not inhibit either of these enzymes. (D) Celecoxib is a selective COX-2 inhibitor and is not used in the treatment of reactive airway disease. Montelukast does not inhibit COX-2. (E) Zileuton inhibits lipoxygenase to decrease the amount of leukotriene synthesized. Montelukast prevents leukotrienes from binding to their receptors but does not inhibit their synthesis.

97 **The answer is B: Inhibits H_1 receptors.** Itchy, watery eyes with runny nose in spring is likely allergic rhinitis, commonly called hay fever. These symptoms are caused primarily by histamine acting on H_1 receptors. Histamine is released from mast cells when they encounter the antigen to which they have been sensitized. Interrupting histamine release (i.e., cromolyn), blocking H_1 receptors (diphenhydramine, cetirizine, and hydroxyzine), and physiologically antagonizing the effects of histamine (epinephrine) are all methods employed to reduce symptoms of allergic rhinitis. The H_1 antagonists are divided into first-generation (diphenhydramine, hydroxyzine) and second-generation (cetirizine) drugs. The second-generation drugs are more specific for the H_1 receptor and do not cross the blood–brain barrier as readily so they have fewer side effects (such as drowsiness). (A) Nonselective β-blockers can antagonize β_2-receptors and lead to bronchoconstriction. Cetirizine does not inhibit β_2-receptors.(C) Ephedrine is an example of a drug that stimulates α_1-receptors. It can be used to decrease nasal congestion. Cetirizine does not stimulate α_1-receptors. (D) Albuterol is a drug that stimulates β_2-receptors. This leads to relaxation of bronchial smooth muscles to make breathing easier in reactive airway diseases such as asthma. Cetirizine does not stimulate β_2-receptors. (E) Histamine stimulation of H_1 receptors is responsible for this patient's symptoms. An antihistamine such as cetirizine will prevent the stimulation of these receptors and reduce his symptoms.

98 **The answer is B: Hepatitis.** Mitoxantrone, a cytotoxic anthracycline analog that can kill T cells, may also be used. The major target of these medications is to modify the body's immune response through inhibition of white blood cell–mediated inflammatory processes that eventually lead to myelin sheath damage and a decreased or inappropriate axonal communication between cells. Adverse effects of these medications may include depression, local injection or infusion reactions, increased hepatic enzyme, flulike symptoms such as fever and myalgias, and leukopenia. (A) Depression is a common side effect of mitoxantrone. (C) Fever is a common side effect of mitoxantrone. (D) Muscle weakness and myalgia is a common side effect of mitoxantrone. (E) Leukopenia is a common side effect of mitoxantrone.

99 **The answer is E: Sedation.** At low doses, the barbiturates produce sedation (have a calming effect and reduce excitement). At higher doses, the drugs cause hypnosis, followed by anesthesia (loss of feeling or sensation) and, finally, coma and death. Thus, any degree of depression of the CNS is possible depending on the dose. Barbiturates do not raise the pain threshold and have no analgesic properties. They may even exacerbate pain. Chronic use leads to tolerance. (A) Anesthesia is a higher dose effect of barbiturates. (B) Coma is the highest dose effect of barbiturates. (C) Death is the highest dose effect of barbiturates. (D) Hypnosis is a higher dose effect of barbiturates.

100 **The answer is B: Lorazepam.** It is important to treat the seizures associated with alcohol withdrawal. Benzodiazepines, such as chlordiazepoxide, diazepam, or the shorter acting lorazepam, are effective in controlling this problem. They are less sedating than pentobarbital or phenytoin. (A) Buspirone can cause hypothermia but cause minimal sedation. (C) Pentobarbital is used to induce anesthesia and is not indicated in this patient. (D) Phenytoin can cause significant sedation. (E) This patient who is a chronic alcoholic should be treated for withdrawal symptoms.

101 **The answer is E: Sirolimus.** Sirolimus forms a complex with FKBP, which then inhibits the mammalian target of rapamycin (mTOR). mTOR is a protein kinase necessary for signal transduction leading to cell proliferation. Without functional mTOR, the cell cycle is arrested and proliferation cannot occur, and the body is unable to mount an effective immune reaction to the foreign tissue. (A) Azathioprine impairs the DNA and RNA synthesis necessary for cell function. It does not inhibit mTOR. (B) Cyclosporine forms a complex with protein called cyclophilin. This complex then binds the calcium-calmodulin-calcineurin complex to inhibit it from dephosphorylating NF-AT, which remains trapped in the cytoplasm and unable to influence gene transcription necessary for T- and B-cell activation. (C) Methotrexate is a folate antimetabolite. It blocks cell proliferation by inhibiting DNA synthesis, not by modulating calcineurin. (D) Prednisolone is not known to modify calcineurin's activity. It is a glucocorticoid and inhibits many pathways necessary for inflammation and immune system function.

102 **The answer is C: Lowers pressure by increasing aqueous humor outflow.** Glaucoma usually involves an increase in intraocular pressure. Physostigmine increases the effects of endogenous acetylcholine by inhibiting acetylcholinesterase, which increases the half-life of acetylcholine in the synaptic cleft. This leads to a decrease in intraocular pressure by stimulating contraction of the ciliary muscle, which opens

the trabecular meshwork, increasing outflow of the aqueous humor. (A) Some β-blockers can be used to treat open-angle glaucoma by lowering pressure through inhibition of aqueous humor secretion. Physostigmine does not decrease aqueous humor secretion. (B) Some α-adrenergic agonists can be used to treat open-angle glaucoma by lowering pressure through the inhibition of aqueous humor synthesis. Physostigmine does not decrease aqueous humor synthesis. (D) Raising intraocular pressure would not be useful in treating glaucoma. Physostigmine does not decrease aqueous humor outflow. (E) Raising intraocular pressure would not be useful in treating glaucoma. Physostigmine does not inhibit aqueous humor secretion.

103 **The answer is C: Inhibits neuraminidase.** Oseltamivir is a neuraminidase inhibitor used in the treatment of influenza A and B. To be most effective, it must be given within 48 h of the initial symptoms. (A) The mechanism of action of amantadine is blocking viral uncoating inside infected cells by acting on M_2 proteins. M_2 proteins are mutated in most strains of influenza A, making it a resistant strain. (B) The mechanism of action of ribavirin is inhibiting IMP dehydrogenase, which decreases the amount of GTP that is needed for the formation of nucleic acids. (D) Inhibiting reverse transcriptase is the mechanism of action of nucleoside and nonnucleoside HIV medications. (E) The mechanism of action of foscarnet is inhibiting viral DNA polymerase. It is commonly used for CMV retinitis and acyclovir-resistant herpetic infections.

104 **The answer is A: Decrease in fatigue.** The caffeine contained in one to two cups of coffee (100 to 200 mg) causes a decrease in fatigue and increased mental alertness as a result of stimulating the cortex and other areas of the brain. Consumption of 1.5 g of caffeine (12 to 15 cups of coffee) produces anxiety and tremors. The spinal cord is stimulated only by very high doses (2 to 5 g) of caffeine. Tolerance can rapidly develop to the stimulating properties of caffeine, and withdrawal consists of feelings of fatigue and sedation. (B) One to two cups of coffee consumed will cause an increase in mental awareness. (C) Tolerance develops over years of chronic consumption. (D) Tremors develop with consumption of 1.5 g of caffeine. (E) Withdrawal consists of feelings of fatigue and sedation.

105 **The answer is A: Cyclooxygenase.** The two key players here are the eicosanoids thromboxane A_2 (TXA_2), which stimulates aggregation, and prostaglandin I_2 (PGI_2 or prostacyclin), which inhibits platelet aggregation. TXA_2 synthesis occurs in platelets themselves and begins with phospholipase A_2 cleaving membrane phospholipid to release arachidonic acid. This arachidonic acid is converted to prostaglandin H_2 (PGH_2) by platelet cyclooxygenase (COX) enzymes. PGH_2 is then converted to TXA_2 by platelet thromboxane synthase. Prostacyclin is synthesized in endothelial cells. It also starts with arachidonic acid, which is converted to PGH_2 by endothelial COX enzymes. PGH_2 in endothelial cells is then converted to prostacyclin by endothelial prostacyclin synthase. Aspirin inhibits COX enzymes in both platelet and endothelial cells; but under chronic aspirin use, endothelial cells can produce new COX enzymes. Platelets cannot replace deactivated enzymes because they lack a nucleus. Therefore, with chronic aspirin exposure, platelets are unable to make TXA_2; but endothelial cells can still make PGI_2 even though the same enzyme is inhibited in both cell types. (B) Lipoxygenase is an enzyme found in mast cells (and others) and is used to convert arachidonic acid into leukotrienes, which cause bronchoconstriction. Lipoxygenase is not found in platelets nor is it an enzyme involved platelet aggregation. (C) Phospholipase A_2 is necessary for the production of both TXA_2 and PGI_2 but is not inhibited by aspirin. Glucocorticoids indirectly inhibit phospholipase A_2. (D) Prostacyclin synthase makes prostacyclin, which inhibits platelet aggregation. This is not the intended target of aspirin for this patient nor does aspirin inhibit this enzyme. (E) Thromboxane synthase is not inhibited by aspirin. Ifetroban is an example of a thromboxane synthase inhibitor.

106 **The answer is A: Binds to CD3 on T cells.** Muromonab is a monoclonal antibody that binds to CD3 on T cells, preventing T-cell activation. It is commonly used to prevent the acute rejection of organs after transplant. (B) The mechanism of action of tacrolimus is binding to FK-binding protein, which inhibits the secretion of IL-2. (C) The mechanism of action of daclizumab is a monoclonal antibody that binds to IL-2 receptors on T cells. (D) The mechanism of action of sirolimus is inhibiting the T cells' response to IL-2 by binding to mTOR. This is similar to cyclosporine, except it inhibits calcineurin. (E) The mechanism of action of cyclosporine is inhibiting the T cells' response to IL-2 by inhibiting calcineurin. This is similar to sirolimus, except it binds to mTOR.

107 **The answer is B: Deferoxamine.** The boy most likely ingested the mother's prenatal vitamins containing iron. He is experiencing the acute symptoms of iron overdose: abdominal pain, nausea, vomiting, and gastric bleeding. The antidote for iron poisoning is deferoxamine, which chelates the iron from the blood. If this fails, the next option is dialysis. (A) Aminocaproic acid is used as the antidote for tPA and streptokinase

overdose. (C) Dimercaprol chelates many metals, including lead, mercury, arsenic, and copper. (D) Penicillamine is a chelating agent used as the antidote for lead, copper, arsenic, and gold. (E) Succimer is a chelating agent used as the antidote for lead, mercury, arsenic, and gold.

108 **The answer is E: Sodium bicarbonate.** She is most likely suffering from an overdose of tricyclic antidepressants. Her symptoms of seizures, confusion, and cardiac arrhythmias are characteristics. Other symptoms include dry mouth, urinary retention, respiratory depression, nausea, and vomiting. The antidote is alkalinizing the urine with sodium bicarbonate and supportive care. Sodium bicarbonate helps with the cardiotoxicity and metabolic acidosis. If this fails, the next option is dialysis. (A) Ammonium chloride is used to acidify the urine as an antidote for amphetamine overdose. (B) Atropine is used as an antidote for anticholinergic and organophosphate overdose. (C) Flumazenil is used as an antidote for benzodiazepine overdose. (D) *N*-acetylcysteine is used as an antidote for acetaminophen overdose.

109 **The answer is A: Lethargy.** Moderate doses of caffeine cause insomnia, anxiety, and agitation. A high dosage is required for toxicity, which is manifested by emesis and convulsions. The lethal dose is 10 g of caffeine (about 100 cups of coffee), which induces cardiac arrhythmias. Death from caffeine is, therefore, highly unlikely. Lethargy, irritability, and headache occur in users who routinely consumed more than 600 mg of caffeine per day (roughly six cups of coffee per day) and then suddenly stop. (B) General headache, not migraine is common with caffeine withdrawal. (C) Irritability, not nausea is a common side effect of caffeine withdrawal. (D) Tinnitus would not be expected to occur in this patient. (E) Lethargy, headache, and irritability are common side effects of caffeine withdrawal.

110 **The answer is A: Eyes remain open.** Phencyclidine, an analog of ketamine, causes dissociative anesthesia (insensitivity to pain without loss of consciousness) and analgesia. In this state, it produces numbness of extremities, staggered gait, slurred speech, and muscular rigidity. Sometimes, hostile and bizarre behavior is seen. At increased dosages, anesthesia, stupor, and coma may result but, strangely, the eyes may remain open. Increased sensitivity to external stimuli results, and the CNS actions may persist for a week. (B) Loss of consciousness occurs at lower doses of phencyclidine. (C) Numbness of extremities occurs at lower doses of phencyclidine. (D) Staggered gait can be observed in patients who use phencyclidine. (E) Slurred speech can be observed in patients who use phencyclidine.

111 **The answer is D: Suicidal tendencies.** It is important for physicians to be aware of particular warnings for certain medications. Sertraline is associated with mania, hypomania, and suicidal tendencies. Hepatic dysfunction can also result. (A) Sertraline is not associated with the development of hepatic carcinoma. (B) Patients can become depleted with this medication. (C) This medication can potentiate the diazepam or tolbutamide.

112 **The answer is C: Headache.** Fexofenadine is used in the treatment of allergic rhinitis. In adults, common adverse effects include headache, back pain, viral infection, GI upset, and sinusitis. (A) Anxiety is not a common side effect of fexofenadine. (B) Cough is a common side effect of this medication when used in children. (D) Otitis media is a common side effect of this medication when used in children. (E) Upper respiratory infection is a common side effect of this medication when used in children.

113 **The answer is E: Tinnitus.** Aspirin or acetylsalicylic acid is an anti-inflammatory salicylate. Its primary therapeutic effects are caused by its ability to inhibit cyclooxygenase (COX) enzymes to prevent production of proinflammatory prostaglandins and platelet aggregation factors. Chronic use of high doses of salicylates such as aspirin, however, can lead to salicylate toxicity. Often, some of the primary symptoms of salicylate toxicity are tinnitus and hearing loss. These usually resolve with cessation of aspirin therapy. (A) Angina is not a known side effect of aspirin. Aspirin is used to reduce the risk of repeat myocardial infarction by inhibiting platelet aggregation. (B) Insomnia is not a known side effect of aspirin. Insomnia is a common side effect of the reverse transcriptase inhibitor abacavir. (C) Aspirin does not affect clotting factors. It does have antiplatelet activity because it prevents platelet synthesis of thromboxane A_2. (D) Nephrolithiasis or kidney stones are not known to be caused by aspirin. Nephrolithiasis may be caused by many chemotherapy drugs.

114 **The answer is E: Ketorolac.** Ketorolac is a nonsteroidal anti-inflammatory drug (NSAID) that inhibits cyclooxygenase (COX) enzymes to block prostaglandin synthesis. This is useful for mild pain management because prostaglandins are pain sensitizers and cause inflammation. But prostaglandins serve other functions as well, one of which is to maintain a patent ductus arteriosus in the fetus. NSAIDs are contraindicated in late pregnancy because they will inhibit production of fetal PGE_2, allowing this physiologic shunt to close prematurely. (A) Acetaminophen, like NSAIDs, relieves pain by inhibition of COX enzymes but only centrally. Acetaminophen does not inhibit peripheral prostaglandin synthesis and would not

cause premature closure of the ductus arteriosus. (B) Codeine is an opioid analgesic. It may cause CNS depression in the fetus but does not inhibit prostaglandin synthesis and would not cause premature closure of the ductus arteriosus. (C) Hydrocodone is an opioid analgesic. It may cause CNS depression in the fetus but does not inhibit prostaglandin synthesis and would not cause premature closure of the ductus arteriosus. (D) Morphine is an opioid analgesic. It may cause CNS depression in the fetus but does not inhibit prostaglandin synthesis and would not cause premature closure of the ductus arteriosus.

115 **The answer is B: Acetylcysteine.** Acetaminophen metabolism follows one of two pathways in the liver. Most (more than 90%) undergoes phase II metabolism directly and is excreted renally. The remainder undergoes phase I metabolism by CYP1A2 or CYP2E1 to produce NAPQI, the toxic metabolite of acetaminophen. NAPQI requires glutathione for its next step of metabolism. Excess acetaminophen in the body produces so much NAPQI that liver glutathione (a natural, endogenous antioxidant) is depleted, allowing oxidative damage to occur. Treatment with acetylcysteine within 8 h of acetaminophen exposure preserves liver glutathione stores by providing an alternative substrate for the toxic metabolite. (A) Acetylsalicylic acid, or aspirin, would offer the liver no protection against acetaminophen toxicity. Aspirin is used for mild pain and as an antiplatelet drug. (C) Bicarbonate would offer the liver no protection against acetaminophen toxicity. Bicarbonate may be useful in mitigating toxic effects of acids such as salicylates by ion trapping them in the urine. (D) Fomepizole would offer the liver no protection against acetaminophen toxicity. It is used to treat toxicity of alcohols such as methanol and ethylene glycol by inhibiting the enzyme that converts these into toxic metabolites. (E) Penicillamine would offer the liver no protection against acetaminophen toxicity. Penicillamine is used to chelate certain metals such as copper to treat metal toxicity.

116 **The answer is D: Injection site reaction.** The IL-1ra (interleukin-1 receptor antagonist) is a natural blocker of the IL-1 receptor. As an antagonist, IL-1ra blocks the effects of IL-1. In rheumatoid arthritis, these effects include bone and cartilage destruction in the joints. Anakinra is a recombinant form of IL-1ra. It must be administered daily and mimics the effects of IL-1ra, blocking IL-1 signaling. The most common adverse effect of anakinra administration is an injection site reaction (inflammation and ecchymosis), occurring in about 70% of patients. (A) Anakinra has not been reported to cause blurry vision. Atropine is a drug that can cause blurred vision secondary to cycloplegia. (B) Diarrhea has been reported following anakinra administration, but the incidence is much lower than an injection site reaction. Diarrhea is a significant side effect of many antibiotics and cholinomimetics. (C) Headache has been reported following anakinra administration, but the incidence is much lower than an injection site reaction. Headaches commonly accompany the use of vasodilators such as nitroglycerin and nitroprusside. (E) Nausea has been reported following anakinra administration, but the incidence is much lower than an injection site reaction. Chemotherapy drugs are notorious for causing nausea.

117 **The answer is D: Inhibition of TNF-α signaling.** Etanercept is a recombinant human IgG molecule fused to a recombinant TNF-α receptor molecule. The TNF-α receptor moiety binds up endogenous TNF-α to prevent it from stimulating its normal downstream effects. TNF-α is a signaling molecule that stimulates leukocyte activation, bone reabsorption, and cartilage degradation. Blocking TNF-α significantly improves symptoms of rheumatoid arthritis. (A) This response describes the action of capsaicin. Capsaicin depletes substance P from neurons, which is an important molecule in the transmission of pain signals. (B) NSAIDs reduce inflammation by inhibition of cyclooxygenase (COX) enzymes. Etanercept does not inhibit COX enzymes. (C) Colchicine is a drug that binds neutrophil microtubules in order to inhibit chemotaxis. It is used to treat gouty arthritis but not rheumatoid arthritis. (E) Glucocorticoids cause inhibition of phospholipase A_2, the enzyme that makes arachidonic acid. Arachidonic acid can then be used to make inflammatory prostaglandins.

118 **The answer is C: β-Blockers.** Cocaine is a potent vasoconstrictor. When β-blockers are added, all β-receptors become blocked, leaving only α-receptors active. The activation of α-receptors leads to additional vasoconstriction, decreasing myocardial perfusion. (A) ACE inhibitors cause vasodilation through the inhibition of angiotensin II. (B) Aspirin is an antiplatelet that does not have vasoconstrictive properties. (D) Calcium channel blockers decrease cardiac contractility and cause vasodilation. (E) Nitroglycerin causes vasodilation of coronary arteries.

119 **The answer is D: Inhibited by fomepizole.** The first step in ethanol metabolism involves conversion by alcohol dehydrogenase into acetaldehyde. Methanol is also metabolized into toxic products by this enzyme; fomepizole can be used to inhibit the enzyme in cases of methanol ingestion to avoid toxicity. Acetaldehyde is then converted to acetate by aldehyde dehydrogenase. This enzyme can be inhibited by disulfiram, resulting in nausea and headache and discouraging alcohol consumption. Acetate is later converted to acetyl CoA and enters the citric acid cycle. (A) Aldehyde dehydrogenase is responsible for converting acetaldehyde into acetate. Alcohol dehydrogenase acts in ethanol to produce acetaldehyde. (B) Acetate produced by aldehyde dehydrogenase is converted into acetyl CoA by acetyl-CoA synthetase. Alcohol dehydrogenase does not act on acetate. (C) Acetaldehyde dehydrogenase is inhibited by disulfiram, causing a rise in acetaldehyde levels, which results in nausea and headache and discourages alcohol consumption. Alcohol dehydrogenase is not inhibited by disulfiram. (E) Acetate is produced by aldehyde dehydrogenase from acetaldehyde. Alcohol dehydrogenase does not produce acetate.

120 **The answer is D: Vasoconstriction.** Cocaine's peripheral effects are mediated by norepinephrine. Once released, norepinephrine binds to postsynaptic receptors. To halt signaling, norepinephrine is taken up into the presynaptic cell or diffuses away from the synapse to be degraded by COMT and MAO. Cocaine inhibits the reuptake of norepinephrine into the nerve terminals and causes some degree of norepinephrine release. Excess norepinephrine in the synaptic cleft leads to vasoconstriction. (A) Cocaine has not been shown to appreciably alter coagulability. A major effect of cocaine increasing norepinephrine in the synaptic cleft is vasoconstriction. (B) Cocaine has not been shown to appreciably alter coagulability. A major effect of cocaine increasing norepinephrine in the synaptic cleft is vasoconstriction. (C) Cocaine-mediated vasoconstriction may actually lead to an increase in body temperature. This occurs from hindering the body's ability to lose heat through vasodilation. (E) Cocaine increases the amount of norepinephrine in the synaptic cleft. Norepinephrine stimulates α_1-adrenergic receptors, causing vasoconstriction.

121 **The answer is D: Psychogenic.** Patient reports of allergic reactions to local anesthetics are fairly common, but investigation shows that most of these are of psychogenic origin. Psychogenic reactions are often misdiagnosed as allergic reactions and may also mimic them, with signs such as urticaria, edema, and bronchospasm. True allergy to an amide is exceedingly rare, whereas the ester procaine is somewhat more allergenic. (A) The most likely allergic association for lidocaine is psychogenic. (B) There is likely a minimal mast cell–mediated component. (C) This allergic response is not neurogenic. (E) This allergic response is not vascular induced.

122 **The answer is C: Seizures.** Bupropion also assists in decreasing the craving and attenuating the withdrawal symptoms for nicotine in tobacco users trying to quit smoking. Side effects may include dry mouth, sweating, nervousness, tremor, a very low incidence of sexual dysfunction, and an increased risk for seizures at high doses. Bupropion is metabolized by the CYP2B6 pathway and is considered to have a relatively low risk for drug–drug interactions. (A) Dry mouth can occur at low doses of bupropion. (B) Nervousness can occur at low doses of bupropion. (D) Sexual dysfunction can occur at low doses of bupropion. (E) Sweating can occur at low doses of bupropion.

123 **The answer is C: Respiratory depression.** Morphine causes respiratory depression by reduction of the sensitivity of respiratory center neurons to carbon dioxide. This can occur with ordinary doses of morphine in patients who are opioid-naïve and can be accentuated as the dose is increased until, ultimately, respiration ceases. Respiratory depression is the most common cause of death in acute opioid overdoses. Tolerance to this effect does develop quickly with repeated dosing, which allows the safe use of morphine for the treatment of pain when the dose is correctly titrated. (A) Morphine does not cause congestive heart failure. (B) Morphine does not cause hepatitis. (D) Morphine does not cause pulmonary edema. (E) Morphine does not cause pulmonary embolism.

124 **The answer is C: Morphine.** Heroin does not occur naturally. It is produced by diacetylation of morphine, which leads to a threefold increase in its potency. Its greater lipid solubility allows it to cross the blood–brain barrier more rapidly than morphine, causing a more exaggerated euphoria when the drug is injected. Heroin is converted to morphine in the body, but its effects last about half as long. It has no accepted medical use in the United States but is used therapeutically in other countries for the severe pain of cancer. That is delivered to the gastrointestinal system after swallowing. (A) Heroin is not converted to dopamine. (B) Heroin is converted to morphine. (D) Heroin is not converted to a catecholamine. (E) Heroin is not converted to serotonin. However, if it were, the symptoms of flushing, sweating, and diarrhea may preclude its abuse.

125 **The answer is B: Celecoxib.** Celecoxib is not a recommended choice for this patient who has back pain and gastrointestinal upset. This agent will make his GI symptoms worse and thus is not recommended. (A) Choline magnesium trisalicylate has a long half-life and some antiplatelet activity. (C) Ketorolac is not recommended for this patient. (D) Naproxen sodium can have some cardiovascular toxicity in this patient. (E) Salsalate should be given with precaution in patients with hepatic and renal dysfunction.

126 **The answer is B: Headache.** Typical adverse effects of fexofenadine include headache, back pain, viral infection, gastrointestinal upset, sinusitis, and otitis media in children. (A) Low back pain would be typical in patients taking fexofenadine. (C) Otitis media can occur with fexofenadine use in children. (D) Pulmonary bacterial infections are not expected with fexofenadine. (E) Headache is much more common than tinnitus in patients taking fexofenadine.

127 **The answer is C: Rifampin.** Singulair is a leukotriene receptor antagonist. This agent has shown promise in the treatment of seasonal allergic rhinitis. Important interactions with this medication include concomitant use of other CYP450 inhibitors such as phenobarbital and rifampin. (A) Ampicillin can be administered with Singulair. (B) Chloramphenicol can be administered with Singulair. (D) Tetracycline can be administered with Singulair.

128 **The answer is D: Fexofenadine.** Fexofenadine is a second-generation reversible inhibitor of H_1 receptors used for the treatment of allergic reactions. Unlike first-generation antihistamines, second-generation antihistamines are much less sedating. (A) Chlorpheniramine is a first-generation antihistamine that causes sedation. (B) Dimenhydrinate is a first-generation antihistamine that causes sedation. (C) Diphenhydramine is a first-generation antihistamine that causes sedation. (E) Ipratropium is an anticholinergic, not an antihistamine, used for the treatment of asthma.

129 **The answer is D: Long-acting β_2-agonist.** Salmeterol is a long-acting β_2-agonist. β_2-Receptors are found on bronchial smooth muscle and activation leads to relaxation of the muscles. This dilates the airways and opposes the bronchoconstriction caused by asthma. (A) Salmeterol is an agonist of β_2-receptors, not β_1-receptors. (B) Salmeterol is an agonist, not an antagonist. Salmeterol also acts on β_2-receptors, not β_1-receptors. (C) β_2-Receptors are found on bronchial smooth muscles and their activation leads to salmeterol's beneficial effects on asthma. β_1-Receptor activation would not affect bronchial smooth muscles. (E) Salmeterol is an agonist, not antagonist, of β_2-receptors.

130 **The answer is E: Zafirlukast.** The first-line treatment of aspirin-induced asthma is desensitization to aspirin. The next treatment options are steroids or leukotriene inhibitors. Zafirlukast blocks leukotriene receptors and is used in the treatment of aspirin-induced asthma. (A) Albuterol is used for asthma exacerbations but is not traditionally used for aspirin-induced asthma. (B) Cromolyn is a mast cell stabilizer that is rarely used to treat asthma. (C) Ipratropium is a muscarinic antagonist used for asthma and COPD, but it is not traditionally used for aspirin-induced asthma. (D) Theophylline is a phosphodiesterase inhibitor used to treat asthma and COPD, but it is not traditionally used for aspirin-induced asthma.

131 **The answer is A: Aspirin.** Ethanol undergoes zero-order elimination, meaning the same amount is eliminated per unit time regardless of its concentration in the blood. Most drugs undergo first-order elimination in which proportionately higher amounts of drug are eliminated when their blood concentration is higher. The duration of first-order type drugs is therefore explained by their half-life or the time it takes for half of the drug to be eliminated. A drug undergoing zero-order elimination cannot be described in terms of half-lives, because its duration of action depends only on the absolute amount of drug in the body (twice as much drug will last twice as long). All drugs would likely undergo zero-order metabolism at high enough concentrations because their eliminating enzymes would be saturated. However, only a few drugs saturate their respective metabolic enzymes at therapeutic concentrations. These include phenytoin, ethanol, and aspirin. (B) Ibuprofen undergoes first-order elimination. Its half-life is between 2 and 4 h. (C) Simvastatin undergoes first-order elimination. Its half-life is approximately 2 h. (D) Tolbutamide undergoes first-order elimination. Its half-life is between 4.5 and 6.5 h. (E) Valproic acid undergoes first-order elimination. Its half-life is between 6 and 16 h.

132 **The answer is A: Ammonium chloride.** Symptoms of amphetamine intoxication may include formication (the feeling of insects on or under skin), diaphoresis, agitation, chest pain, palpitations, xerostomia, and altered mental status. This patient's symptoms are consistent with amphetamine intoxication, and this suspicion is supported by the mother's presentation of an empty ADHD medicine bottle (many contain amphetamine salts). Because amphetamines are weak bases, administration of a weak acid such as ammonium chloride will acidify the urine and trap the amphetamine salts in the tubules to hasten removal. (B) Epinephrine is an adrenergic agonist. It stimulates the sympathetic nervous system and is used to treat anaphylactic shock. It would significantly hasten removal of amphetamines from this patient's system. (C) Flumazenil is used as an antidote for benzodiazepine overdose. It binds to the same receptors as benzodiazepines but does not stimulate the receptors. (D) Pilocarpine is a muscarinic cholinergic agonist. It would cause an increase not only in saliva but also in sweat and tears. It would not address the amphetamine toxicity directly and would be a poor choice for treating this patient. (E) Theophylline is structurally similar to caffeine. It is used to treat and prevent bronchospasm.

133 **The answer is C: Paralytic ileus.** This patient is taking amitriptyline and Ditropan, an anticholinergic agent. This medication combination can produce paralytic ileus, which is what this patient likely has. There is no evidence of bowel function because he cannot pass flatus or a bowel movement. (A) There is no evidence to suggest alcoholic hepatitis in this patient. No information is given that this patient is an alcoholic. (B) This patient is not an alcoholic nor does he have evidence of gallstones so pancreatitis is unlikely. (D) This complication is not caused by overdose; rather, it is caused by drug interaction. (E) Paralytic ileus is not a normal finding.

134 **The answer is B: Digoxin immune Fab.** In the severely poisoned patient, reduction of digoxin plasma concentrations is paramount and can be accomplished with administration of antidigoxin antibodies. (A) Amiodarone would enhance digoxin intoxication both by displacing digoxin from tissue protein–binding sites and by competing with digoxin for renal excretion. (C) Antiarrhythmics such as lidocaine are useful if there is need, but not in this case. (D) Potassium concentrations, if low, can be increased. (E) Verapamil would increase heart rate.

135 **The answer is C: *N*-Acetylcysteine.** The patient overdosed on acetaminophen and the antidote is *N*-acetylcysteine. A toxic metabolite, *N*-acetyl-*p*-benzoquinone imine (NAPQI), of acetaminophen is bound by glutathione in the body; however, once these stores are used up, the toxic metabolite damages the liver. *N*-Acetylcysteine binds to the toxic metabolite, preventing liver damage. (A) Ammonium chloride is used to acidify the urine as an antidote for amphetamine overdose. (B) Flumazenil is used as an antidote for benzodiazepine overdose. (D) Naloxone is used for the treatment of opioid overdose. (E) Sodium bicarbonate is used to alkalinize the urine for the treatment of amphetamine and tricyclic antidepressant overdose.

136 **The answer is A: Alcoholism.** Heparin is contraindicated for patients who are hypersensitive to it; have bleeding disorders; are alcoholics; or are having or have had recent surgery of the brain, eye, or spinal cord. (B) Drug abuse is not a contraindication to heparin. (C) Hypertension is not a contraindication to heparin. (D) Immune deficiency state is not a contraindication to heparin. (E) Recent surgery to the brain, eye, or spinal cord represents a contraindication to heparin therapy.

137 **The answer is A: Fresh frozen plasma.** The best way to convert warfarin in an emergency is with fresh frozen plasma. This patient's vital signs show that she is probably hypovolemic. Fresh frozen plasma will replace the coagulation factors deficient (II, VII, IX, and X) from the use of warfarin and the lack of vitamin K. (B) A transfusion of platelets would not replenish the deficient clotting factors II, VII, IX, and X. (C) Protamine sulfate is used for the reversal of heparin, not warfarin. (D) Vitamin K is used in the reversal of warfarin, but it takes a couple of days for the vitamin K to replenish the deficient clotting factors. This patient needs immediate reversal. (E) A whole blood transfusion is rarely necessary. Fresh frozen plasma has a greater concentration of clotting factors, which is needed in the reversal of warfarin.

138 **The answer is B: Permanent darkening of the irises.** Bimatoprost is a prostaglandin analog often used to treat glaucoma and hypotrichosis. An increase in length and amount of eyelashes occurs with use by an unknown mechanism and may be accompanied by a darkening of the iris. The mechanism for this side effect is caused by an increase in melanosomes in iridal melanocytes. Once darkened by bimatoprost, the irises often never regain their original color even after the use has ceased. (A) Latanoprost is a prostaglandin analog and increases the outflow of aqueous humor from the eye. This decreases intraocular pressure and thus can be used to treat glaucoma. (C) Stevens–Johnson syndrome is a rare but potentially fatal side effect of some drugs. Sulfonamides are an example, but bimatoprost is not known to cause Stevens–Johnson syndrome. (D) Drugs known for causing weight gain include many atypical antipsychotics such as quetiapine and olanzapine. Bimatoprost is not known to cause weight gain. (E) Bimatoprost is not known to increase either the frequency or duration of migraines. Nonmigraine headaches have been reported as a side effect of bimatoprost use, but bimatoprost is not contraindicated in patients with migraines.

139 **The answer is B: Irreversibly inhibits cyclooxygenases 1 and 2.** The boy is suffering from Reye's syndrome caused by taking aspirin for a viral infection. The mechanism of action of aspirin is the irreversible inhibition of cyclooxygenases 1 and 2. The exact reason for aspirin causing Reye's syndrome has not been discovered. (A) Inhibiting phospholipase A_2 is the mechanism of action of glucocorticoids, which does not cause Reye's syndrome. (C) The mechanism of action of NSAIDs is the reversible inhibition of cyclooxygenases 1 and 2. NSAIDs do not cause Reye's syndrome. (D) The mechanism of action of celecoxib is the reversible inhibition of cyclooxygenase 2. Celecoxib does not cause Reye's syndrome. (E) The mechanism of action of diphenhydramine is the reversible inhibition of H_1 histamine receptors. Antihistamines do not cause Reye's syndrome.

140 **The answer is A: Inhibits microtubule polymerization.** The mechanism of action of colchicine is the inhibition of microtubule polymerization by binding to and stabilizing tubulin. This impairs leukocyte chemotaxis. Colchicine and indomethacin are the first-line treatments for an acute gout attack. (B) Probenecid inhibits the reabsorption of uric acid in the proximal convoluted tubules. (C) Allopurinol inhibits xanthine oxidase, which decreases the production of uric acid. (D) Aspirin irreversibly inhibits cyclooxygenase. It should not be used in gout attacks because it can increase uric acids by preventing its clearance. (E) Indomethacin reversibly inhibits cyclooxygenase, but it also decreases the motility of leukocytes like colchicine. Therefore, it is also used as a first-line treatment for acute gout attacks.

141 **The answer is D: Respiratory depression.** A major concern with opioid use during birthing is respiratory depression of the newborn. All opioids cause respiratory depression to some degree because they act on μ-receptors, and it is the activation of the μ-receptors that is responsible for respiratory depression. An opioid antagonist such as naloxone or a respiratory stimulant such as doxapram may be administered to the infant following birth to restore normal respiration. (A) Chronic opioid use can cause constipation and withdrawal from opioids can cause diarrhea, but these effects would not likely be seen after the short course given in this case. Respiratory depression is more of a concern. (B) It would be difficult to assess hallucinations in a newborn. Second, hallucinations are not life threatening. Respiratory depression is more of a concern in this case. Last, although opioids can cause hallucinations, this occurs mostly with high doses and would not be likely here. (C) Symptoms of opioid withdrawal can include chills and perspiration, but opioids generally do not otherwise cause temperature disturbances. Respiratory depression in the newborn is the concern in this case. (E) Symptoms of opioid withdrawal can include insomnia and anxiety, but a single dose of opioids as in this case is unlikely to lead to restlessness in the newborn. Respiratory depression in the newborn is the concern in this case.

142 **The answer is B: Constipation.** Tolerance develops as a person chronically uses opioids; however, tolerance never occurs with constipation and miosis. Patients are commonly prescribed stool softeners and laxatives as prophylaxis for constipation when opioids are taken. (A) Tolerance does develop to CNS depressions. (C) Tolerance does develop to nausea caused by opioids. (D) Tolerance does develop the patients' pain response. Increased doses of opioids are needed to treat chronic users' pain. (E) Tolerance does develop to respiratory depression.

143 **The answer is E: Simvastatin.** This patient's altered mental status was caused by high levels of ammonia in his blood. Normally, the liver converts excess ammonia into water-soluble urea to be excreted by the kidneys; but in patients with impaired liver function, this may not happen. When ammonia cannot be converted to urea, it will build up in the body to toxic levels and can lead to mental status changes. This condition is called hepatic encephalopathy and may be fatal if left untreated. Simvastatin is absolutely contraindicated in all cases of hepatic disease, including hepatic encephalopathy. (A) Alprostadil is prostaglandin E_1. It can be used to treat erectile dysfunction. It is not hepatotoxic and is not contraindicated in hepatic encephalopathy. (B) Ascorbic acid or vitamin C is given as an antioxidant or simply as a general nutritional supplement. It is not hepatotoxic and is not contraindicated in hepatic encephalopathy. (C) Bimatoprost is a synthetic prostaglandin used to reduce intraocular pressure in patients with glaucoma. It is not hepatotoxic and is not contraindicated in hepatic encephalopathy. (D) Lisinopril is an angiotensin-converting enzyme (ACE) inhibitor used to treat hypertension. It is not hepatotoxic and is not contraindicated in hepatic encephalopathy.

144 **The answer is B: Corneal deposits.** Chlorpromazine is a typical antipsychotic that has been known to accumulate in the eyes. It is phototoxic when exposed to light and can lead to permanent blindness if not stopped once deposits or symptoms develop. (A) Agranulocytosis is a common side effect of clozapine, not chlorpromazine. (C) Diabetes insipidus is a common side effect of lithium, not chlorpromazine. (D) Hypertension is a common side effect of venlafaxine, not chlorpromazine. (E) Hypothyroidism is a common side effect of lithium, not chlorpromazine.

145 **The answer is A: Dimenhydrinate.** This boy's complaint is most consistent with motion sickness. This is a sensation that occurs when visual stimuli do not seem to agree with information from the vestibular system of the inner ear. Dimenhydrinate can be used to interrupt signals from the vestibule in order to prevent the disagreement between visual and vestibular messages. Although the mechanism is not completely clear, it has been proposed that the anticholinergic activity possessed by dimenhydrinate blocks signals from the vestibule. (B) Droperidol is a neuroleptic similar to haloperidol and antagonizes multiple CNS receptors but not cholinergic receptors. Its antinausea activity is likely caused by antagonism at dopaminergic receptors. (C) Medical marijuana is currently indicated for nausea only when arising from chemotherapy regimens. Its actions are thought to relate primarily to stimulation of CB receptors, not inhibition of cholinergic receptors. (D) Ondansetron works both centrally and peripherally by blocking serotonin receptors in the vagal nerve and in the chemoreceptor trigger zone. It does not have significant anticholinergic activity. (E) Palonosetron works both centrally and peripherally by blocking serotonin receptors in the vagal nerve and in the chemoreceptor trigger zone. It does not have significant anticholinergic activity.

146 **The answer is C: Flatulence.** Varenicline is a commonly used agent to assist with smoking cessation. This agent can cause nausea, flatulence, vomiting, sleep disturbance, abnormal dreams, and insomnia. (A) This agent does not cause attention deficit disorder. (B) This agent does not cause diarrhea; rather, it causes nausea and vomiting. (D) This agent does not induce hepatitis. (E) This agent does not have pulmonary side effects.

147 **The answer is C: Mast cell stabilizer.** Cromolyn is a mast cell stabilizer preventing the release of inflammatory mediators. It is dosed many times throughout the day and does not offer much benefit. For this reason, cromolyn is rarely used to treat asthma. (A) Zafirlukast blocks leukotriene receptors and is used in the treatment of aspirin-induced asthma. (B) Bosentan inhibits endothelin-1 receptors and is used in the treatment of pulmonary hypertension. (D) Ipratropium is a muscarinic antagonist used in the treatment of asthma and COPD. (E) Theophylline is a phosphodiesterase inhibitor used to treat asthma and COPD.

148 **The answer is D: Letter D.** This agent, salmeterol, has long duration of action—approximately 12 h—and would be most efficacious for this athlete who is going to complete a marathon in 6 h. It does take approximately 1 h for bronchodilation to occur. (A) Letter A represents epinephrine with a rapid onset and short duration of action. (B) Letter B represents isopreterenol with a rapid onset and a longer duration of action. (C) Letter C represents albuterol with a rapid onset and a duration of action of 4 h. (E) Letter E represents terbutaline with a very rapid onset of action and a 3.5-h duration of action.

149 **The answer is B: Figure B.** Figure B represents nicotine gum. If two pieces of nicotine gum are chewed, a steady state concentration of nicotine will be achieved for approximately 2 h. (A) Figure A represents smoking 1.5 cigarettes with an abrupt rise in blood nicotine level and then a drop off. (C) Figure C represents the transdermal patch with elevated blood nicotine levels over time. (D) This information can be determined from the graphs.

150 **The answer is A: Letter A.** Letter A represents the excitation of the postsynaptic receptor, causing depolarization and calcium influx. (B) Letter B represents the elevation of calcium levels, which stimulate the release of endocannabinoids. (C) Letter C represents the binding of endocannabinoids to receptors on the presynaptic neuron. (D) Letter D represents the release of inhibitory neurotransmitters such as GABA.

151 **The answer is D: Inhibition of xanthine oxidase.** Xanthine oxidase is the enzyme responsible for urate production as the final step in purine metabolism. Urate or uric acid can accumulate in susceptible people and cause flares of gout as in this patient. The level of uric acid in the blood is not a reliable predictor of who will suffer a gout attack—some patients have relatively high levels of serum urate but may never have an attack, whereas others with relatively low levels can suffer an attack. Regardless of the baseline serum urate level, patients who are symptomatic may find relief from lowering the amount of urate in the blood. Febuxostat is a drug that lowers serum urate by inhibiting xanthine oxidase. (A) NSAIDs are common anti-inflammatory drugs used for acute gout attacks. They can help with the pain and inflammation associated with an attack but will not increase urate excretion. (B) Colchicine is a drug used in gout to inhibit leukocyte migration. Specifically, colchicine interferes with microtubules. It has no effect on urate excretion. (C) Probenecid works on the renal tubules by interfering with organic acid secretion and reabsorption. Its exact mechanism is not known, but probenecid inhibits urate reabsorption to lower blood urate levels. (E) Humans lack a uricase enzyme which can be found in other animals allowing them to break down urate. There is to pathway for urate metabolism in humans.

152 **The answer is A: Blurry yellow vision.** Blurry yellow vision is a side effect experienced during digoxin toxicity. The exact reason for the yellow vision is unknown. It was believed that Van Gogh may have had digoxin toxicity during his "Yellow Period" of paintings. (B) Impotence is a common side effect of β-blockers, not digoxin. (C) Lupus-like syndrome is a common side effect of procainamide, not digoxin. (D) Prolongation of the AV refractory period is a common side effect of Class 1c antiarrhythmics, like flecainide, encainide, and propafenone, not digoxin. (E) Amiodarone has several well-known side effects, including pulmonary fibrosis, hepatotoxicity, and thyroid imbalances.

153 **The answer is C: C.** Misoprostol stimulates the prostaglandin receptor. This is represented by letter C in the diagram. (A) Letter A represents where dicyclomine would block the cholinergic receptor. (B) Letter B represents where cimetidine would block the H_2 histamine receptor. (D) Letter D represents where omeprazole would block the proton pump.

154 The answer is D: Penicilloic acid. This is the most important adverse effect of the penicillins. The major antigenic determinant of penicillin hypersensitivity is its metabolite, penicilloic acid, which reacts with proteins and serves as a hapten to cause an immune reaction. Approximately 5% of patients have some kind of reaction, ranging from maculopapular rash (the most common rash seen with ampicillin hypersensitivity) to angioedema (marked swelling of the lips, tongue, and periorbital area) and anaphylaxis. (A) Penicillin anaphylaxis is caused by the metabolite penicilloic acid. (B) Eosinophils play a role in the anaphylactic reaction. (C) Penicilloic acid, not penicillin, is the metabolite causing this reaction. (E) Xanthine oxidase does not cause anaphylaxis in patients taking penicillin.

155 The answer is A: Destroyed hair cells in the organ of Corti. Ototoxicity (vestibular and cochlear) is directly related to high peak plasma levels and the duration of treatment. The antibiotic accumulates in the endolymph and perilymph of the inner ear, and toxicity correlates with the number of destroyed hair cells in the organ of Corti. Deafness may be irreversible and has been known to affect fetuses in utero. Patients simultaneously receiving another ototoxic drug, such as cisplatin or the loop diuretics furosemide, bumetanide, or ethacrynic acid, are particularly at risk. (B) The pinnae are expected to be intact in this patient. (C) Peak plasma levels of gentamicin would be expected to be high. (D) The mechanism of ototoxicity does not involve otitis externa. (E) Hearing loss does not involve vestibular dysfunction.

Index

Page numbers followed by "*f*" denotes figures.

B

D

N

O

P

T